Complementary and Alternative Medicine

Complementary and Alternative Medicine

Second edition

Edited by

Steven B Kayne

PhD, MBA, LLM, MSc(SpMed), DAgVetPharm, FRPharmS, FCPP,
FIPharmM, FFHom, MPS(NZ), FNZCP
Honorary Consultant Pharmacist, Glasgow Homeopathic Hospital, UK
Honorary Lecturer, University of Strathclyde School of Pharmacy, UK

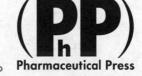

London • Chicago

Published by the Pharmaceutical Press
An imprint of RPS Publishing

1 Lambeth High Street, London SE1 7JN, UK
100 South Atkinson Road, Suite 200, Grayslake, IL 60030-7820, USA

© Pharmaceutical Press 2009

(**P.P**) is a trade mark of RPS Publishing
RPS Publishing is the publishing organisation of the
Royal Pharmaceutical Society of Great Britain

First edition published in 2001
Second edition published in 2009

Typeset by J&L Composition, Filey, North Yorkshire
Printed in Great Britain by TJ International, Padstow, Cornwall

ISBN 978 0 85369 763 3

A catalogue record for this book is available from the British Library.

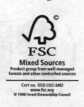

Contents

Preface vii
About the editor ix
Contributors x
Abbreviations xii

**Part 1 Introduction to complementary and
alternative medicine** 1

1 Introduction to the complementary concept of healthcare 3
2 Integrative medicine – incorporating complementary and
alternative medicine into practice 23
3 Delivering complementary and alternative medicine 43
4 Complementary and alternative medicine in the USA 93
5 The evidence base for complementary and alternative
medicine 121
6 Pharmacovigilance of complementary medicines 145

Part 2 Therapies involving use of medicines 185

7 Homeopathy and anthroposophy 187
8 Medical herbalism 269
9 Aromatherapy 341
10 Flower remedy therapy 383

Part 3 Traditional medicine 393

11 The traditional healthcare environment 395
12 Traditional Chinese medicine 415
13 Indian ayurvedic medicine 449

Part 4 Other therapies and diagnostic techniques 473

14 Naturopathy and its associated therapies 475

15   Diagnostic therapies   511
16   Manual therapies   517
17   Mind and body therapies   561

Index   597

Preface

Much has happened since the first edition of this book appeared in 2002. Despite the continuing paucity of robust scientific evidence to support most of its constituent therapies, complementary and alternative medicine (CAM) remains popular with clients who appreciate the holistic approach and have a belief in its effectiveness. Some elements of CAM such as aromatherapy and herbalism have acquired a more dedicated following, whereas others including homeopathy have been subjected to a campaign of scepticism in the UK in recent years, resulting in a reduction in the services available under the country's National Health Service. Interest in traditional medicine, in particular Chinese and Indian medicine has increased both by the arrival of immigrants, making it important for health providers to have some knowledge of the principles and treatments involved, and by host communities, resulting in the opening of Chinese herbal medicine shops on the high streets of British cities.

Among healthcare providers there is an increasing realisation that CAM is here to stay and must at least be acknowledged as a credible option in appropriate circumstances. The concept of integrative medicine is gaining ground. As statutory control of practitioners in many CAM therapies and licensing of medicines becomes established full recognition must surely follow.

This second edition has been reorganised and expanded with three important new chapters covering integrative medicine, pharmacovigilance and the marketing of CAM products in the USA. I am grateful to three highly experienced colleagues from New Zealand and the USA for agreeing to contribute to these chapters, thus strengthening the content. The book also provides an introduction to a much wider range of CAM therapies. It is divided into four parts:

1. The first part serves as an introduction and deals with the concepts that underpin CAM practice
2. The second part looks at therapies that generally, but not exclusively, involve the use of medicines after a consultation or through self-treatment

3. The third part gives information on traditional medicine
4. The fourth part covers a range of other therapies and diagnostic procedures.

An abbreviated *FASTtrack* version of this book, covering the major topics and providing self-assessment exercises, was also published by the Pharmaceutical Press in 2008. It has been designed as a resource to assist students preparing for examinations

Steven B Kayne
Glasgow, August 2008
steven.kayne@nhs.net

About the editor

Dr Steven B Kayne practised as a Community Pharmacist in Glasgow for more than 30 years before retiring from active practice in 1999. He is currently Honorary Consultant Pharmacist at Glasgow Homeopathic Hospital and Honorary Lecturer in CAM at the University of Strathclyde School of Pharmacy. Steven was a member of the UK Advisory Board on the Registration of Homeopathic Products from its formation in 1994 until he retired in 2008, and currently serves on two other UK Government Expert Advisory Bodies: the Herbal Medicines Advisory Committee and the Veterinary Products Committee. He has also acted as an adviser to the WHO Collaborating Centre for Traditional Medicine and chaired the European Committee on Homeopathy Pharmacy sub-committee. Steven's current interests are in patient communication and the application of CAM in sports care and veterinary medicine

He has written numerous papers and journal articles and has presented as an invited speaker at conferences around the world on a variety of topics associated with complementary and alternative medicine. Steven is a member of the editorial advisory board of several journals and has authored, edited and contributed chapters to many books.

Contributors

Joanne Barnes, BPharm, PhD, MRPharmS, MPS (NZ)

Joanne Barnes is Associate Professor in Herbal Medicines at the School of Pharmacy, Faculty of Medical and Health Sciences, University of Auckland, New Zealand (since November 2005). Previously, she was Lecturer in Phytopharmacy (2002–5) and Research Fellow (1999–2002) in the Centre for Pharmacognosy and Phytotherapy, School of Pharmacy, University of London, UK, and Research Fellow in Complementary Medicines, Department of Complementary Medicine, University of Exeter, UK (1996–99).

Joanne's research explores the utilisation, safety and efficacy of herbal medicines. In particular, this has focused on examining issues relevant to the pharmacovigilance of herbal medicines, e.g. investigating methods for the safety monitoring of herbal medicines and communication of information on herbal safety concerns. Joanne is a member of the editorial boards of the journals *Drug Safety*, *Phytotherapy Research*, *International Journal of Pharmacy Practice* and *Current Clinical Pharmacology*, and is immediate past co-editor of *Complementary Therapies in Medicine* and was editor (1996–99) and one of the founders of *FACT* (*Focus on Alternative and Complementary Therapies*). She is lead co-author of the reference text *Herbal Medicines* (third edition published 2007), published by the Pharmaceutical Press, UK, and a co-author of the reference text *Fundamentals of Pharmacognosy and Phytotherapy* (Churchill Livingsone, 2004). Joanne is an honorary consultant to the World Health Organization's Collaborating Centre for International Drug Monitoring, a member of Health Canada's Natural Health Products Directorate's Expert Resource Group and, until moving to New Zealand, was a member of the UK Medicines and Healthcare products Regulatory Agency's Independent Review Panel on Classification of Borderline Products (1999–2005). Joanne is an elected member of the executive committee of the International Society of Pharmacovigilance (2006 to present) and was appointed as a Fellow of the Linnean Society of London in 2003.

Iris R Bell, MD, PhD

Iris Bell is Professor of Family and Community Medicine, Psychiatry, Psychology, Medicine, and Public Health at the University of Arizona College of Medicine. Dr Bell received her AB degree from Harvard University, magna cum laude in biology, PhD in Neuro- and Biobehavioral Sciences, and MD from Stanford University. After psychiatry residency at the University of California – San Francisco, she served as a faculty member at the University of California – San Francisco and, later, Harvard Medical School. She is Board certified in Psychiatry, with added qualification in Geriatric Psychiatry. She is also certified in biofeedback (Biofeedback Certification Institute of America) and a fellow of the American College of Nutrition. Dr Bell has published over 100 peer-reviewed articles, a dozen book chapters and a monograph on environmental chemical sensitivity. She has received grant funding from the National Institutes of Health, Department of Veterans Affairs, and numerous private foundations to study topics including biofeedback and psychophysiology, nutrition in dementia and depression, the neurobiology of environmental illness, and individual difference predictors of classic homeopathy outcomes. Her current research interests focus on synthesising complexity science and homeopathic theory in understanding the healing process at the whole person level of organisation.

JP Borneman, BS, MS, MBA, PhD

JP Borneman is the chairman and chief executive officer of Standard Homeopathic Company and Hyland's Inc. He holds master's degrees in chemistry in business from St Joseph's University, Philadelphia, and a Doctorate in health policy at University of Sciences in Philadelphia, with a research interest in patient perceptions and patterns of use of complementary and alternative medicine (CAM). He serves as emeritus director of the National Center for Homeopathy, director of the Consumer Healthcare Products Association (CHPA), as well as a director, editor and chairman of the Council on Pharmacy for the Homeopathic Pharmacopoeia of the USA. He is also chairman of the regulatory affairs committee for the American Association of Homeopathic Pharmacists, the industry trade association, and serves on the advisory board of the St Joseph's University College of Arts and Sciences and as an adviser to the board of the National Association of Chain Drug Stores.

Abbreviations

95%CI	95% confidence interval
AAPS	Arable Area Payments Scheme
ADHD	attention deficit hyperactivity disorder
ADROIT	Adverse Drug Reaction On-line Information Tracking
ADR	adverse drug reaction
AIDS	acquired immune deficiency syndrome
AOR	adjusted odds ratio
ANZTPA	Australia New Zealand Therapeutic Products Authority
ARGCM	Australian Regulatory Guidelines for Complementary Medicines
ATC	anatomical–therapeutic–chemical
ATCM	Association of Traditional Chinese Medicine
AVM-GSL	Authorised Veterinary Medicine – General Sales List
BAHM	British Association of Homeopathic Manufacturers
BHomP	*British Homeopathic Pharmacopoeia*
BHMA	British Herbal Medicine Association
CAM	complementary and alternative medicine
CFCs	chlorofluorocarbons
CFR	Code of Federal Regulation
cGMP	current good manufacturing practice
CHM	Chinese herbal medicine
CHM	Commission on Human Medicine
CHPA	Consumer Healthcare Products Associations
CONSORT	Consolidated Standards of Reporting Trials
CPPE	Centre for Pharmacy Postgraduate Education
CRISP	Computer Retrieval of Information on Scientific Projects
CSM	Committee on Safety of Medicines (since 2005 CHM)
DHA	docosahexaenoic acid
DSHEA	Dietary Supplement Health and Education Act

EBM	evidence-based medicine
EFA	essential fatty acid
ESCOP	European Scientific Cooperative on Phytotherapy
EU THMPD	European Union Traditional Herbal Medicinal Products Directive
FAO	Food and Agriculture Organization
FDA	US Food and Drug Administration
FDCA	Food, Drug and Cosmetic Act
FM	Feldenkreis method
FTC	Federal Trade Commission
GGHOS	Glasgow Homeopathic Hospital Outcome Scale
GHP	*German Homeopathic Pharmacopoeia*
GMP	good manufacturing practice
HA	health authority
HBM	Health Belief Model
HIV	human immunodeficiency virus
HMP	herbal medicinal product
HMPWG	Heads of European Medicines Agencies Homeopathic Medicinal Product Working Group
HRQoL	health related quality of life
HPCUS	Homeopathic Pharmacopeia Convention for the United States
HPUS	*Homeopathic Pharmacopeia of the United States*
HUFA	highly unsaturated fatty acid
IM	integrative medicine
IOM	Institute of Medicine
LOC	locus of control
MA	marketing authorisation
MAOI	monoamine oxidase inhibitor
MHLC	Multidimensional Health Locus of Control
MHRA	Medical and Healthcare products Regulatory Agency
MRSA	meticillin-resistant *Staphylococcus aureus*
NAHAT	National Association of Health Authority and Trusts
NCCAM	National Center for Complementary and Alternative Medicine
NCRs	non-conventional remedies
NDA	new drug application
NES	NHS Education for Scotland
NHIS	National Health Information Survey
NHP	Nottingham Health Profile or natural health product

NHS	National Health Service
NIH	National Institutes of Health
NIMH	National Institute of Medical Herbalists
NMQP	non-medically qualified practitioner
NSAID	non-steroidal anti-inflammatory drug
NVNM	non-vitamin, non-mineral
NZFSA	New Zealand Food Safety Authority
OAM	Office of Alternative Medicine
OM	orthodox medicine
OR	odds ratio
OTC	over the counter
PEM	prescription event monitoring
PHLC	powerful others health locus of control
QALY	quality-adjusted life-years
QoL	quality of life
RCHM	Register of Chinese Herbal Medicine
RCT	randomised controlled trial
RMT	rhythmical massage therapy
RPSGB	Royal Pharmaceutical Society of Great Britain
RR	response rate
SSRI	selective serotonin reuptake inhibitor
TCM	traditional Chinese medicine
TDS	total dissolved solid
TGA	Therapeutic Goods Administration
TM	traditional medicine
UMC	Uppsala Monitoring Centre
VMD	Veterinary Medicines Directorate
WHO	World Health Organization
WWF	Worldwide Fund for Nature or World Wildlife Fund (US & Canada)

Part 1

Introduction to complementary
and alternative medicine

1

Introduction to the complementary
concept of healthcare

Steven B Kayne

Definitions

Trying to construct a definition that covers a large heterogeneous group
of complementary and alternative therapies is difficult. Many therapies
are well known whereas others may be exotic, mysterious or even dangerous. Some relaxation techniques, massage therapies, special diets and
self-help groups could be considered to be lifestyle choices rather than
true therapeutic interventions, although it could be argued that an
enhanced feeling of well-being is sufficient to warrant the inclusion of a
procedure in the latter.

Support for the complementary notion of healthcare is far from
universal. Saks rejects the term complementary and alternative
medicine (CAM) because, in his view, it 'excludes therapies such as
homoeopathy which in their purest form are based on philosophies that
fundamentally conflict with medical orthodoxy'.[1] He opts for the term
'alternative medicine' and defines it thus:

> Alternative Medicine can be taken to encompass all the health care prac-
> tices that at any specific point in time generally do not receive support
> from the medical establishment in the British context, whether this be
> through such mechanisms as orthodox medical research funding, sympa-
> thetic coverage in the mainstream medical journals or routine inclusion in
> the mainstream medical curriculum. (page 4)

The term 'alternative' is used widely in the USA, the point being
made that not all alternative therapies complement allopathic
medicine.[2] The opposite approach has been expressed by a paper in
which the authors' aim was to determine the association between the
use of non-conventional and conventional therapies in a representative
population survey.[3] A total of 16 068 people aged 18 years or older
were involved in the study. Participants were asked about their visits to

non-conventional and conventional practitioners during the past year. From the resulting data it was estimated that:

- 6.5% of the US population had visited both types of practitioner during the year studied
- 1.8% visited only non-conventional practitioners
- 59.5% visited only conventional practitioners
- 32.2% visited neither type of practitioner.

It appeared, therefore, that unconventional therapies were being used to complement orthodox treatments rather than to replace them.

In fact, CAM is often used alongside orthodox medicine (OM) to treat different aspects of a disease. Rarely are the two therapies used to treat exactly the same symptoms. In fact evidence suggests that many Americans use CAM in addition, rather than as an alternative to, OM.[4]

The following definition has been suggested by colleagues working at Harvard Medical School:[5]

> Alternative medicine refers to those practices explicitly used for the purpose of medical intervention, health promotion or disease prevention which are not routinely taught at US Medical Schools nor routinely underwritten by third-party payers within the existing US health care system. (page 5)

Lannoye has suggested that it may be misleading to make a firm distinction between the terms 'complementary' and 'alternative', because it is the precise context within which a therapy is being used that will determine just how it should be defined at any one time.[6]

Not all proponents of complementary medicine agree with the terms 'complementary' and 'alternative'. They believe that the use of such terminology serves to emphasise the gap between the OM and CAM approaches. They would prefer to see the various CAM therapies referred to as *specialities* within an integrated medical system of practice (see Chapter 2) and not grouped together under a separate label.

Complementary and alternative medicine is frequently described by what it is *not*, rather than what it is. Thus, it may be described as being 'not taught formally to health professionals' or 'not having a robust evidence base'. Current definitions often obscure the debate about holism and integrative care and give therapies and therapists precedence over patients in the design of healthcare systems, for example:[7]

> CAM is a group of non-orthodox and traditional therapies that may be used alone, or to complement orthodox or other non orthodox therapies,

in the treatment and prevention of disease in human and veterinary patients. (pages 413–16)

The term 'traditional therapy' is defined in Chapter 11. Ernst et al have proposed the following definition:[8]

> Complementary medicine is a diagnosis, treatment and/or prevention which complements mainstream medicine by contributing to a common whole, by satisfying a demand not met by orthodoxy or by diversifying the conceptual framework of medicine.

This definition poses at least two questions:

1.   What is meant by 'mainstream'?
2.   Whom does complementary medicine seek to satisfy?

A rather more comprehensive definition by the Cochrane Collaboration was reported by Zollman and Vickers in 2000.[9] The Cochrane Collaboration is an international organisation that aims to help people make well informed decisions about healthcare by preparing, maintaining and promoting the accessibility of systematic reviews of the effects of healthcare interventions. The main output of the Collaboration is through the Cochrane Library an electronic database that is updated quarterly and distributed on CD-Rom and via the Internet.

The Cochrane definition is as follows:

> CAM is a broad domain of healing resources that encompasses all health systems, modalities and practices and their accompanying theories and beliefs, other than those intrinsic to the politically dominant health systems of a particular society or culture in a given historical period.
>
> CAM includes all such practices and ideas self-defined by their users as preventing or treating illnesses or promoting health and well-being. Boundaries within CAM and between the CAM domain and that of the dominant system are not always sharp or fixed.

The definition of CAM differs slightly from country to country. For example, in Japan, Japanese herbal medicine (part of Kampo medicine) and acupuncture are covered by public health insurance, so Japanese practitioners of Kampo and acupuncture would object to their inclusion in CAM and would rather regard themselves as belonging to the authentic traditional medicine. However, these treatments are categorised as CAM in Europe and the USA.

The following definition is preferred by the author because it implies a greater degree of flexibility:

> CAM is a group of non-orthodox and traditional therapies that may be used alone, or to complement orthodox or other non-orthodox therapies,

in the treatment and prevention of disease in human and veterinary patients.

It would be appropriate to offer two further definitions at this stage.

Patients: by convention anyone who is unwell is usually called a patient derived from the Latin *patior* – 'to suffer'. Throughout this book this generic term will be used to identify people who are unwell, whether they are to be treated by orthodox or complementary medicine. This is not meant to imply that other words such as 'client' or 'customer' are inappropriate in certain circumstances, merely that one word is being used to prevent confusion.

Disease is used in its orthodox sense to mean the following related items, collectively recognised as having a separate coexistence and origin:

- A group of subjective problems reported by the patient (symptoms)
- Objective alterations in body functions, usually identified by a trained observer (signs)
- The results of various investigations or procedures (investigations).

It has been pointed out that disease and health are commonly thought of as distinct opposites.[10] In fact, both may be considered to be facets of healthy functioning, each necessary for the other and each giving rise to the other. Thus, disease may be thought of as a manifestation of health – it is the healthy response of an individual striving to maintain equilibrium within his or her body. Disease can be viewed as a meaningful state that can inform health professionals how to help patients heal themselves. People's problems then become 'diseases of meaning'.

The art and science of medicine

Throughout history there have been two separate traditions in the practice of medicine. One is the so-called 'art of healing' and usually involves its own specialised brand of training and relies mainly on a prescriber's intuition and patient perceptions of successful outcomes. The tradition should not be confused with the art of healing programme, an initiative that aims to use the arts as a form of therapy to soothe patients' minds and bodies and help them on their path to recovery[11] (see Chapter 18). The second tradition, the 'science of healing', is based on technological and scientific ideas and leaves much less opportunity for practitioners to express an innovative and intuitive approach to medicine.

In the past, the phrase 'art of medicine' was often applied to the practice of CAM. Practitioners have used the phrase to cover up a good deal of muddled thinking and uncritically accepted prejudices. The term is perhaps most misleading when applied to aspects of medical practice that are amenable to empirical study but about which sufficient data have not been accumulated. Practitioners commonly used the word 'philosophy' in a similar context, e.g. 'My philosophy for using antihistamines to treat allergies is . . .'. Implicit in such usage is the erroneous assumption that what has been labelled a matter of philosophy or personal opinion is thereby exempt from rigorous evaluation. This view has hampered the progress of CAM. However, the situation is being forced to change with the growing importance of evidence-based medicine to purchasers, providers and patients alike.

There has not always been a clear and strict division between art and science.[12] The purpose of anatomical images from the Renaissance until the nineteenth century had as much to do with aesthetics and disclosing the 'divine architecture' as with the intention of medical illustration. Medical science was more closely linked with a 'naturalistic observation' than with 'intervention', and this was the dominant view until well into the nineteenth century. Since then scientific medicine and non-scientific medicine have interacted. In some cases this interaction has had positive results, with one supplying features that the other has lacked, e.g. homeopathic remedies may be used alongside orthodox medicines to treat different aspects of the same disease. Complementary therapies usually stress the idea of restoring a patient's overall wellness rather than merely seeking a reduction in any particular clinical symptom.

Unfortunately, there has been considerable suspicion, and scepticism, voiced by members of the scientific and medical community when referring to CAM. Orthodox medicine insists that the evidence supporting CAM is flimsy or absent.[13,14] Some treatments are not supported by any randomised clinical trials at all. In other cases there are trials that are methodologically flawed with inappropriate conclusions. Sceptics go on to claim that the inability to explain mechanisms of action of most complementary disciplines equates to a simple placebo response at best, and quackery at worst. CAM proponents point out that many orthodox interventions are not proven to be effective beyond reasonable doubt nor can their mechanisms be adequately explained, yet they still remain in routine use. Further a placebo effect is evident in orthodox medicine. A study testing pain relief from analgesics showed that merely telling people that a novel form of codeine that they were taking (actually a placebo) was worth $US2.50 (£1.25 or €1.58) rather than

10 cents increased the proportion of people who reported pain relief from 61% to 85.4%.[15] When the 'price' of the placebo was reduced, so was the pain relief.

Modern scientific thinking believes that knowledge should be pursued by the following criteria:[16]

- *Objectivism*: the observer is separate from the observed
- *Reductionism*: complex phenomena are explainable in terms of simpler component phenomena
- *Positivism*: all information can be derived from physically measurable data
- *Determinism*: phenomena can be predicted from scientific laws and environmental conditions.

Complementary medicine just does not fit into this mould. Most complementary disciplines have developed from patient-oriented studies – observational and anecdotal information assembled over hundreds and, in some cases, even thousands of years. This does not answer the very real criticisms about lack of detailed evidence of effectiveness or concerns over possible dangers.

Complementary and alternative approaches to healthcare

Complementary and alternative medicine is a term applied to over 700 different treatments and some diagnostic methods. A distinction is sometimes made between CAM (involving the use of medicines or other products) and complementary and alternative therapies (including interventions that rely on procedures alone). In this book the term 'complementary and alternative medicine' (CAM) is used to describe all types of non-orthodox medicine.

The words *complementary* and *alternative* are often used interchangeably. In the UK, health professionals prefer to use the former because it implies an ability to complement or complete other treatments. There is evidence to show that this is what happens in practice. Users of CAM are not so much seeking alternatives as a result of direct dissatisfaction, but are more probably using complementary therapies in parallel,[17] except in the case of purchasing homeopathic medicines over the counter in a pharmacy.[18] Alternative, on the other hand, implies 'instead of' or a choice between two courses of action, e.g. whether to treat a patient with orthodox (or 'allopathic') medicine or with homeopathy. In fact there are many instances where patients can benefit from using the best of both worlds. It is not unusual for homeopathic doctors in the UK to prescribe an antibiotic and a homeopathic medicine (e.g. Belladonna) on the same prescription form. In some cases CAM practitioners may use more than one complementary discipline concurrently. Asthma, for example, may be treated by a whole range of therapies, including relaxation, breathing exercises, yoga, as well as neutraceuticals, homeopathy and acupuncture.[19]

It is significant that the 1986 BMA report was entitled 'Alternative medicine',[20] whereas 6 years later in its next report it was using the title 'Complementary medicine'. A similar trend in the literature can be observed over the same period of time. In the early 1990s a British pharmacy launched an involvement in what it initially called alternative medicine, quickly changing its promotional material to use the term 'complementary medicine' within some months (see also Chapter 2).

Perceptions of the OM and CAM approaches to healing

The following terms have been applied to describe the OM and CAM approaches to healing:[21]

OM	CAM
Orthodox	Unorthodox, unconventional
Conventional	Alternative
Established	Fringe
Scientific	Natural
Proven	Unproven

All of these words communicate a particular viewpoint, some betraying the preconceptions of people who apply them to the practice of medicine.

The words 'orthodox' and 'conventional' clearly imply a certain correctness in the approach to healing. 'Established' similarly suggests that a degree of authority has been applied, perhaps by learned bodies or even society as a whole. 'Scientific' and 'proven' imply an expected, almost guaranteed, successful outcome.

By contrast, in the other column we find 'unorthodox' defined as *being irregular, unwanted* or *unusual*. From a sociological viewpoint unconventional therapy refers to medical practices that are not in conformity with the accepted standards of the medical community and therefore not taught at medical schools. 'Alternative' is a neutral word meaning *presenting a choice*. 'Fringe' and 'unproven' are words associated with a wish to marginalise the subject. Used in this context 'natural' could mean unstandardised.

Over recent years OM has become better at curing and helping with diseases but worse at relieving illness and sickness, and providing comfort. One of the key roles of CAM is in the management of illness and sickness and the provision of human comfort.[22]

The healing response

What does *healing* mean? In the minds of many CAM practitioners healing means restoring an unwell patient to his or her own particular state of wellness – not simply seeking to treat a condition in isolation. Does the term mean *actively treating*, i.e. a meaningful intervention provided by a practitioner during a consultation? Reilly[23] has suggested that the healing response begins long before the consultation and ends long after it finishes. A potential for change is inherent – and a creative 'meeting' may be the potent agent of its release – with or without prescriptions.

Self-healing

One aspect of healing that is common to all the therapies that collectively make up CAM is the belief that they work by stimulating the body to heal itself.

This response can be initiated by administering carefully chosen interventions – medicines or a physical procedure by the practitioner alone during a well-structured consultation. The quality of the consultation can be an important element in initiating a positive response in human patients[24] and perhaps in animals too. It is an interesting argument that, if this is indeed the case, i.e. if the interaction is so important, then self-treating with CAM including the purchase of over-the-counter (OTC) medicines without advice, might exclude a major source of the healing process. Not being able to see the wood for the trees might be the appropriate expression!

One could consider whether a definition of healing should include a reference to a person's intrinsic genetic or acquired ability to withstand disease itself, without external intervention. There are many examples of the body's ability to heal itself if given the chance.

Hippocrates was born on the Greek island of Kos, now a popular holiday destination. During his lifetime it is said that people came to him in their thousands to seek his advice for their ills. They found a Temple of Healing dedicated to the god Asclepius. Inside the stone walls of the Temple and beside bubbling mineral springs, the medical pilgrims experienced a ritual relaxation programme called incubation or temple sleep. Hippocrates made little use of drugs, relying on fomentations, bathing and diet. The last was very simple and included vinegar and honey. Above all he did not attempt to interfere with nature; he made no attempts to modify or block biochemical pathways. He knew that many diseases were self-limiting. He is said to have believed that:

Our natures are physicians of our diseases.

Further examples come from modern times. Proportionally more soldiers died of their wounds in Vietnam than in the Falkland Islands conflict between the UK and Argentina. In Vietnam helicopter evacuation was quick, and casualties were given blood transfusions and kept warm. In the Falklands, evacuation was often impossible because of the appalling weather. Doctors could not reach soldiers on exposed moorland to administer transfusions. Many casualties survived despite injuries that could have been expected to kill them. Without transfusion natural clotting mechanisms were not disturbed and haemorrhage was less severe. The cold weather complemented the normal effects of shock, slowing the body mechanisms.

A second example comes from an African sex worker. Despite the fact that over the past 20 years 1 or 2 of the 8 men she serviced each day at a cost of less than 50p ($US1) had HIV, the girl has never become infected. While many people are dead and dying of AIDS in Africa, there are about 200 sex workers, all of whom appear to be disease free. Are these girls genetically protected? When these girls give up their repeated exposure to the deadly virus they seem to lose their immunity. The spiritually minded might say that divine providence is at work offering protection during the working life of these girls.

A final example of what might be called intrinsic self-treatment is provided by the treatment of asthma. The UK has one of the highest prevalence rates for asthma in the world, along with New Zealand, Australia and Ireland. The 2001 Asthma Audit by the National Asthma Campaign provided a higher estimate of the number of people suffering with asthma in the UK than ever before. The audit estimated that 5.1 million people – 1 in 13 adults and 1 in 8 children – were being treated for asthma.[25] By contrast, it is almost unheard of in parts of Africa where there is more exposure to germs in childhood, and families are bigger. Research has found that young children in a family are less likely to develop asthma in later childhood than their older siblings.[26] Fewer babies would develop asthma, hayfever and other allergic diseases in the first place if they were exposed to dirt. Parents who are over-concerned with hygiene may be weakening their children's resistance. This comes as good news to grubby little boys and girls everywhere!

The foregoing is by way of providing evidence that there does seem to be an intrinsic ability – genetic or acquired – to self-heal one's body. Stimulating or encouraging this ability in some way might therefore be a reasonable approach to healing. This is the aim for most CAM disciplines.

The holistic approach to healing

The term 'holistic' has traditionally been understood to refer to CAM. In fact the concept is being increasingly adopted by OM.[27,28]

Definition

The origin of the word 'holism' is attributed to Jan Christian Smuts (1870–1950), a South African botanist and philosopher with the distinction of having the international airport at Johannesburg named in his memory. Smuts, who was Prime Minister of his country after World War I, wrote a book entitled *Holism and Evolution*[29] in which he described holism as:

> . . . the principle which makes for the origin and progress of wholes in the universe.

He further explained his idea thus:

- Holistic tendency is fundamental in nature.
- It has a well-marked ascertainable character.
- Evolution is nothing but the gradual development and stratification of progressive series of wholes, stretching from the inorganic beginnings to the highest levels of spiritual creation.

The concept of holism is much, much older, dating back to Cicero (106–43 BC), to whom the following has been attributed:

> . . . a careful prescriber before he attempts to administer a remedy or treatment to a patient must investigate not only the malady of the person he wishes to cure, but also his habits when in health, and his physical condition.

The precise definition of what is now understood by a 'holistic approach' seems to vary between practitioners according to Rosalind Coward.[30] She found that some practitioners consider holism as the ability to integrate different treatments for different needs, such as using herbal medicine for a specific ailment, acupuncture for chronic pain or hypnosis to stop smoking. A small minority stressed that holism implied links between individual and environment, and suggested treatments that would balance not only the internal parts of an individual but also the relationship between the individual and the environment. More generally, however, practitioners and patients define holism as the treatment of the whole person, an approach that considers body, mind and spirit as a single unit.

Pietroni has described holistic medicine in the following terms:[31]

- Responding to the person as a whole entity (body, mind and spirit) within that person's own environment (family, culture and ecological status)
- Willingness to use a wide continuum of treatments ranging from surgery and drugs to nutrition and meditation
- An emphasis on a participatory relationship between practitioner and patient
- An awareness of the impact of the health of the practitioner on the patient.

The World Health Organization defines health as follows: 'Health is a state of complete physical, mental and social well being, and not merely the absence of disease or infirmity.' (Preamble to the Constitution of the World Health Organization as adopted by the International Health Conference, New York, 19–22 June, 1946; signed on 22 July 1946 by the representatives of 61 States (Official Records of the World Health Organization, no. 2, p. 100) and entered into force on 7 April 1948.)

The WHO Commission on Social Determinants of Health has called for a new global agenda for health equity. In a report entitled 'Closing the health gap in a generation' the Commission points out that our children have dramatically different life chances depending on where they were born. In Japan or Sweden they can expect to live more than 80 years; in Brazil, 72 years; India, 63 years; and in several African countries, fewer than 50 years. And within countries, the differences in life chances are dramatic and are seen worldwide. the poorest of the poor have high levels of illness and premature mortality. But poor health is not confined to those worst off. In countries at all levels of income, health and illness follow a social gradient: the lower the socio-economic position, the worse the health. The report cites the example of the Carlton area of Glasgow, Scotland, where a boy growing up can expect to live 28 years less than if he was born around eight miles away in the more privileged area of Lenzie. The report published in 2008 may be viewed online at http://tinyurl.com/5qnyu9.

It is difficult to see how this could possibly be achieved without a holistic approach to health delivery as detailed above.

CAM and the holistic approach

Virtually all CAM practices claim to be holistic, i.e. treating the whole person rather than a condition in isolation. This in turn leads to a highly individual approach, which means that patients with apparently similar symptoms may be treated in a very different manner. Conversely it also means that particular treatments may be used to treat widely different conditions.

When a patient visits a complementary practitioner for the first time, the consultation may well extend to over an hour, although about 40 minutes is more usual. During this time a complete picture of the patient will be built up. The aim is to obtain the best therapeutic outcomes for patients, by integrating clinical expertise and knowledge with patients' needs and preferences, using the most current information available in a systematic and timely way.

The CAM community has tended historically to understand something important about the experience of illness and the ritual of practitioner–patient interactions. It has been suggested that the rest of medicine might do well to acknowledge the benefits of this approach.[32] Many people may be drawn to CAM practitioners because of the holistic concern for their wellbeing that they are likely to experience, and many may also experience appreciable placebo responses. Why should OM not try to understand what alternative practitioners know and do, because this may help explain why so many patients are prepared to pay to be treated by them, even when many of the treatments are unproven?

Gathering information from the patient   In providing holistic care the CAM practitioner needs to obtain information on how the patient functions in a normal state of wellbeing, in addition to hearing about symptoms that prompted the visit so that they may be returned to their own state of good health. Environmental and social factors also have to be considered. To obtain this information patients are often asked a list of seemingly unrelated questions on their first visit including the following:

- What type of food do you like – sweet, salty, spicy or bland?
- What type of weather conditions do you prefer – hot, cold, wet, dry, etc.?

- Do you like to be with other people or do you like to be alone?
- Are you a gregarious extravert type of person or are you quiet and introverted?
- Do you dream and if so can you remember the main subjects involved?

Patients' style of handwriting and colour preferences could be useful in establishing various personality traits, and therefore in choosing an appropriate therapy.[33] Personality and demeanour are important because they can determine how a patient is treated. This procedure is known in OM, but is usually practised covertly. For example, in an American study, medical staff were found to have given placebos to unpopular patients who were suspected of exaggerating their pain or had failed to respond to traditional medication.[34] The holistic practitioner acknowledges that people have different personalities and treats them, taking this fact into consideration overtly.

Practitioners may be interested in any modalities – what makes the condition feel better or worse, or whether the condition is better or worse at certain times of the day. The exact site of the problem will be identified. In response to the patient's statement 'I have a sore throat' the practitioner may ask is it worse 'on the right or left side?' Individualised treatment appropriate to the patient can then be chosen, the aim being to return him or her to his or her own particular state of good health.

The consultation   It is probably not possible to define a typical consultation even within one discipline, let alone generalise across all CAM consultations. Essentially the difference lies in the focus of the approach to healthcare. CAM seeks to focus on overall health, whereas the focus of OM is essentially disease oriented (see Chapter 3).

Consultations are so varied that any differences are only stereotypical, misleading or meaningless. Table 1.1 speculates as to how a consultation with a CAM practitioner might differ from one with a conventional healthcare provider.

The time taken for an initial consultation in which the practitioner seeks to establish a picture of the patient's whole health status with detailed questioning, as outlined above, and a sympathetic unhurried manner establishes a beneficial rapport. Kaptchuk and colleagues[35] undertook a dismantling approach to the examination of placebo effects. In 262 adults with irritable bowel syndrome, they examined the effects of placebo acupuncture in circumstances that involved observation only,

Table 1.1 Speculative differences between complementary and alternative medicine (CAM) and orthodox medicine (OM) consultations

Component	CAM	OM
Time	More	Less
Touch	More	Less
History-taking	Holistic, expansive	Specific, behavioural
Patient's role	Conscious, participatory	Passive
Decision-making	Shared with patient	Practitioner tends to make decisions (paternalistic)
Bedside manner	Empathic, warm	'Professional', cool
Language used	Subjective, simple words	Objective, uses jargon

sham acupuncture alone and sham procedure together with a 45-minute consultation with the treating doctor. The consultation involved questions about the patient's symptoms and beliefs about them, and was conducted in a 'warm, friendly manner', with empathy and communication of confidence and positive expectations. The second group improved significantly more than the first group but significantly less than the third, who improved by 37%. As the authors of a linked editorial conclude, the work shows that a constructive doctor–patient relationship can tangibly improve patients' responsiveness to treatment, be it placebo or otherwise.

Social considerations In the early days of the current wave of interest in CAM, some researchers were of the opinion that the holistic approach was inappropriate, because it provided an individualistic solution to problems of health, rather than seeking to alter the social structure that promoted an unhealthy environment.[36] The sociological literature often highlights the fact that, in concentrating on an individual, the needs of the wider community may be overlooked.[37] When responsibility is shifted to a single person, the social structures that constrain individual behaviour and lifestyle choices may be obscured. It has been suggested that this emphasis on such weaknesses in the holistic view may be one reason for its lack of acceptance by orthodox practitioners in the past.

Notwithstanding this opinion, the idea of individualising treatments is gaining acceptance and it is likely that modern biotechnology will provide the opportunity for future orthodox medicines to be tailored to patients' specific requirements.[38]

Change of emphasis   Many practitioners are becoming concerned that the special holistic nature of CAM is becoming eroded by the modern trend towards a more disease-centred approach. The increasing appearance of over the counter (OTC) products that contain multiple ingredients and make the limited claims of efficacy (allowed under newly enacted legislation) promotes self-treatment without consultation. This is in contrast to orthodox medicine which, in many therapeutic areas, is moving to a more focused approach made possible by the advent of gene therapy noted above.

Classification of CAM

The British Medical Association report in 1986 identified 116 complementary medical treatments that were used 'reasonably often' in the UK;[20] this number has increased considerably by now. It also includes an uncertain number of traditional ethnic therapies. Many are well known, others are exotic or mysterious, and some may even be dangerous.

Pietroni presented an early classification of the different approaches in CAM:[39]

- Complete systems of healing including acupuncture, chiropractic, herbalism, homeopathy, naturopathy and osteopathy
- Specific therapeutic methods including aromatherapy, massage and reflexology
- Psychological approaches and self-help exercises including relaxation, meditation and exercise
- Diagnostic methods including hair analysis, iridology and kinesiology.

In their report published in 2000[40] the House of Lords Select Committee on Science and Technology divided CAM therapies into three groups (Table 1.2):

1.   Group 1 embraces disciplines that have an individual diagnostic approach and well-developed self-regulation of practitioners. Research into their effectiveness has been established, and they are increasingly being provided on the NHS. The report says that statutory regulation of practitioners of acupuncture and herbal medicine should be introduced quickly and that such regulation may soon become appropriate for homeopathy. Some progress has been made in establishing statutory control over the practice of certain CAM disciplines.

Table 1.2 House of Lords' classification of complementary and alternative medicine (CAM) disciplines[7]

Group 1	Group 3A
Acupuncture	Anthroposophical medicine
Chiropractic	Ayurvedic medicine
Herbal medicine	Chinese herbal medicine
Homeopathy	Eastern medicine
Osteopathy	Naturopathy
	Traditional Chinese medicine
Group 2	**Group 3B**
Alexander technique	Crystal therapy
Aromatherapy	Dowsing
Flower remedies	Iridology
Hypnotherapy	Kinesiology
Massage	Radionics
Meditation	
Nutritional medicine	
Reflexology	
Shiatsu	
Spiritual healing	
Yoga	

2. Group 2 covers therapies that do not purport to embrace diagnostic skills and are not well regulated.
3. Group 3 covers other disciplines that either are long established but indifferent to conventional scientific principles (3A) or lack any credible evidence base (3B).

There were criticisms of the Lords' classification, in particular the lowly status given to Chinese herbal medicine (CHM) by placing it in category 3A. Lambert complained in a letter to the *Lancet*[41] that the classification ignored the existence of research that has shown the usefulness of CHM in many disorders. Evidence supports its provision in state hospitals throughout China, alongside conventional medicine.[42] It is suggested that, although the research is of variable quality, it should still not be ignored. Furthermore, promising trials have been carried out in the west, including two successful, double-blind, placebo-controlled trials of a Chinese formula for atopic eczema which concluded that 'there is substantial clinical benefit to patients who had been unresponsive to conventional treatment'.[43,44]

The US National Center for Complementary and Alternative Medicine (NCCAM) classifies CAM in five domains:[45]

1.   Alternative medical systems
2.   Mind–body interventions
3.   Biologically based therapies
4.   Manipulative and body-based methods
5.   Energy therapies.

In this book the therapies are divided into the following categories:

* Therapies principally involving the use of remedies (e.g. homeopathy)
* Therapies based on traditional use (e.g. traditional Chinese medicine)
* Complete complementary systems (e.g. naturopathy)
* Diagnostic procedures (e.g. iridology and jinesiology)
* Manual therapies (e.g. massage and reflexology)
* Mind body therapies (e.g. meditation and reiki).

References

1.   Saks M, ed. *Alternative Medicine in Britain.* Oxford: Clarendon Press, 1992: 4.
2.   Lin JH. Evaluating the alternatives. *JAMA* 1998;**279**:706.
3.   Druss BG, Rosenheck RA. Association between use of unconventional therapies and conventional medical services. *JAMA* 1999;**282**:651–6.
4.   Eisenberg DM, Kessler RC, Foster C et al. Unconventional medicine in the United States. *N Engl J Med* 1993;**328**:246–52.
5.   Micozzi M. *Fundamentals of Complementary & Alternative Medicine.* New York: Churchill Livingstone, 1996: 5.
6.   Lannoye MP. Amendments to the Explanatory Statement (Part B-A3-0291/94-26.4.94) for the Report on the status of complementary medical disciplines to the European Parliament's Committee on the Environment, Public Health and Consumer Protection. In: Richardson J. *Complementary Therapy in the NHS: A service evaluation of the first year of an outpatient service in a local district general hospital.* London: Health Services Research and Evaluation Unit, Lewisham Hospital NHS Trust. 1994.
7.   Leckridge B. The Future of complementary and alternative medicine – models of integration. *J Alt Comp Med* 2004;**10**:413–16.
8.   Ernst E, Resch KL, Miller S et al. Complementary medicine – a definition. *Br J Gen Pract* 1985;**35**: 506.
9.   Zollman C, Vickers A. ABC of complementary medicine. What is complementary medicine? *BMJ* 2000;**319**:693–6.
10.   Jobst KA, Shostak D, Whitehouse PJ. Diseases of meaning: manifestations of health and metaphor (Editorial). *J Alt Comp Med* 2000;**5**:495–502.
11.   Friedrich MJ. The arts of healing. *JAMA* 1999;**281**:1779–81.
12.   Van Haselen R. Reuniting art with science: impossibility or necessity? *Proceedings of the Third International Conference.* London: RLHH & Parkside Health, 22–23 February 2001: 7.

13. Ernst E. Quadruple standards? (Editorial). *Focus Alt Comp Ther* 2000;**5**:1–2.
14. Colquhoun D. Head to head. Should NICE evaluate complementary and alternative medicines? *BMJ* 2007;**334**:507.
15. Waber RL, Shiv B, Carmon Z, Ariely D. Commercial features of placebo and therapeutic efficacy. *JAMA* 2008;**299**:1016–17.
16. Micozzi M. *Fundamentals of Complementary & Alternative Medicine*. New York: Churchill Livingstone, 1996: 3.
17. Sharma U. *Complementary Medicine Today: Practitioners and patients*. London: Routledge, 1992
18. Kayne SB, Beattie N, Reeves A. Buyer characteristics in the homoeopathic OTC market. *Pharm J* 1999;**263**:210–12.
19. Huntley A, White A, Ernst E. Complementary medicine for asthma. *Focus Alt Comp Ther* 2000;**5**:111–16.
20. British Medical Association. *Alternative Therapy: Report of the Board of Science and Education*. London: BMA, 1986.
21. Buckman R, Sabbagh K. *Magic or Medicine?* London: Macmillan, 1993.
22. Dieppe P. The role of complementary medicine in our society and the implications that this has in research. (Editorial) *Focus Alt Comp Ther* 2000;**5**:109–10.
23. Reilly D. The therapeutic encounter. In: Kayne SB (ed.), *Homeopathic Practice*. London: Pharmaceutical Press, 2008: 98.
24. Howie JGR, Heaney DJ, Maxwell M, Walker JJ, Freeman GK, Rai H. Quality at general practice consultations: cross sectional survey. *BMJ* 1999;**319**: 738–43.
25. National Asthma Campaign (Asthma UK). Survey. London: Asthma UK, 2001.
26. Ball TM, Castro-Rodriguez JA, Griffith KA, Holberg CJ, Martinez FD, Wright AL. Siblings, day-care attendance, and the risk of asthma and wheezing during childhood. *N Engl J Med* 2000;**343**:538–43.
27. Mitchell CA, Adebajo A. Managing osteoarthritis of the knee: Holistic approach is important. (Letter) *BMJ* 2005;**330**:673.
28. Ventegodt S, Kandel I, Merrick J. A short history of clinical holistic medicine. *Sci World J* 2007;**7**:1622–30.
29. Smuts JC. *Holism and Evolution*. New York: Macmillan, 1926: 84–117.
30. Coward R. *The Whole Truth. The myth of alternative health*. London: Faber & Faber, 1989.
31. Pietroni PC. Holistic medicine: new lessons to be learned. *Practitioner* 1987;**231**:1386–90.
32. Spiegal D. What is the placebo worth? (Editorial) *BMJ* 2008;**336**:967–8.
33. Mueller J. Handwriting as a symptom. *Allgemeine Homöopathische Zeitung* 1993;**238**:60–3.
34. Goodwin JS, Goodwin JM, Vogel AV. Knowledge and use of placebos by house officers and nurses. *Ann Intern Med* 1979;**91**:112–18.
35. Kaptchuk TJ, Kelley JM, Conboy LA et al. Components of placebo effect: randomised controlled trial in patients with irritable bowel syndrome. *BMJ* 2008;**336**: 999–1003.
36. McKee J. Holistic health and the critique of Western medicine. *Soc Sci Med* 1988;**26**:775–84.

37. Labonte R, Penfold PS. *Health Promotion Philosophy. From victim blaming to social responsibility.* Vancouver: Western RO Health & Welfare, 1997: 7.

38. Davies M. From genomics to the clinic: the challenge for molecular science. *Pharm J* 2000;**265**:411–15

39. Pietroni PC. Alternative medicine. *Practitioner* 1986;**230**:1053–4.

40. House of Lords Select Committee on Science and Technology. Complementary and alternative medicine, 6th report 1999–2000 [HL123]. London: The Stationery Office, 2000.

41. Lampert N, Ernst E, Moss RW. Complementary and alternative medicine. (Letter) *Lancet* 2001;**357**:802.

42. Dharmananda S. *Controlled Clinical Trials of Chinese Herbal Medicine: A review.* Oregon: Institute for Traditional Medicine, 1997.

43. Sheehan MP, Rustin MHA, Atherton DJ et al. Efficacy of traditional Chinese herbal therapy in adult atopic dermatitis. *Lancet* 1992;**340**:13–17.

44. Bensoussan A, Menzies R. Treatment of irritable bowel syndrome with Chinese herbal medicine. *JAMA* 1998;**280**:1585–9.

45. National Center for Complementary and Alternative Medicine. *CAM Basics.* Available at: http://tinyurl.com/2jhwml (accessed 14 October 2007).

2

Integrative medicine – incorporating complementary and alternative medicine into practice

Iris R. Bell

Introduction

The purpose of this chapter is to provide an introduction to the concepts, practice and controversies of integrative medicine.[1-4] The terms 'complementary and alternative medicine' (CAM) and 'integrative medicine' (IM) are often used interchangeably in professional and lay discussions of healthcare. However, CAM and IM are labels for overlapping but not identical ways of considering and practising a wide range of clinical interventions. 'CAM' as a term refers more to what type of (CAM) treatment and how a provider prescribes the treatment (in a complementary or alternative way relative to conventional care), whereas IM describes a type of clinical practice by a conventional medical provider who adds CAM to his or her total toolkit of conventional therapies (Table 2.1).

Features of IM

One influential group of physicians who describe their practices as integrative offers a much broader definition of their clinical field, which goes beyond merely employing CAM modalities as clinical tools. The Consortium of Academic Health Centers for Integrative Medicine,[5] for example, defines IM on its website as follows:

> Integrative Medicine is the practice of medicine that reaffirms the importance of the relationship between practitioner and patient, focuses on the whole person, is informed by evidence, and makes use of all appropriate therapeutic approaches, healthcare professionals and disciplines to achieve optimal health and healing.

Table 2.1 Definitions of complementary, alternative and integrative medicine[a]

Label	Status relative to western conventional medicine	Comments
Alternative medicine	Used instead of conventional medicine	A form of healthcare often, but not always, with a lengthy historical tradition. Leading whole system forms of alternative medicine, such as traditional Chinese medicine, classic homeopathy, ayurveda, naturopathy and various indigenous healing systems, usually have philosophical, diagnostic and therapeutic approaches that differ significantly from those of western medicine and from each other. Treatment addresses the alternative medical diagnosis, not necessarily the western medical diagnosis
Complementary medicine	Used as adjunct to and in combination with conventional medicine	Examples – a single herb, acupuncture or a homeopathic remedy, often taken out of its usual full diagnostic and therapeutic context from an alternative medical system and prescribed or used in addition to conventional drugs to treat a western diagnosis or side effect(s) of conventional pharmaceutical drugs
Integrative medicine	Blended medicine provided by mainstream healthcare providers, primarily medical doctors, employing and/or referring patients to both conventional and CAM modalities to treat conventionally diagnosed conditions	A metasystem of systems of care created by each provider who assembles an individualised package of care drawn from conventional and CAM options. The choices are more idiosyncratic to the provider and patient rather than driven by a specific alternative theory of health and disease

Table 2.1 *Continued*

Label	Status relative to western conventional medicine	Comments
		Some IM physicians follow a general philosophy of stimulating self-healing within the patient and providing care as a partner rather than an authority figure. However, the diagnoses are still typically western medical labels with an overlay of focus on global healing rather than cure, quality of life, biopsychosocial issues and spirituality

[a]The politically dominant form of healthcare, western/allopathic/mainstream/conventional medicine, defines other forms of healthcare in relation to itself, using the terms in the table. CAM, complementary and alternative medicine; IM, integrative medicine.

Thus, IM for some providers involves a strong reorientation to patient-centred rather than disease-centred care and the role of the primary provider as partner and educator rather than as authority figure. The principle of starting with the lowest risk options (which are often from CAM rather than pharmaceutical/surgical models of care) is also foremost in certain forms of IM.[1] Detractors of the broad definition of IM often question what differentiates an IM practitioner from any good primary care provider. The answer to the latter question often refers to the inclusion of CAM modalities in routine IM practice and the reliance on treatments to stimulate the self-organised healing capacity from within the patient, rather than on the treatments themselves, to cure disease from outside the individual.[1,6]

Practice models and roles

Medical physicians see IM as their domain, often with themselves as the most influential hubs for orchestrating overall care – with CAM practitioners as lesser members of a multidisciplinary team. Interestingly, Boon et al.[7] described seven different possible conceptual models for team provision of both conventional and CAM treatments in Canada, i.e. parallel, consultative, collaborative, coordinated, multidisciplinary, interdisciplinary and integrative practice. In preliminary follow-up research, conventional physicians prefer models similar to current biomedical practice situations, in which a medical physician directs overall care and refers patients to CAM providers as multidisciplinary team members. Many CAM practitioners prefer a more distinct role with autonomy from MDs, involving parallel practice models in which CAM and conventional providers offer separate lines of care to patients.[8–10]

The risks for treatment interactions and poorer outcomes from inadequate communication and coordination among providers caring for the same patient are obvious even in conventional care teams. Patients often do not tell providers about other providers whom they see or other drugs that they take,[11] nor do they routinely recognise the importance of insisting on professional communication among all of their providers for their own safety. Anecdotal problems from communication failures in CAM and IM include cases of adverse interactions and/or side effects between herbs (e.g. *Gingko biloba*) or nutrients (e.g. high-dose vitamin E) and drugs, leading to, for example, impaired platelet aggregation and poor coagulation during surgeries.[12–14]

History-taking in IM

As a result of the IM emphasis on patient-centred and preventive care through lifestyle modification, intake and follow-up clinical histories are typically broader and less focused in scope than contemporary conventional care visits. IM providers tend to spend more time with each patient during a clinic visit (e.g. 1–2 hours for intake), a non-specific factor known to improve patient satisfaction levels in both conventional and CAM studies.[4,15–18]

The overarching goal of IM care is generally healing (restoring the individual's capacity for wholeness and resilience in the face of change and challenge) rather than, necessarily, a defined cure of a specific condition (though conventional medical 'cure' outcomes can and do occur).[18] Consequently, history-taking encompasses a comprehensive review with the patient not only of a full conventional medical and medication history, but also of biopsychosocial and spiritual aspects of the individual's life and context for the presenting complaint. Details include history of customary diet, exercise and habits, social network and support history, spiritual beliefs and practices, as well as specific information on all non-drug interventions such as nutritional and herbal supplements, homeopathic treatments, and self- and provider-administered forms of CAM.[1,2]

Complementary versus alternative uses of therapies in IM

As defined by the Cochrane Collaboration,[19] complementary therapies are treatments that fall outside acceptance by the politically dominant form of medicine (variously termed western, allopathic, mainstream or conventional medicine), but used adjunctively, with mainstream western medicine, to treat conditions diagnosed within the conceptual framework of western medicine. An example of complementary care would be the addition of self-hypnosis or provider-administered acupuncture as an adjunct to the usual standard care with physician-prescribed analgesic drugs and standard wound care for management of post-surgical pain. As another example, some cancer patients use CAM supplements, such as ginger-based products or Chinese herbs, for chemotherapy- or radiation-induced nausea and vomiting, i.e. a complementary use of an unconventional treatment to address side effects of a mainstream treatment for a life-threatening disease.

In contrast, alternative therapies are treatments falling outside acceptance by the politically dominant western form of medicine and used to modify the primary disease, thereby replacing or eliminating western medicine for a given clinical problem. For instance, some providers of traditional Chinese medicine (TCM, which is a multi-faceted intervention with thousands of years of history far exceeding that of modern western medicine) would use complex, coordinated packages of care, including acupuncture, mixtures of multiple Chinese herbs, dietary changes, tai chi or qi gong and other modalities, to treat a patient with, for example, chronic hepatitis, for the imbalances underlying vulnerability to expressing the disease itself. Providers of TCM would also assert the necessity to perform their own diagnostic procedures to determine the proper treatment package, leading to different types of aetiological labels for patients with the 'same' western medical diagnosis.[20]

Thus, a group of patients with a seemingly homogeneous western diagnosis would probably receive a heterogeneous range of TCM diagnoses, based on TCM theory. Each TCM diagnosis would guide development of multi-faceted, individualised packages of care, rather than a one-size-fits-all standardised treatment for each patient.[21,22] An underlying assumption in many forms of CAM, especially whole systems, such as TCM, homeopathy and ayurveda, would be that the multiple treatment components are necessary to work together towards a common goal of catalysing healing in the person as a whole intact network or complex system,[23] as opposed to prescribing a single 'magic bullet' drug or purified agent to foster a good outcome for each separate body part. Similarly, some IM physicians see the overall treatment package that draws on multiple approaches to healing as an interrelated, whole system with an impact that is greater than the sum of the separate parts.

Even when a healthcare professional tries to offer patients guidance from an 'evidence-based' point of view, the data on real-world outcomes of individualised packages of care are almost non-existent. Most available evidence, influenced by the reductionistic pharmaceutical trial model for randomised controlled trials (RCTs), addresses only isolated efficacy trials of single interventions, one by one, rather than the effectiveness of combined complex interventions characteristic of real-world practice. Reports from some pragmatic and observational trials on large samples of patients, cost-effectiveness studies and intensive self-report interview data from qualitative research may end up filling clinicians' need for information on how real patients fare under treatment with such multi-faceted interventional programmes.[9,24–34]

Individualised care

Complementary and alternative researchers have formalised recognition of the diagnostic differences between western and CAM practices by introducing a dual selection procedure into their clinical trial designs.[35] In acknowledgement of the dominance of western medicine, they first identify a group of patients who are homogeneous by western diagnosis, and then permit the CAM providers to make their own individualised diagnoses within their system of care, thereby generating multiple, highly heterogeneous subgroups carrying both western and CAM labels.[20] The data from at least one study of Chinese herbal combinations for treatment of irritable bowel syndrome support the importance of determining the individualised CAM diagnosis and treatment plan. In a double-blind trial published in the *Journal of the American Medical Association*, both standardised and individualised herbal combinations were superior to placebo in reduction of symptoms after 16 weeks, but only the subgroup receiving individualised herbs maintained improvements 14 weeks after the end of the trial.[36]

Interestingly, other researchers reported that acupuncture, when taken out of context from the rest of TCM (e.g. with herbal mixtures and other treatments), was effective only for some recurrent cystitis patients who met criteria for one of several different TCM diagnoses.[20] The latter study, taken together with other emerging research of individual differences, suggests that IM practitioners may be able to draw on

CAM diagnostic systems and other types of clinical research of individual differences to triage patients clinically to the care programmes most likely to help them.[37–39] Not only do patients with a given western medical diagnosis differ from each other within other (CAM) types of diagnostic frameworks, but they also may differ in their capacity to respond to an isolated CAM modality taken out of its own context for inclusion in an 'integrative' medical treatment package.

For clinicians, research designs may seem too remote from everyday practice to be relevant. Even in mainstream medical practice, primary providers acknowledge great difficulty in applying results of idealised RCTs on single drugs to the average complex patient in their surgeries.[40] Some investigators in both mainstream[41,42] and CAM[28,33,43,44] clinical research have begun to point out the advantages of performing good observational and/or pragmatic rather than RCT studies to assess treatments in a more real-world context of practical relevance to actual clinical circumstances, i.e. practising clinicians encounter many complex patients with multiple conditions, multiple treatments, differential treatment responsivity and side-effect profiles, individual preferences and tolerances, and cultural/familial/social modifying factors for effectiveness (even when a treatment has itself demonstrated efficacy).[1]

Moreover, for any clinician attempting to implement 'evidence-based' IM practice, it is crucial to understand the significant methodological problems and challenges that arise in interpreting even 'high-quality' CAM-related research papers, in order to put the findings of any given study into appropriate perspective, i.e. 'high quality' refers to the quality for internal validity from a conventional medical design and reporting perspective, assuming that the intervention can be standardised and administered to allopathically homogeneous patient populations. Both the assumption of treatment standardisation, which is fair to evaluate purified pharmaceutical drugs, and the assumption of patient sample homogeneity based on western medical diagnosis are often inappropriate for meeting external validity requirements in studies of complex CAM and IM interventions requiring individualised CAM-based diagnoses and multidimensional treatment plans. As IM practice usually involves more than one treatment approach, the emergence of IM brings to a head the necessity of developing better ways of generating high-quality study data useful to clinicians.[45–47]

Even in mainstream medicine, it is a rare clinician who can use only one intervention in a patient, at least in an individual with chronic diseases and the need for multiple drugs for multiple health problems and side effects. Survey data demonstrate that CAM users constitute from a third to a half or more of the population. Many surveys have also shown even higher prevalence of CAM utilisation in people with existing chronic conditions for which mainstream care either has failed to produce benefit or offers risks that patients find unacceptable. As CAM users rely a great deal on natural products for self-care in both acute and chronic health problems (e.g. 19% of the US population use supplements that have the potential to interact with pharmaceutical drugs[48]), mainstream clinicians must expand their knowledge base of CAM, whether or not they practise IM.

Emergent properties of natural products and coordinated packages of care

Apart from the question of individualised diagnosis and treatment, another major claim within IM is the importance of leaving natural products intact rather than seeking to extract and prescribe purified components. The actual evidence for the presumed value of leaving natural products intact (i.e. using the whole herb rather than a purified extract) and/or combining treatments for presumed positive synergy is mixed.

A recent basic science study,[49] for instance, demonstrated that a purified extract of curcuminoids from the spice turmeric exert a strong anti-inflammatory effect in an experimental animal model for arthritis. In contrast, the crude intact turmeric inhibited such benefits, suggesting that, for this specific situation, a conventional pharmaceutical drug development approach may be more helpful than a CAM-derived reliance on an intact natural agent. On the other hand, data suggest that multiple vitamins and minerals together, i.e. inherently complex mixtures of nutritional supplements that naturally work together in the body's biochemical networks, may be beneficial for preventive care,[50] whereas high doses of individual vitamins – used pharmaceutically by themselves as drugs at non-physiological doses – may be harmful under certain conditions.[51]

A lesson from the available research is that IM providers need to be cautious in assuming that they can take CAM treatments out of their original context to assemble blended treatment programmes designed from a western medical perspective. Any given CAM treatment may originate as part of a package of care geared to treat the CAM diagnosis in the person as a whole, not the western diagnosis. An IM physician runs the risk of using CAM as though it were a drug. Unintended outcomes could include no benefit, where some might otherwise be possible in a proper context, or even adverse effects from imbalanced use of treatments in isolation from each other.

Who practises IM versus CAM?

Healthcare professionals

The term 'integrative medicine' refers more to a form of practice by western-trained and -licensed physicians and allied health professionals who add CAM treatments into an otherwise 'conventional' practice than it does to any specific type of intervention as such. IM providers are typically medical doctors or nurse practitioners, whereas CAM practitioners could be licensed conventional providers or naturopaths, acupuncturists or doctors of oriental medicine, chiropractors, osteopaths, hypnotherapists, professional homeopaths, or laypeople performing self-care or alternative healthcare for clients. CAM providers may or may not practise under regulated licensing boards or certification bodies, depending on their field and location of practice. As many CAM providers are not licensed physicians or conventional allied health professionals, they offer CAM therapies to patients, but not necessarily IM ones. Treatments become 'complementary' or 'integrative' by the patient's actual use of both conventional and unconventional therapies.

Patients as integrators

At present, IM itself is a meta-system of systems of care that is poorly delineated.[3] There are no widely accepted standards of practice or credentials for IM providers. Meanwhile, with or without an IM provider, patients who use both conventional and CAM interventions are developing their own idiosyncratic, 'integrated' treatment programmes, often without overall professional guidance as to potential benefits and risks of the total package of care. Numerous studies demonstrate that the vast majority of CAM-using patients also use conventional western care, when available to them. In fact, over half of CAM users in the USA indicated a belief that combining conventional and CAM treatments would help.[48]

Some findings reveal distinct differences in decision-making processes among patients who use conventional-only, CAM-only or combined conventional and CAM treatments.[52] Moreover, patients who have ever used a high number of different CAM modalities and/or certain types of CAM (e.g. energy medicine or whole systems such as homeopathy and TCM) exhibit individual baseline differences in cross-culturally consistent personality traits such as greater openness to experience, or the related genetically based trait – absorption in internal and external experiences.[53,54] Thus, it is important to recognise that, even among people who seek out and use IM treatment, individual patients – and providers – differ in their attitudes towards specific aspects of IM and preferences for specific CAM modalities.[55]

Integrating IM into healthcare systems

Some CAM training leads to formal licensing and/or government-issued credentials, but not necessarily. Countries and municipalities differ markedly in their laws and regulations concerning the credentials of doctors and various types of CAM practitioners. Thus, in 4-year accredited US naturopathic colleges, students would take courses relevant to mainstream medicine, such as anatomy, physiology, biochemistry, pharmacology, but people obtaining a naturopathic degree from a non-accredited programme could have entirely different educational experiences. Moreover, the teaching of basic medical sciences for CAM providers might focus more on concepts and findings of clinical relevance to the CAM practice rather than to western medicine. In short, CAM providers may or may not practise western medicine in any way and therefore, by definition, are not offering IM as such to their patients. A medical doctor diagnoses and treats disease as defined by western medicine. Legally, CAM providers are not practising medicine without a licence if they avoid using western medical diagnoses and treatments. Some clinical training programmes in IM have developed at academic health centres in the USA, including forging proposed competency models for IM education.[17]

Again, the theme running consistently through use of the terms 'CAM' and 'IM' is the implicit assumption that mainstream western conventional medicine and its practitioners are 'superior' to other types of therapy. Implicit in such use of language is the assumption that western medical doctors and allied health professionals are still the final authorities on health and healthcare. If their form of science (i.e. double-blind, placebo-controlled RCTs, originally developed in the mid-1900s to test pharmaceutical drug agents) 'proves' the efficacy of an unconventional therapy to act in a drug-like manner in treatment of a western diagnosis, IM providers will accept the unconventional treatment as a drug surrogate – and assimilate it into their practices. If a treatment does not behave like a drug in an RCT, however, IM practitioners may find themselves rejecting treatments that could help specific individuals not recognised as a subgroup within an RCT design.[20]

Furthermore, CAM philosophies and some approaches to IM raise other issues, e.g. the question of the goals of the care as such. In the CAM and IM worlds, providers emphasise the World Health Organization's definition of health as follows:

> Health is a state of complete physical, mental and social well-being, and not merely the absence of disease or infirmity.

At a practical level, does the nurturance of wellness, not merely the removal of disease, fall within the mission of the health professions? Should third party payers, including government healthcare services, pay for a person without disease to enhance their wellness? Many IM clinics in North America have failed to find viable financial models under which to offer their care programmes. Some have found unusual compromise solutions by offering the high-tech, conventional, western diagnostic and treatment services that generate revenue in order to support the low-tech, health-promoting, CAM-derived care that does not.

What are the unique risks of IM to the patient?

It is striking that the relatively rare instances of serious adverse effects from a given natural product supplement or a CAM therapy receive widespread attention in both the professional and the lay media. The consistently worrisome reports of severe morbidity and mortality from western medical tools, including properly prescribed drugs, as well as the risks of improperly prescribed drugs (e.g. antibiotics for viral infections, leading to emergence of drug-resistant strains of bacteria) lead many IM providers to favour CAM modalities with better safety track records in widespread community use as the first, rather than secondary or tertiary, line of treatment.[1] Some data suggest that inclusion of certain types of CAM in an IM practice can, in certain settings, reduce overall patient care costs, generate higher patient acceptability and adherence, and lower incidence of adverse events.[56–58] Concerns about possible interference of dietary supplements with effectiveness of chemotherapeutic agents persist, but evidence for harm is not definitive. In fact, many studies suggest potential improved survival outcomes in cancer patients who add antioxidants during conventional oncology treatments with chemo- or radiotherapy.[59]

Nevertheless, for any provider who includes CAM in practice, certain risks and potential liabilities exist, e.g. the lack of regulatory oversight in many countries has led to manufacturing failures and abuses. Numerous nutritional and herbal supplements do not necessarily contain the amounts of ingredients listed on the labels. Some introduce dangerous contaminants and toxicants into the supplements themselves, such as lead, hormones and pharmaceutical drugs in variable amounts. Previous problems with tryptophan supplements stemmed, at least partly, from a contaminant produced by the manufacturing process itself in a major supplier. More recently, kava-kava products, originally touted as valuable for treating mild anxiety and related problems, caused notable, albeit fairly rare cases of fulminant liver damage, perhaps because of the use of alcoholic extracts in western processing (differing from traditional preparation methods). The herbal mixture PC-SPES, found initially helpful for treating men with prostate cancer,[60,61] turned up with significant oestrogenic and other contaminants in some batches.[62]

Apart from contaminants, excessive long-term use of high-dose vitamin B6 (pyridoxine) can lead to peripheral neuropathy that may or may not reverse upon discontinuation. In certain cases, the herbal St John's wort, used for mild-to-moderate depression, can adversely affect levels and/or activity of oral contraceptives, and anti-HIV and some cancer chemotherapy agents, among others. Several excellent reviews summarise specific concerns for monitoring drug–herb and drug–nutrient interactions.[63-67] For example, a recent Canadian review noted that patients who are female, older, in the lower socioeconomic levels, and already treated for diabetes or hypertension have elevated risk of at least one such reaction. However, the clinical significance of the potential interactions is not as yet established. In the UK, similarly, older individuals – who often take multiple prescription drugs – carry an increased risk of drug interactions with dietary supplements.[68]

Both pharmacokinetic and pharmacodynamic interactions are risks in IM involving natural supplements, albeit at an apparently low incidence, from available data. Although other forms of CAM also can cause adverse effects at a low rate (e.g. cases of increased anxiety in certain panic attack patients trying to meditate, serious spinal cord injury in occasional chiropractic patients and lung needle punctures in rare acupuncture patients), the incidence and usually severity of CAM risks are relatively much lower than those of pharmaceutical drugs in the hands of properly trained clinicians.

Complementary and alternative medicine modalities such as homeopathic remedies have a generally excellent safety record, and several countries have greater standardisation guidelines for homeopathic manufacturing than they do for herbal or nutritional supplements.[66-68] Notably, both healthcare professionals and laypeople sometimes confuse or mistake herbal and other supplement products with homeopathic remedies. The preparation procedures and standards for homeopathic remedies, even though they derive from animal, mineral and plant sources, differ substantially from those of herbal or nutritional products. Only homeopathic products undergo systematic dilution and succussion steps as a requisite of their manufacture. The dilution/succussion process places 24x or 12c and higher potencies at concentrations beyond Avogadro's number of molecules, but with measurable evidence of biological activity and altered physical chemical properties.[69-77]

Mainstream providers often worry that patients will defer time-sensitive conventional treatments, e.g. in cancer, when late failure of CAM and initiation of conventional care may not be as effective in reducing mortality as earlier intervention. However, the prevalence data on the latter scenario across CAM users are not compelling. Most CAM users are already using conventional care and are satisfied with their own primary care provider, but find that the tools of mainstream medicine are insufficient for their own personal health goals.[48,78]

As noted earlier, even when a product reliably provides the ingredients claimed on the label and nothing more, adverse reactions could occur from interactions with other treatments involving drugs, herbs or nutrients. Even drinking grapefruit juice can interfere with drug metabolism. One of the more commonly reported problems is heightened anticoagulant effects of high-dose vitamin E or *Ginkgo biloba*. Patients in the USA taking coumadin (Warfarin Sodium tablets USP; warfarin in the UK), for example, must receive close monitoring for necessary stabilisation of polypharmacy components, selection of different agents with less risk of pharmacological interactions and readjustments of drug doses.

Conclusions

Although controversial among CAM proponents, the regulatory environment clearly favours the structured culture of western mainstream medicine. For patient safety, the trend towards basic standards of training, professionalisation and providing credentials for CAM providers is a practical and desirable development.[79] At the same time, the nature of consumer-directed healthcare choices highlights the urgency of implementing formal continuing educational requirements on the potential beneficial and harmful interactions of western medical and CAM treatments, not only for conventional physicians, nurses, pharmacists and other allied health professionals, but also for CAM providers and consumers.[80]

The shift towards regulation of consumable CAM products, such as nutritional and herbal supplements, is a more complex and controversial area. Undoubtedly, it is in the best interests of public health in every country that dangerous products containing toxic contaminants, drugs and hormones be detected swiftly and removed from accessibility. The generation and enforcement of good manufacturing standards for supplements also meet the public's needs for safe and reliable over-the-counter products. However, the specifics of how to set and enforce the standards for CAM providers and for products become a difficult challenge.

One risk is that regulators will seize upon, for example, standardisation of a herbal product to a single constituent on the assumption that the constituent is the only meaningfully active component of the herb. In some situations, this assumption may be correct and appropriate. However, many herbalists argue that a single constituent strategy could distort the true medicinal effectiveness of the intact herb and prematurely exclude products with greater potential for higher benefit and lower risk.

Another risk of regulation in CAM is that the detractors would use their political control over setting and enforcing standards to block certain CAM practices, practitioners and products from availability to the public. The history of science and healthcare is replete with well-documented and anecdotal instances of the effects of mainstream power-holder biases on preventing challengers to the status quo beliefs making their case and/or from offering their services.[81–83] Recent examples where science eventually supported the 'outrageous' claims of medical mavericks were in the role of *Helicobacter pylori* in causation of peptic ulcers and the importance of elevated homocysteine levels as an independent risk factor for cardiovascular disease.

On the one hand, the assumed superiority of western medicine falls mainly in the areas of benefits, the presumption of scientific evidence-based practice and regulatory standards for products and provider credentials. On the other, long-term historical use and safety records in real-world contexts, as well as high levels of patient acceptability within certain cultural and/or ethnic communities, actually favour many CAM therapies over more modern western approaches.

In short, whether or not a mainstream provider favours, disfavours, uses or does not use CAM for themselves or their patients,[84,85] the consumer-based reality is that all providers are thrown into dealing with patients who use both CAM and conventional medicine in most healthcare settings. All responsible healthcare professionals must seek continuing education in CAM and monitor the literature for appropriately designed and implemented studies of packages of care in IM. IM, as a field, is in its infancy, but the extent of consumer expectations requires rapid maturation at the clinical, educational and research levels.

References

1. Rakel D. *Integrative Medicine*, 2nd edn. Philadelphia, PA: Saunders Elsevier, 2007.
2. Kliger B, Lee R. *Integrative Medicine: Principles for practice*. New York: McGraw-Hill, 2004.
3. Bell IR, Caspi O, Schwartz GE et al. Integrative medicine and systemic outcomes research: issues in the emergence of a new model for primary health care. *Arch Intern Med* 2002;**162**:133–40.
4. Gaudet TW. Integrative medicine: the evolution of a new approach to medicine and to medical education. *Integr Med* 1998;**1**(2):67–73.
5. Consortium of Academic Health Centers for Integrative Medicine. *Integrative Medicine*, 2005. Available at: www.imconsortium.org/cahcim/about/home.html (accessed 27 September 2007).
6. Snyderman R, Weil AT. Integrative medicine: bringing medicine back to its roots. *Arch Intern Med* 2002;**162**:395–7.
7. Boon H, Verhoef M, O'Hara D, Findlay B. From parallel practice to integrative health care: a conceptual framework. *BMC Health Services Research* 2004;**4**(1):1.
8. Hollenberg D. Uncharted ground: patterns of professional interaction among complementary/alternative and biomedical practitioners in integrative health care settings. *Soc Sci Med* 2006;**62**:731–44.
9. Kaptchuk TJ, Miller FG. Viewpoint: what is the best and most ethical model for the relationship between mainstream and alternative medicine: opposition, integration, or pluralism? *Acad Med* 2005;**80**:286–90.
10. Thompson TD, Weiss M. Homeopathy – what are the active ingredients? An exploratory study using the UK Medical Research Council's framework for the evaluation of complex interventions. *BMC Compl Altern Med* 2006;**13**(6):37.
11. Eisenberg DM, Davis RB, Ettner SL et al. Trends in alternative medicine use in the US, 1990–1997. Results of a follow-up national survey. *JAMA* 1998; **280**:1569–75.

12. Busato A, Donges A, Herren S, Widmer M, Marian F. Health status and health care utilisation of patients in complementary and conventional primary care in Switzerland – an observational study. *Fam Pract* 2006;**23**(1):116–24.

13. Agdal R. Diverse and changing perceptions of the body: communicating illness, health, and risk in an age of medical pluralism. *J Altern Compl Med* 2005;**11**(suppl 1):S67–75.

14. Chang LK, Whitaker DC. The impact of herbal medicines on dermatologic surgery. *Dermatol Surg* 2001;**28**:759–63.

15. Tai-Seale M, McGuire TG, Zhang W. Time allocation in primary care office visits. *Health Serv Res* 2007;**42**:1871–94.

16. Lin CT, Albertson GA, Schilling LM et al. Is patients' perception of time spent with the physician a determinant of ambulatory patient satisfaction? *Arch Intern Med* 2001;**161**:1437–42.

17. Kligler B, Maizes V, Schachter S et al., Education Working Group, Consortium of Academic Health Centers for Integrative Medicine. Core competencies in integrative medicine for medical school curricula: a proposal. *Acad Med* 2004;**79**:521–31.

18. Bikker AP, Mercer SW, Reilly D. A pilot prospective study on the consultation and relational empathy, patient enablement, and health changes over 12 months in patients going to the Glasgow Homoeopathic Hospital. *J Altern Compl Med* 2005;**11**:591–600.

19. Zollman C, Vickers A. ABC of complementary medicine: what is complementary medicine? *BMJ* 1999;**319**:693–6.

20. Alraek T, Baerheim A. The effect of prophylactic acupuncture treatment in women with recurrent cystitis: kidney patients fare better. *J Altern Compl Med* 2003;**9**:651–8.

21. Caspi O, Bell IR. One size does not fit all: aptitude-treatment interaction (ATI) as a conceptual framework for outcome research. Part I. What is ATI research? *J Altern Compl Med* 2004;**10**:580–6.

22. Caspi O, Bell IR. One size does not fit all: aptitude-treatment interaction (ATI) as a conceptual framework for outcome research. Part II. Research designs and their application. *J Altern Compl Med* 2004;**10**:698–705.

23. Bell IR, Koithan M. Models for the study of whole systems. *Integr Cancer Ther* 2006;**5**:293–307.

24. MacPherson H, Thorpe L, Thomas K. Beyond needling – therapeutic processes in acupuncture care: a qualitative study nested within a low-back pain trial. *J Altern Compl Med* 2006;**12**:873–80.

25. Paterson C, Britten N. Acupuncture for people with chronic illness: combining qualitative and quantitative outcome assessment. *J Altern Compl Med* 2003;**9**:671–81.

26. van Wassenhoven M, Ives G. An observational study of patients receiving homeopathic treatment. *Homeopathy* 2004;**93**(1):3–11.

27. Witt CM, Luedtke R, Baur R, Willich SN. Homeopathic medical practice: long-term results of a cohort study with 3981 patients. *BMC Public Health* 2005;**5**(1):115. epub

28. Verhoef MJ, Mulkins A, Boon H. Integrative health care: how can we determine whether patients benefit? *J Altern Compl Med* 2005;**11**(suppl 1):S57–65.

29. Pelletier KR, Astin JA. Integration and reimbursement of complementary and alternative medicine by managed care and insurance providers: 2000 update and cohort analysis. (Comment) *Altern Ther Hlth Med* 2002;**8**(1):38–9, 42, 4 *et seq.*
30. Herman PM CB, Caspi O. Is complementary and alternative medicine (CAM) cost-effective? A systematic review. *BMC Compl Altern Med* 2005;**5**:11.
31. Paterson C, Dieppe P. Characteristic and incidental (placebo) effects in complex interventions such as acupuncture. *BMJ* 2005;**330**:1202–5.
32. Paterson C, Britten N. Acupuncture as a complex intervention: a holistic model. *J Altern Compl Med* 2004;**10**:791–801.
33. Linde K, Streng A, Hoppe A, Weidenhammer W, Wagenpfeil S, Melchart D. Randomized trial vs. observational study of acupuncture for migraine found that patient characteristics differed but outcomes were similar. *J Clin Epidemiol* 2007;**60**:280–7.
34. Maxion-Bergemann S, Wolf M, Bornhoft G, Matthiessen PF, Wolf U. Complementary and alternative medicine costs – a systematic literature review. *Forsch Komplementarmed 2006*;**13**(suppl 2):42–5.
35. Vincent C, Furnham A. *Complementary Medicine: A research perspective.* New York: John Wiley & Sons, 1997.
36. Bensoussan A, Talley NJ, Hing M, Menzies R, Guo A, Ngu M. Treatment of irritable bowel syndrome with Chinese herbal medicine: a randomized controlled trial. (Comment) *JAMA* 1998;**280**:1585–9.
37. Bell IR, Lewis DA, 2nd, Brooks AJ et al. Individual differences in response to randomly assigned active individualized homeopathic and placebo treatment in fibromyalgia: implications of a double-blinded optional crossover design. *J Altern Compl Med* 2004;**10**:269–83.
38. Bell IR, Lewis DAI, Schwartz GE et al. Electroencephalographic cordance patterns distinguish exceptional clinical responders with fibromyalgia to individualized homeopathic medicines. *J Altern Compl Med* 2004;**10**:285–99.
39. Owens JE, Taylor AG, Degood D. Complementary and alternative medicine and psychologic factors: toward an individual differences model of complementary and alternative medicine use and outcomes. *J Altern Compl Med* 1999;**5**:529–41.
40. Freeman AC, Sweeney K. Why general practitioners do not implement evidence: qualitative study. *BMJ* 2001;**323**:1100–2.
41. Concato J, Shah N, Horwitz RI. Randomized, controlled trials, observational studies, and the hierarchy of research designs. *N Engl J Med* 2000;**342**:1887–92.
42. Concato J. Observational versus experimental studies: what's the evidence for a hierarchy? *NeuroRadiology* 2004;**1**:341–7.
43. Verhoef MJ, Lewith G, Ritenbaugh C, Boon H, Fleishman S, Leis A. Complementary and alternative medicine whole systems research: Beyond identification of inadequacies of the RCT. *Compl Ther Med* 2005;**13**:206–12.
44. Fonnebo V, Grimsgaard S, Walach H et al. Researching complementary and alternative treatments – the gatekeepers are not at home. *BMC Med Res Methodol* 2007;**7**(1):7.
45. Frei H, Everts R, von Ammon K et al. Randomised controlled trials of homeopathy in hyperactive children: treatment procedure leads to an

unconventional study design. Experience with open-label homeopathic treatment preceding the Swiss ADHD placebo controlled, randomised, double-blind, cross-over trial. *Homeopathy* 2007;**96**(1):35–41.

46. Verhoef MJ, Casebeer AL, Hilsden RJ. Assessing efficacy of complementary medicine: adding qualitative research methods to the 'Gold Standard'. *J Altern Compl Med* 2002;**8**:275–81.

47. Verhoef M, Lewith G, Ritenbaugh C, Thomas K, Boon H, Fonnebo V. Whole systems research: moving forward. *Focus Altern Compl Ther* 2004;**9**(2): 87–90.

48. Barnes PM, Powell-Griner E, McFann K, Nahin RL. *Complementary and Alternative Medicine use among Adults: United States, 2002.* Hyattsville, MD: National Center for Health Statistics, 2004.

49. Funk JL, Oyarzo JN, Frye JB et al. Turmeric extracts containing curcuminoids prevent experimental rheumatoid arthritis. *J Natural Products* 2006;**69**: 351–5.

50. Huang HY, Caballero B, Chang S et al. The efficacy and safety of multivitamin and mineral supplement use to prevent cancer and chronic disease in adults: a systematic review for a National Institutes of Health state-of-the-science conference. *Ann Intern Med* 2006;**145**:372–85.

51. Lee DH, Folsom AR, Harnack L, Halliwell B, Jacobs DR Jr. Does supplemental vitamin C increase cardiovascular disease risk in women with diabetes? *Am J Clin Nutr* 2004;**80**:1194–200.

52. Caspi O, Koithan M, Criddle MW. Alternative medicine or 'alternative' patients: a qualitative study of patient-oriented decision-making processes with respect to complementary and alternative medicine. *Medical Decision Making* 2004;**24**(1):64–79.

53. Honda K, Jacobson JS. Use of complementary and alternative medicine among United States adults: the influences of personality, coping strategies, and social support. *Prev Med* 2005;**40**(1):46–53.

54. Owens JE, Taylor AG, Degood D. Complementary and alternative medicine and psychologic factors: toward an individual differences model of complementary and alternative medicine use and outcomes. *J Altern Compl Med* 1999;**5**:529–41.

55. Schneider CD, Meek PM, Bell IR. Development and validation of IMAQ: Integrative Medicine Attitude Questionnaire. *BMC Med Educ* 2003;**3**:5.

56. Riley D, Fischer M, Singh B, Haidvogl M, Heger M. Homeopathy and conventional medicine: an outcomes study comparing effectiveness in a primary care setting. *J Altern Compl Med* 2001;**7**:149–59.

57. Guthlin C, Lange O, Walach H. Measuring the effects of acupuncture and homoeopathy in general practice: an uncontrolled prospective documentation approach. *BMC Public Health* 2004;**4**(1):4.

58. Haidvogl M, Riley DS, Heger M et al. Homeopathic and conventional treatment for acute respiratory and ear complaints: a comparative study on outcome in the primary care setting. *BMC Compl Altern Med* 2007;**2**(7):7.

59. Simone CB, Simone NL, Simone V, Simone CB. Antioxidants and other nutrients do not interfere with chemotherapy or radiation therapy and can increase kill and increase survival, Part 2. *Altern Ther Health Med* 2007;13(2):40–7.

60. Shabbir M, Love J, Montgomery B. Phase I trial of PC-Spes2 in advanced hormone refractory prostate cancer. *Oncol Rep* 2008;**19**:831–5.

61. Oh WK, Kantoff PW, Weinberg V et al. Prospective, multicenter, randomized phase II trial of the herbal supplement, PC-SPES, and diethylstilbestrol in patients with androgen-independent prostate cancer. *J Clin Oncol* 2004; **22**:3705–12

62. Sovak M, Seligson AL, Konas M et al. Herbal composition PC-SPES for management of prostate cancer: identification of active principles. *J Natl Cancer Inst* 2002;**94**:1275–81.

63. Bressler R. Herb-drug interactions: interactions between kava and prescription medications. *Geriatrics* 2005;**60**(9):24–5.

64. Bush TM, Rayburn KS, Holloway SW et al. Adverse interactions between herbal and dietary substances and prescription medications: a clinical survey. *Altern Ther Hlth Med* 2007;**13**(2):30–5.

65. Charrois TL, Hill RL, Vu D et al. Community identification of natural health product-drug interactions. *Ann Pharmacother* 2007;**41**:1124–9.

66. Singh SRLM. Potential interactions between pharmaceuticals and natural health products in Canada. *J Clin Pharmacol* 2007;**47**:249–58.

67. Gabardi S, Munz K, Ulbricht C. A review of dietary supplement-induced renal dysfunction. *Clin J Am Soc Nephrol* 2007;**2**:757–65.

68. Canter PH, Ernst, E. Herbal supplement use by persons aged over 50 years in Britain: frequently used herbs, concomitant use of herbs, nutritional supplements and prescription drugs, rate of informing doctors and potential for negative interactions. *Drugs Aging* 2004;**21**:597–605.

69. Bornhoft G, Wolf U, Ammon K et al. Effectiveness, safety and cost-effectiveness of homeopathy in general practice – summarized health technology assessment. *Forsch Komplementärmed* 2006;**13**(suppl 2):19–29.

70. Dantas F, Rampes H. Do homeopathic medicines provoke adverse effects? A systematic review. *Br Homoeopath J* 2000;**89**(suppl 1):S35–8.

71. Borneman JP, Field RI. Regulation of homeopathic drug products. *Am J Health Syst Pharm* 2006;**63**(1):86–91.

72. Chaplin MF. The memory of water: an overview. *Homeopathy* 2007;**96**: 143–50.

73. Roy R, Tiller W, Bell IR, Hoover MR. The structure of liquid water: novel insights from materials research and potential relevance to homeopathy. *Materials Research Innovation* 2005;**9**:557–608.

74. Elia V, Napoli E, Germano R. The 'memory of water': an almost deciphered enigma. Dissipative structures in extremely dilute aqueous solutions. *Homeopathy* 2007;**96**:163–9.

75. van Wijk R, Wiegant FAC. *Cultured Mammalian Cells in Homeopathy Research. The Similia principle in self-recovery.* Utrecht, The Netherlands: Universiteit Utrecht, 1994.

76. van Wijk R, Bosman S, van Wijk EP. Thermoluminescence in ultra-high dilution research. *J Altern Compl Med* 2006;**12**:437–43.

77. Rey L. Thermoluminescence of ultra-high dilutions of lithium chloride and sodium chloride. *Physica A: Statistical mechanics and its applications* 2003;**323**:67–74.

78. Kroesen K, Baldwin CM, Brooks AJ, Bell IR. US military veterans' perceptions of the conventional medical care system and their use of complementary and alternative medicine. *Family Pract* 2002;**19**(1):57–64.
79. Walker LA, Budd S. UK: the current state of regulation of complementary and alternative medicine. *Compl Ther Med* 2002;**10**(1):8–13.
80. Kelner M, Wellman B, Welsh S, Boon H. How far can complementary and alternative medicine go? The case of chiropractic and homeopathy. *Soc Sci Med* 2006;**63**:2617–27.
81. Barber B. Resistance by scientists to scientific discovery. *Science* 1961;**134**: 596–602.
82. McCully KS. *The Homocysteine Revolution*. New York: McGraw-Hill, 1999.
83. Hellman H. *Great Feuds in Medicine: Ten of the liveliest disputes ever*. Chichester: Wiley, 2002.
84. Baugniet J, Boon H, Ostbye T. Complementary/alternative medicine: comparing the view of medical students with students in other health care professions. *Family Med* 2000;**32**:178–84.
85. White ARR, Ernst K-LE. Complementary medicine: Use and attitudes among GPs. *Family Pract* 1997;**14**:302–6.

3

Delivering complementary and
alternative medicine

Steven B Kayne

The demand for complementary medicine

Patients' requirements for healthcare

Patients require the following four features of a healthcare system.[1]

Treatment and care that work

Patients' perceptions of what constitutes 'better' or 'improved' may differ from the opinion of their healthcare provider and is taken into consideration in complementary and alternative medicine (CAM) by the use of patient-oriented outcome measures.

Good relationship with practitioner

Patients put their relationship with their doctors as second only to that with their families.[2] This includes such features as 'a feeling of comfort', 'getting support and sympathy', being told the truth, getting valid explanations, being treated as a person', etc. It would appear that the relationship between the patient and prescriber is a highly significant factor in determining whether or not patients adhere to treatment regimens and to what extent they improve.[3] Patients need empathy and understanding in order to express their preferences, values and fears. Evidence is not enough: healthcare providers need to communicate with patients, listen to their concerns, elicit their values, be involved and really care about them. They also need to integrate the evidence with patients' values and preferences.[4] Building concordant relationships may depend on practitioners developing strategies to establish individuals' preferences for involvement in decision-making as part of the ongoing prescriber–patient relationship.[5] The holistic basis to CAM practice requires extended consultations that may in themselves contribute to the healing process. The building of a good relationship is instrumental in obtaining the requisite amount of information.

Provision of information

Giving information about the condition and treatment on the condition for which advice is being sought is important. Safety issues and interactions need to be discussed. McIver[1] reviewed a number of studies and found that better outcomes were achieved when patients had received more information. Treatment with CAM often involves complicated dose regimens and necessitates the provision of information to the patient.

Remaining in control of treatment

Health professionals have found themselves in the position of having to respond reactively to requests for advice and treatment. Governments have begun to acknowledge that patients have the right to be treated as they wish.

Patient involvement in decision-making is widely regarded as an important feature of good-quality healthcare. Policy-makers have been particularly concerned to ensure that patients are informed about and enabled to choose between relevant treatment options, but it is not clear how patients understand and value involvement. It should be acknowledged that a decision on what constitutes best evidence may well differ in the opinion of the healthcare provider and the patient, and careful and sensitive discussion should ensue to ensure that the patient's best interests are considered. CAM practitioners make treatment choices on the basis of all aspects of a condition, not just the physical symptoms. Research suggests that practitioners who aspire to facilitate patient involvement should attend to the ethos that they foster in consultations and the way that they discuss problems, as well as to the provision of information about treatment options and the scope that patients have to influence decisions.[6] As CAM practitioners arrive at a course of treatment through negotiation the patient remains in control.

Why do people choose to be treated with CAM?

In addition to the main principles of healthcare that need to be satisfied, there are other specific multifactorial reasons that motivate consumers to seek out CAM. There is no doubt that orthodox medicine (OM) is important in the care of many physical ailments, particularly those related to trauma, emergency medicine and terminal disease. However, it is less effective in preventing the development of disease, in altering the course of chronic physical disease, and in addressing the mental, emotional and spiritual needs of an individual. Efforts at prevention have generally focused on screening programmes designed to detect early disease such as cervical smear programmes, mammography clinics, and cholesterol and blood pressure checks, rather than on primary prevention. The non-specific symptoms and signs that are the frequent forerunner to many major diseases are given less attention.[7]

Vincent and Furnham[8] studied patients receiving homeopathy at three London clinics and sought to identify reasons why they chose this particular complementary therapy. A total of 268 patients took part in the study, of whom 201 (74.9%) were female; 89 patients were attending the British School of Osteopathy, 92 a large acupuncture centre in London and the remaining 87 the Royal London Homoeopathic Hospital.

The following were identified as being the most common across the three groups.

• 'Because the emphasis was on treating the whole person.'
• 'Because I believe complementary medicine will be more effective for my problem than OM.'
• 'Because I believe that CAM will enable me to take a more active part in maintaining my health.'
• 'Because OM was not effective for my particular problem.'

In fact a total of 20 reasons were identified and the authors classified them into five groups:

1. Value of CAM
2. OM ineffective
3. Adverse effects of OM
4. Communication between patient and practitioner
5. Cost and availability.

Overall, it would seem that the swing towards CAM is a result of patients' requirements for healthcare being satisfied to a large extent rather than for the other reasons in McIver's list.

An Australian study involving a convenient sample of 158 clients attending a clinic demonstrated that clients access CAM practitioners not only for improvement of physical symptoms, with 54% of clients indicating a desire for counselling for general health issues and 50% wanting dietary and nutritional treatment.[9] Of the participants 36% sought increased self-insight and benefit from a wider perspective of healing. In addition 55% of respondents indicated that the quality of the relationship between the CAM and the client has a major impact on compliance and continuity of treatment, which in turn affects the overall success of the treatment.

Knowing why people choose to use homeopathic medicines is useful as a basis for understanding the source of future demand.[10] From a marketing perspective, these factors can be divided into 'push' and 'pull' factors. *Push factors* are essentially clinical in nature, so they relate to the perceived dangers of using conventional medicines, such as drug toxicity, which may encourage patients to seek safer alternatives. *Pull factors* are those that encourage people to use complementary treatments (usually for particular complaints). These may be social (advice from family and friends), financial (considered to be good value for money) or resulting from patients' beliefs that CAM is a good form of treatment.

Safety concerns – the risk–benefit ratio

At a time when conventional medicine continues to achieve spectacular successes in understanding and treating a plethora of new diseases with ever more ingenuity, there is an undertone of public dissatisfaction with orthodox medicine. With a growing emphasis on quality of healthcare, iatrogenic illnesses and adverse events, significant professional and public attention has been focused on the issue of drug safety and the risk–benefit ratio. A recent meta-analysis estimated that, in the USA, 6.7% of hospitalised patients experience serious adverse drug reactions and that more than 100 000 Americans die annually from drug-induced conditions. One leading hospital spends more than $US5m each year as a result of adverse drug events. These and other similar studies are described in a book by Sharpe and Faden that details many aspects of medical harm.[11]

It has been suggested that some patients may think of unconventional therapies as a type of risk-free supplementary insurance that buys a higher state of wellness and a symptom-free, stress-free existence.[12]

In 1985 the public was assured that:

Drugs are remarkably safe. Few patients would refuse an elective surgical operation with a risk of less than 1:10,000. Yet for medicines much greater safety is demanded and achieved.[13]

In fact the seeds of discontent with orthodox medicine predated this statement by some 30 years. The most significant event affecting complementary medicine was the terrible tragedy of thalidomide. Although the first child afflicted by thalidomide damage to the ears was born on Christmas Day 1956, it took about four and a half years before an Australian gynaecologist, Dr WG McBride of Huntsville, NSW, suspected that the drug was the cause of various abnormalities in three children whom he had seen at a local hospital and brought the matter to the notice of his colleagues in a short letter to *The Lancet*.[14] Until then patients picked up prescriptions from their doctors, visited their local pharmacy to obtain the medicines and went home fully expecting to get better. Adverse drug reactions – called 'side effects' – were relatively unknown, at least to patients. However, after thalidomide, regulatory authorities the world over became aware of the dangers of approving drugs without adequate testing procedures. From this time on consumers began asking questions about the risks as well as the benefits of a particular drug.

Perceptions of unacceptable drug risks have been known to affect people's choice of treatment for some time.[15] There is considerable evidence that the public consider complementary medicines to offer a more satisfactory health benefit ratio.

The attitudes and perceptions of a sample of Swedish adults with respect to a number of common risks have been studied by Slovak et al.[16] Respondents characterised themselves as people who disliked taking risks and who resisted taking medicines unless forced to do so. Prescription drugs (except for insomnia and antidepressant treatments) were perceived to be generally high benefit and low risk. The results for herbal medicine and acupuncture showed an extremely low perceived risk (only slightly higher than vitamins) and a perceived benefit (approximately equal to vitamins, oral contraceptives and aspirin).

In a survey of patients from the UK, Germany and Austria, it was found that the two most frequent reasons for using CAM were a desire to use all options in healthcare and the hope of being cured without any side effects.[17]

Thirty-nine per cent of 465 Canadian men recently diagnosed with prostate cancer chose to use CAM therapies, with the most common being herbal supplements (saw palmetto), vitamins (vitamin E) and minerals (selenium),[18] in order to boost their immune system and prevent recurrence.

General disenchantment with OM

In a period of hyperdifferentiation in biomedicine, when medicine is practised in large bureaucratic structures where there is minimal attention to the individual and her or his social and psychological needs, CAM provides a non-invasive, holistic alternative that is increasingly attractive to many, in particular to those who are better educated, richer and residents of urban centres.

The new approach to healthcare In the period after World War II, health for most people was something that became an important issue only when they fell ill.[19] Health and illness were beyond one's control. Health was dispensed by the doctor and the local chemist, whereas illness was the result of either an unfortunate chance meeting with some passing bacterium or virus, or a genetic predisposition. The mood was almost fatalistic. There was, of course, a general view that people should protect their health by maintaining appropriate standards of hygiene, but the overall responsibility for promoting wellbeing was seen as resting with the state.

In the last few decades there has been a move from paternalism to consumerism in health policy.[20] Patients are now being treated more as consumers who make demands and have individual needs that must be satisfied. The UK health reforms in recent years have served to define consumerism in terms of:

- the maximisation of patient choice
- the provision of adequate information about proposed treatment plans
- taking patients' preferences into account
- carrying out surveys on patient satisfaction.

Patients are given information and encouraged to complain if services do not meet their expectations. The Patients' Charter published by the Ministry of Health in 1991 implied that people should be treated as healthcare *customers*.[19] Important considerations are issues such as communication, staff attitudes and consultation environments. With widespread discussion of these matters in the media, it is not surprising that OM should become a target for discontent in some people's minds, and that they should demand other types of treatments. As early as 1978 patients are thought to have turned to homeopathy as a result of a dissatisfaction with allopathic medicine.[21] The medical establishment is well aware of the growing demand for CAM. As long ago as 1994, an editorial in the *British Medical Journal* referred to patients as 'sophisticated consumers who are challenging the unique authority of doctors'.[22] It went on: 'Patients cannot be treated as passive fodder of medical practice. Increasingly, patients are as educated as their doctors.'

Bakx[23] has summarised some of the possible reasons for the development of widespread discontent with OM among users of CAM:

- OM has culturally distanced itself from the consumers of its services.
- OM has failed to match its promises with real breakthroughs in combating disease created by modern lifestyles.
- OM has alienated patients through unsympathetic or ineffectual practitioner–patient interaction.

With the advent of healthcare consumerism, and as a result of a finite health budget, the public are now encouraged to be largely responsible for their own health. And that does not apply to self-treating trivial ailments alone. It means having a 'responsible' lifestyle too. If you smoke 60 cigarettes a day, you are likely to go to the very back of the queue for bypass surgery, if indeed you are considered at all. It is indicative of the responsibilities now expected of the population. If the public accept this argument, should healthcare professionals not respond accordingly? Healthcare should be a two-way dialogue in many people's minds. This notion has always been part of the CAM doctrine.

The reasons for CAM use were examined by Sirois and Gick.[24] They divided complementary medicine clients into two groups, based on the frequency and length of their use of complementary therapies, and compared them with conventional medicine clients as well as with each other. New/infrequent CAM clients ($n = 70$), established CAM clients ($n = 71$) and OM clients ($n = 58$) were distinguished on the basis of health beliefs, sociodemographic, medical and personality variables. Different patterns of predictors of CAM use emerged depending on which client groups were compared. In general, health-aware behaviours and dissatisfaction with conventional medicine were the best predictors of overall and initial/infrequent CAM use, and more frequent health-aware behaviours were associated with continued CAM use. Medical need also influenced the choice to use CAM, and was the best predictor of committed CAM use, with the established CAM clients reporting more health problems than the new/infrequent CAM group.

A Danish study found that patients before seeking homeopathic consultations for asthma and allergy had experienced inappropriate healthcare within the conventional healthcare system.[25] The results of the study also indicate that, if the homeopathic patients experienced inappropriate healthcare within homeopathic treatment, they terminated the treatment. A group of cancer patients in Hawaii generally perceived CAM as an effective and less harmful alternative to conventional treatment.[26] Some participants reported that their discovery of CAM contributed to their decision to decline conventional treatment. Most participants also felt that conventional treatment would not make a difference in disease outcome, and some but not all participants perceived an unsatisfactory or alienating relationship with healthcare providers.

A study by Berg and Arnetz[27] found that dermatological patients using alternative medicine in general did not differ with regard to personal characteristics from non-users. Rather, it appeared that patients with long-standing skin disease turn to alternative medicine as a complement to orthodox treatment.

Dissatisfaction with the OM consultation   The holistic approach to treatment offers a quality of personal attention and care. A whole range of aspects of an individual's life is considered – aspects that a GP conducting a busy surgery with limited resources would normally ignore. Furthermore, it gives an individual a feeling of participating in health decisions and thus allows some measure of control over his or her care. Indeed this latter point is being accepted by OM if rather slowly. Legal opinion is moving towards the position that doctors and other healthcare providers should discuss healthcare decisions with patients, inviting them to indicate preferences where options are available.

Furnham et al.[28] asked three groups of CAM patients and an OM group to compare the consultation styles of GPs and CAM practitioners. CAM practitioners were generally perceived as having more time to listen. Ernst et al.[29] tested the hypothesis that patients judge the manner of non-medically trained complementary practitioners more favourably than that of their GPs. A questionnaire was sent out to 3384 individuals suffering from symptoms described as being arthritis, who had responded to a feature in a popular women's magazine. A little under 30% of the questionnaires were returned and of these 333 respondents said that they had consulted both a complementary practitioner and a GP. In answer to the question 'Were you satisfied or dissatisfied with your treatment?' the former scored more highly. As far as friendliness was concerned, however, the GPs appeared to be ahead of the complementary practitioners.[30] Professor Ernst acknowledged in the paper that the group was self-selected and therefore could be considered to be biased in favour of CAM.

Consultations with CAM practitioners are often patient led and loosely structured, as opposed to the usually highly structured, time-constrained, physician-led OM consultation. The patient's problem is often explored at length by the former, with a mutually acceptable approach being fully explained before being chosen. This approach has been frequently described by patients as being 'far more sympathetic than OM'. Furthermore, CAM practitioners tend to be more relaxed, less formal in their approach and more casually dressed, to try to encourage a sense of rapport with their patients. All this does not necessarily mean that patients will receive a more accurate diagnosis or a more successful outcome. However, experience shows that a participatory type of consultation is generally more acceptable to the patient and often leads to improved compliance with the treatment regimone.

A consistent patient concern is the concealment of information about diagnosis and treatment by OM doctors. Katz[31] has pointed out that such practices date back to Hippocrates, who instructed physicians:

> ... to perform duties calmly and adroitly, concealing most things from the patient while you are attending to him ....

Old habits die hard!

The growing emphasis on a systems approach to medical treatment may reduce the potential conflict between patient and a practitioner's reputation, as well as the escalating costs to the funder. Responsibility for a patient's welfare may no longer rest with a single physician but with a team of healthcare providers, each dealing with a different aspect of medicine. In general, complementary practitioners tend to take total ownership of a problem, giving a heightened sense of security to the patient who then has only one person to whom they have to tell their story.

Belief in the value of CAM as an appropriate approach to healthcare   It may be that the discontent results not from just the failings of conventional medicine itself, but also from a new consciousness of the value of involving the individual in his or her wellbeing and a new sense of the value of being 'natural'. Patients are no longer willing to be treated in a paternalistic 'I know best' manner with standardised medication. They want a sensitive recognition of themselves as unwell people, rather than accepting treatment for a disease in isolation.

Helman[32] has shown that laypeople's views of medicine may vary from the theories generally accepted by practitioners of orthodox medicine. Furnham[33] has argued that such beliefs may well influence their choice of healthcare.

Finnegan[34] studied in depth the motives of 38 patients for attending a centre specialising in CAM. A high proportion of the patients had long-term chronic diseases and had been unable to find satisfactory relief using OM. Some were uninterested in the philosophy of CAM and were keen to get better by whatever means available, whereas others were more interested in the techniques by which their health was to be improved.

In a two-part study, also by Finnegan,[35] an attempt was made to measure the depth of commitment to CAM quantitatively using factor analysis and correlation measures. In the first study, a total of 79 undergraduates were asked to consider 35 statements, of which 12 were sympathetic to CAM and 23 expressed antagonism or scepticism towards it. The statements were arranged beside a Likert scale, ranging from 1 (strongly agree) to 6 (strongly disagree). In the second study, the number of statements was reduced to 19, and the responses of 24 students recorded. Subsequently a further 5 statements were removed, leaving a 14-statement scale requiring clinical validation.

It has been said that CAM, in particular homeopathy, appeals to patients who feel that attention should be paid to underlying causes of ailments rather than just the symptoms.[36] Furnham and Smith[37] carried out a study concerned with the different health and illness beliefs of patients choosing traditional and alternative medicine. Two groups of patients, one visiting a GP and the other a homeopath, were matched in physical and social characteristics. They were invited to complete a questionnaire measuring several items including perceived susceptibility to disease and illness, their own control over health, perceived efficacy of traditional (by which the authors meant orthodox) versus alternative health. The major difference between the two groups was that the homeopathic group were much more critical and sceptical about the efficacy of orthodox medicine.

Decreased efficacy of orthodox drugs It is known that some drugs appear to become less efficacious the longer they are used to treat a particular condition. Skin conditions treated with steroids fall into this category: as time proceeds patients often claim that the efficacy of the various topical preparations falls.

A study in Southampton by Moore et al.[38] determined that the failure of OM was almost always the main reason given for the sample of 56 patients attending a CAM centre.

In one of a series of studies that contrasted the beliefs, behaviours and motives of users of OM and CAM, Furnham and Kirkcaldy[39] have examined different attitudes towards health and illness among an adult working German population. A group of 202 individuals recruited from several OM and CAM therapeutic centres completed a questionnaire that assessed a number of beliefs, including control over one's health and perceived efficacy of OM versus CAM treatment. Overall the CAM group, compared with the OM group, were more critical and sceptical of the effectiveness of orthodox medicine; they were likely to express less satisfaction with their orthodox doctor's treatment, felt that their doctors were less concerned with their wellbeing, listened to them less and viewed their GPs as being less effective in their treatment

Perceived effectiveness

Vincent and Furnham[40] examined the perceived effectiveness of acupuncture, herbalism, homeopathy, hypnosis and osteopathy in the treatment of 25 complaints ranging from cancer to the common cold. They showed that conventional medicine was clearly seen by most respondents as being more effective in the treatment of most major illnesses. On the other hand, CAM was seen to be most useful in specific conditions, including depression, stress and smoking cessation (where hypnosis was considered to be superior to conventional medicine), and in the treatment of common colds and skin problems. Among those people with a strong belief in CAM, herbalism and homeopathy were seen as being valuable in chronic and psychological conditions; homeopathy was favoured in the treatment of allergies. Acupuncture and osteopathy were both perceived as valuable in the treatment of back pain, whereas hypnosis was seen as useful in the treatment of a variety of psychological problems, and considered to be superior to orthodox procedures. Overall, herbalism appeared slightly more popular than homeopathy and acupuncture. It has been suggested that rheumatological patients perceive CAM to have certain advantages over OM. Between 64% and 94% of people attending North American rheumatology clinics use some form of CAM.[41]

The fact that people are able to specify which complementary therapies are likely to be effective in which conditions should make researchers cautious about using 'CAM' as an umbrella term.

Table 3.1 gives referral guidelines that were created for staff working in the Lewisham Hospital NHS Trust in south London, and published in a report on the first year of providing complementary services.[42] The guidelines reflected ongoing evaluation and other sources of effectiveness data for the four disciplines offered by the Trust, and gave an indication of those interventions likely to be the most successful for a given condition.

Financial reasons

There are two issues; the cost of CAM when prescribed under the NHS or at the expense of another third party and that available as an out-of-pocket expense to the final consumer.

Cost of prescribed CAM   CAM often claims to offer therapies that are good value for money. Hard evidence of this is sparse; many of the figures that do exist suffer from considerable limitations. Pharmacoeconomic methodology has only recently evolved and few studies have applied the principles rigorously to CAM.

Economic evaluations such as cost-effectiveness analyses (CEAs) are intended to inform decision-makers about the relative efficiency of different interventions, including CAM.[43] To be generalisable, economic

Table 3.1 Lewisham Hospital NHS Trust complementary referral guidelines[29]

Condition	Treatment
Arthritis	Acupuncture, homeopathy, osteopathy
Back and neck pain	Acupuncture, osteopathy
Digestive disorders	Acupuncture, homeopathy
Gynaecological (dysmenorrhoea)	Acupuncture, homeopathy
Headaches, migraine	Acupuncture, homeopathy
Musculoskeletal (pain and functional problems)	Acupuncture, osteopathy
Upper respiratory tract disease, asthma and hayfever	Acupuncture, homeopathy

evaluations should use the same metric to assess health benefits, e.g. quality-adjusted life-years (QALYs). However, the recurrent conditions for which CAM is typically used suggest that the health benefits of CAM will manifest themselves primarily as quality-of-life improvements that appear in CEA as 'utilities' attached to health states. Therefore, appropriate utility measures will be critical to the production of valid CEAs of CAM therapies.

As competition for healthcare expenditure grows, the importance of economic and therapeutic evaluation to healthcare providers and purchasers is becoming more evident. CAM must provide the necessary data to facilitate comparison with orthodox therapies. In measuring the costs of any therapy, both direct and indirect costs should be included; in orthodox medicine the costs of the latter are usually significantly greater than of the former. Indirect costs include days lost at work and the cost of providing caregivers during rehabilitation. White et al.[44] have investigated existing methods of assessing CAM costs and considered some potential outcome measures for CAM in a wide-ranging review article. Four methods for the economic evaluation of treatment have been developed for orthodox medical care and could be applied to CAM:

1.   Cost minimisation: to compare cost of alternative methods of healthcare
2.   Cost-effectiveness: to relate costs to outcome measured as days lost at work and similar physical units
3.   Cost utility: to relate cost to QALY
4.   Cost–benefit: to relate cost to outcome in economic benefits.

Examples of studies in the *cost minimisation* area include the following. Swayne[45] showed that 22 homeopathic GPs working within the UK NHS issued 12% fewer prescriptions than the average for the area and that the mean cost of ingredients was reduced by 20p per item. Unfortunately, there were several serious limitations to the study, not the least being that the sample was too small to allow generalisations to be made. No allowance was made for extended consulting time. When it was published Swayne's survey gained widespread attention in the media and the results certainly contributed to discussions on widening the availability of homeopathy in the NHS.

The cost of a consultation (which can last six times longer than an orthodox consultation[46]) is considerably more expensive to the NHS than the standard 4-minute OM consultation. In a retrospective study of treating a sample group of 89 rheumatoid arthritis patients with CAM, van Haselen et al.[47] concluded that the costs of using CAM appear to be most sensitive to the time spent with the patient by the doctor.

Savings have also been identified among German dental surgeons after the use of homeopathic Arnica 12x before dental surgery.[48] Unfortunately no time period was stated. Savings of about £45 per patient were reported by Myers after the use of acupuncture rather than drugs.[49]

An example of work in the *cost-effectiveness* category is that of Carey et al. in the USA.[50] A total of 208 practitioners involved in primary care of back pain were recruited. The group comprised physicians, chiropractors, orthopaedic surgeons and nurse practitioners. The practitioners treated 1633 consecutive patients who presented with untreated back pain of less than 10 weeks' duration. Use of medication was significantly lower and patient satisfaction significantly higher among the patients treated by chiropractors than in all other groups. There was no difference between the groups in time to functional recovery.

In order to determine *cost utility*, effective outcome measures are necessary, but there are certain difficulties in measuring quality of life and calculating its financial value.

The Nottingham Health Profile (NHP) provides one method of gathering the required data. The NHP uses a questionnaire comprising 38 questions covering patients' energy, physical mobility, emotional reactions, social isolation, pain and sleep. This tool was used by Johannson et al.[51] to study the effects of acupuncture in stroke patients in an open controlled study. There was a clear trend in favour of acupuncture improving the quality of life with respect to mobility and emotion.

Cost–benefit measures, in purely financial terms, what a treatment costs and what it achieves. In the study carried out by Johannson et al. cited above, it was calculated that hospital costs were on average $US26 000 less for the patients treated with acupuncture than for the controls.

White et al.[44] conclude that the systematic economic evaluation of CAM is still in its infancy. It is vital that appropriate standardised outcomes are developed so that an accurate picture of costs of treatment can be provided. It is unlikely that CAM will be integrated into the main stream of therapeutics until such action has been taken.

In England there is some advantage to the patient of having been prescribed homeopathic medicines as part of an NHS treatment, because in almost all cases the cost of the medicine will be less than the prescription charge (currently about £7 [€9; $13] per item in England) and pharmacists will generally invite the 20% of patients who are liable to pay the charge to buy the remedies over the counter at the lower retail price. In other parts of the UK this situation will not arise: in Wales there is no prescription charge and in Scotland the government has pledged to reduce the charge to zero by 2010.

Out-of-pocket purchase   The average cost of a CAM medicine is generally below the average orthodox over-the-counter (OTC) medicine purchase in a community pharmacy or health store. This can act as an incentive to the purchaser. Medicines bought by pet owners for veterinary use are similarly perceived as being good value, especially as the vet's fees are avoided.

There does not appear be to any literature on how costs of attending CAM practitioners affect the demand, although the classic buyer profile would seem to indicate that people with higher disposable income are more likely to purchase private treatment.

The 'green' association

Bakx[23] has argued that a heightened awareness of green issues has resulted in an increasing dissatisfaction with traditional orthodox cures. Many of the CAM disciplines are considered to be 'natural' and the medicines made from non-synthetic sources. This appeals to the sensitivities of the environmentalist lobby.

Encouragement by media and self study materials

Almost every popular journal and most newspapers have run features on CAM in the last 5 years. Many relate in graphic detail almost magical cures achieved by people who had given up on ever feeling well again.

A rich source of written patient education material comes from publications with more focused readerships than the popular magazines. They are self-help oriented and may be directed towards issues involving gender or age group, or medical problems. Several doctors and other health professionals have taken a lead in offering consumer guides to healthcare. Disciplines such as aromatherapy, herbalism, homeopathy, exercise and relaxation all readily lend themselves to use in self-treatment.

Cultural reasons

The mobility across national borders of people whose cultural backgrounds emphasise the use of holistic forms of medicine is another reason for increased demand for homeopathic medicines. Thus, migrants from the Indian subcontinent and China bring their customs with them when they migrate. Either from an inherent mistrust of western medicine or from a misunderstanding of what it can achieve, such people prefer to continue using traditional methods that have proved successful over many centuries.

The effect of opinion leaders

It is likely that role models have a significant effect in leading people to use CAM. Film stars and royalty are particularly active in promoting their particular discipline by taking on some capacity either within an organisation or in newspaper and magazine articles. The British royal family, especially HM The Queen Mother, who was Patron of the British Homeopathic Association for many years before her death in 2002, have used homeopathy widely and the spin-off has been noted.

Why do people choose not to be treated with CAM?

Among the possible reasons for not selecting CAM as a favoured method of treatment are the following:[52]

- Concern about lack of scientific evidence that complementary therapies work
- A strong belief in the value of 'scientific medicine'
- Conventional medicine works, so why try something else?
- No belief in complementary therapies: 'old wives' tales', 'myth', 'superstition'
- Strong trust in orthodox doctors: 'the doctor knows best'
- Lack of awareness of or interest in complementary therapies
- No complementary therapy use within personal social networks
- Financial cost of private complementary therapies
- Uncertainty about quality and safety of OTC complementary treatments.

The use of CAM

Fulder and Munro[53] conducted an early survey of the prevalence of CAM in the UK. It showed that there were approximately 13 million visits to an estimated 7500 practitioners annually, about 30% of the number of GPs. Zollman and Vickers[54] have reviewed some later surveys carried out to study the users of complementary medicine in the UK. Their data, together with examples of other studies, are reproduced in Table 3.2.

However, relying on market research data is not always appropriate, because there are often shortcomings in the way in which the data are collected.[55] As reporting methods may vary significantly, it can be difficult to compare the results of CAM surveys effectively. Surveys may differ in their target populations and their time frame of use, and the way in which questions are asked can influence the type of response received. Even the definition of 'complementary' medicine can vary, as some therapies and OTC medicines may be excluded from questioning.[56] The study by Thomas et al.,[57] adjudged by Zollman and Vickers to be the most rigorous investigation, provides an estimate for lifetime use of acupuncture, chiropractic, herbal medicine, homeopathy and hypnotherapy in England of more than one in four adults. If reflexology

Table 3.2 Examples of surveys on use of complementary and alternative medicine (CAM) in the UK

Survey	Percentage sample ever used CAM	Percentage sample used CAM in past year	No. of therapies surveyed
Gallup 1986[45]	14%	No data	6
Which? 1986[45]	No data	14%	5
MORI 1989[45]	27% (including OTC medicines)	No data	13
Thomas 1993[45]	16.9% (33% if OTC is included)	10.5%	6
Ernst and White 2000[58]	No data	20%	6 most popular
Thomas et al. 2001[57] (England)	46.6% (including OTC medicines)	13.6% (28.3% if OTC medicines included)	8
Shakeel et al. 2008[58] (Scotland)	68%	46%	No data

OTC, over the counter.

and aromatherapy are included, the figure moves up to one in three. In any year it is estimated that 11% of the adult population visit a CAM therapist for one of the named therapies.

A survey was carried out for the BBC in 2000 by Ernst and White.[59] Of the 1204 interviewees, 254 (20%) reported using CAM within the preceding year. Herbal medicine was the most commonly used therapy (34%), followed by aromatherapy (21%) and homeopathy (17%). Acupuncture and acupressure ranked fourth, with 14% of adults having used it in the past year. Osteopathy (5%), massage (4%), reflexology(3%) and chiropractic (2%) completed the list. Overall, use of complementary therapies was higher among females (24%) than among males (17%), with the greatest percentage of CAM use occurring among people between the ages of 35 and 64 (26%). When asked why they used complementary therapies, most respondents cited the perceived effectiveness of CAM, the user's liking it and the therapy's 'relaxing effects'. Interestingly, 11% of the respondents said that they used complementary therapies because their doctor had either recommended them or referred them to an alternative health practitioner. Participants were also asked to estimate the amount of money that they spent each month on complementary therapies. According to the survey, the average user spent £13.62 (€17; $24) on CAM per month.

Shakeel et al. found that 68% of a sample of 430 patients attending general, vascular and cardiothoracic units at a regional Scottish centre had ever used CAM and 48% had used CAM in the preceding year.[58]

Figure 3.1 shows the actual and predicted market value for herbalism, aromatherapy and homeopathy in the UK over a 15-year period collated from different reports.[60] These data demonstrate that herbalism continues to outstrip the other two therapies in its popularity.

If the popularity of four examples of CAM is compared across several countries, some interesting differences emerge.[61] There is likely to be some disparity in the definitions of what is meant by CAM and the selection of therapies assessed. Table 3.3 shows that consumer surveys carried out in the early 1990s demonstrated positive public attitudes to CAM in many European countries, with France and Germany leading the way. In Spain, the UK and the USA, the most popular treatments appear to be the manipulative disciplines. Herbal medicine is more popular than homeopathy in the UK.

Zollman and Vickers' review[54] shows a rather different result for the UK. Four of the five studies that they considered placed the popularity of the disciplines in the order: acupuncture, chiropractic, herbalism,

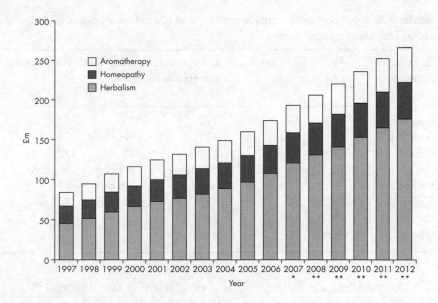

Figure 3.1 Market values for complementary and alternative medicine (CAM) sectors 1998–2012.
*Estimated, **projected.

homeopathy and osteopathy. The remaining study by MORI in 1989 did not ask about herbalism and recorded faith healers as third choice, but was otherwise identical. Zollman and Vickers[54] also list the following recognised patterns of use of CAM:

- Earnest seekers: these users have an intractable health problem for which they try many different forms of treatment
- Stable users: people who use one type of therapy for most of their healthcare problems or have one main problem for which they use a regular portfolio of CAM therapies
- Eclectic users: people who choose different therapies depending on individual circumstances
- One-off users: people who use CAM for limited experimentation.

A study by Furnham and Bond[62] examined whether people thought neurotic individuals were more likely to 'get better' when using CAM rather than orthodox medicine. Homeopathy was perceived as being more effective for treating patients with unstable psychological characteristics and OM was seen as more effective for treating patients with stable psychological characteristics.

Table 3.3 A comparison of complementary and alternative medicine (CAM) usage (percentage population)[55]

Percentage population using	All CAM	Acupuncture	Chiropractic/ osteopathy	Herbalism	Homeopathy
Belgium	31	19	19	31	56
Denmark	23	12	23	No data	28
France	49	21	7	12	32
Germany	46	No data	No data	No data	No data
Netherlands	20	16	No data	No data	31
Spain	25	12	48	No data	15
UK	26	16	36	24	16
USA	34	3	30	9	3

In the USA, the estimated number of visits made during 1990 to providers of unconventional therapy was greater than the number of visits to all primary care medical doctors nationwide, and the amount spent on CAM was comparable to the amount spent by Americans for all hospitalisation.[63] There were limits to the representative nature of the sample used in this study, which was carried out by telephone. People living in houses without a telephone and non-English speakers were excluded. The sample was largely made up of white people. Extrapolations from a further survey carried out in 1997 suggested a 47.3% increase in total visits to alternative medicine practitioners from 427 million in 1990 to 629 million in 1997, thereby exceeding total visits to all US primary care physicians.[64] The authors concluded that the substantial increase in use and expenditure between 1990 and 1997 was attributable primarily to an increase in the proportion of the population seeking alternative therapies rather than increased visits per patient.

The profile of a CAM user in the USA has been defined by Astin[65] following a 1998 survey that included a total of 1035 individuals randomly selected from a panel who had agreed to participate in mail surveys and who lived throughout the USA and had used CAM in the previous year. Astin concluded that CAM users tend to:

- be better educated
- be of poorer health status
- have a belief in body, mind and spirit in health
- have had a transformational life experience

- have a commitment to values of environmentalism, feminism, personal growth psychology and spirituality, love of the foreign and exotic
- be reporting anxiety, back problems, chronic pain or urinary tract problems.

Outstanding questions still exist about:

- the relationship between CAM use and health status
- the role played by the media and the internet in influencing choice to use CAM
- whether CAM users were more likely to be psychologically distressed
- the extent of CAM use among minority ethnic populations.

Astin's study was criticised because it did not test respondents' views on dissatisfaction with orthodox medicine. Lord Baldwin,[66] a member of the Parliamentary Group for Alternative and Complementary Medicine, suggested that it could be implied from the results that patients' choices have little to do with dissatisfaction with conventional healthcare. He did not believe that this was the case.

The extent to which demographic and health-related variables are related to visits to a CAM practitioner was also investigated by Bausell et al.[67] Overall visits to CAM providers (9%) were lower than reported in other surveys. Gender, education, age, geographical location and race (Hispanic and African–American individuals proved to be less likely to visit CAM providers than white people) were statistically significant predictors of visits to CAM providers. Individuals in poorer health and those suffering from mental, musculoskeletal or metabolic disorders also tended to be more likely to have visited a CAM provider. Although the choice of alternative versus orthodox treatment appears to be a complex phenomenon, these data suggest that the heaviest users of CAM therapies tend to be individuals with comorbid, non-life-threatening health problems.

An interesting study in Hawaii estimated the prevalence of CAM use and its relation to quality of life (QoL) among cancer patients from diverse ethnic backgrounds.[68] Given the ethnically diverse population in Hawaii, it provided an excellent model for the study. CAM use was highest among Filipino and white patients, intermediate for native Hawaiians and Chinese, and significantly lower among Japanese. Some ethnic preferences for CAM followed ethnic folk medicine traditions, e.g. herbal medicines by Chinese, Hawaiian healing by native

Hawaiians and religious healing or prayer by Filipinos. CAM users reported lower emotional functioning scores, higher symptom scores and more financial difficulties than non-users. This study detected ethnic differences in CAM use, in particular a low use among Japanese patients, and supports the importance of cultural factors in determining the frequency and type of CAM therapies chosen.

In 1995 the percentage of the Canadian population who saw an alternative practitioner during the previous year was estimated at 15%.[69]

By 2006 54% of a sample of 2000 adult Canadians reported using at least one form of complementary or alternative medicine or treatment during the previous year. The most commonly used complementary and alternative medicines and therapies reported were massage (19%), prayer (16%), chiropractic care (15%), relaxation techniques (14%) and herbal therapies (10%).[70]

In both Canada[71] and the United States[72] CAM use appears higher in western regions than in other areas. In Canada, western provinces are much more likely than those in the east to cover CAM in their health programmes.[73]

In Australia approximately half the population have used CAM,[74] whereas in Israel the figure was around 6% in the mid-1990s.[75] With substantial immigration from eastern Europe in recent years, this figure is likely to have increased by now. In Israel CAM users tend to report worse health.[76] With CAM becoming a mainstream, although somewhat luxurious, medical practice, pain and affective–emotional distress are the main drivers of CAM use.

What sort of conditions are most often treated with CAM?

Comprehensive applications are given under each therapy in the rest of the book; some general examples of conditions for which CAM has been used are given below.

Long et al.[77] determined which complementary therapies are believed by their respective representing professional organisations to be suited for which medical conditions. For the study, 223 questionnaires were sent out to CAM organisations representing a single CAM therapy. The respondents were asked to list the 15 conditions that they felt benefited most from their CAM therapy, the 15 most important contraindications, the typical costs of initial and any subsequent treatments, and the average length of training required to become a fully qualified practitioner. Of the 223 questionnaires sent out, 66 were completed and returned. Taking undelivered questionnaires into account, the response rate was 34%. Two or more responses were received from CAM organisations representing 12 therapies: aromatherapy, Bach flower medicines, Bowen technique, chiropractic, homeopathy, hypnotherapy, magnet therapy, massage, nutrition, reflexology, reiki and yoga. The top seven common conditions deemed to benefit from all 12 therapies, in order of frequency, were: stress/anxiety, headaches/ migraine, back pain, respiratory problems (including asthma), insomnia, cardiovascular problems and musculoskeletal problems. Aromatherapy, Bach flower medicines, hypnotherapy, massage, nutrition, reflexology, reiki and yoga were all recommended as suitable treatments for stress/anxiety. Aromatherapy, Bowen technique, chiropractic, hypnotherapy, massage, nutrition, reflexology, reiki and yoga were all recommended for headache/migraine. Bowen technique, chiropractic, magnet therapy, massage, reflexology and yoga were recommended for back pain.

In the USA high levels of CAM use tend to occur among individuals with chronic conditions, particularly where pain is a central component (such as arthritis, low back problems and headaches), mental health problems (particularly anxiety, depression and insomnia), cancer and AIDS. A substantial amount of CAM use also appears to be for health maintenance, wellness and prevention of disease.

Asthma

The most commonly used therapies in the UK for asthma are homeopathy, herbal medicine, relaxation, acupuncture and aromatherapy. A review of evidence supporting the use of CAM may be found on the CAM Specialist Library website http://tinyurl.com/4eb5rb.

Cancer management

Complementary and alternative medicine is increasingly popular with cancer patients and yet information provision or discussion about CAM by health professionals remains low. Previous research suggests that patients may fear clinicians' 'disapproval' if they raise the subject of CAM, and turn to other sources to acquire information about CAM. As a result of the lack of CAM information from health professionals, men in a study carried out in Bristol, England, became either 'proactive seekers' or 'passive recipients' of such information.[78] Their main information resource was the 'lay referral' network of family, friends and acquaintances, especially females. 'Traditional' information sources, including books, magazines, leaflets and the media, were popular, more so in fact than the internet.

Little is known about the use of CAM in paediatric oncology. A Dutch study to determine which medical and demographic characteristics distinguish users from non-users was conducted in a paediatric oncology sample of children with different survival perspectives.[79] The parents of 84 children with cancer (43 patients in first continuous remission and 41 patients who had suffered a relapse or second malignancy) participated in the study and were surveyed with respect to the use of CAM. The survival perspective appeared to be the most important variable distinguishing users of CAM from non-users. Twenty-six families (31%) had used or were using alternative treatment, of which 19 were families of children with cancer who had suffered a relapse (46%), and 7 were families of children with cancer in remission (16%). The most common types of CAM used were based on homeopathy and anthroposophy.

Influenza

A review by Guo et al.[80] assessed the evidence for the effectiveness of CAM for preventing or treating influenza or influenza-like illness, including avian influenza. Systematic literature searches were conducted in five databases until June 2006; other data sources included bibliographies of located articles, manufacturers of commercially available preparations and experts in the field. Randomised clinical trials (RCTs), controlled against placebo or active comparator, were included. Fourteen RCTs testing seven preparations were included. For *Panex quinquefolium* extract, *Sambucus nigra*, and the herbal combination Kan Jang and the French homeopathic OTC product known as Oscillococcinum, two or more trials reporting some encouraging data were identified. The authors concluded that current evidence from RCTs is sparse and limited by small sample sizes, low methodological quality or clinically irrelevant effect sizes. The effectiveness of any CAM for treating or preventing seasonal influenza was not established beyond reasonable doubt.

Musculoskeletal conditions

Over three-quarters of patients presenting to practitioners of the major CAM disciplines have musculoskeletal problems as their main complaint. Neurological, psychological and allergic disorders are also common.[54] Homeopathy and herbalism are used more often by patients with asthma, skin conditions and menstrual problems. Acupuncture, osteopathy and Alexander technique are used by rheumatologists.[81]

Stroke

A paper by Bell[82] presents an overview of nutritional, herbal and homeopathic treatment options from CAM as adjuncts in stroke prevention, treatment and rehabilitation. Despite many promising leads, the evidence does not favour recommendation of most of these treatments from a public health policy perspective. However, simple preventive interventions, such as use of a high-quality multivitamin/multimineral supplement in patients with undernutrition, may improve outcomes with minimal long-term risk. Natural agents such as the antioxidant α-lipoic acid, certain traditional Asian herbal mixtures and some homeopathically prepared medicines show promise for reducing infarct size and associated impairments. A number of nutrients and herbs may assist in treatment of stroke-related complications such as pressure sores, urinary tract infections and pneumonia. Individualised homeopathy may even play a helpful adjunctive role in treatment of aspain. However, a great deal of systematic research effort lies ahead before most of the options discussed would meet mainstream medical standards for introduction into routine treatment regimens.

The provision of CAM

In the UK the common law right to choose one's own treatment for illness has been barely constrained by law.[83] It is currently legal for anyone in the UK to practise complementary medicine without any training (except in the areas of osteopathy and chiropractic, which are protected by statute). This position will change in the foreseeable future with other disciplines becoming statutorily controlled. Non-medical practitioners must not claim to be statutorily registered in protected professions such as dentistry, medicine or pharmacy, supply medicines classified as limited to prescription or claim cures for certain medical conditions.

By contrast, in many other European Union countries, as well as the USA, there are few healthcare activities that are allowed without some type of certification. Acupuncturists, herbalists, naturopaths and osteopaths have been prosecuted for practising without medical qualifications, and the technical illegality of much complementary practice has meant that it has been pursued informally and disparately, with less opportunity for professional organisations to develop.[84] One of the recommendations of the House of Lords Report (see below) was that standardised training courses and accreditation by professional bodies should be developed in CAM.

Any effort to increase the understanding of CAM by healthcare professionals requires an interdisciplinary and collaborative approach. Between 2000 and 2002, the US National Institutes of Health National Center for Complementary and Alternative Medicine funded 15 educational institutions to develop curricular models for educating allopathic medical and nursing learners in CAM literacy.[85] Four of these 15 programmes – Tufts University School of Medicine, University of California at San Francisco School of Medicine, Oregon Health and Sciences University School of Medicine and University of Washington School of Nursing – formed collaborative partnerships with nearby academic institutions that train CAM practitioners. Among the other institutions barriers to acceptance included: resistance by teaching staff; the curriculum being perceived as too full; presenting CAM content in an evidence-based and even-handed way; providing useful, reliable resources; and developing teaching and assessment tools.[86]

The various routes for delivery of CAM are summarised in Figure 3.2. It includes the factors influencing the decision to choose CAM discussed earlier in this chapter. These are clinical considerations, social and financial reasons, and beliefs in holistic therapies. It also shows the progression from self-treating to medical practitioner, and the part played by various intermediaries who may be consulted directly or in a chain of consultations as the condition being treated progresses.

Medically qualified physician

This is a person who has undergone training at a medical school and is a registered medical practitioner. Doctors may use complementary medicine exclusively, or more probably as an adjunct to their orthodox practice. They may hold a formal postgraduate qualification, have a lesser course of training or no training at all. In the UK untrained doctors may issue NHS prescriptions for homeopathic medicines quite legally without having any real knowledge of the subject. This usually occurs as a reactive response to requests from patients. An editorial in the *British Medical Journal* has noted that CAM is no longer an obscure issue in medicine.[87] Patients are using alternative therapies in addition to conventional care and sometimes do not share this information with

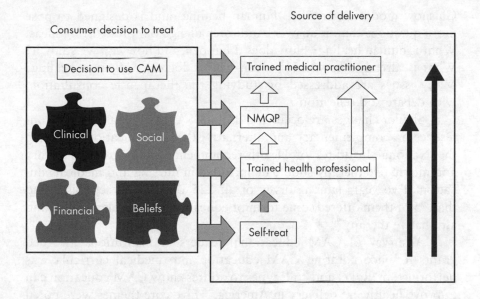

Figure 3.2 Representation of delivery of complementary and alternative medicine (CAM). Grey and black arrows represent consumer decisions; white arrows represent referral of other healthcare providers, NMQP non medically qualified practitioner (also known as 'professional health provider').

their GP, but, even if they did, would conventional doctors know how best to advise them about safety issues or the effectiveness of a particular therapy for their problem? Although many medical schools and training programmes now include teaching on CAM, the approaches are variable and often superficial. This situation is likely to be responsible for resistance among some doctors to embrace CAM.

Owen et al.[88] have posed a number of questions about physicians' attitudes and behaviour towards complementary and alternative therapy, including the following:

• If the care is provided on a delegated or referred basis, how much does a doctor need to know to make appropriate referrals and supervise delegated treatment?
• If doctors are to treat patients with CAM what training do they require?

They describe initiatives to include CAM therapy in medical education provided at Southampton Medical School and by other bodies in the UK. Teaching in Glasgow has also developed in recent years.[89] The

Glasgow module is entitled 'Human healing' and is designed to pose more questions than it answers and to challenge our pre-existing ideas. What is human healing? How does it happen, and how can we study it? What is already known? How can we, as doctors, influence healing? Many issues are addressed by studying the therapeutic consultation, with debate and reflection.

Similar changes are occurring in the USA. In 1995 a national conference on complementary and alternative therapy education involving the National Institutes of Health recommended that complementary and alternative therapy should be included in nursing and medical education. Two years later a survey of all 125 US medical schools found that 75 of them offered some form of education on complementary and alternative therapy.[90]

A survey of CAM educational leaders at institutions awarded grants for incorporating CAM education into medical curricula was performed by Rakel and colleagues to address how CAM education can improve healthcare delivery in America.[91] Five core themes were noted to be successful in achieving this goal. These included:

- Education on the importance of relationship-centred care
- Understanding holism
- The promotion of self-reflection and self-care
- Collaboration with CAM providers to enhance communication
- The need for faculty development in CAM.

In discussing these themes the authors explore how a shift in medical education towards a focus of understanding what is needed for the creation of health (salutogenesis) can bring balance to a curriculum that is currently weighted in teaching about the creation of disease (pathogenesis). They identify potential benefits, including reduced healthcare costs and improved quality of life for learners.

Attitude of GPs to CAM

Resistance to information that directly contradicts conventional 'wisdom' has a long history. Apparently it was not unusual for well-known physicians to get up and leave when medical papers were being read that emphasised the germ theory of disease in 1919![92]

Many physicians still dismiss a patient's questions concerning CAM because they believe that it is 'quackery', without any proof to support this claim.[93] This violates the patient's right to full disclosure of all possible treatment options and encourages patients to use these

therapies without their physician's knowledge. As a result, it is estimated that 46% of those using alternative medicine do so without the
supervision of their primary care doctors or alternative medicine practitioners. An Italian study found that CAM knowledge among GPs is
not as widespread as the public demand seems to require, and the
scarce evidence of CAM effectiveness hinders its professional use
among a considerable number of GPs.[94]

Over the years there has been a change in the attitude of the medical profession towards those practising CAM. In 1980 an editorial in
the *British Medical Journal* suggested that some aspects of chiropractic
ought to be as extinct as 'divination of the future by examination of a
bird's entrails' whereas other CAM practitioners' beliefs were described
as being 'irrational'.[95] By 1999 attitudes had changed such that 'a new
dawn' was being welcomed and acknowledgement given that CAM was
not 'unproved', there being increasing evidence to show the effectiveness
of some treatments in some conditions.[96]

The attitude of the British GP to CAM may have a significant
influence on whether it is made available to patients under the NHS or
whether the full cost of treatment has to be borne by the patient.

Several studies have been carried out to investigate doctors' attitudes to CAM. Hunter[97] studied a random selection of 77 GPs in the
Tayside area of Scotland, and a cohort of 95 medical students at
Dundee University. The disciplines covered in the survey were acupuncture, chiropractic, homeopathy, herbalism, hypnosis and osteopathy. It
was found that one in six of the GPs had undertaken training in one or
more complementary therapies and a further 47% would like to
arrange training in at least one CAM technique. Twenty per cent of GPs
used CAM in their surgeries, and most thought that the techniques studied in this survey were useful. Most students showed an interest in
CAM: 75% would like the subject included in the curriculum.
Generally the two groups were enthusiastic about CAM. They appeared
to be less concerned with the question 'how does it work?' than with
'does it work?'

Researchers from the University of Aberdeen analysed official
prescribing data from 2003–4, covering 1.9 million patients from 323
Scottish medical practices.[98] They found that 60% of the surgeries
prescribed homeopathic or herbal medicines. Children under 12 months
were most likely to be prescribed a homeopathic or herbal medicine
(9.5 per 1000 children in that age group), followed by adults aged
81–90 (4.5 per 1000). Of homeopathic prescribing 16% was to children
under 16.

Reilly[99] found 86 of 100 GP trainees had a positive attitude to non-conventional therapies. In work with other colleagues, he found that 70% of medical students considered non-conventional therapy useful and 63% were in favour of such therapies being made available on the NHS.[100]

A meta-analysis of 12 surveys addressing the subject of what physicians think of CAM was published by Ernst and his colleagues in 1995.[101] The results showed a substantial variability between surveys. On average physicians perceived CAM to be moderately effective. Manipulative therapies were believed to be the most useful and/or effective form of CAM, acupuncture was ranked second and homeopathy third. Young physicians judged CAM more optimistically than their older colleagues.

The attitude varies with geographical location. Of GPs in the English south-western counties of Devon and Cornwall who responded to a survey, 68% had been involved with CAM in some way during the previous week and 16% had actually practised it.[102] The doctors were asked to rate the usefulness of various disciplines on a visual analogue scale. Most of the respondents believed that acupuncture, chiropractic and osteopathy were effective and should be funded by the NHS. Studies in other regions of the UK have shown that the proportion of GPs practising CAM varies from 37% in Avon[103] to 14% in west Dorset, where a total of 11 complementary disciplines was surveyed.[104] Another source states that at least 40% of general practices in the UK provide some complementary medicine services,[105] although the evidence base for their use is limited at best and non-existent at worse. Lewith surveyed members and fellows of The Royal College of Physicians to determine their use of CAM.[106] As a result of a low response rate (23%; $n = 2875$), the results needed to be interpreted with caution, but, nevertheless, 32% of respondents practised CAM and 41% referred patients to CAM. CAM practice and referral appeared to be similar in private practice and in the NHS, and was most common in palliative care and pain. Female respondents had more positive attitudes to CAM than male respondents. Overall, respondents thought that more evaluation of CAM was required, CAM was not just a fad, CAM should not be available on the NHS and it was not necessarily important that physicians knew about their patients' use of CAM treatments.

There was a distinct level of practice of CAM among hospital doctors, and this required an undergraduate and postgraduate educational strategy.

Akhtar and van Haselen[107] investigated the reasons for GPs referring or not referring patients for homeopathy, and concluded that better communication was necessary between the homeopathic community and GPs; this could lead to a provision of better healthcare for patients in the future. Some doctors have appointed CAM practitioners to work alongside their surgery staff. In a project closely linked to the idea of integrative medicine, Francis Treuhertz, the English homeopath, was employed in a general medical practice in the 1990s for a day a week.[108] Using a Glasgow Homeopathic Hospital Outcome Scale (GGHOS), he found that most of the 500 patients picked in order of arrival at the surgery were returning scores in the 0 to +4 range.

In a study of 275 physicians practising at two sites in America and one in southern Israel, Borkan et al.[109] showed that primary care physicians were more likely than other medical specialists to be knowledgeable about, personally subscribe to and refer patients for alternative therapies. Referral rates were similar across the three sites and were based on patient requests, failure of conventional treatment and a belief that the patient had a 'psychological' illness. Physicians who used alternative therapies for themselves and in their practices had higher rates of referrals.

International rates for the practice of CAM by primary care physicians vary from 8% in Israel, 16% in Canada,[110] 30% in New Zealand[111] to an impressive 95% in Germany.[112]

Owen et al.[88] have asked their colleagues to consider a number of provocative issues:

- How do you feel about your patients using CAM? What do you think their expectations or assumptions about your knowledge of CAM might be?
- Are you mostly interested in fundamental questions about whether CAM works and its mechanism of action, or more curious about its safety, cost-effectiveness and how to optimally combine it with conventional treatments?
- Can you recall the last time a patient mentioned that he or she was using CAM? What was your attitude to this? Do you think your attitude has changed in the past 5–10 years. If so, why?
- Reflecting on your undergraduate training, were opportunities there to challenge basic assumptions and values of medicine to prepare you for a changing working environment?
- Why do you think some doctors choose to do a 3-year part time training in CAM? If you were to undertake such a course, would

you think it would be a challenging experience and would you be well supported by your peers?

- If you had undertaken training in CAM, how might it change your current working practice? Would your current professional organisations be adequate for your ongoing training, regulation and representation needs?

- With an increased proportion of undergraduate teaching in CAM occurring in optional modules, how will those who choose not to do them compensate for these lost opportunities in education? Will it be as part of their specialist or general practice training or through continuing professional development?

Recognising the increasing demand for CAM in modern healthcare, more than 80% of medical students may like further training in these areas.[113]

In the USA a new medical school panel has been established at Harvard to develop a new Division of Complementary and Alternative Medicine.[114] Its aim will be to pursue research in and evaluation of alternative medicine and to enable Harvard physicians to be well informed about any 'offbeat therapies they may encounter'. Medical schools across the USA are likely to follow this lead. More than 70 US universities now offer some sort of CAM programme.

Attitude of pharmacists to CAM

Pharmacy has had a long association with herbal medicine. Indeed it was as a result of concerns about herbal adulteration that regulation came to the profession in Great Britain in the mid-1800s. However, its contact with other CAM therapies has been less harmonious. Homeopathy was the target of much opposition for many years with reports of acrimonious debates at Council in the 1960s. Following the publishing of an article in the *Pharmaceutical Journal* in 1991,[115] a correspondence on the topic continued for many months. The situation has changed considerably. Appropriate CAM therapies are now accepted by The Royal Pharmaceutical Society of Great Britain (RPSGB) as a potential adjunct to the pharmacists' armamentarium, and training in the particular disciplines being offered by its members is considered to be mandatory. The Pharmaceutical Press (the publishing arm of RPSGB) has built a portfolio of commissioned books on CAM topics (www.pharmpress.com).

The first in a series of factsheets on complementary and alternative therapies, produced by the Society's Science Committee's working group on complementary medicine, was launched at the British Pharmaceutical Conference in Birmingham in September 2000 by Professor William Dawson (chairman of the Science Committee and of the complementary medicine working group).[116] All participants at the Conference received a copy of the factsheet, which was also distributed to pharmacists with the *Pharmaceutical Journal*. The factsheet provided key information for pharmacists on various aspects of essential oils and aromatherapy preparations containing them. Sections on the use and administration of essential oils, and how essential oils should be packaged and stored, are included, together with a summary of clinical research involving essential oils, and aspects of quality and safety relating to their use. Other factsheets on complementary medicine cover aromatherapy, herbal medicine and homeopathy, and are available at the Society's website (www.rpsgb.org) and are updated from time to time.

Support for CAM has been carefully screened. In 1997 the Statutory Committee of the RPSGB ruled that any pharmacist who was practising Spagynk therapy was liable to a charge of misconduct and to be struck off the register.[117] In Spagynk therapy patients provide a sample of blood or urine that undergoes a steam distillation process. The residue is heated and it is claimed that subsequent microscopic examination allows the recognition of certain patterns that can be 'read' by a trained practitioner.

A survey of community pharmacists commissioned by the RPSGB on the use of CAM showed that 99% of respondents reported that one or more types of complementary medicines, including vitamin and mineral supplements, were sold in the pharmacy in which they practise.[118] There does not seem to be any assessment of the number of trained pharmacists who actually offer CAM on their premises proactively. In the past any treatment received in a pharmacy was likely to be a reactive response, given at the request of the patient, rather than proactive at the instigation of the practitioner. With improved availability of training at both postgraduate and undergraduate levels, this situation is changing slowly, and health professionals are beginning to use complementary therapies alongside OM. In a pharmacy this has generally been confined to herbalism, homeopathy and aromatherapy, although Chinese and Indian medicine are being offered on a limited scale by pharmacists of Asian origin (see below).

There is a trend in the UK (as with some GP surgeries) towards refitting pharmacies to include facilities for practitioners trained in the main CAM disciplines (homeopathy, herbalism, aromatherapy, reflexology, chiropractic).

There has been some penetration into the hospital pharmacy, with pharmacists encouraging the inclusion of various herbal, homeopathic and aromatherapy products in pharmacy inventories.

In England, training for pharmacists is provided by the Centre for Pharmacy Postgraduate Education (CPPE), funded by the Department of Health and based at the Department of Pharmacy, Manchester University. CPPE has a distance learning workbook and tape package on CAM. A similar body serving Wales and NHS Education for Scotland (NES) also provide training on CAM, some by video link to remote communities. Articles on various aspects of CAM appear in the pharmacy press on a regular basis. A survey funded by the RPSGB of 1337 community pharmacists, to which 67% responded, 40% of pharmacists reported that they had received or undertaken some type of training in complementary medicine at either postgraduate or undergraduate level.[119] Most schools of pharmacy in the UK offer exposure to CAM.[120]

Although most pharmacists involved in CAM use their skills as an adjunct to orthodox pharmacy practice, a few colleagues have pursued their studies through bodies providing professional qualifications and conduct consultations on their premises. Postgraduate qualifications in homeopathy are available through the Faculty of Homeopathy (http://tinyurl.com/2okuqj).

Attitude of nurses to CAM

The nursing profession may be considered as being 'a combination of art and science' and provides the ideal situation for supporting the essential components of holism that form such an important part of CAM practice.[121] The benefits of using CAM in nursing and midwifery have been identified by Hamilton and Tomlinson.[122] It has been suggested that, although nurses value complementary and alternative therapies, many may lack the knowledge about their application.[119] An American study investigated the knowledge and attitudes of 40 undergraduate nurses and found that familiarity was highest for massage therapy (100%), spiritual healing (95%) and megavitamins/nutritional supplements (95%).[123] Most students had used spiritual healing (85%), massage therapy (85%) and music therapy (75%). None had used reiki and the vast majority had not used ayurveda (95%) or homeopathy (92.5%). Laurenson et al.[124] investigated the knowledge and attitudes that student nurses have to CAM therapies and their use in cancer and palliative care. The findings demonstrated the respondents' acknowledgement of their limited knowledge of CAM therapies, and the study highlighted the need to continue working towards integrated CAM education into the pre-registration nursing curriculum.

Other health professionals

This group comprises people statutorily registered in the various professions allied to medicine including dentistry, physiotherapy and podiatry, who offer complementary disciplines in addition to their orthodox skills. There is also a growing acceptance of CAM in veterinary medicine, until now the most resistant profession to accepting it. Postgraduate training in homeopathy is available from the British Faculty of Homeopathy (http://tinyurl.com/2okuqj).

Complementary Practitioners

> Sharing responsibility for the care of patients by integrating properly trained and registered complementary therapists alongside what are considered to be more conventional practitioners could, I believe, provide exciting long-term benefits. *HRH The Prince of Wales speaking in 1994.*

In common with most European countries and the USA, a group of professional health providers (also called non-medically qualified practitioners or NMQPs) whose living is derived from the practice of their chosen discipline is the main provider of CAM in the country.[125] In 1981 there were only about 13 500 registered practitioners working in the UK.[44] By 1997 this figure had reached about 40 000, with aromatherapy, healing and reflexology accounting for over half of all registered CAM practitioners. A survey of voluntary regulatory bodies for complementary therapies, commissioned by the Department of Health and published in 2000, indicated that there were then about 50 000 CAM practitioners in the UK.[126] These practitioners are therapists who have completed a course of training that may vary from a few days to several years. University degrees are also available in some disciplines. At present there are no statutory regulations or minimal education requirements for CAM practitioners in the UK (with the exception of chiropractic and osteopathy) and thus it is difficult to assess individuals' medical knowledge and limits of competence. Depending upon the way in which the particular profession is organised, practitioners may or may not be registered with an appropriate professional body which can act in a regulatory capacity. However, this position is likely to change in the foreseeable future, particularly in relation to herbal practitioners.

There was a substantial use of practitioner-provided complementary therapies in England in 1998 with an estimated 22 million visits to practitioners of the main therapies being funded privately by users. Annual out-of-pocket expenditure on any of the six best-established therapies was estimated at £450 million. Further research into the cost-effectiveness of different CAM therapies for particular patient groups is now urgently needed to facilitate equal and appropriate access via the NHS.

The British Medical Association has published a report that highlights the need for 'good practice' among what it terms 'discrete clinical disciplines' which include acupuncture, chiropractic, homeopathy, herbalism and osteopathy:[127]

For all therapies, good practice would demand that each body representing a therapy demonstrate:[127]

- An organised structure
- A single register of members
- Guidelines on relationships with medical practitioners
- Sound training at accredited institutions
- An effective ethical code
- Agreed levels of competence
- A proven commitment to research.

The National Association of Health Authority and Trusts (NAHAT) has also addressed the problem. It has published a list of guidelines, stating that NMQP should be selected from membership lists of professional bodies with codes of conduct, ethics and discipline, and who have appropriate indemnity insurance.[128] In the UK there has been considerable progress towards the establishment of statutory controls for some complementary therapies.

Part of the problem that keeps health professionals and complementary practitioners apart concerns the approach to treatment. The former see the advantage of using non-orthodox therapies to complement their extensive orthodox armamentarium, whereas the latter adopt an alternative approach using non-orthodox therapies alone, either by choice or because of a lack of training in orthodox techniques. There is always a suspicion that patients suffering from conditions that would benefit from orthodox treatments are not being offered this option, e.g. with one or two notable exceptions, bacterial infections are not thought to respond to homeopathy alone. Homeopathy cannot be used alone to treat vitamin or hormone deficiencies. The BMA report mentioned above reiterates the need for complementary practitioners to be well versed in medical sciences, and to show an awareness of their limits of competence and the scope of their particular therapy, so that they know when to refer cases to the GP. However, disquiet still exists and relationships between CAM practitioners and medically qualified practitioner, although improving, are often strained.

In Canada it has been suggested that consultations with alternative care providers occur as an adjunct to, rather than a replacement of, visits to physicians. Particular types of medical conditions as well as psychosocial and spiritual factors are determinants of concurrent use of physicians and alternative practitioners.[129]

In Germany there is a group of professional health providers known as 'Heilpraktikers'.[130] These practitioners are required to pass a test conducted by the local health authority that emphasises alternative diagnostic procedures. The *Heilpraktikers* are empowered to use injectables. They tend to use several complementary disciplines concurrently.

Lay practitioners

According to Helman[131] there are certain individuals who tend to act as a source of health advice more often than others:

- Those with first-hand knowledge of a long-standing chronic illness or different types of treatment
- Those with considerable experience of certain life experiences such as caring for elderly parents or raising children
- The organisers of self-help groups
- The members of certain healing cults or churches
- The spouses and staff of health professionals.

Any of these people, self-taught mainly through experience rather than formal study, may be viewed as lay practitioners depending on the frequency with which they offer advice or treatment.

Self-treatment[132]

People who become ill typically follow a 'hierarchy of resort',[32] beginning with self-medication, leading on to consultation with relations, friends or lay practitioners in the groups outlined above, perhaps more self-medication, and finally consultation with a doctor or other health professional. However, they do not always follow this logical pathway. They may return to previous treatments if later ones fail, try different methods simultaneously or consult CAM practitioners along the way. This makes the assessment of certain treatment outcomes extremely difficult.

Self-treatment may encompass proprietary drugs, patent medicines, aromatherapy oils, herbal or homeopathic medicines, as well as changes in diet or lifestyle. Increasingly government policy is to drive patients away from the NHS for simple self-limiting type conditions and to encourage self-treatment. The switching of certain high-powered drugs from a prescription-only category to allow sale in a pharmacy has facilitated this. In the UK about 75% of abnormal symptoms are dealt with outside the NHS. The GP sees around 20% of patients, 16% take no action, 63% self-medicate and 1% go directly to hospital. Thus the influence of the pharmacist or health shop assistant is often important in recommending what medicines patients should purchase.

Integrating CAM into the UK healthcare system

Integrated (or integrative) medicine is practising medicine in a way that selectively incorporates elements of CAM into comprehensive treatment plans alongside solidly orthodox methods of diagnosis and treatment.[133] As explained in Chapter 2 the term is not simply a synonym for complementary medicine. Integrated medicine has a larger meaning and mission, its focus being on health and healing rather than on disease and treatment. It views patients as whole people with minds and spirits as well as bodies, and includes these dimensions in diagnosis and treatment. It also involves patients and practitioners to maintain health by paying attention to environmental and lifestyle factors such as quality of housing, diet, exercise, amount of rest and sleep, and the nature of relationships (Figure 3.3).

Homeopathy has been available theoretically under the NHS in both primary and secondary care environments since the service was set up in 1948. The medicines may be prescribed on standard prescription forms throughout the UK and are fully reimbursable. Ryan[134] has sug-

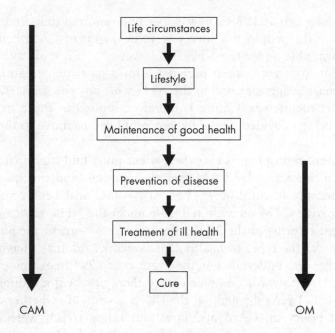

Figure 3.3 Representation of the factors involved in complementary and alternative medicine (CAM) and orthodox medicine (OM) healthcare systems.

gested that integrating homeopathy into general practice, rather than pursuing it as a career in itself, is 'straightforward'. Other therapies are available through the NHS via physiotherapy departments and pain clinics (acupuncture and mind–body therapies) as well as forming an essential and effective element of palliative care within hospices (mind–body therapies, reflexology, massage and aromatherapy).[135]

The Department of Health's stated aim was:

> ... to give patients wherever they live in the UK better health care and greater choice of the services available.

The availability of other disciplines under the NHS has been limited and the provision of CAM and orthodox medicine has largely developed along separate pathways. The call for integration of the two systems of medicine has grown considerably in recent years. However, at the time of writing in England, primary care trusts are withdrawing funding from homeopathy. Tunbridge Wells Homeopathic Hospital will close[136] and The Royal London Homeopathic Hospital is said to be in great danger.[137]

As long ago as 1989 a newspaper poll reported that almost three-quarters of the people in a survey were in favour of CAM being more widely available under the NHS.[138] However, it is not always possible for patients to exercise their preference for a particular treatment. It is the purchasing agencies within the NHS who buy the services, not the consumers themselves. Choice is therefore limited to those treatments that are being provided or the patient is obliged to move to the private sector.

A second problem is that the patient must find a sympathetic GP trained in the particular CAM therapy required, and this may not be easy, especially in rural areas. Presently some local health authorities (HAs) provide CAM on a limited scale under the NHS, some not at all. The recent reforms of the NHS offered an environment for purchasers to reconsider the types of health care available. Adams[139] has reported a study that was undertaken in the summer of 1994 to examine the attitudes of HAs towards complementary therapies. A questionnaire was sent to all 171 HAs throughout the UK to investigate whether they had a formal policy on CAM and how purchasing trends were likely to develop in the future; 57% of the HAs responded. The results showed that 67% of the HAs that responded were purchasing one or more complementary therapies. Only 10 HAs had an established policy on CAM; a further 10 were developing a policy and 77 had no formal policy. The survey suggested that a lack of information about scientific evaluation of the therapies was the most frequent reason for the last point. Of the HAs that did have a policy four had decided to purchase CAM in limited and specific circumstances, three had agreed to purchase only those therapies that they considered well established and the remaining three had not yet purchased any CAM. Current HA purchasing varies greatly across individual therapies, with some considerably more popular than others. Whether this is a result of the nature of the therapies or local availability is unclear.

Although formal policies on CAM were the exception and fairly limited where they did exist, it is significant that as many as 20 HAs were considering establishing a policy. Decisions are being made that are based on issues of scientific efficacy. This suggests that the potential for CAM to be made more widely available by HAs depends on resolving the problems of testing and evaluation.

A report on the future role of CAM and how therapies can be more fully integrated into the NHS was published in October 1997 by the Foundation for Integrated Medicine.[140] The 70-page document was entitled *'Integrated health care – a way forward for the next five years?'*

and summarised the conclusions of four working groups set up at the request of the Prince of Wales under the guidance of a Steering Committee. The culmination of 18 months' work, it was designed to stimulate debate on the possible role of CAM within the healthcare system. The document, which formed part of the Prince of Wale's Initiative on Integrated Medicine, was designed to stimulate debate on the possible role of complementary medicines within the healthcare system. It contains 28 specific proposals and highlights research, professional regulation, education and training, and effective delivery of integrated healthcare as priority areas.[141] Speakers at a meeting held to discuss the proposals some months later identified a lack of both evidence-based material and good quality research as being the main barriers to progress. The deans of all medical schools in the UK were asked to comment on the initial draft of this document, and those who responded highlighted the need for more research in association with an appropriate structure to carry such a policy forward. If the best of conventional medicine and CAM are to be combined in a truly integrative approach to healthcare, the latter must be research led and evidence based.

The key issues involved in the provision of CAM have been studied in a survey of the 481 primary care groups (PCGs) in England and Wales.[142] In 58% of the 60% of groups that responded CAM was available through primary care services. The most commonly used therapies were acupuncture (73%), osteopathy (43%), chiropractic (23%), homeopathy (38%) and hypnotherapy (12%).

A number of models exist of the provision of CAM in primary care in England,[143] including the Glastonbury Health Centre (acupuncture, osteopathy, herbalism and massage), St Margaret's Surgery, in Wiltshire (homeopathy), South Norfolk PCG (acupuncture) and Somerset Coast PCG (chiropractic). In London the Marylebone Health Centre provides access to acupuncture, homeopathy, osteopathy and massage for its population of 6000 patients. Secondary homeopathic care is provided by hospitals in London, Bristol and Glasgow where the first phase of a new purpose-built homeopathic hospital – the first in the UK for more than 100 years – opened in Glasgow in January 1998, replacing an older facility that had served the west of Scotland for more than 50 years. The Hospital seeks to integrate several complementary therapies into its portfolios of disease management.

There are some excellent examples of midwives who have introduced CAM into clinical practice and who are providing an enhanced service to women as a result.[144] Overall, however, service provision remains patchy and ad hoc with little evidence of a robust integration into the maternity services. Views appear to be positive, with increasing consumer satisfaction, promotion of normal childbirth and a reduction in medical intervention being seen as the main benefits.[139]

CAM and veterinary medicine

The Veterinary Surgeon's Act 1966 states, subject to a number of exceptions, that only registered members of The Royal College of Veterinary Surgeons (RCVS) can practise veterinary surgery in the UK.

Veterinary surgery is defined as:

> ... encompassing the art and science of veterinary surgery and medicine which includes the diagnosis of diseases and injuries in animals, tests performed on animals for diagnostic purposes, advice based upon a diagnosis ....

The exceptions include:

*   Veterinary students and veterinary nurses – governed by various amendments to the Veterinary Surgeons Act.
*   Farriers, although farriers have their own Farriers Registration Acts they are also governed by the Veterinary Surgeons Act and are not allowed to perform acts of veterinary surgery.

The other exceptions (including CAM) are governed by the Veterinary Surgery (Exemptions) Order 1962. With the movement of complementary therapies into the field of animal treatment, this Order was introduced to amend the Veterinary Surgeons Act to take such legitimate therapies into account.

As far as complementary therapies are concerned, this Order refers to four categories:

1. Manipulative therapies: this covers only physiotherapy, osteopathy and chiropractic and allows these therapies where a vet has diagnosed the condition and decided that this treatment would be appropriate.
2. Animal behaviourism: behavioural treatment is exempt, unless medication is used where permission must again be sought from the vet.
3. Faith healing: according to the *RCVS Guide to Professional Conduct*, faith healers have their own code of practice which indicates that permission must be sought from a vet before healing is given by the 'laying on of hands'.

4.   Other complementary therapies: according to the *RCVS Guide to Professional Conduct*:[146]

It is illegal, in terms of the Veterinary Surgeons Act 1966, for lay practitioners however qualified in the human field, to treat animals. At the same time it is incumbent on veterinary surgeons offering any complementary therapy to ensure that they are adequately trained in its application.

Thus, apart from the manipulative therapies, behavioural treatment and faith healing, all other forms of complementary therapy are illegal in the treatment of animals in the UK when practised by non-vets.

In the UK, herbal and homeopathic medicines registered by the Veterinary Medicines Directorate under the Veterinary Medicines Regulations are available.

References

1.   McIver S. *Obtaining the Views of Primary and Community Health Care Services.* London: King's Fund Centre, 1993.
2.   Pincock S. Patients put their relationship with their doctors as second only to that with their families. *BMJ* 2003;**327**:581.
3.   Nolan P, Badger F. Aspects of the relationship between doctors and depressed patients that enhance satisfaction with primary care. *J Psychiatr Ment Health Nurs* 2005;**12**:146–53. PubMed
4.   Hunink MGM. Does evidence based medicine do more good than harm? *BMJ* 2004;**329**:1051.
5.   Garfield S, Smith F, Francis SA, Chalmers C. Can patients' preferences for involvement in decision-making regarding the use of medicines be predicted? *Patient Educ Couns* 2007;**66**:361–7. PubMed
6.   Entwistle V, Prior M, Skea ZC, Francis JJ. Involvement in treatment decision-making: Its meaning to people with diabetes and implications for conceptualisation. *Soc Sci Med* 2007;**66**: 362–75.
7.   Watkins AB Contemporary context of complementary and alternative medicine. Integrated mind-body medicine. In: Micozzi MS (ed.), *Fundamentals of Complementary and Alternative Medicine.* New York: Churchill Livingstone, 1996: 49–63.
8.   Vincent CA, Furnham A. Why do patients turn to complementary medicine? An empirical study, *Br J Clin Psychol* 1996;**35**:37–48.
9.   D'Crus A, Wilkinson JM. Reasons for choosing and complying with complementary health care: an in-house study on a South Australian clinic. *J Altern Compl Med* 2005;**11**:1107–12.
10. Kayne SB. *Homoeopathic Pharmacy: An introduction and handbook.* Edinburgh: Churchill Livingstone, 1997: 10–12.
11. Sharpe VA, Faden AI. *Medical Harm.* New York: Cambridge University Press, 1998.
12. Campion EW. Why unconventional medicine? Editorial. *N Engl J Med* 1993;**328**:282–3.

13. Asscher W. Risk benefit analysis in medical treatment. *BIRA J* 1985;**4**:54–6.
14. McBride WG Thalidomide and congenital abnormalities. (Letter) *Lancet* 1961;**ii**:1358.
15. Von Wartburg WP. Drugs and perception of risks. *Swiss Pharmaceutica* 1984;**6**:21–3.
16. Slovak P, Kraus N, Lapps H, Major M. Risk perception of prescription drugs: report on a survey in Sweden. *Pharm Med* 1989;**4**:43–65.
17. Ernst E. Willoughby M, Weihmayr Th. Nine possible reasons for choosing complementary medicine. *Perfusion* 1995;**11**:356–9.
18. Eng J, Ramsum D, Verhoef M, Guns E, Davison J, Gallagher R. A population-based survey of complementary and alternative medicine use in men recently diagnosed with prostate cancer. *Integr Cancer Ther* 2003;**2**:212–16.
19. Department of Health. *The Patients' Charter*. London: HMSO, 1991.
20. Klein R. *The Politics of the National Health Service*, 2nd edn. Harlow: Longman, 1989.
21. Avina RL, Schneiderman LJ. Why patients choose homoeopathy. *West J Med* 1978;**128**:366–9.
22. Morrison I, Smith R. The future of medicine (Editorial). *BMJ* 1994;**309**: 1099–100.
23. Bakx K. The 'eclipse' of folk medicine in western society. *Society of Health and Illness* 1991;**13**:17–24
24. Sirois FM, Gick ML. An investigation of the health beliefs and motivations of complementary medicine clients. *Soc Sci Med* 2002;**55**:1025–37. PubMed
25. Jørgensen V, Launsø L. Patients' choice of asthma and allergy treatments. *J Altern Compl Med* 2005;**11**:529–34.
26. Shumay DM, Maskarinec G, Kakai H, Gotay CC. Why some cancer patients choose complementary and alternative medicine instead of conventional treatment. *J Family Pract* 2001;**50**:1067.
27. Berg M, Arnetz B. Characteristics of users and nonusers of alternative medicine in dermatologic patients attending a university hospital clinic: a short report. *J Altern Compl Med* 1998;**4**:277–9.
28. Furnham A, Vincent C, Wood R. The health beliefs and behaviours of three groups of complementary medicine and a general practice group of patients. *J Altern Compl Med* 1995;**1**:347–59.
29. Ernst E, Resch KL, Hill S. Do complementary medicine practitioners have a better bedside manner? *J R Soc Med* 1997; **80**:118–19.
30. Resch KL, Hill S, Ernst E. Use of complementary therapies by individuals with 'arthritis'. *Clin Rheumatol* 1997;**16**:391–5.
31. Katz J. *The Silent World of Doctor and Patient*. New York: The Free Press, 1984: 4.
32. Helman C. *Culture, Health and Illness*, 2nd edn. Oxford: Butterworth-Heinemann, 1990.
33. Furnham A. The A type behaviour pattern, mental health and health locus of control beliefs. *Soc Sci Med* 1983;**17**:1569–72.
34. Finnegan M. The Centre for the Study of Complementary Medicine: An attempt to understand its popularity through psychological demographic and operational criteria. *Compl Med Res* 1991;**5**:83–8.

35. Finnegan M. Complementary medicine: attitudes and expectations, a scale for evaluation. *Compl Med Res* 1991;**5**:79–81.

36. English JM. Homoeopathy. *Practitioner* 1986;**230**:1067–71.

37. Furnham A, Smith C. Choosing alternative medicine: A comparison of the beliefs of patients visiting a general practitioner and a homoeopath. *Soc Sci Med* 1988; **26** 685–9.

38. Moore J, Phipps K, Mercer D, Lewith G. Why do people seek treatment by alternative medicine? *BMJ* 1985;**290**:28–9.

39. Furnham A, Kirkcaldy B. The health beliefs and behaviours of orthodox and complementary medicine clients. *Br J Clin Psychol* 1996;**35**:49–61.

40. Vincent C, Furnham A. The perceived efficacy of complementary and orthodox medicine: preliminary findings and development of questionnaire. *Compl Ther Med* 1994;**2**:128–34.

41. Boisset M, Fitzeharles MA. Alternative medicine use by rheumatology patients in a universal health care setting. *J Rheumatol* 1994;**21**:149–52.

42. Richardson J. *Complementary Therapy in the NHS: A service evaluation of the first year of an outpatient service in a local district general hospital.* London: Health Services Research and Evaluation Unit, the Lewisham Hospital NHS Trust, 1994.

43. Meenan R Developing appropriate measures of the benefits of complementary and alternative medicine. *J Health Serv Res Policy* 2001;**6**:38–43. PubMed CAM

44. White AR, Resch KL, Ernst E. Methods of economic evaluation in complementary medicine. *Forsch Komplmenternmed* 1996;**3**:196–203.

45. Swayne J. The cost and effectiveness of homoeopathy. *Br Homeopath J* 1992;**81**:148–50.

46. Fulder SJ, Munro RE. Complementary medicine in the United Kingdom: Patients, practitioners and consultations. *Lancet* 1985;**2**:542–5.

47. van Haselen RA, Graves NB, Dahiha S. The costs of treating rheumatoid arthritis patients with complementary medicine: exploring the issue. *Compl Ther Med* 1999;**7**:217–21.

48. Feldhaus H-W. Cost-effectiveness of homoeopathic treatment in a dental practice. *Br Homeopath J* 1993;**82**:25–8.

49. Myers CP. Acupuncture in general practice: effect on drug expenditure. *Acupunct Med* 1991;**9**:71–2.

50. Carey TS, Garrett J, Jackman A et al. The outcomes and costs of care for acute low back pain among patients seen by primary care practitioners, chiropractors and orthopedic surgeons. *N Engl J Med* 1995;**333**:913–17.

51. Johansson K, Lindgren I, Widner H et al. Can sensory simulation improve the functional outcome in stroke patients? *Neurology* 1993;**43**:2189–92.

52. Shaw A, Thompson E, Sharp D. Complementary therapy use by patients and parents of children with asthma and the implications for NHS care: a qualitative study. *BMC Health Services Res* 2006;**6**:76. Available at: http://tinyurl.com/2njdcg (accessed 8 December 2007).

53. Fulder SJ, Munro RE. Complementary medicine in the United Kingdom: patients, practitioners and consultants. *Lancet* 1985;**2**:542–5.

54. Zollman C, Vickers A. Users and practitioners of complementary medicine. *BMJ* 1999;**319**:836–8.

55. Vickers A (1994) Use of complementary therapies. *BMJ* 1994;**309**:1161.
56. Devitt M. Complementary care in the UK. *Acupunct Today* 2000;**1**(9). Available at: http://tinyurl.com/3yunaz (accessed 8 December 2007).
57. Thomas KJ, Coleman P, Nicholl JP. Use and expenditure on complementary medicine in England – a population based survey. *Compl Ther Med* 2001; 9:2–11.
58. Shakeel M, Bruce J, Jehan S et al. Use of complementary and alternative medicine by patients admitted to a surgical unit in Scotland. *Ann R Coll Surg Engl* 2008; Aug 12. [Epub ahead of print] PubMed Available at: http://www.ncbi.nlm.nih.gov/pubmed/18701007?dopt=Abstract (accessed 25 August 2008).
59. Ernst E, White A. The BBC survey of complementary medicine use in the UK. *Compl Ther Med* 2000;**8**:32–6.
60. Mintel International Group. *Complementary Medicines.* London: Mintel International Group Ltd, 2007.
61. Fisher P, Ward A. Complementary medicine in Europe. Report from complementary research: an international perspective. COST and RCCAM Conference. Luxembourg: EU Science Research and Development Directorate, 1994: 29–43.
62. Furnham A, Bond C The perceived efficacy of homeopathy and orthodox medicine: a vignette-based study. *Compl Ther Med* 2000;**8**:193–201. PubMed
63. Eisenberg DM, Kessler RC, Foster C et al. Unconventional medicine in the United States. *N Engl J Med* 1993;**328**:246–52.
64. Eisenberg DM, Davis RB, Ettner SL et al. Trends in alternative medicine use in the United States 1990–1997. *JAMA* 1998;**280**:1569–75.
65. Astin JA Why patients use alternative medicine: results of a national study. *JAMA* 1998;**279**:1548–53.
66. Baldwin, Lord. Why patients use alternative medicine. (Letter) *JAMA* 1998;**280**:1659.
67. Bausell RB, Lee WL, Berman BM. Demographic and health-related correlates to visits to complementary and alternative medical providers. *Med Care* 2001;**39**:190–6. PubMed
68. Maskarinec G, Shumay DM, Kakai H, Gotay C. Ethnic differences in complementary and alternative medicine use among cancer patients. *J Altern Compl Med* 2000;**6**:531–8.
69. Millar WJ. Use of alternative health care practitioners by Canadians. *Can J Public Health* 1997;**88**:154–8.
70. Esmail N. *Complementary and Alternative Medicine in Canada: Trends in use and public attitudes, 1997–2006.* Vancouver BC: The Fraser Institute, 2007.
71. Millar WJ. Use of alternative health care practitioners by Canadians. *Can J Public Health* 1997;**88**:154–8. PubMed
72. Druss BG, Rosenheck RA. Association between use of unconventional therapies and conventional medical services. *JAMA* 1999;**282**:651–6. PubMed
73. Achilles R, Adelson N, Antze P, et al. *Complementary and Alternative Health Practices and Therapies. A Canadian overview.* Toronto, Ontario: York University Centre for Health Studies, 1999.

74. MacLennan AH, Wilson DH, Taylor AW. Prevalence and cost of alternative medicine in Australia. *Lancet* 1996;**347**:569–73.
75. Berenstein JH, Shmuel A, Shuval JT. Consultations with practitioners of alternative medicine. *Harefuah* 1996;**130**:83–5.
76. Amir Shmueli A, Shuval J. Are users of complementary and alternative medicine sicker than non-users? *Evidence-based Compl Altern Med* 2007;**4**:251–5.
77. Long L, Huntley A, Ernst E. Which complementary and alternative therapies benefit which conditions? A survey of the opinions of 223 professional organizations. *Compl Ther Med* 2001;**9**:178–85.
78. Evans M, Shaw A, Thompson EA et al. Decisions to use complementary and alternative medicine (CAM) by male cancer patients: information-seeking roles and types of evidence used. *BMC Compl Altern Med* 2007;**7**:25.
79. Grootenhuis MA, Last BF, de Graaf-Nijkerk JH, van der Wel M. Use of alternative treatment in pediatric oncology. *Cancer Nurs* 1998;**21**:282–8.
80. Guo R, Pittler MH, Ernst E. Complementary medicine for treating or preventing influenza or influenza-like illness. *Am J Med* 2007;**120**:923–9. e3 (PubMed)
81. Pal B. Complementary medicine. (Letter) *BMJ* 1996;**313**:1080.
82. Bell I. Complementary and alternative medicine modalities in stroke treatment and rehabilitation. *Top Stroke Rehabil* 2007;**14**:30–9.
83. Stone J, Matthews J. *Complementary Medicine and the Law*. Oxford: Oxford University Press, 1996.
84. Mills SY. Regulation in complementary and alternative medicine. *BMJ* 2001; **322**:158–60.
85. Nedrow AR, Heitkemper M, Frenkel M, Mann D, Wayne P, Hughes E. Collaborations between allopathic and complementary and alternative medicine health professionals: four initiatives. *Acad Med* 2007;**82**:962–6. PubMed
86. Sierpina VS, Schneeweiss R, Frenkel MA, Bulik R, Maypole J. Barriers, strategies, and lessons learned from complementary and alternative medicine curricular initiatives. *Acad Med* 2007;**82**:946–50. PubMed
87. Berman BM Complementary medicine and medical education. (Editorial) *BMJ* 2001;**322**:121–2.
88. Owen DK, Lewith G, Stephens CR. Can doctors respond to patients' increasing interest in complementary and alternative medicine? *BMJ* 2001;**322**: 154–8.
89. Bryden H. Commentary: Special study modules and complementary and alternative medicine – the Glasgow experience. *BMJ* 2001;**322**:158.
90. Wetzel MS, Eisenberg DM, Kaptchuk TJ. Courses involving complementary and alternative medicine at US medical schools. *JAMA* 1998;**280**:784–7.
91. Rakel DR, Guerrera MP, Bayles BP, et al. CAM Education: Promoting a salutogenic focus in health care. *J Alt Compl Med* 2008;**14**:87–93.
92. Kao FF, Kao JJ, eds. *Recent Advances in Acupuncture Research*. New York: Institute for Advanced Research in Asian Science and Medicine, 1979.
93. Clark PA The ethics of alternative medicine therapies. *J Public Health Policy* 2000;**21**:447–70. PubMed

94.   Giannelli M, Cuttini M, Da Frè M, Buiatti E. General practitioners' knowledge and practice of complementary/alternative medicine and its relationship with life-styles: a population-based survey in Italy. *BMC Family Pract* 2007; **8**:30. PubMed

95.   Anon. The flight from science. (Editorial) *BMJ* 1980;**280**:1–2.

96.   Anon. An ABC of complementary medicine: a new dawn (Editor's choice). *BMJ* 1999;**319**:ii.

97.   Hunter AJ. Attitudes to complementary medicine: A survey of general practitioners and medical students in the Tayside area. *Comm Br Homeopath Res Grp* 1988;**17**:34–44.

98.   Ross S, Simpson C R, McLay J S. Homeopathic and herbal prescribing in general practice in Scotland. *Br J Clin Pharmacol* 2006; **62**:647–52.

99.   Reilly DT. Young doctors' views on alternative medicine. *BMJ* 1983;**287**: 337–9.

100.   Halliday J, Taylor M, Jenkins A, Reilly DT. Medical students and complementary medicine. *Compl Ther Med* 1993;**1**(suppl 1):32–3.

101.   Ernst E, Resch KL, White AR. Complementary medicine. What physicians think of it: A meta-analysis. *Arch Intern Med* 1995;**155**:2405–8.

102.   White AR, Resch KL, Ernst E. Complementary medicine: use and attitudes among GPs. *Family Pract* 1997;**14**:302–6.

103.   Wharton R, Lewith G. Complementary medicine and the general practitioner. *BMJ* 1986;**292**:1498–500.

104.   Franklin D. Medical practitioners' attitudes to complementary medicine. *Compl Med Res* 1992;**6**:69–71.

105.   Thomas K, Fall M, Parry G, Nichol J. National survey of access to complementary health care via general practice. Sheffield: University of Sheffield, 1995.

106.   Barnes J. Can alternative medicine be integrated into mainstream care? Report on RCP/NCCM Conference, London 23–24 Jan 2001. *Pharm J* 2001;**286**:367–9.

107.   Akhtar S, van Haselen R. Why GPs refer or do not refer patients for homeopathy. *Proceedings of the Third International Conference on Homeopathy.* London: RLHH & Parkside Health, 22–23 February 2001: 62.

108.   Treuhertz F. Homeopathy in general practice: a descriptive report of work with 500 consecutive patients. *Br Homeopath J* 2000; (suppl 1):S43.

109.   Borkan J, Neher J, Anson O, Smoker B. Referrals for alternative therapies. *J Family Pract* 1994;**39**:545–50.

110.   Verhoef MJ, Sutherland LR. General practitioners' assessment of and interest in alternative medicine in Canada. *Soc Sci Med* 1995;**41**:511–15.

111.   Marshall RJ, Gee R, Dumble J et al. The use of alternative therapies by Auckland general practitioners. *NZ Med J* 1990;**103**:213–15.

112.   Himmel W, Schulte M, Kochen MK. Complementary medicine: are patients' expectations being met by their general practitioners? *Br J Gen Pract* 1993;**43**:232–5.

113.   Halliday J, Taylor M, Jenkins A, Reilly D. Medical students and complementary medicine. *Compl Ther Med* 1993;**1**:32–3.

114.   Anon. News focus – bastions of traditional adapt to alternative medicine. *Science* 2000;**288**:1571.

115. Kayne SB. Demand and scepticism. *Pharm J* 1991;**247**:602–4.
116. Anon. The Conference. *Pharm J* 2000;**265**:403.
117. Anon. Statutory committee statement on Spagnyck therapy. *Pharm J* 1997; **259**:250–1.
118. Barnes J. *Uncovering Potential Problems Associated with Complementary Remedies: A survey of community pharmacists*. London: Royal Pharmaceutical Society of Great Britain, 1999.
119. Hessig R, Arcand L, Frost M. The effects of an educational intervention on oncology nurses attitude, perceived knowledge, and self-reported application of complementary therapies. *Oncol Nursing Forum* 2004;**31**: 71–8.
120. Kayne SB. Survey on the teaching of complementary medicine in British schools of pharmacy. *Br Hom J* 1993;**82**:172–3.
121. Langley P, Fonseca J, Iphofen R. Psychoneuroimmunology and health from a nursing perspective. *Br J Nursing* 2006;**15**:1126–9.
122. Hamilton ET, Tomlinson K. The application of homeopathy in nursing and midwifery. In: Kayne SB (ed.), *Homeopathic Practice*. London: Pharmaceutical Press, 2008: Chapter 12.
123. Keimig TJ, Braun CA. Student nurses? Knowledge and perceptions of alternative and complementary therapies. *J Undergrad Nursing Scholarship* 2004;6. Available at http://tinyurl.com/2rs3ls (accessed 10 December 2007).
124. Laurenson M, MacDonald J, McCready T, Stimpson A. Student nurses' knowledge and attitudes toward CAM therapies. *Br J Nurs* 2006;**15**:612–5.
125. Fisher P, Ward A. Complementary medicine in Europe. *BMJ* 1994;**309**: 107–11.
126. *A Survey of Voluntary Regulatory Bodies for Complementary Therapies*. London: Department of Health, 2000.
127. British Medical Association. *Complementary Medicine: New approaches to good practice*. Oxford: Oxford University Press, 1993.
128. NAHAT. *Guidelines to Employment of Complementary Therapists in the NHS*. London: NAHAT, 1995.
129. Muhajarine N, Neudorf C, Martin K. Concurrent consultations with physicians and providers of alternative care: results from a population-based study. *Can J Public Health* 2000;**91**:449–53.
130. Ernst E. Towards quality in complementary health care: is the German 'Heilpraktiker' a model for complementary practitioners? *Int J Qual Health Care* 1996;**8**:187–90.
131. Helman C. *Culture, Health and Illness*, 2nd edn. Oxford: Butterworth–Heinemann, 1990.
132. Vincent C, Furnham A. *Complementary Medicine*. Chichester: Wiley & Sons, 1998: 29–30.
133. Rees L Weil A. Integrated medicine. (Editorial) *BMJ* 2001;**322**:119–20.
134. Ryan K. Career focus. Medical homoeopathy. *BMJ* 1998;**316**:2.
135. Lewith GT. What to do about CAM? (Letter) *BMJ* 2007;**335**:961.
136. Anon. NHS trust stops homeopathy funds. BBC News 24, 27 September 2007. Available at http://tinyurl.com/33rznn (accessed 17 November 2007).

137.   Campbell D, Fitzgerald M. Royals' favoured hospital at risk as homeopathy backlash gathers pace. *The Observer* Sunday 8 April 2007. Available online at http://tinyurl.com/3yfnfw (accessed 17 November 2007).
138.   MORI poll. *The Times* 13 November 1989.
139.   Adams J. With complements. *Health Serv J* 1995;June 1:23.
140.   London Foundation for Integrated Medicine. *Integrated Health Care. A way forward for the next five years?* London: London Foundation for Integrated Medicine, 1997.
141.   Kmietowicz Z. Complementary medicine should be integrated into the NHS. *BMJ* 1997;**315**:1111–16.
142.   Bonnet J. *Complementary Medicine in Primary Care – what are the key issues?* London: NHS Executive. 2000.
143.   Department of Health. *Complementary Medicine. Information pack for primary care groups.* London. Department of Health/NHS Alliance, 2000: 19–21.
144.   Ager C. A complementary therapy clinic, making it work. *RCM Midwives J* 2002;**5**:198–200.
145.   Williams J, Mitchell M. Midwifery managers' views about the use of complementary therapies in the maternity services. *Compl Ther Clin Pract* 2007;**13**:129–35.
146.   Royal College of Veterinary Surgeons. *RCVS Guide to Professional Conduct: Treatment of animals by non-veterinary surgeons.* London: RCVS, 2000.

4

Complementary and alternative medicine in the USA

JP Borneman

Introduction

Sales of non-food natural and complementary and alternative medicine (CAM) products in the USA exceeded $US29.97 billion in 2006, growing at an annual rate of 9.7%.[1] The most recent (2004) National Health Information Survey (NHIS) estimated that 36% of Americans over the age of 18 used some form of CAM during the previous 12 months.[2] Furthermore, a recent Institute of Medicine (IOM) Report, *Complementary and Alternative Medicine in the United States*, esti mates that Americans are now spending more on CAM than primary care, that more than 15 million Americans routinely use herbal medicines and that spending now exceeds $US27bn per year on CAM and CAM-related products.[3] Although it is estimated that Americans made more visits to CAM providers (629 million) than primary care providers (386 million) in 1997,[3,4] data indicate that many consumers of CAM do not discuss their CAM use with their physician,[3-5] a situation that has impacts on health policy, best practices, healthcare funding and the doctor–patient relationship. What are the drives for CAM use in the USA? Who is the 'typical' CAM user? What are the psychosocial attributes of those who use CAM?

Institutionalising CAM: NIH and NCCAM

Increasing amounts of tax dollars are being spent on CAM research. The budget for the National Institutes of Health's (NIH's) National Center for Complementary and Alternative Medicine (NCCAM), formerly the Office of Alternative Medicine (OAM), grew from its initial allocation of $US2m in 1992 to a high of $US121.1m in fiscal 2005,[6] a 60-fold increase over 13 years – an average 466% increase each year (Figure 4.1).

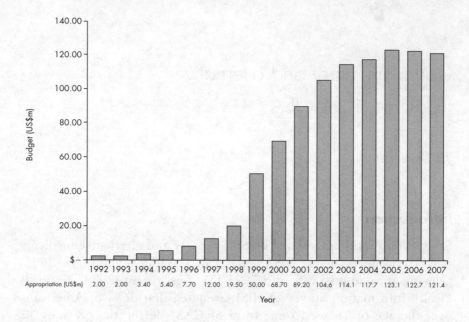

Figure 4.1 NCCAM appropriations 1992–2007.

The increase in CAM in the literature, as well as the increasing federal money spent on CAM at NIH, tend to indicate that CAM is slowly entering the mainstream of biomedical research and attracting an increasing amount of attention.

The ambiguity in the definition of CAM has a practical problem. To illustrate this, a review of the Computer Retrieval of Information on Scientific Projects (CRISP)[7] database at the NIH was undertaken.[8] CRISP was searched for the 50 CAM modalities identified in the literature for grants made by NIH as a whole, and by NCCAM specifically, for the periods 1992–6, 1997–2001 and 2002–4. This search was confounded by a lack of precision in CAM terminology, duplication of records and a strategy at NCCAM before 1997 of using other institutes' grant-making authority to fund CAM projects. Consequently, for comparison purposes, data were limited to the periods 1997–2001 and 2002–4. For specific CAM modalities, Table 4.1 shows a comparison of rank by mention in the literature, with grants identified at NIH as a whole and with NCCAM specifically for the two periods. In some cases, e.g. herbs and diet, there was an alignment between NCCAM funding and mentions in the literature. However, in other cases, notably homeopathy and mind–body disciplines (hypnosis, guided imagery, biofeedback, relaxation), there were

Table 4.1 Comparison of modality ranking in the literature with NIH funding

Modality	Rank by mentions[a]	NIH Ranking by grants 1997–2001[b]	NCCAM Ranking by grants 1997–2001[c]	NIH Ranking by grants 2002–2004[d]	NCCAM Ranking by grants 2002–2004[e]
Herbal	1	9	1	7	1
Homeopathy	1	22	10	25	12
Massage	1	25	9	15	9
Acupuncture	4	11	2	10	3
Chiropractic	5	17	4	16	5
Hypnosis	6	16	21	20	22
Diet	7	1	3	1	2
Guided imagery	8	22	27	32	29
Prayer	8	31	15	30	17
Vitamins	8	40	27	40	34
Biofeedback	11	8	17	9	20
Relaxation	11	26	27	30	34
Folk medicine	13	12	7	12	4
Spirituality	13	15	13	11	11
Support groups/self-help	13	10	27	13	34
Energy medicine	16	37	27	33	20
Exercise	16	2	6	2	7
Naturopathy	16	29	10	21	10
Reflexology	19	40	27	37	34
Aromatherapy	20	32	27	35	34
Meditation	21	13	5	14	6
Commercial weight loss	22	40	27	40	34
Magnets	22	37	21	36	29
Tai c'hi	22	20	12	19	17
Therapeutic touch	22	30	27	25	14
Traditional Chinese medicine	22	19	8	17	8
Counselling	27	3	15	3	24
Yoga	27	26	17	23	13
Art	29	37	21	37	32
Ayurveda	29	40	27	37	32
Chelation	29	7	27	8	24
Curanderismo	29	35	27	40	34
Faith healing	29	40	27	40	34
Healthfood	29	28	27	40	34
Humour	29	40	27	40	34
Light	29	14	21	18	24
Music	29	24	21	24	22
Osteopathy	29	18	17	22	17

Table 4.1 *continued*

Modality	Rank by mentions[a]	NIH Ranking by grants 1997–2001[b]	NCCAM Ranking by grants 1997–2001[c]	NIH Ranking by grants 2002–2004[d]	NCCAM Ranking by grants 2002–2004[e]
Ozone	29	40	27	40	34
Psychotherapy	29	5	14	5	14
Reiki	29	32	20	28	16
Acupressure	42	35	27	33	24
Astrology	43	40	27	40	34
Behavioural therapy	43	6	27	6	24
Colonic irrigation	43	40	27	40	34
Cranial sacral therapy	43	40	27	40	34
Drama	43	32	27	27	34
Electrostimulation	43	21	27	28	34
Metabolic	43	40	27	40	34
Native American healing	43	4	21	4	29

[a] Ranked by number of mentions in 25 CAM surveys analysed
[b] Ranked by raw number of grants across NIH listed by keyword in the NIH CRISP database 1997–2001
[c] Ranked by raw number of grants for NCCAM listed by keyword in the NIH CRISP database 1997–2001
[d] Ranked by raw number of grants across NIH listed by keyword in the NIH CRISP database 2002–2004
[e] Ranked by raw number of grants for NCCAM listed by keyword in the NIH CRISP database 2002–2004
NICCAM, National Center for Complementary and Alternative Medicine; NIH, National Institutes of Health.

wide differences between the prevalence of modalities appearing in the literature and NIH's grant making.

NCCAM domains of CAM

In an attempt to resolve the ambiguity, NCCAM has attempted to organise CAM modalities into five domains:[9]

1. Alternative medical systems (homeopathy, naturopathy, traditional Chinese medicine, ayurveda)
2. Mind–body medicine
3. Energy medicine (magnets, therapeutic touch)
4. Biologically based medicine (dietary supplements)

5.   Manipulative therapies (chiropractic, osteopathy, massage therapies).

The rationale was to impose some form of order on the field while maintaining flexibility within each domain. Clearly the domains have different attributes and varying levels of acceptance by the consumer and practitioner communities. In addition, although numerous researchers have attempted to estimate CAM use by consumers, a common theme is a lack of discussion of their CAM use with their health-care providers. Eisenberg and colleagues[4] found in 1998 that 63–72% of consumers of CAM do not discuss their use of these products with their doctor. It is evident that better understanding of patient use patterns of CAM, particularly in populations with specific health needs, is essential in informing the dialogue between doctor and patient.

CAM prevalence: emerging picture

Complementary and alternative medicine, by many of its definitions, has entered into the domain of public health and health policy. In the preface of a special issue of the *American Journal of Public Health* specifically dedicated to CAM, guest editor Vincent Silenzio wrote:

> Although in different ways, complementary and alternative health care and healing practices represent a vast and as yet unrealized sector of the public health systems of developed and developing nations. Moreover, the limits of our current biomedical knowledge and capabilities cannot be denied. We do not, as yet, have all the answers, or even, for that matter, know all the questions. There are more things in heaven and earth than can be dreamt of in our current biomedical philosophies. Stagnant biomedical orthodoxy cannot achieve the fullness of public health's potential and has no role to play in human progress. Maintaining an openness to this reality may serve to help marshal the resources of indigenous, complementary, and alternative health practices in the service of public health, now and in the future.[10]

This statement is more practical than visionary. Recently, in an article marking the twenty-fifth anniversary of Starr's social transformation of American medicine,[11] UCLA sociologist Michael Goldstein held that Starr might have it wrong.[12] The medical profession was not as cleanly consolidated as Starr would have held. The sectarians, in the main the practitioners of CAM, were not eliminated; rather they were driven underground to re-emerge in a different political time and place. Goldstein writes:

Starr's hesitancy to be more critical in assessing the relationship of med-ical practice to scientific rationality is important because it allows him to neglect or dismiss other forms of healthcare such as CAM. That many types of alternative healers have maintained, and recently expanded, their presence within the American health care scene is not solely due to their ability to survive as deviants within the corpus of medicine. Rather, the public remains attracted to what they have to offer; a greater willingness and ability to provide care to the chronically ill; attention to the individ-ual needs of their clients; an appreciation of the interplay of mind, body and spirit as they affect health and illness; and a hesitancy to apply 'heroic' measures that often are useless or have disastrous side effects.[12]

As an example, Goldstein cites Oncolink, a website run by the University of Pennsylvania and underwritten by a host of conventional pharmaceutical companies. On the site is information about CAM. Public health must find what healthcare practices work, and then be willing to implement them. The first part of the process is to determine what is happening in the field.

CAM prevalence in the USA: who uses it?

Cross-sectional surveys of the general population tend to indicate that CAM use has become common, both in self-care and in seeking the assistance of a provider.[2,4,5,13,14] The first national survey of the use of CAM by the American public, conducted by Eisenberg and colleagues, estimated that, in 1991, 34% of adults in the USA had used at least one CAM modality during the previous 12 months. Furthermore, of those who had used at least one modality, one-third had seen a CAM provider.[5] In 1997, a follow-on survey by the same team using similar methods found that the proportion seeking out a practitioner had changed from 36.3% to 46.3%.[4] For example, of the 18 CAM modal-ities listed in 1991, a quarter of respondents used exercise and prayer, whereas 1–3% used herbal products, diet or homeopathy.[5] Use of these modalities increased across the board by 1997, with approximately one-half having statistically significant increases.[4] By 2002, usage had increased further. The National Health Information Survey (2002) reported that 74.6% of those surveyed had used a CAM modality at least once, and that 62.1% had used at least one CAM modality in the previous year.[2]

From an ecological perspective, repeating the methodology first published in 1961,[15] Green and colleagues used Gallup telephone survey data of 1000 civilian, non-institutionalised individuals who had experienced health events in 1996. The purpose was to determine surgery visits, hospitalisations, illness and injuries. Their surprising finding was that although 113 participants reported visiting a primary care provider and 21 reported visiting an outpatient clinic, 65 (6.5%) reported visiting a CAM provider. It is also noteworthy that out-of-pocket (unreimbursed) expenditures were incurred in most of these visits.[13] McFarland and colleagues[16] compared prevalence of use of CAM in the USA and Canada using the 1996 US Medical Expenditure Panel Survey ($n = 16\,400$; response rate [RR] 78%) and the 1996 Canadian National Population Health Survey ($n = 70\,884$; RR 83%). They noted that, although the US and Canadian populations had essential differences, especially related to ethnicity and access to care and insurance, CAM use was in many ways similar. They reported that, in both countries, CAM seemed to be an adjunctive (add-on) therapy as opposed to essential care. Some differences of note were that 16% of Canadians vs 5% of Americans used 'any CAM provider', whereas 2% of Canadians vs 1% of Americans used a CAM provider exclusively. Canadians were more than three times as likely to use CAM in addition to conventional providers.[16]

Drivers to CAM use in the USA

Sociodemographic drivers

Numerous studies have been undertaken to characterise CAM use in smaller specific population samples.[17-20] These studies tend to show higher CAM utilisation rate than in larger cross-sectional measures, with 37–58% of respondents having used at least one CAM therapy on the list in the previous year. Burge and Albright[19] found that only 43% had told their health professional about their CAM use. Rafferty et al.[20] used data from the Behavioural Risk Factor Surveillance System to survey 3764 Michigan residents in 2001. They found that 49.7% of adults had used at least one CAM therapy in the previous year, the most common being herbal therapies (20.5%), special diets (12.6%) and chiropractic (12.2%). Of this sample, women were more likely to use CAM than men.

Gender differences associated with CAM use are found in the literature. Salmenpera[21,22] found that women (59%) were more likely than men (44%) to 'seriously consider' CAM use in the past year. Among those who considered CAM but did not use it, reasons included insufficient scientific evidence (women 57%, men 77%) or conventional treatments worked 'well enough' (women 45%, men 70%). Of those who started to use CAM for their illness, the reasons given were 'to restore hope in their future' (women 36%, men 36%), and 'to do as much as they can for themselves' (women 46%, men 29%). Both of these findings are of interest because they support the hypotheses of the effects of internal locus of control on CAM use (discussed later).

Thus, the sociodemographic data around CAM use tend to indicate that the most common factors are gender, age, ethnicity, education level and income.[14,23–26]

These investigations cannot be compared with each other as such. However, they show clearly that CAM is being used in the USA as in other countries. However, the limitations of these reports are clear: sample sizes are small, populations are generally limited, the definition of CAM is variable (from 3 to over 20 modalities) and methodological quality is highly variable. With the widespread use of CAM established, at least to the limits of the literature, what are the variables related to use?

Psychosocial drivers to CAM use

Other factors for CAM use have been found in the literature. They can be divided into psychosocial and other possible factors.

The literature tends to indicate that psychosocial and health behaviour factors may be associated with CAM use. These factors include ratings of health, advice satisfaction and a variety of factors associated with beliefs about health and locus of control. For the purposes of this discussion, the locus of control theory is defined in its original meaning, which effectively separates the population into a continuum between two poles: on the one extreme, those with internal locus of control who believe that they have control over outcomes in their lives and, on the other, people with external locus of control, who believe that outcomes in their lives are controlled by external forces or people.[27]

In a sample of college students ($n = 913$) in 2003, Chng and colleagues[24] found that, in addition to the common factors, health locus of control and 'holistic attitude' were associated with CAM use. They found that internal locus of control was highly correlated ($r = 0.25$, $p = 0.01$) with CAM use. Sturm[25] had a similar finding. Using a 1998 US national household survey ($n = 9585$) and CAM use in the previous year as the dependent variable, risk-taking behaviour was found to be a factor. There was a difference between CAM self-care and doctor-provided CAM. Sturm found that individuals using only CAM self-care (as opposed to seeing a CAM provider) rated themselves as 'more cautious' (odds ratio [OR] 1.08), not statistically different from the general population.

The relationship of health locus of control and patient behaviour has been explored in the literature with inconsistent findings. In early work, Schlenk and Hart[28] conducted structured interviews with patients who had diabetes. They found a statistically significant relationship between compliance and social support, 'powerful others health locus of control' (PHLC) and 'internal health locus of control'. They found that social support and PHLC accounted for at least 50% of the variance in compliance scores. The multiple R of the independent variables with compliance reached a significance level of $p < 0.005$. However, only the two variables of social support and PHLC added significantly ($p < 0.05$) to prediction accuracy.

Contrary findings were reported by Ramos-Remus and colleagues.[29] They administered the Multidimensional Health Locus of Control (MHLC) instrument as well as structured interviews to determine use of non-conventional remedies (NCRs) to 200 patients with rheumatological conditions. They found that over half of the patients used NCRs for treatment of their rheumatic disease, NCRs were costly and the MHLC scale scores alone did not explain all the variance in health behaviours. Other contributing factors may have included perceived severity of the disease, health motivation or previous behaviour. Furnham et al.[30] evaluated 250 patients who were currently using CAM practitioners in the UK. Patients completed a seven-part questionnaire that evaluated demographic data, medical history, familiarisation with complementary therapies, health beliefs and lifestyle, health locus of control (LOC), scientific health beliefs, and their perceptions of the consultation style of general and complementary practitioners. Sociodemographic differences were not found between those who used CAM and those who did not. However, LOC was not found to be primarily associated. In fact, the investigators reported the following:

> ... that patients of complementary practitioners are not a homogeneous group, but do differ in their views on satisfaction with GPs, healthy life-style, global environmental issues, confidence in prescribed drugs, faith in medical science, importance of a 'healthy mind,' harmful effects of medical science, and scientific methodology.[30]

Clearly, the literature varies because it relates locus of control to CAM use. However, it appears that a relationship could exist given the manner in which it is measured as well as the co-variates in the models.

The Health Belief Model (HBM) appears to be a construct that could unify these findings and give a clearer explanation as to why some patients choose to use CAM and others do not. The HBM was developed by three psychologists – Hochbaum, Kegels and Rosenstock – in the 1950s for the Public Health Service.[31] The developers had backgrounds in social psychology with phenomenological orientation and were probably influenced by their knowledge of the phenomenologically oriented theories of Kurt Lewin.[31] Originally, the model was designed to predict behavioural response to the treatment received by acutely or chronically ill patients, but in more recent years the model has been used to predict more general health behaviours.[32] In general, the HBM attempts to predict health-related behaviour in terms of certain belief patterns including individual perceptions, modifying behaviours and likelihood of action.

The key factors in the HBM model are:

- Perceived susceptibility: the perception of the likelihood of experiencing a condition that would adversely affect one's health.
- Perceived seriousness: the effects that a given disease or condition would have on the patient's life at the time.
- Perceived benefits of taking action: the perceived benefit of prevention of disease or dealing with an illness.
- Barriers to taking action: characteristics of a treatment or prevention that may prevent action, e.g. unpleasant side effects, difficulty obtaining convenient treatment.
- Cues to action: the cost–benefit of the action to the individual.

The HBM is built around the perceptions of the individual and how those perceptions affect their behaviour. It suggests that individuals who take control of their health (internal LOC) assess the likelihood of the illness (perceived susceptibility) and the seriousness of the illness (perceived seriousness). The potential utility of CAM (perceived benefit) is then assessed, as well as the risks associated with CAM (barriers to taking action). The cost–benefit decision (cues to action) could result in the decision whether or not to utilise CAM.

This HBM cost–benefit approach is not limited to the general population, e.g. Boon[33] discusses the 'push' and 'pull' influences of CAM use on men with prostate symptoms. Men were 'pushed' by negative perceptions of conventional treatment and 'pulled' by positive perceptions of CAM.

These factors are consistent with the findings of Borneman[8] who, in an analysis of the Kaiser-Permanente Member Health Survey

($n = 34\ 000$), found that respondents who reported that 'stress and emotional troubles were associated with health' were twice as likely to use CAM than respondents who did not associate stress, emotions and health. Statistically significant factors associated with CAM use in the previous 12 months in the population included: being white (adjusted odds ratio [AOR] 1.39, 95% confidence interval [95%CI] 1.32–1.47), being a college graduate (AOR 1.85, 95%CI 1.75–1.95), being a non-smoker (AOR 1.41, 95%CI 1.27–1.57), having poor health rating (AOR 1.12, 95%CI 1.07–1.17) and less satisfaction with health advice (AOR 1.08, 95%CI 1.04–1.33). In women, sociodemographic factors were similar.

In addition to an individual's beliefs about his or her healthcare, researchers have found that personality traits may also affect healthcare usage. Honda and Jacobson[34] reported that the personality trait of openness was associated with CAM use, particularly with the use of mind–body therapies. Furnham et al.[35] found that CAM users were more likely to believe that their therapy would be efficacious, but neither Lewith et al.[36] nor White[37] found an association between 'belief' in CAM and positive clinical outcomes as compared with non-belief in the therapies studied. Owens et al.[38] found that higher CAM use could be associated with the psychological trait identified as 'absorption' ('openness to experience'[34]), a finding similar to that of Honda, but these psychological 'traits' can be distinguished from 'belief'. Wyatt et al.[39] found that 'optimism' was a significant associated variable of CAM use. Thus, although the literature has examples of the potential relationship of personality traits to CAM use, there is little specific research linking these types of factors to CAM use, and little agreement on the definitions of specific traits.

Other factors may have an influence on the choice to use CAM. An early evaluation of factors of CAM use was conducted by Astin in 1998.[14] Using a random sample of 1035 surveys from a panel who had agreed to participate in a mail survey and who live throughout the USA, Astin hypothesised that CAM use could be predicted by: dissatisfaction with conventional treatment, need for personal control and philosophical congruence. In addition, health status and demographic variables were measured. Astin found that more education, poorer health status, holistic orientation to health, having had a 'transformational event that changed the person's worldview' and belonging to a cultural group characterised by 'commitment' (feminism, environmentalism, personal growth) were associated with increased CAM use. Although CAM use was predicted by anxiety, back problems, chronic pain and urinary tract problems, it was not predicted by dissatisfaction with conventional medicine.

Other drivers: reimbursement and other effects

Insurance reimbursement tends to have an impact on CAM use.[26,40] Gordon and Lin,[40] using data from the Kaiser-Permanente Members' survey in 1999, compared members who had a chiropractic reimbursement benefit with members who did not. They determined that chiropractic coverage had a larger impact on use in men than in women. Logistic regression modelling showed that, controlling for age, education and income, having a chiropractic benefit were associated with CAM use among men but not among women. These findings are similar to those of Wolsko et al.[26] who conducted a secondary analysis on the 1997 Eisenberg data. Wolsko et al. found that 'a small minority of persons accounted for more than 75% of visits to CAM providers. Extent of insurance coverage for CAM providers and use for wellness are strong correlates of frequent use of CAM providers.' They found that factors independently associated with seeing a CAM provider were: having been in the upper quartile of visits to conventional providers in the last year, female gender, and having used the therapy to treat diabetes, cancer, or back or neck problems. Factors independently associated with frequent use (eight or more visits a year) of a CAM provider were: full or partial insurance coverage of the CAM provider, having used the therapy for wellness and having seen the provider for back or neck problems.

Although data in the literature tend to indicate that reimbursement may increase CAM use, lack of reimbursement may not decrease CAM. As Eisenberg et al.[4,5] and Wolsko et al.[26] have shown, patients are willing to pay out of pocket. In fact, Pagan and Pauly[41] have reported that it is likely that CAM may be used by uninsured users because of the lack of reimbursement.

Delivery of CAM in the USA

Methods for receiving CAM services in the USA are a direct reflection of the diversity in CAM modalities and reimbursement status, e.g. although the professional delivery of some modalities including homeopathy, osteopathy, naturopathy, chiropractic and psychology fall under the licensed practice of the therapy, other modalities, including massage, prayer, herbs, biofeedback and megavitamins, are unregulated. Other therapies, including acupuncture, fall into both categories. Consequently, the array of providers of CAM in the USA fall along a continuum of informal ad hoc interventions by laypeople, all the way to Centers for Integrative Medicine at more than 20 university medical centres throughout the country.[3]

The delivery of CAM products is almost as complicated. CAM products can be classified as dietary supplements, foods and drugs. In addition, the same product can have more than one status depending on how it is labelled. The situation is sufficiently complex that the Food and Drug Administration (FDA) has been forced to issue proposed guidance on the matter that has been exceedingly controversial.[42] With such confusion in the market place, a significant focus has shifted to regulation.

Regulation of CAM products and services

In the USA, the delivery of medical services is a matter of state regulation, whereas the regulation of products falls under federal statutes. This difference result from the structure of laws under the constitution, which restrict federal laws to only a limited number of areas, including interstate commerce. It is from the interstate commerce clause that the FDA derives its authority to regulate food and drugs. As services are generally offered within an individual state, regulations fall to state law, and more specifically state-constituted boards of medicine and other professional services (e.g. psychology, naturopathy, acupuncture, homeopathy).

CAM products

At present, CAM products that are intended for ingestion such as herbs and dietary supplements, as opposed to procedures such as acupuncture and massage, are subject to one of three regulatory mechanisms, depending on whether they are classified as drugs, dietary supplements or homeopathic drugs. The regulatory scheme for conventional drug products based on pre-marketing clinical trials is widely discussed in public policy debates. The mechanism for dietary supplements relies primarily on post-marketing regulation and covers the vast majority of CAM products. The process by which homeopathic drugs are regulated is similar to the allopathic drug regulatory scheme, but has significant differences.

The sales of prescription drugs and dietary supplements represent multi-billion dollar industries in the USA. Although sales of homeopathic drug products are at least an order of magnitude smaller, they are among the top ten, best-selling, over-the-counter (OTC) drugs in the specialty analgesics, oral analgesics for children and cough/cold/flu categories in the USA, out of several hundred products currently tracked.[43]

Industry estimates suggest sales of homeopathic drugs in the USA in 2006 of between $US500m and $US600m, with a compound average growth rate of approximately 8% per year.[44]

Homeopathy

The example of homeopathy is now considered. Homeopathy is a system of medicine that dates back more than 200 years. Its use is based on the observation that high doses of pharmacologically active substances cause symptoms when administered to healthy individuals. Those same substances, when prepared in very dilute form, may relieve similar symptoms in conditions resulting from different aetiologies.[45] The clinical use of certain drugs according to this 'like cures like' observation is called the 'principle of similars' (similia principle) and forms the theoretical basis for homeopathy. Vaccines and the use of some conventional medications, such as nitroglycerin for angina, stimulants for attention deficit hyperactivity disorder and digitalis for congestive heart failure, have been compared in effect to homeopathic use.[45] Homeopathy is covered in detail in Chapter 7.

Since 1938, homeopathic medicines have been classified as drugs within the meaning of the federal Food Drug and Cosmetic Act (FDCA).[46] Official homeopathic drugs are those that have monographs, official listings of drug data, in the *Homeopathic Pharmacopeia of the United States* (HPUS). The HPUS is prepared by a non-governmental organisation, the Homeopathic Pharmacopeia Convention for the United States (HPCUS), which is made up of scientists and clinicians trained in the medical specialty of homeopathic medicine.[47,48] As most homeopathic drugs are sold on a non-prescription basis, very few are subject to reimbursement by insurance.

Homeopathy's introduction into the USA is credited to an American of Danish descent who was trained in Copenhagen, Hans Burch Gram, in 1826.[49] By 1871, sectarians, practitioners who were not members of the American Medical Association including homeopaths, represented at least 13% of practitioners in the USA. By 1880, homeopaths operated 14 medical schools, compared with the 76 operated by conventional physicians.[11] However, by the middle of twentieth century, the professional practice of homeopathy was all but over.[50] The last pure homeopathic medical college closed in 1920, although Hahnemann Medical College in Philadelphia taught homeopathic electives until mid-century. The author's great-grandfather was a professor at Hahnemann from 1904 to 1948, teaching homeopathic pharmacy and pharmacognosy. The last of the homeopaths, Garth Boericke, retired in 1964.

Nevertheless, the influence of the homeopaths was not completely gone. In 1938, Senator Royal Copeland of New York, a physician trained in homeopathy and a principal author of the FDCA, included within the law's definition of 'drugs' articles monographed in the HPUS.[46] Whether Congress's acceptance of this definition was a personal concession to Copeland or an attempt by reformers to regulate homeopathic drugs more closely is not clear.[51,52] The effect was to include homeopathic drugs as a formal component of food and drug law in the USA.

Allopathic drugs, homeopathic drugs and dietary supplements

It is important to understand the status of allopathic drugs and dietary supplements in terms of clinical use and regulation. From the perspective of clinical use, allopathic drugs are used to treat symptoms, provide prophylaxis and induce structural or biochemical changes in a biological system. By contrast, homeopathic medicines are used principally for treatment of symptoms, Consistent with the similia principle, the body must first exhibit symptoms before the correct homeopathic drug may be chosen and rarely for prophylaxis, although there are some case reports in the literature showing the successful use of homeopathic drugs in epidemic disease.[53,54] Dietary supplements include an array of substances, such as vitamins, enzymes, herbs and functional foods.[55] Thus, clinical use of dietary supplements is highly variable. As a result, in addition to content and deficiency of nutrients and approved health claims, manufacturers are limited to making claims that their products cause the body to maintain 'healthy function'.[55] In practice, however, dietary supplement manufacturers routinely make claims that could be interpreted by the public as relating to the structure or function of physiological systems or to the relief of symptoms, e.g. claims have been made that dietary supplements 'help the body maintain natural sleep'. The allopathic drug claims for 'sleep-aid' are effectively the same. Consequently, from a clinical perspective, dietary supplements and allopathic drugs share the goals of prophylaxis and biochemical change, whereas homeopathic and allopathic drugs share the goal of symptom relief.

The regulatory differences among allopathic drugs, homeopathic drugs and dietary supplements are no less complicated. Table 4.2 shows a comparison of regulation of the three categories. For ease of discussion, it is helpful to contrast controlling law according to whether it addresses pre-market approval, post-market regulation (manufacturing, marketing and sales), advertising regulation or reimbursement status for the three types of products.

As discussed, allopathic drugs are governed by the federal FDCA and related regulations, published in Title 21 of the Code of Federal Regulation (CFR). Pre-market approval is administered by the FDA through the new drug application (NDA) process for new drugs, whereas certain non-prescription drugs that are available for purchase directly by consumers on an OTC basis are subject to a separate OTC review process. Post-market regulation is principally specified in 21 CFR and includes current good manufacturing practices (cGMPs) and reporting of adverse drug events. The cGMPs specify the methods and conditions under which drugs must be produced, including validation

Table 4.2 Comparison of regulatory schemas for allopathic drugs, homeopathic drugs and dietary supplements

	Enabling legislation	Pre-market approval	Good manufacturing practices (cGMPs)	Labelling guidelines	Indications for use	Advertising guidelines
Allopathic	FDCA	New drug application or drug monograph	21 CFR	21 CFR	Required	Rx-FDA; OTC-FTC
Homeopathic	FDCA	HPCUS monograph process	21 CFR	21 CFR	Required	Rx-FDA; OTC-FTC
Dietary supplements	DSHEA	None	Implementing	DSHEA	Drug claims impermissible, 'Strucuture-function' claims only	FTC

CFR, Code of Federal Regulation; DSHEA, Dietary Supplement Health and Education Act 1994; FDA, Food and Drug Administration; FTC, Federal Trade Commission; OTC, over the counter; Rx, treatment; HPCUS, Homeopathic Pharmacopeia Convention for the United States.

of equipment and processes, and training of staff. The FDA regulates drug claims that are included in labelling. OTC drugs are limited to making claims for self-limiting conditions that do not require medical diagnosis or monitoring.[56]

Advertising for prescription allopathic drugs is regulated by the FDA, whereas advertising for non-prescription allopathic drugs is regulated by the Federal Trade Commission (FTC). Although reimbursement patterns for allopathic drugs vary, the general rule is that prescription drugs are reimbursed by most private health insurance plans and may be deducted as a medical expense for federal tax purposes; however, OTC drugs are generally not reimbursable but are subject to coverage under qualifying tax-advantaged flexible-spending plans.[57]

Dietary supplements are regulated under the Dietary Supplement Health and Education Act 1994 (DSHEA), which was enacted as an amendment to the FDCA. As a practical matter, no pre-market approval has applied to supplements currently on the market because no new chemical entities have been approved since the passage of DSHEA. All products marketed since the inception of DSHEA are either single supplements or combinations of products that existed at the time of DSHEA's implementation. Claims for the products must be reported to the FDA before marketing,[58] and products may be freely sold unless and until the agency objects. Until recently, there was little federal oversight of the manufacturing of dietary supplements. Supplements have become subject to recently promulgated GMP standards of their own;[59] however, some critics point out that dietary supplement GMPs are less rigorous that their drug cGMP counterparts.

Manufacturers of dietary supplements may not make claims that their products act like drugs. Claims about effects on physiological structures and functions, 'structure–function' claims, are permissible, if they do not fall into one of the categories of drug claims outlined by the FDA. Among those categories are products claiming to have an effect on a specific disease or class of diseases, or on one or more signs or symptoms that are characteristic of a specific disease. Also proscribed are implicit disease claims through the name of the product, a statement about the formulation of the product, a claim that the product contains an ingredient that has been regulated by the FDA as a drug and is well known to consumers for its use in preventing or treating a disease, or citation of a publication or reference. Also prohibited are claims that a supplement belongs to a class of products that is intended to diagnose, mitigate, treat, cure or prevent a disease, or that is a substitute for a product that is a recognised therapy for a disease.[60] However, even with the great specificity of regulation recently developed by the FDA, as previously noted, the line between a drug claim and a dietary supplement claim can be difficult to draw, and advertising of dietary supplements is regulated solely by the FTC. This practice is a result of an agreement between the FDA and FTC in 1971 under which the FDA took responsibility for enforcement of regulations concerning prescription drug advertising, leaving the FTC with the responsibility for non-prescription articles including dietary supplements and OTC drugs.[61]

By contrast, homeopathic drugs are subject to the FDCA and regulations issued by the FDA. Instead of the NDA process, pre-market approval for homeopathic drugs is by way of monograph approval by HPCUS. Although homeopathic drugs are also subject to the FDA OTC review, the FDA has not yet used this authority. However, manufacturing, labelling, marketing and sales of homeopathic drugs are subject to FDA compliance rules. With the exception of provisions for expiration dating, tablet imprinting and finish product testing, they are functionally identical to their allopathic counterparts. GMP standards for homeopathic and allopathic drugs are the same, and advertising oversight and reimbursement for homeopathic and allopathic drugs are also identical.

Bringing a homeopathic OTC drug to market

The decision to enter the OTC market comes as the result of an interconnected analysis of a number of factors.

Development of need

For its size, the OTC marketplace in the USA is fairly crowded. In addition 'time to success' – the period of time that a new product demonstrates economic viability – for the introduction of a new product into the drug store and mass market channels has compressed from 1–2 years several years ago to 90–210 days. This means that a new introduction needs to sell well from inception and has no time to find a market. These factors put added pressure on the selection of products for the market. 'Me-too' introductions generally fare poorly, so it is important not only that the successful new product has a significant value proposition, but also that this value is immediately understandable to the consumer.

Successful products are generally the result of a gap analysis in the market. Gaps can be clinical (no existent products fill an identified clinical need), economic (current offerings are too expensive) or product driven (a product improvement is possible). From the perspective of the homeopathic offering, matching the gap analysis with homeopathic capabilities generally yields an array of possible novel product entries.

Formulation

A principal component of formula development is the analysis of whether the target product will be a single entity or combination, and whether the component drugs are existent in the HPUS or will be new drugs. Intellectual property protection, patents and trademarks will be a consideration. Although trademarks are a relatively straightforward matter, patents are much more difficult to obtain; they are granted only for novel entities or improvements, meaning that new drugs are eligible, but new combinations of old drugs are not. Novel use of old drugs may warrant a new patent. If the decision is to enter the market with a novel entity, the approval process to be granted a monograph in the HPUS requires 1–2 years from submission for complete review by the HPUS working committees.

Literature review

The first step in drug development is a formal review of the literature. This study can be undertaken from a number of perspectives: clinical indication (repertory), drug family (material medical) and state of the existing science (environmental scan), as well as a review of existing trials in the literature. The last is a critical step because it reveals opportunities from a perspective of not only the existing science, but also a market opportunity point of view.

Clinical data collection

Upon completion of a literature review, an array of potential formulations can be developed. Standard clinical trial techniques can then be applied to study of the efficacy of the proposed formula. If a novel entity is involved, a trial of the single entity may be undertaken for regulatory purposes. Trial data contribute to the development of a proof of claims document as well as elucidating the optimal dosage and posology for the formula. Methodologies for the trials follow standard best practices: safety, followed by a pilot randomised trial to assess effect size and finally a full-scale trial. Novel entities may require a 'proving' trial, a pathogenic study on healthy individuals to determine the homeopathic effect of the novel drug.

Formula selection

After development of the market need and collection of clinical data, the final formulation for the product can be determined. As important as clinical effectiveness and safety is intellectual property protection. Novel substances can obtain patents that have a 20-year duration. New product improvements may also be eligible for protection.

Claims development

Claims development for the product is a natural outgrowth of the needs analysis and clinical data collection. Claims are subject to FDA oversight pursuant to relevant sections of 21CFR and the specific Compliance Policy Guide for Homeopathy 400.400 (formerly 7132.15) – 'Conditions Under Which Homeopathic medicines May be Marketed'. Under these regulations, claims for OTC products are limited to self-limiting conditions that do not require medical diagnosis or monitoring. Claims developed at this juncture should be referred to council for legal review and to the company's medical officer for clinical review.

Claims should be supported by a file that contains all relevant data from the literature review as well as company-sponsored trials. This file, called a 'Proof of Claims Document', should be available for review by regulators at any time. Legal review should include filing the relevant Drug Listing Form FDA2657 with FDA for the assignment of a NDC number. The NDC number will appear on the principal display panel of the label pursuant to FDA and HPCUS regulations.

Dosage form selection

The appropriate dosage form for the new entry should be determined as a result of the needs analysis and clinical data collection. Research and development in this area focus on manufacturing scale and supply chain for the products, as well as requisite stability studies and preservative challenges (if applicable), pursuant to the relevant portions of Section 210 of 21CFR. Accelerated studies may be undertaken if the dosage form is well understood. Conventional studies will be required if the dosage form is novel. Although homeopathic medicines are generally exempted from expiration dating in the USA pursuant to 21CFR 211.137, expiry dates may be required on certain topical or parenteral dosage forms.

Marketing plan

The marketing and roll-out plan for the new entity will be driven by the needs and clinical analyses. Typically, focus groups are used to develop the language, package and label for the product, as well as marketing positioning. Advertising and sales plans follow from relevant sections of the sales plan.

Reviews

Once all the planning has been completed, the new entity should be returned to relevant stakeholders for reviews. These analyses include: legal and regulatory, clinical, manufacturing and supply chain (including forecasting), and sales (including retailer feedback). At this juncture, a roll-out plan can be developed that is consistent with the planogram update calendar of the relevant retailers.

Feedback loop

Once the product is on the shelf, a feedback loop of data is critical to success of the product. This loop includes consumer feedback, retailer feedback, reported adverse events, sales turn rate, advertising efficiencies and promotional efficiencies. These data are merged to make adjustments to forecasting, promotions and advertising. If the product is successful, these data will also be used to determine possible line extensions and future planning.

Figures 4.2 and 4.3 show examples of homeopathic OTC drugs.

Reimbursement

As discussed, the reimbursement schemes for CAM products are subsumed within the highly fragmented general reimbursement system in the USA. There is wide variability in payments, e.g. healthcare services provided by a licensed provider may be reimbursed if the condition for which the service is rendered *and* the service itself are both covered in the private health plan, or under the federal (Medicare) or state (Medicaid) schemes. For example, some preventive care (non-reimbursed condition), psychological interventions and alternative practices (e.g.

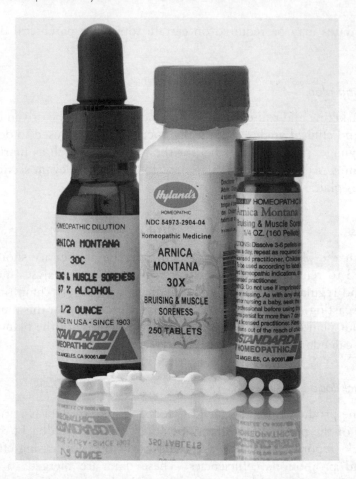

Figure 4.2 Examples of homeopathic medicines packaged for over-the-counter sale.

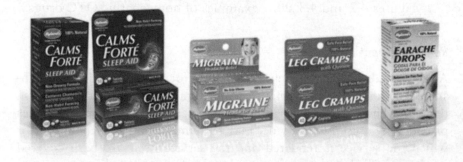

Figure 4.3 Examples of homeopathic product labels.

acupuncture), both non-reimbursed services, are not covered. Services that are provided by a non-licensed practitioner are generally not reimbursed. The net result is that, as Eisenberg reported, most CAM services in the USA are paid out of pocket.[4,5,62]

Reimbursement for CAM products falls under a different scheme. In general, only approved drugs available on prescription are reimbursable. Further restrictions may be applied to certain prescription drugs on restricted formularies. All other OTC drugs and dietary supplements are not reimbursed. As previously discussed, the costs of certain of these products may be deducted from taxes as healthcare expenses, or reimbursed if the individual has a Section 125 Flexible Spending Account.

The way forward

Without doubt CAM has become part of the healthcare landscape in the USA. Its future depends on the relative success of individual modalities. This future will turn on:

- Continued focus on data collection demonstrating safety and effectiveness
- Development of a stable regulatory scheme
- Implementation of safety practices, including cGMPs, for dietary supplements and mandatory adverse event reporting for all products
- Development of best practices
- Oversight of certain unregulated practices to ensure public safety.

The evolution of CAM will not occur in a vacuum. As public policy evolves concerning access to healthcare in the USA, with all of its subparts – including quality, best practices, reimbursement and evidence-based practice – CAM will doubtlessly be affected, for better or worse. It is hope that CAM practices can positively contribute to accessible high-quality healthcare in the USA.

Further reading

Institute of Medicine (US) Committee on the Use of Complementary and Alternative Medicine. *Complementary and Alternative Medicine in the United States*. Washington DC: National Academic Press, 2005.

References

1. Spencer MT. NFM's market overview. *Natural Foods Merchandiser* June 2007.
2. Barnes PM, Powell-Griner E, McFann K, Nahin RL. Complementary and alternative medicine use among adults: United States, 2002. *Advance Data* 2004;**343**:1–19.
3. Bondurant S, Anastasi JK, Berman B et al. *Complementary and Alternative Medicine in the United States.* Washington DC: Institute of Medicine, 2005.
4. Eisenberg DM, Davis RB, Ettner SL et al. Trends in alternative medicine use in the United States, 1990–1997: results of a follow-up national survey. *JAMA* 1998;**280**:1569–75.
5. Eisenberg DM, Kessler RC, Foster C, Norlock FE, Calkins DR, Delbanco TL. Unconventional medicine in the United States. *N Engl J Med* 1993;**328**: 246–52.
6. NCCAM. *Appropriations History.* Available at: http://nccam.nih.gov/about/appropriations/index.htm (accessed 3 June 2008).
7. CRISP (Computer Retrieval of Information on Scientific Projects). Searchable database of US federally funded biomedical research projects. Available at: http://crisp.cit.nih.gov (accessed 3 June 2008).
8. Borneman J. *Use and Prevalence of Complementary and Alternative Medicine (CAM) by Populations with Specific Needs: Patients with cancer, breast cancer, benign prostatic hyperplasia and asthma.* Philadelphia: Department of Health Policy and Public Health, University of the Sciences in Philadelphia, 2007.
9. National Center for Complementary and Alternative Medicine. *Back to Health Information – What is CAM?* National Center for Complementary and Alternative Medicine. Available at: http://nccam.nih.gov/health/whatiscam (accessed April 2008).
10. Silenzio VM. What is the role of complementary and alternative medicine in public health? *Am J Pub Hlth* 2002;**92**:1564.
11. Starr P. *The Social Transformation of American Medicine.* New York: Basic Books, 1982.
12. Goldstein MS. The persistence and resurgence of medical pluralism. *J Hlth Politics Policy Law* 2005;**29**:929.
13. Green LA, Fryer GE, Yawn BP. The ecology of medical care revisited. *N Engl J Med* 2001;**344**:2021–5.
14. Astin JA. Why patients use alternative medicine: results of a national study. *JAMA* 1998;**279**:1548–53.
15. White KL, Williams TE, Greenberg BG. The ecology of medical care. *N Engl J Med* 1961;**265**:885–92.
16. McFarland B, Bigelow D, Zani B, Newsom J, Kaplan M. Complementary and alternative medicine use in Canada and the United States. *Am J Public Hlth* 2002;**92**:1616–18.
17. Ashton EN. *Community Receptiveness to Complementary and Alternative Medicine (CAM): Attitudes, usage, and perceived resource needs of nurses and the public at large.* Research report. Spalding University, Louisville, Kentucky, 2001: 77.

18. Lewis D, Paterson M, Beckerman S, Sandilands C. Attitudes toward integration of complementary and alternative medicine with hospital-based care. *J Altern Compl Med* 2001;**7**:681–8.
19. Burge SK, Albright TL. Use of complementary and alternative medicine among family practice patients in south Texas. *Am J Public Hlth* 2002;**92**:1614–16.
20. Rafferty AP, McGee HP, Miller CE. Prevalence of complementary and alternative medicine use: state specific estimates from the 2001 behavioural risk factor surveillance system. *Am J Pub Hlth*. 2002;**92**:1598–600.
21. Salmenpera L. The use of complementary therapies among breast and prostate cancer patients in Finland. *Eur J Cancer Care* 2002;**11**:44–50.
22. Salmenpera L, Suominen T, Lauri S, Puukka P. Attitudes of patients with breast and prostate cancer toward complementary therapies in Finland. *Cancer Nursing* 2001;**24**:328–34.
23. Wallstrom P, Elmstahl S, Hanson BS et al. Demographic and psychosocial characteristics of middle-aged women and men who use dietary supplements. *Eur J Public Hlth* 1996;**6**:188–95.
24. Chng CL, Neill K, Fogle P. Predictors of college students' use of complementary and alternative medicine. *Am J Hlth Educ* 2003;**34**:267–71.
25. Sturm R. Patient risk-taking attitude and the use of complementary and alternative medical services. *J Altern Compl Med* 2000;**6**:445–8.
26. Wolsko PM, Eisenberg DM, Davis RB, Ettner SL, Phillips RS. Insurance coverage, medical conditions, and visits to alternative medicine providers: results of a national survey. *Arch Intern Med* 2002;**162**:281–7.
27. University of South Florida Community and Family Health. *Health Locus of Control*. Tampa, FL: University of South Florida Community and Family Health, 1999.
28. Schlenk EA, Hart LK. Relationship between health locus of control, health value, and social support and compliance of persons with diabetes mellitus. *Diabetes Care* 1984;**7**:566–74.
29. Ramos-Remus C, Watters CA, Dyke L, Suarez-Almazor ME, Russell AS. Assessment of health locus of control in the use of nonconventional remedies by patients with rheumatic diseases. *J Rheumatol* 1999;**11**:2468–74.
30. Furnham A, Vincent C, Wood R. The health beliefs and behaviours of three groups of complementary medicine and a general practice group of patients. *J Altern Compl Med* 1995;**4**:347.
31. University of Twente. Health Belief Model. University of Twente, The Netherlands. Available at: http://tinyurl.com/9vats (accessed January 2006).
32. Ogden J. *Health Psychology: A textbook*, 4th edn. Milton Keynes, Bucks: McGraw Hill/Open University Press, 2007.
33. Boon H. Men with prostate cancer: Making decisions about complementary/alternative medicine. *Med Dec Making* 2003;**23**:471–9.
34. Honda K, Jacobson J. Use of complementary and alternative medicine among United States adults: the influences of personality, coping strategies, and social support. *Prev Med* 2005;**40**:46–53.
35. Furnham A, Kircady B. The health beliefs and behaviours of orthodox and complementary medicine clients. *Br J Clin Psychol* 1996;**35**(Pt1):49–61

36.   Lewith GT, Hyland ME, Shaw S. Do attitudes toward and beliefs about complementary medicine affect treatment outcomes? *Am J Public Hlth.* 2002;**92**: 1604–6.

37.   White P. Attitude and outcome: Is there a link in complementary medicine? *Am J Public Hlth* 2003;**93**:1038.

38.   Owens J, Taylor A, Degood D. Complementary and alternative medicine and psychologic factors: toward an individual differences model of complementary and alternative medicine use and outcomes. *J Altern Compl Med* 1999;**5**:529–41.

39.   Wyatt GK, Friedman LL, Given CW, Given BA, Beckrow KC. Complementary therapy use among older cancer patients. *Cancer Practice.* 1999;**7**:136–44.

40.   Gordon NP, Lin TY. Use of complementary and alternative medicine by the adult membership of a large Northern California health maintenance organization, 1999. *J Ambulatory Care Man* 2004;**27**(1):12–24.

41.   Pagan JA, Pauly M. Access to conventional medical care and the use of complementary and alternative medicine. *Health Affairs* 2005;**24**(1):255.

42.   US Department of Health and Human Services FaDA. *Guidance for Industry: Complementary and alternative medicine products and their regulation by the Food and Drug Administration.* Washington DC: US Department of Health and Human Services, 2006.

43.   ScanTrack. *12 months trailing December 31, 2004.* New York: AC Nielsen, 2004.

44.   Lewith GT, Broomfield J, Prescott P. Complementary cancer care in Southampton: a survey of staff and patients. *Compl Ther Med* 2002;**10**: 100–6.

45.   Kayne SB. *Homeopathic Pharmacy: An introduction and handbook*, 2nd edn. Edinburgh: Elsevier Churchill Livingstone, 2006.

46.   US Federal Food, Drug and Cosmetic Act 1938. Available at: http://tinyurl.com/dgff3 (accessed 3 June 2008).

47.   Baker C, Borneman J, Abecassis J, Foxman E, eds. *The Homeopathic Pharmacopeia of the United States.* Homeopathic Pharmacopeia Convention for the United States, 2002.

48.   Homeopathic Pharmacopoeia Convention for the United States. *General Information.* Available at: www.hpcus.com (accessed 3 June 2008).

49.   Coulter H. *Divided Legacy: The conflict between homeopathy and the American Medical Association.* Berkeley: North Atlantic Books, 1973.

50.   Creighton University School of Medicine. *History of Homeopathy*, homeopathy tutorial. Available at: http://altmed.creighton.edu/Homeopathy/history.htm (accessed 3 June 2008).

51.   Junod S. An alternative perspective: Homeopathic drugs, Royal Copeland, and Federal Drug regulation. *Food, Drug Law J* 2000;**55**:161–84.

52.   Robins N. *Copeland's Cure.* New York: Knopf, 2005.

53.   Winston J. Influenza – 1918. *N Engl J Homeopathy* 1998;**7**(1).

54.   Hoover T. *Homeopathic Prophylaxis: Fact or fiction.* Available at: www.homeopathic.org/crtoddh.htm (accessed 27 February 2005).

55.   US Food and Drug Administration. *Overview of Dietary Supplements.* Available at: http://www.cfsan.fda.gov/~dms/ds-oview.html (accessed 3 June 2008).

56. Section 400.400. *Conditions Under Which Homeopathic Medicines May be Marketed.* Washington DC: Food and Drug Administration, Office of Regulatory Affairs.

57. GMC Educational Foundation. *New Developments in Flexible Spending Accounts Open Opportunities. Paying for OTCs with pre-tax dollars.* New York: GMC Educational Foundation. Available at: www.chpa-info.org/web/for_consumers/otcs_pretax.aspx (accessed 3 June 2008).

58. Koh H, Teo H, Ng H. Pharmacists' patterns of use, knowledge, and attitudes toward complementary and alternative medicine. *J Altern Compl Med* 2003; **9**:51–63.

59. Neergaard L. *FDA Takes Stand on Dietary Supplements.* New York: Associated Press, 2003.

60. Regulations on Statements Made for Dietary Supplements Concerning the Effect of the Product on the Structure or Function of the Body. FR 65:4 1001. January 6, 2000.

61. Working Agreement Between FDA and FTC, 3 Trade Reg. Re. (CCH) 9850.01; 1971.

62. Eisenberg D, Pelletier KR. Update on CAM coverage in the USA. *Focus on Alternative and Complementary Therapies* 2002;**7**:266–7.

5

The evidence base for complementary and alternative medicine

Steven B Kayne

Evidence associated with the use of complementary and alternative medicine (CAM) therapies is discussed in detail in Chapter 7. Here a brief overview of CAM research is given.

Historically, there has been little scientific research into CAM, largely because of its place as a 'fringe' profession. Complementary medicine in general is deeply rooted in a tradition where experience comes first and science second. The arguments usually claim that hundreds of years of experience on thousands of patients are innumerably stronger than scientific studies, which normally include only a few patients and are far removed from 'real life' anyway.[1] Most research is funded by private sector interests which might see the economic benefit of a certain procedure or product. The research culture that has developed has been one that emphasises an evidence-based approach to establishing the efficacy of single herbs and nutrients, which overlooks the way that complementary therapists use these substances.

There is no doubt that many CAM disciplines suffer greatly from an inability to provide robust evidence acceptable to orthodox observers. In particular, homeopathy, which commonly uses dilutions of medicine that are well beyond Avogadro's number, is the subject of much scepticism. At this dilution level there are no molecules of drug left in solution – at least none that can be measured with methods currently available.

The House of Lords Report

In a letter dated 28 July 1999 the British House of Lords Science and Technology Committee (Sub Committee 111) issued a 'call for evidence' to numerous organisations and individuals related to complementary medicine. The call for evidence related to six areas: evidence, information, research, training, regulation and risk, as well as provision within the NHS. The 140-page Report was published in November 2000.[2] It set out major recommendations for action that will have a far-reaching impact on the development of integrated conventional and complementary health services in the UK. Some critics of the report argued that the House of Lords was calling for tougher regulation – a 'crackdown' – on alternative medicine. Others interpreted the report as an endorsement for complementary therapies. An editorial in *The Lancet* suggested that the report was 'thin on data, but replete with opinion – opinion that could be taken any way one wished'.[3] A CAM practitioner said that while the report was overall a good one, it did contain some 'sceptical and patronising turns of phrase'.[4] Despite these comments most CAM proponents thought that the report provided a reasonable basis for future progress in integrating the major disciplines into mainstream medicine.

The report included the recommendation that in the interests of public safety the complementary medicine sector should be properly regulated and more research carried out into its effectiveness. Fragmentation, disagreement between groups and concentration on differences rather than common aims have been identified as frequent problems with existing professional bodies for complementary medicine.[5]

The report found that complementary medicine in the UK suffers from a poor research infrastructure and a lack of high-quality work. Common reasons given for this were a lack of understanding of research ethics and methodology, an unwillingness to evaluate evidence and a shortage of resources.

The committee recommended two strategies to address these issues. A central mechanism for coordinating, advising and training on research into CAM was suggested, using government and charitable resources. Second, it asked the government NHS Research and Development Directorate and the Medical Research Council to provide dedicated research funding to create centres of excellence for complementary medicine research based on the National Center for Complementary and Alternative Medicine in the USA. The committee also stated that accredited training of complementary practitioners was vital to ensure consistently good standards. There has been some progress on regulation (notably osteopathy and chiropractic) but little on the other recommendations.

Types of outcome measures

There are two terms commonly used to describe the outcome of any given treatment: efficacy and effectiveness.

Efficacy is measured under standard scientific conditions (usually a randomised clinical trial – RCT). It is the normal requirement before regulatory authorities will consider granting a licence for the release of a medicine to the market.

Effectiveness is based on a patient-oriented outcome determined under 'field' conditions. Thus, if a homeopathic medicine is given to a patient who is then seen to improve, one would say that the medicine was effective rather than efficacious. Theoretical justification is not usually an issue. The perception that an intervention is 'effective' differs widely between patients, and in many cases between patient and prescriber too. Part of this divergence may result from the fact that it is possible to identify two treatment outcomes. The first, an improvement in the clinical characteristics of the condition being treated, can be assessed in terms of any or all the following:

- resolution of symptoms
- reduction in severity of symptoms with less discomfort
- a need to take less medication
- better quality of life.

The second outcome concerns the patient's overall feeling of wellness. This is largely subjective and may vary from day to day. Patients differ in their ability to deal with disease and this may be reflected in the success or otherwise of treatment.

Objective outcome measurements have been developed to obtain some idea of the extent of positive or negative outcome. Examples include the visual analogue scale, the Overall Progress Interactive Chart and the Glasgow Homoeopathic Hospital Outcome Scale. These measures were developed for use in studying outcomes resulting from homeopathic treatment and are mentioned again in Chapter 7.

Some CAM disciplines are more difficult than others to assess; determining a mechanism of action may be impossible. This topic is discussed further when each therapy is described in future chapters.

The quality of evidence

Definition

The Grading of Recommendations Assessment, Development and Evaluation (GRADE) Working Group (www.gradeworkinggroup.org) provides a specific definition for the quality of evidence in the context of making recommendations. The quality of evidence reflects the extent to which confidence in an estimate of the effect is adequate to support a particular recommendation. This definition has two important implications. First, guideline panels must make judgements about the quality of evidence relative to the specific context in which they are using the evidence. Second, as systematic reviews do not – or at least should not – make recommendations, they require a different definition. In this case the quality of evidence reflects the extent of confidence that an estimate of effect is correct.[6]

Factors affecting the quality of evidence

Study design

An eight-point hierarchy of evidence continuum exists to rank the quality of evidence. This leads from strictly controlled randomised trials, systematic reviews and meta-analyses at one end (efficacy) to observational studies, including anecdotal case reports, case series and comparison with historical groups (effectiveness) at the other.[7,8]

The widespread use of hierarchies of evidence that grade research studies according to their quality has helped to raise awareness that some forms of evidence are more trustworthy than others. Glasziou et al.[9] believe that several issues should be considered in any revision or alternative approach to helping practitioners to find reliable answers to important clinical questions, including the following.

Systematic reviews of research should always *be preferred* because they should give the most robust evidence. However, the outcome of a systematic review relies to a large extent on the methods employed to locate, include and evaluate the RCT in the literature.

Different types of clinical situations require different types of evidence
There may be issues other than clinical outcomes that need to be investigated to prove that an intervention is beneficial to the patient, e.g. pragmatic questions associated with the effective use of an intervention

in day-to-day practice According to the BMJ Clinical Evidence website, of about 2500 treatments supported by 'good' evidence, only 15% of treatments are rated as beneficial, 22% as likely to be beneficial, 7% as part beneficial and part harmful, 5% as unlikely to be beneficial and 4% as likely to be ineffective or harmful, and in the remaining 47% the effect of the treatment was 'unknown'. The figures suggest that the research community has a large task ahead and that most decisions about treatments still rest on the individual judgements of clinicians and patients.[10] This shows that many orthodox interventions are in common use despite uncertainty about their overall effectiveness.[11]

The use of the prospective randomised therapeutic study, does not necessarily ensure quality research or reporting. Critical analysis of scientific work is important regardless of the study design.[12] Was the experiment well performed and are the outcomes reliable enough for acceptance? Was there adequate measurement of side effects and toxicity?[13] Confidence in recommendations decreases if studies have major limitations that may bias their estimates of the treatment effect.[14] Other problems with RCT evidence are noted below (page 133).

There may be a confirmation bias: researchers may evaluate evidence that supports their prior belief differently from that apparently challenging these convictions. Despite the best intentions, everyday experience and social science research indicate that higher standards may be expected of evidence, contradicting initial expectations.[15] Although parallel group randomised trials will remain the principal means of obtaining reliable evidence about the average effects of treatments, there are some circumstances in which treatment effects can be inferred from well-designed case series.[16] A poorly designed and badly implemented RCT is, as a rule, less valuable than well-conducted studies using other designs, and sometimes even non-randomised studies can produce more reliable and useful information than a well-conducted randomised study. Observational studies have their place, although the results often depend crucially on the type of analysis used to generate them[17] and should be interpreted with caution.[18]

Balanced assessments should draw on a variety of types of research
The value of stringently conducted RCTs is undisputed because they have great internal validity.[19] However, the crucial question is whether their results have relevance to everyday decision-making. In RCTs patients are randomly assigned to standard and investigational arms and are followed up over a defined period. The final results of the randomised groups are often compared, irrespective of whether the positive

result of one treatment arm was induced in part by using the alternative treatment principle (the intent-to-treat principle[20]) as a result of crossover. The best and most appropriate evidence for each outcome is required from the perspective of both healthcare provider and patient. This cannot be provided by a single outcome study. An RCT is not the best way to determine rare side effects of a treatment: a case–control or observational study is better. The ethical basis for entering patients in RCTs is under debate.[21] Research into causes of illnesses and prognoses is usually best done with cohort studies – lower in the hierarchy of levels of evidence but vital to an understanding of disease.[22]

Walach et al.[23] have argued for a broader, circular view that illustrates the equivalence of research methods in non-pharmacological interventions. They state that there is no such thing as a single, inherently ideal methodology. There are different methods to answer different questions, all of which come together in a multidimensional mosaic or evidence profile.[24] Jonas has proposed the framework of an 'evidence house' for addressing many of the challenges associated with providing evidence for CAM.[25]

Evidence-based medicine

Evidence-based medicine (EBM) reflects a particular perception of how medical decisions ought to be made. The movement towards evidence-based practice underscores the division between orthodox biomedicine and CAM.

Evidence-based medicine is defined as 'the conscious, judicious use of current best evidence in making decisions about the care of individual patients'.[26] It is about getting the best therapeutic outcomes for patients, by integrating clinical expertise and knowledge with patients' needs and preferences, using the most current information available in a systematic and timely way. Figure 5.1 represents this graphically and Figure 5.2 shows the position in CAM where the amount of robust evidence is limited.

Advocates of EBM have criticised the adoption of interventions evaluated by using only observational data. In 2003 Smith and Pell[27] published an entertaining but profound article in which they pointed out that, as with many interventions intended to prevent ill health, the effectiveness of parachutes in preventing death after jumping from an aeroplane has not been subjected to rigorous evaluation by using RCTs.

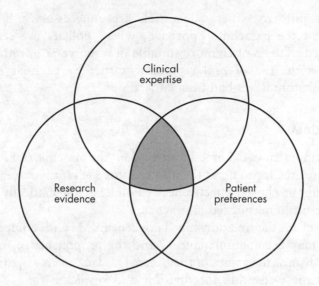

Figure 5.1 Graphical representation for EBM in orthodox medicine.

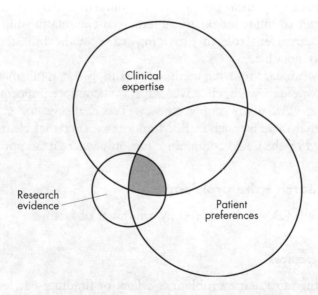

Figure 5.2 Graphical representation for EBM in complementary and alternative medicine.

Situations still exist where such trials are unnecessary.[27] It has been argued that the parachute approach, where policies are set without randomised trials, is often more suitable in resource-poor settings.[28] An example is the use of oral replacement therapy to treat childhood diarrhoea before RCTs had been carried out.[29]

EBM and CAM

It is important that CAM practitioners adopt the principle of EBM sooner rather than later. It promotes the idea that for each form of treatment the evidence about clinical effectiveness should be systematically reviewed and the results implemented in practice.

However, the relationship between EBM and complementary medicine may become unbalanced, and the proponents of one system ignore or dismiss the values of the other. This lack of cross-paradigmatic respect is the wellspring for division and suspicion that is currently permeating the arranged marriage between CAM and EBM.[30]

Rational, quantitative decision-making is important, but patients and healthcare providers are human beings, and human beings are by no means always rational. Focusing too much on the rational and quantitative aspects of clinical problems – an inherent danger in EBM – can have a negative influence on the doctor–patient relationship and can erode the caregiver's role in providing 'care' in the fullest and most human way possible.[22]

Many standard research methods are simply not applicable to CAM and, even where they are, effectiveness is a much more important means of assessing CAM than simply efficacy. The challenge for CAM is to recognise that there is much in EBM and its practice that clearly should be emulated by the CAM community but only where it is appropriate.[31]

CAM research – the problems

Research into CAM is hampered by a number of factors.

Financial resources

Probably the most acute problem is a lack of funding – at least in the UK.[32] Funding bodies are often unwilling to make grants in unorthodox areas. It has been claimed that only about 0.08% of NHS research funding goes to CAM.[33] Lewith et al.[34] have pointed out that much CAM research originates from the UK but, without appropriate support, this embryonic academic discipline will certainly flounder. They claim that public sources of funding should be responsive to patient need and therefore, with increasing use, more should be made available to develop research structures within CAM. British researchers cast their eyes enviously across the Atlantic.

A second problem with research into CAM in the UK is that much of it is performed without prioritising those projects with the best chance of success.

In the USA the National Center for Complementary and Alternative Medicine (NCCAM) was established in 1999, following on from its predecessor. The Office of Alternative Medicine, set up in 1992, is the federal government's lead agency for scientific research on CAM. The centre is one of the 27 institutes and centres that make up the National Institutes of Health (NIH) within the US Department of Health and Human Services. NCCAM sponsors and conducts research using scientific methods and advanced technologies to study CAM (http://nccam.nih.gov/research). It also trains researchers. The centre's resources were $US121.4m (£65m; €83m) in 2007. Research priorities currently include:

• mechanisms of action
• exploratory clinical studies and phase I and phase II clinical trials
• areas of special interest
• areas subject to a short 'pause' in new funding.

Lack of research skills

Many early clinical trials investigating CAM have had serious flaws. Research is not included in many homeopathic courses although attempts are being made among educationalists to interest students in this important aspect of CAM.

Research design

Lack of a suitable hypothesis to test   Most scientific research sets out to provide evidence for or against a hypothesis. Most CAM research does not have a formal hypothesis to test.

Placebo design   There are difficulties in designing placebo for many CAM disciplines to enable placebo-controlled trials, e.g. sham acupuncture or sham reflexology is extremely difficult to achieve. Research design is further confounded by the wide variation in how many forms of CAM are practised, e.g. there are many different approaches to the practice of chiropractic and acupuncture.

Inappropriate extrapolation of results Despite the emphasis on multi-modality treatment regimens in many CAM disciplines, most research has examined only one, or perhaps two, interventions taken from a whole treatment system, e.g. there are hundreds of small studies examining the efficacy of acupuncture needling alone for treating asthma, pain, hypertension or nausea. Yet in practice, acupuncture needling would be just one of a portfolio of interventions used by an acupuncturist including herbal medicines, dietary changes, exercise therapy, etc. (see Chapter 7). This makes forming an opinion as to the effectiveness of a particular intervention in isolation difficult.

Standardisation The number and length of treatments and the specific treatment used may vary both between individuals and for an individual during the course of treatment, e.g. when designing an RCT for acupuncture, the investigator is faced with choices concerning the selection of points, the depth of needle insertion, and the frequency and scheduling of treatment. Lack of standardisation of herbal medicines also makes comparisons between trials difficult.[35]

Lack of patients

There is an unfortunate catch-22 situation where lack of evidence means lack of patients from the NHS and therefore lack of evidence again. Other problems include difficulties in retaining patients.

Despite these complexities, rigorously designed clinical trials are possible, including pragmatic studies of complete CAM systems. The quantity of applied health research on complementary medicine is growing rapidly, and the quality is improving. The number of randomised trials of complementary treatments has approximately doubled every 5 years,[36] and by 2004 the Cochrane Library contained 145 CAM-related systematic and an additional 340 non-Cochrane CAM-related systematic reviews.

CAM research – the criticisms

It has been made clear that claims of clinical effectiveness will be universally accepted only when interventions have been subject to the same rigorous tests as those required in orthodox medicine (OM).

The stance of many orthodox practitioners is illustrated in the following editorial from *The Lancet*:[37]

> If a claim of clinical efficacy cannot be put in a way that allows it to be corroborated or refuted, and its efficacy is challenged by a substantial group of well-informed observers, that claim belongs to the world of metaphysical discussion rather than medical practice.

The two main criticisms applied to CAM, in general, concern the quality of the research and that the outcome is a placebo response.

Variable quality of the research

Outcome measures

Many of the studies demonstrating the clinical benefit of complementary techniques have reported improvements in subjective measures of disease activity. Subjective improvement in symptoms, or an increased sense of wellbeing, is a valid therapeutic goal, just like objective improvements. In fact, objective benefits might not actually be perceived by the patient. In a study of 82 individuals with asthma, 15% of patients were unable to perceive a 50% reduction in their capacity to exhale rapidly.[38] Notwithstanding this possibility, it is likely that, until CAM therapies are able to show consistent objective benefits, they will not achieve full promotion to mainstream medicine.

One possible explanation for how complementary therapies could produce objective benefit is by first producing a subjective benefit. Such subjective, perceptual improvements might promote objective improvements. Perception is an evaluative process involving a number of higher cognitive and limbic emotional centres of the brain. These centres are thought to be capable of regulating virtually all aspects of the immune system, with the involvement of neuropeptides and cytokines, having a profound effect on health and illness.[39,40] Thus the immune system, perception and pathology are all closely interlinked.[41]

Statistical significance

Much of the evidence involves small numbers of patients and is of poor methodological quality, but some high-quality systematic reviews of complementary medicine have been published recently that provide a reliable basis for making healthcare decisions. The specific areas of study are dealt with under each of the disciplines covered in this book. What follows is a general account of research activities common to CAM as a whole.

Inappropriate focus

Caspi[42] has observed that, currently, much of the research effort in CAM is in the form of treatment X for a disease. Almost no systematic research is taking place on the delivery, organisation and financing of different integrative healthcare models, or on the appropriateness, quality, availability and cost of CAM modalities in the current healthcare system. At a time when there is much interest in marketing, to ignore this line of research would undoubtedly be counterproductive in the long run, simply because money is easier to measure and relate to than healing. Only by combining both types of research – biomedical that looks mainly at mechanisms of effect and health services that look mainly at modes of delivery – will true integration beyond the mere expansion of therapeutic tools be possible.

Publishing bias

CAM practitioners often complain about bias against their research. Pittler et al.[43] have studied what the effect of journal quality has on published controlled clinical trials on CAM. They concluded that more positive than negative trials of CAM therapies are published except in high-impact mainstream medical journals. In CAM journals positive studies were of poorer methodological quality than in corresponding negative studies. The authors stress that location of trials in terms of journal type and impact factor should be taken into account when the literature on CAM is being consulted.

However, it is necessary to acknowledge that bias for CAM does exist too. Of the many explanations for a positive response to complementary medicine, perhaps the most acceptable in many sceptics' minds is that the patient was taking a conventional therapy at the same time, but did not mention it, underemphasised it, did not think that it was important or perhaps did not realise what it was. Such circumstances will be very familiar to healthcare providers interviewing patients before prescribing medicines for acute self-limiting complaints. Frequently questions about specific drugs, e.g. oral contraceptives, need to be asked before the whole picture slowly emerges.

Penny Brohn,[44] a co-founder of the Cancer Help Centre in Bristol, England, wrote a book entitled *Gentle Giants* in which she described her experiences while suffering from breast cancer. The implication is that a range of complementary therapies was successful in effecting a remission in her condition. In fact her cancer was found to be of a type that was likely to respond to hormone therapy and the drug tamoxifen was prescribed by orthodox doctors and indeed taken by Ms Brohn for 7 years. It is at least worth considering the fact that the orthodox drug, which has a high success rate when given for this type of cancer, was responsible.

Practitioner bias is another factor that can lead to credit for an apparently successful outcome being misplaced. It may be that practitioners can communicate to patients in some way a belief that one or other therapies is likely to be more successful in given sets of circumstances, e.g. in a study by Gracely et al.[45] the doctors' beliefs about the treatment were found to have influenced patients' experience of placebo-induced pain reduction.

Source of evidence on CAM

In a review of recent advances in the status of CAM, Vickers[46] states that the quantity of applied health research is growing rapidly and the quality is also improving. As stated earlier the number of randomised trials of CAM has approximately doubled every 5 years and the Cochrane Library now includes over 50 systematic reviews of CAM interventions.

The evidence currently available may be considered under four headings: RCTs, clinical audit, observational studies and searching the literature.

Randomised clinical trials

The initial BMA report on alternative therapy[4] dismissed alternatives to conventional medicine as flawed or fraudulent. Much of the criticism was based on the belief that the randomised, double-blind, clinical trial was the gold standard in demonstrating the value of a particular intervention. Indeed there have been few innovations that have influenced clinical practice more than the development of such sophisticated methodology. There are RCTs supporting the use of CAM and many are cited in the relevant chapters in this book; however, generally they are of less than robust quality.

As implied above the RCT is far from being a gold standard.[47] Most – but not all – results come from large groups of people and cannot easily be used to assist prediction of an outcome in any given individual. Others including chemotherapeutic agents may be $n = 1$ trials. There are few paediatric trials. It is difficult to design a suitable placebo for physical interventions such as exercise therapy, massage or acupuncture. Patient (and operator) blinding is difficult in such therapies. Studies involving relaxation or meditation provide similar difficulties.

Leibrich[48] points out that, in standardising the treatment to satisfy RCT procedures, the trial may remove from the treatment some elements that are an essential part of it. In a review of the use of acupuncture for the treatment of asthma, Aldridge and Pietroni[49] conclude that there is a disparity between the claims of acupuncturists as to positive clinical benefits and the findings of clinical trials, which demonstrate little 'objective' change but emphasise 'subjective' change. They argue that clinical trials have not investigated acupuncture as a therapy, but as a 'needling' technique.

In some cases a response resulting from the administration of a placebo in an RCT may mask the expected nil reaction. Another disadvantage of the RCT is that it measures reaction under standard conditions, rather than under real or field conditions. The results produce statistical probabilities rather than an absolute prediction as to what will happen with every patient. There are even examples of drugs being licensed on the basis of RCT results only to be withdrawn at a later date as a result of unacceptable adverse reactions.

It should be noted that bias is an important possibility. Sackett[50] alerts medical researchers to the 56 known potential sources of bias in clinical research.

In many instances, depending on the discipline involved, evaluation of CAM poses both paradigmatic and procedural difficulties. Manual therapies and herbalism are relatively easy to accept by OM and can be shown to be of benefit. Understanding acupuncture or homeopathy may involve changes to the conventional view of medicine. OM cannot easily make use of procedures that are seen to contradict its paradigmatic base.

Clinical audit

This is the systematic evaluation of clinical activity – the effectiveness of a particular intervention. It involves the identification of a problem and its resolution as part of an audit cycle. Audit is about ultimately improving a procedure. Rarely is this work carried out as part of an audit cycle. Usually, practitioners conduct an uncontrolled observational study by recording an outcome in isolation without any recommendations or a commitment to improving clinical practice.

Abbot and Ernst[51] quote three examples of what they consider to be good CAM audit studies:

1. The first was an audit of acupuncture practice in a rheumatology unit that arose from a need to improve and standardise treatment, and ensure that patient referrals were appropriate and that measurements of outcome were sensitive and meaningful.[52]
2. The second described how a service offering osteopathy for back pain was rapidly adapted to meet the requirements of local GPs.[53]
3. The third, involving an extensive audit of a German hospital specialising in Chinese medicine, resulted in improvements in the hospital's efficiency.[54]

Observational studies

Patient-oriented outcome measures such as those mentioned above may contribute to evidence of effectiveness of CAM interventions.

Anecdotal evidence

This type of evidence is the basis of many CAM procedures. It usually refers to single episode reports collected in the literature over many years. This traditional bibliographical evidence is acceptable to regulatory authorities for certain licensing procedures. From an orthodox point of view such observations are interesting but do not necessarily mean that the next patient will respond in the same manner. To be acceptable to orthodox colleagues, anecdotal reports must be well documented and outline new findings in a defined setting. There is a requirement for information on the disease and its extent, and information about any other patients who did not recover after being administered similar treatment. Such detailed anecdotal reports are usually called 'case studies'. In fact several orthodox medicines, especially in the field of psychiatry, are administered on the basis of case studies, although the acceptability of such justification is often challenged by orthodox colleagues.

Complementary and alternative medicine reports rarely include this detail and tend to be statistically non-significant because of the small sample size. Of course if one had enough anecdotal reports then the probability of success might be more predictable, but one is still faced with an inability to answer the question: 'Would they have responded positively without treatment?' One often hears patients saying: 'Yes, I got better, but I am unsure as to whether it was the treatment that did it or whether I got better on my own.'

Searching the literature

The evidence-based approach seeks to gather the information necessary to support clinical intervention.[55] It involves three stages:

1. Formulating a clear clinical question to be investigated
2. Searching for the evidence
3. Appraising the evidence.

Formulating a clinical question

The well-built clinical question has four elements summarised by the acronym PICO:

Patient, Population or Problem: a description of the discrete group of patients and/or the problem being investigated (e.g. depression in menopausal women)

Intervention, Prognostic Factor, or Exposure: what is the main intervention, prognostic factor or exposure? (e.g. use of St John's wort)

Comparison or Intervention (if appropriate): what is the main alternative to compare with the intervention? (e.g. use of orthodox drug)

Outcome you would like to measure or achieve : what can I hope to accomplish, measure, improve or affect? (reduction in symptoms)

These elements may be used to formulate a question on which a search strategy can be built. Given the examples above, this might be: 'In pregnant women suffering from depression, does the use of St John's wort, when compared with an orthodox drug, provide a reduction in symptoms?' This in turn facilitates organised database searching to find the most relevant highest quality evidence that can inform a particular clinical decision.

There are some limitations to the procedure, including occasions when evidence is unavailable or insufficient to answer the question effectively and when practitioner skills are inadequate to interpret the literature. However, it may be particularly useful where the practitioner has some gaps in his or her knowledge that need to be filled.

Searching for the evidence

The relatively small number of robust studies on CAM in the literature preclude firm recommendations on one or more sources of reliable data.[56] The large proportion of positive articles published in CAM journals appears not to reflect adequately the best available effectiveness evidence.[57] This has implications for those using CAM journals as their main source of information in this area. A range of different sources is required for identifying relevant studies. Examples include the following:

• The Cochrane Data Base of Systematic Reviews: a resource known as the Cochrane Collaboration was established in 1993. The Cochrane Collaboration publishes critical summaries known as systematic reviews that focus upon healthcare interventions by continually collating and appraising all the evidence (clinical trials and other studies of interventions) on any given clinical question. The reviews bring together a number of separately conducted studies, sometimes with conflicting findings, and synthesising their results. Data from 2004 showed that there are more than 11 500 people working within the Cochrane Collaboration in over 90 countries, half of whom are authors of Cochrane Reviews. The number of people has increased by about 20% every year for the last 5 years (http://tinyurl.com/yqcvgr)
• PubMed, Medline: http://tinyurl.com/2gjcwh
• The Research Council for Complementary Medicine: http://tinyurl.com/ywcry8
• HerbNed: www.herbmed.org/
• Complementary and Alternative Medicine Specialist Library: http://tinyurl.com/q86oe
• Internet search engines (e.g. Google at www.google.com).

Appraising the evidence

When critically appraising the literature there are three key issues:

1. Validity: are results of the study valid?
2. Importance: do the results matter clinically?
3. Relevance: are the results likely to assist in caring for my patient?

Two resources that can help with the appraisal process are: Critical Appraisal Skills Program (CASP) provided by the UK NHS at http:// tinyurl.com/2qkkn3 and the Oxford Centre for Evidence Based Medicine site (CEBM) at www.cebm.net. Other tools and guides are available through Google.

Having obtained answers to the PICO question(s), the prescriber may move on to the second stage in gathering information and integrate all the data into clinical practice.

Safety

It is generally perceived by the public that CAM is entirely safe. In fact many interventions have the potential to do harm if used inappropriately, e.g. herbalism has medicines with a potential risk of intrinsic toxicity as well as possible dangerous interactions with orthodox drugs being taken concurrently.[58] Certain manipulative therapies can also cause damage if not performed correctly.

Barnes and Abbot[59] conducted a study aimed to explore UK community pharmacists' experiences with complementary medicines, in particular to determine if pharmacists identify or receive reports from patients/consumers of suspected adverse drug reactions (ADRs) to complementary medicines and if, in the course of their work, pharmacists routinely question patients/consumers specifically about their use of complementary medicines, e.g. when counter prescribing. The study was a postal questionnaire survey of community pharmacists in six areas of England: Devon, Cornwall, Bradford, Leeds, Manchester and Stockport. Overall, 90 pharmacists (11.0% of respondents) provided 107 reports of suspected ADRs to complementary medicines where minimum details were provided. Where the source of the report was stated (n = 99), 25.3% were identified by pharmacists, 72.7% were reported to pharmacists by patients/consumers and 2% by other sources. Most of the reports were of non-serious suspected ADRs, but at least three reports could be considered serious.

The general dangers of using CAM may be categorised under two headings: direct and indirect risks.

Direct risks

* Allergic reactions or other adverse reactions to medicines or diagnostic agents used during the practice of CAM
* Use of adulterated or poor quality preparations

- Interaction between CAM medicines and existing medication
- Manipulative or other damage caused by inexperienced practitioners.

Indirect risks

- Patient's condition deteriorates due to inaccurate diagnosis and/or inappropriate treatment
- Serious illness not detected through lack of knowledge or experience of practitioner
- Discontinuation of prescribed orthodox medication without permission (or knowledge) of patient's doctor
- Application of alternative approach to CAM preventing consideration of other orthodox procedures
- Patient attempts to self-treat in response to media pressure when professional advice should be sought.

To study the incidence of adverse effects. Abbot et al.[60] surveyed 1521 GPs, of whom 45% responded. A little over a third of these respondents reported a total of 291 non-serious adverse reactions. Of the respondents 11% reported what they considered to be serious adverse effects, most of which involved damage during manipulative treatment and misadvice or misdiagnosis by homeopaths. In total 12 different disciplines featured in the 'serious' list; there were 52 serious direct effects and 44 serious indirect effects. The information derived from this paper is circumstantial and anecdotal, suffering from similar limitations as the case studies referred to above. It does give an indication of the sorts of problems that can arise. The need for proper training and control is substantial. A formal system for collecting reports on CAM should be established. Practitioners should be aware of their limits of competency and remain within them at all times. The public should be made aware of the potential dangers of using CAM.

Specific dangers will be dealt with under each discipline.

Advances in CAM

The following advances in CAM have been noted by Vickers:[46]

- The quantity of applied research in complementary medicine is growing rapidly and the quality is improving.
- Complementary medicine is increasingly practised in conventional medical settings, particularly acupuncture for pain, and massage,

music therapy and relaxation techniques for mild anxiety and depression.

- There is a more open attitude to complementary medicine among conventional health professionals; this is partly explained by the rise of EBM.

More information

CAM Research Institute: www.camresearch.com

Complementary and Alternative Medicine Specialist Library: www.library.nhs.uk/cam

Complementary and Integrated Medicine Research Unit: www.cam-research-group.co.uk

Databases

Alternative Medicine Resources: www.pitt.edu/~cbw/database.html

The Prince's Foundation for Integrated Health: www.fih.org.uk/

US National Center for CAM: www.nccam.nih.gov

General CAM references: www.forthrt.com/~chronicl/archiv.htm

Further reading

Ernst E. *Understanding Research in Complementary and Alternative Medicine.* London: Holistic Therapy Books, 2001.

Lewith GT, Jonas WB, Walach H. *Clinical Research in Complementary Therapies: Principles, problems and solutions.* London: Elsevier Churchill-Livingstone, 2002.

References

1. Ernst E. The need for an evidence base. In: Kayne SB (ed.), *Homeopathic Practice.* London Pharmaceutical Press, 2008: 33–42.
2. Roach JO'N. News: Lords call for regulation of complementary medicine. *BMJ* 2000;**321**:1365.
3. Anon. Complementary medicine: time for critical engagement. (Editorial) *Lancet* 2000;**356**:2023.
4. Anon. Life after the Lords report on CAM – Report on Meeting, London 29 Jan 2001. *Pharm J* 2000;**265**:808.
5. Mills S, Peacock W. *Professional organisation of complementary and alternative medicine in the United Kingdom: A report to the Department of Health.* Exeter: University of Exeter, 1997.

6. Guyatt GH, Oxman AD, Kunz R, Vist GE, Falck-Ytter Y, Schünemann HJ. Rating quality of evidence and strength of recommendations. *BMJ* 2008; **336**:995–8.

7. Piantadosi S. David Byar as a teacher. *Control Clin Trials* 1995;**16**:202–11. (PubMed)

8. Olkin I. Statistical and theoretical considerations in meta-analysis. *J Clin Epidemiol* 1995;**48**:133–46. (PubMed)

9. Glasziou P, Vandenbroucke J, Chalmers I. Assessing the quality of research. *BMJ* 2004;**328**:39–41.

10. Garrow JS. What to do about CAM? *BMJ* 2007;**335**:951.

11. Tovey DI. Evidence is important but should not be the only consideration: patients' and clinicians' views matter too. *BMJ* 2007;**335**:951.

12. Cowan J, Lozano-Calderón S, Ring D. Quality of prospective controlled randomized trials. Analysis of trials of treatment for lateral epicondylitis as an example. *J Bone Jt Surg Am* 2007;**89**:1693–9. (PubMed)

13. Bent S, Padula A, Avins AL. Brief communication: better ways to question patients about adverse medical events: a randomized, controlled trial. *Ann Intern Med* 2006;**144**:257–61.

14. Guyatt G, Cook D, Devereaux PJ et al., eds. *The Users' Guides to the Medical Literature: A manual for evidence-based clinical practice.* Chicago: AMA publications, 2002.

15. Kaptchuk TJ. Effect of interpretive bias on research evidence. *BMJ* 2003;**326**:1453–5.

16. Glasziou P, Chalmers I, Rawlins M, McCulloch P. When are randomised trials unnecessary? Picking signal from noise. *BMJ* 2007;**334**:349–51.

17. Stukel TA, Fisher ES, Wennberg DE et al. Analysis of observational studies in the presence of treatment selection bias. *JAMA* 2007;**297**:278–85.

18. Anon. News – Shortcuts from other journals. *BMJ* 2007;**334**:179.

19. Grapow MTR, von Wattenwyl R, Guller U, Beyersdorf F, Zerkowski H-R. Randomized controlled trials do not reflect reality: Real-world analyses are critical for treatment guidelines. (Editorial) *J Thorac Cardiovasc Surg* 2006;**132**:5–7.

20. Begg CB. Ruminations on the intent-to-treat principle. *Control Clin Trials* 2000;**21**:241–3.

21. Weijer C, Shapiro SH, Glass KC, Enkin MW. Education and debate: Clinical equipoise and not the uncertainty principle is the moral underpinning of the randomised controlled trial. *BMJ* 2000;**321**:756–8.

22. Hunink MGM. Does evidence based medicine do more good than harm? *BMJ* 2004;**329**:1051.

23. Walach H, Falkenberg T, Fønnebø V et al. Circular instead of hierarchical: methodological principles for the evaluation of complex interactions. *BMC Med Res Methodol* 2006;**6**:29.

24. Reilly D, Taylor MA. The evidence profile. The multidimensional nature of proof. *Compl Ther Med* 1993;**1**(suppl 1):11–12.

25. Jonas WB. Building an evidence house: challenges and solutions to research in complementary and alternative medicine. *Forsch Komplementärmed Klass Naturheilk* 2005;**12**:159–67.

26. Sackett DL, Richardson WS, Rosenberg WMC, Haynes RB. *Evidence-based Medicine: How to practice and teach EBM*, 2nd edn. London: Churchill-Livingstone, 2000:27.
27. Smith G, Pell JP. Parachute use to prevent death and major trauma related to gravitational challenge: systematic review of randomised controlled trials. *BMJ* 2003;**327**:1459–61.
28. Potts M, Prata N, Walsh J, Grossman A. Parachute approach to evidence based medicine. *BMJ* 2006;**333**:701–3.
29. Avery M, Snyder JD. Oral therapy for acute diarrhea. The underused simple solution. *N Engl J Med* 1990;**323**: 89–94.
30. Hunter A, Grant A. Complementary medicine and evidence-based practice: power and control in healthcare – questions about an arranged marriage. *Curr Opin Evidence-Based Integr Med* 2005;**2**:189–94.
31. Coulter ID. Evidence based complementary and alternative medicine: promises and problems. *Forsch Komplementärmed* 2007;**14**:102–8.
32. Ernst E. Funding research into complementary medicine: the situation in Britain. *Compl Ther Med* 1999;**7**:250–3.
33. Ernst E. Regulating complementary medicine. *BMJ* 1996;**313**:882.
34. Lewith GT, Ernst E, Mills S et al. Complementary medicine must be research led and evidence based. (Letter) *BMJ* 2000;**320**:188.
35. Nahin R, Straus SE. Research into complementary and alternative medicine: problems and potential. *BMJ* 2001;**322**:161–4.
36. Vickers AJ. Bibliometric analysis of randomised controlled trials in complementary medicine. *Compl Ther Med* 1998;**6**:185–9.
37. Anon. Alternative medicine is no alternative. (Editorial) *Lancet* 1983; **ii**:773–4.
38. Rubinfield AR, Pain MCF. Perception of asthma. *Lancet* 1976;**i**:882–4.
39. Reichlin S. Neuroendocrine-immune interactions. *N Engl Med J* 1993; **xx**:1246–53.
40. Blalock JE. The immune system: our sixth sense. *Immunology* 1994;**2**:8–15.
41. Watkins AB. Perceptions, emotions and immunity: an integrated homeostatic network. *Q J Med* 1995;**88**:283–94.
42. Caspi O. Bringing complementary and alternative medicine (CAM) into mainstream is not integration. (Letter) *BMJ* 2001;**322**:168.
43. Pittler MH, Abbot NC, Harkness EF, Ernst E. Location bias in controlled clinical trials of complementary/alternative therapies. *J Clin Epidemiol* 2000;**53**:485–9.
44. Brohn P. *Gentle Giants: The powerful story of one woman's unconventional struggle against cancer*. London: Century Hutchinson, 1986.
45. Gracely RH, Dubner R, Deeter WR, Wolskee PJ. Clinical expectations influence placebo analgesia. (Letter) *Lancet* 1985;**i**:43.
46. Vickers A. Recent advances – Complementary medicine. *BMJ* 2000; **321**:683–6.
47. Ernst E, Resch KL. The clinical trial – gold standard or naïve reductionism? *Eur Phys Med Rehabil* 1996;**1**:26–7.
48. Leibrich J. Measurement of efficacy: a case for holistic research. *Compl Med Res* 1990;**4**:21–5.

49. Aldridge D, Pietroni PC. Clinical assessment of acupuncture in asthma therapy: discussion paper. *J R Soc Med* 1997;**80**:222–4.
50. Sackett DL. Bias in analytical research. *J Chronic Dis* 1979;**32**:51–63.
51. Abbot NC, Ernst E. Clinical audit, outcomes and complementary medicine. *Res Compl Med* 1997;**4**:229–34.
52. Camp AV. Acupuncture audit in rheumatology. *Acupunct Med* 1994; **12**:47–50.
53. Peters D, Davies P. Audit of changes in the management of back pain in general practice resulting from access to osteopathy. Executive summary. South and West RHA report of workshop on Research and Development in Complementary Medicine 12 July 1994, Winchester UK.
54. Melchart D, Linde K, Liao JZ et al. Systematic clinical auditing in complementary medicine: Rationale, concept and a pilot study. *Altern Ther* 1997; **3**:33–9.
55. Duncan G, Galbraith K. Evidence based practice and complementary medicines: teaching and learning by example. Report of Session G3 FIP Congress Beijing. *Pharm J* 2007;**279**(suppl): F21.
56. Pilkington K. Searching for CAM evidence: an evaluation of therapy-specific search engines. *J Altern Compl Med* 2007;**13**: 451–9.
57. Coelho HF, Pittler MH, Ernst E. An investigation of the contents of complementary and alternative medicine journals. *Altern Ther Health Med* 2007; **13**:40–4.
58. Brinker F. *Herb Contra-indications and Drug Interactions*, 2nd edn. Sandy, UK: Eclectic Medical Publications, 1998.
59. Barnes J, Abbot NC. Experiences with complementary medicines: a survey of community pharmacists. *Pharm J* 1999;**263**:R37.
60. Abbot NC, Hill M, Barnes J et al. Uncovering suspected adverse effects of complementary and alternative medicine. *Int J Risk Safety Med* 1998; **11**:90–106.

6

Pharmacovigilance for complementary medicines

Joanne Barnes

There is now an increasing awareness at several levels of the need to develop pharmacovigilance practices for complementary medicines and for herbal medicines in particular; the World Health Organization (WHO), for example, has produced guidelines on this.[1] Awareness has arisen not only because of the extensive use of herbal (and complementary) medicines, but also because recently there have been several high-profile safety concerns associated with herbal medicines that have had an impact on public health. In addition, the unique characteristics of complementary medicines, and the ways in which they are utilised, regulated and perceived, raise important issues and underpin the need for safety monitoring.

Definition

Pharmacovigilance is defined by the WHO as:[2]

> ... the science and activities relating to the detection, assessment, understanding and prevention of adverse effects or any other drug-related problems.

Pharmacovigilance developed after the thalidomide tragedy of the 1950s and 1960s when over 10 000 children worldwide were born with phocomelia (limb deformities). As a result, national and international systems were introduced for reporting and monitoring of adverse effects of medicines. Today, pharmacovigilance involves monitoring drug safety and identifying adverse drug reactions (ADRs) in humans, evaluating potential harms and benefits of medicines, and responding to and communicating drug safety concerns. Recently, it has been suggested that there could be more emphasis on extending knowledge of safety rather than focusing on demonstrating harm.[3]

In many countries, there is a regulatory framework for pharma-covigilance, e.g. in the European Union (EU), Directive 2001/83/EC (as amended by Directive 2004/27/EC) provides the legal framework for pharmacovigilance for licensed medicines, including licensed herbal medicines.[4] This legislation requires pharmaceutical companies to demonstrate to the relevant competent authority for licensing medicines the quality, safety and efficacy of their products before marketing. After assessment, the licensing authority may, or may not, grant a marketing authorisation (MA, product licence); licensed products, including licensed herbal medicinal products (HMPs) should comply with regulatory provisions on pharmacovigilance. In summary, these include requirements for MA holders (for their licensed products) to:

- have constant access to an appropriately qualified person responsible for pharmacovigilance
- maintain detailed records of all suspected ADRs occurring worldwide
- record and report all suspected serious ADRs notified to them by a healthcare professional in the EU to the licensing authority within 15 calendar days (this is a two-way process, and the licensing authority is required to notify the MA holder within 15 calendar days of any such reports that it receives)
- include all other ADRs as part of periodic safety update reports submitted to the licensing authority.

The legislation also places obligations on national competent authorities with respect to their pharmacovigilance activities.

The WHO definition of pharmacovigilance makes no distinction between pharmacovigilance of conventional and pharmacovigilance of complementary/traditional medicines. Indeed, there is no need, nor is it desirable, to separate the two; pharmacovigilance should embrace all preparations used medicinally regardless of their regulatory status, pharmaceutical composition, cultural use and philosophical framework. Hence, the same aims and activities of pharmacovigilance apply to complementary medicines. However, the current model of pharmacovigilance and its science and processes have developed in relation to synthetic drugs, and pharmacovigilance activities have largely been focused on conventional medicines. Applying the existing model and its tools to monitoring the safety of complementary medicines presents unique challenges in addition to those described for conventional medicines.[5]

Why is pharmacovigilance necessary for complementary medicines?

Most complementary medicines can be obtained without a prescription from various retail and other outlets, not only pharmacies. Thus, the problems that apply to pharmacovigilance of conventional non-prescription medicines, e.g. that generally their use does not involve a prescriber and is not recorded or monitored through health systems, also apply to complementary medicines. Other problems are specific to complementary medicines and present difficulties additional to those described for conventional prescription and non-prescription medicines.

Utilisation of complementary medicines

The use of complementary medicines with or instead of conventional medicines is a popular healthcare approach among patients and consumers, and extrapolation of estimates of use obtained from cross-sectional studies suggests that large numbers of people are being exposed to complementary medicines. The public health implications of this need to be considered, together with issues relating to access to complementary medicines, users' behaviour towards these products and healthcare professionals' and complementary medicine practitioners' practice, because there is the potential for complementary medicines to be used inappropriately, even unsafely, and for suspected ADRs to go undetected and unreported.

A study involving adults in England found that 19.8% (95% confidence interval or 95%CI 18.3–21.3) had purchased an over-the-counter (OTC) herbal medicinal product and that 0.9% (95% CI 0.6–1.3) had consulted a medical herbalist in the previous year.[6] Studies conducted in other developed countries, such as Australia and the USA, suggest increasing prevalence of use of herbal medicines among the general adult population.[7,8] Complementary medicines are used by a wide range of individuals for both acute and chronic conditions, as well as for maintenance of general health and wellbeing. Use is not necessarily based on evidence, or limited to symptoms and conditions suitable for self-treatment. Some patient groups, such as children and older people, are at increased risk of experiencing ADRs, and this also applies where they use complementary medicines, particularly herbal medicines. Other groups, e.g. pregnant women, may use complementary medicines in preference to conventional medicines because complementary medicines are perceived to be safer; however, little is known about the possible adverse effects of complementary medicines taken during pregnancy.

Typically, users of complementary medicines do not seek professional advice in selecting products, but rather rely on friends' or relatives' recommendations, and information in the popular media.[9,10] Complementary medicines are widely available for purchase over the internet and from retail outlets in which no trained healthcare professional is available.[11] Even where complementary medicines are purchased from pharmacies, a consumer or patient may not have any interaction with a pharmacist or trained pharmacy counter assistant or, if a consultation does occur, pharmacy staff may not have sufficient knowledge to feel confident about providing information and advice on these products.[12] A proportion of users of complementary medicines seeks treatment from complementary medicine practitioners but, at present, in many countries, there is no legal requirement for such practitioners to have undertaken appropriate training or to belong to a relevant professional organisation and, although many complementary medicine practitioners will have taken these steps, some will not have.

A related issue is that some users of complementary medicines may not disclose use to a healthcare professional;[10] equally, healthcare professionals do not ask their patients routinely whether they are using complementary medicines, even when receiving reports from patients of suspected ADRs associated with conventional medicines, and rarely record information on complementary medicine use on patient records.[13–15] It is possible, therefore, that undisclosed complementary medicine use could be an alternative explanation for reports of suspected ADRs associated with conventional medicines.

Disclosure of complementary medicine use to healthcare professionals is particularly important where patients start, stop or are already receiving treatment with conventional medicines and, equally, individuals consulting complementary medicine practitioners should disclose their current use of conventional medicines, because there may be a potential for drug–herb interactions. Information on the extent to which concurrent use of complementary and conventional medicines occurs is limited, although preliminary data suggest that it may be extensive, e.g. in a cross-sectional survey of complementary-therapy use among adults in the USA ($n = 2055$ respondents; 60% weighted overall response rate), 44% were regular users of prescription medicines and, of these, 18.4% were concurrently using a herbal or high-dose vitamin preparation.[8] In a small study conducted in the UK, 59% of herbal medicine users identified in pharmacies and health food stores claimed that they had used herbal medicines together with conventional medicines, mostly prescription medicines, in the previous year.[10]

Characteristics of herbal medicines

Composition

In contrast with most conventional medicines (i.e. single chemical entities), herbal medicines are chemically rich complex mixtures comprising several hundreds of constituents, often more.[16] Many manufactured HMPs contain several herbal ingredients, and medical herbalists usually prescribe combinations of herbal tinctures often supplied as a mixture, in both cases further adding to the chemical complexity of the herbal medicine taken by the patient (see Chapter 8). The chemical complexity of herbal medicines creates difficulties in determining their clinical pharmacokinetics, pharmacodynamics and toxicology; equally, where a safety concern has been identified in association with a particular herbal medicine, establishing which constituent(s), even which herbal ingredient(s) with combination herbal medicines, is implicated is problematic.

For many herbal medicines, the specific chemical constituents, and therefore their safety, are unknown and, even for herbal medicines with well-documented phytochemistry there are few for which the specific constituents responsible for pharmacological activity (including adverse effects) are fully understood.[17] Furthermore, the profile of constituents is not uniform throughout a plant and, for many plants, only a specific plant part, or parts such as roots or leaves, are (or should be) used medicinally. Moreover, the precise profile of constituents is likely to vary both qualitatively and quantitatively between different batches of herbal starting materials because of one or more of the following factors:

- inter- or intraspecies variation in constituents
- environmental factors, such as climate, and growing conditions
- time of harvesting – the profile of constituents can vary even over the course of a day
- post-harvesting factors, such as storage conditions, drying and processing.[17]

There will also be variations in the chemical composition of herbal medicines containing the same herbal ingredient(s) but produced by different manufacturers (see Chapter 8); this will apply to both licensed (authorised) and unlicensed herbal medicines.

Several studies have found important differences in the pharmaceutical quality of herbal products on the US market, e.g. variations in the content of major constituents in St John's wort (*Hypericum perforatum*) products (which in several cases also differed markedly from concentrations stated on the label),[18] and variations in and unacceptably high concentrations (in several cases > 25 000 parts per million or p.p.m.) of ginkgolic acids, which are potentially allergenic, in ginkgo products.[19] Standardisation on content of certain constituents is an approach used by some manufacturers to achieve more consistent pharmaceutical composition, but its usefulness is limited at present because the specific active constituents are known only for a few herbal medicines.

As a result of the variations that can exist between different manufacturers' products and preparations of the same herbal ingredient, evidence of safety (and efficacy) should be considered in this light; strictly speaking, evidence is product or extract specific, and should be extrapolated only to those products or extracts that have been shown to be pharmaceutically equivalent and bioequivalent.[20] This is largely impractical at present, given the limited data available for herbal medicines; nevertheless, the differences between different preparations of a herbal ingredient should not be ignored. As a result of the nature of herbal medicines, a group of related constituents, rather than a single constituent, may be responsible for an observed adverse effect.

Toxic constituents

Contrary to popular belief, herbal medicines are not 'safe' because they originate from natural sources; some plants are highly poisonous, and many others have inherently toxic constituents, e.g. metabolites of unsaturated pyrrolizidine alkaloids, such as senecionine, are hepatotoxic in humans, and carcinogenic and mutagenic in animals.[17] Senecionine is found in liferoot (*Senecio aureus*) and in other *Senecio* species, such as *S. scandens*, which has been reported as an ingredient in a traditional Chinese medicine product qianbai biyan pian found in the UK.[21,22]

Other known intrinsically toxic groups of constituents, their effects and examples of plant sources include aristolochic acids (nephrotoxic and carcinogenic), found in *Aristolochia* species throughout the plant, sesquiterpene lactones (allergenic), found in feverfew (*Tanacetum parthenium*), and other species in the Asteraceae family, and furanocoumarins (phototoxic), found in angelica (*Angelica archangelica*) and other species belonging to the Apiaceae family.[17]

Recent herbal safety problems include hepatotoxic reactions associated with the use of both kava (*Piper methysticum*) and black cohosh (*Cimicifuga racemosa*) root/rhizome preparations,[23,24] and numerous problems relating to the use of poor-quality traditional Chinese and ayurvedic medicines contaminated with conventional prescription medicines, heavy metals, animal parts and other substances.[25-28]

Regulation of herbal medicines and pharmacovigilance requirements

The regulation of complementary medicines varies markedly between countries and even within the same country there are often differences in the regulation of different types of complementary medicines.[29]

The United Kingdom

In the UK until 2004, the regulatory framework for herbal medicines allowed products to be marketed as licensed herbal medicines, herbal medicines exempt from licensing or unlicensed food supplements. Most of the licensed herbal medicines had initially been granted product licences of right (PLRs) because they were on the market when the medicines licensing system was set up in 1971; these products have not undergone the stringent testing required to obtain a full MA today. For herbal medicines sold as products exempt from licensing or as unlicensed food supplements, manufacturers were not required to demonstrate to the competent authority the quality, safety and efficacy of these products before marketing or for these products to comply with regulatory provisions on pharmacovigilance.

The lack of regulation for many HMPs in the UK had important implications for pharmacovigilance, because the range of possible regulatory actions that the licensing authority could take in response to a herbal safety concern was limited for unlicensed HMPs; indeed for some possible regulatory responses, HMPs required the voluntary cooperation of herbal medicine manufacturers. For example, after important interactions between St John's wort and certain prescription medicines emerged around 1999–2000, the MHRA (Medical and Healthcare products Regulatory Agency) took the decision that provision of warnings on St John's wort products was an appropriate part of the regulatory response, but this required the cooperation of manufacturers of unlicensed St John's wort products. At the same time, MA holders of conventional medicines believed to interact with St John's wort products were obliged to make variations to product information for their relevant products. Similarly, when an association between use of kava-kava (*Piper methysticum*) preparations and liver toxicity was being investigated by the UK Committee on Safety of Medicines (CSM), the herbal sector agreed to withdraw kava-kava products from sale. Voluntary withdrawal worked reasonably well initially, but, as the period of evaluation drew on, some retail outlets began selling kava-kava products again. Community pharmacists, however, had a professional and ethical responsibility not to do so.[30]

Other issues relevant to pharmacovigilance arise because manufacturers of unlicensed HMPs are not required to demonstrate to the MHRA the quality, safety and efficacy of their products before marketing. The importance of pharmaceutical quality for the safety (and efficacy) of HMPs is well recognised,[17,31,32] but manufacturers are required to demonstrate pharmaceutical quality standards only for their licensed HMPs. Some manufacturers of unlicensed HMPs may have appropriate quality control and quality assurance procedures for their products, but others do not, and the pharmaceutical quality of many unlicensed HMPs is of real concern. In addition to difficulties with assuring pharmaceutical quality due to the variation in chemical composition, quality problems with unlicensed herbal products include intentional or accidental substitution of species, contamination with restricted or toxic substances, including prescription medicines, and differences between labelled and actual contents.[22,33] It is essential, therefore, when assessing reports of suspected ADRs associated with a particular unlicensed herbal medicine to establish whether the herbal ingredient(s) implicated are what the product actually contains, and whether the product could be adulterated or contaminated. Ideally, a sample of the suspected herbal medicine should be retained for pharmaceutical analysis.

European Union

In 2005, a new EU directive on traditional HMPs was introduced that required each EU member state to set up a new registration scheme for traditional HMPs.[34] In order to obtain a product registration under these schemes, manufacturers must satisfy requirements for bibliographic data on the safety of their products, provide evidence that the herbal product has been used traditionally in the EU for at least 15 years, and manufacture products according to the principles of good manufacturing practice. Manufacturers of products registered under the directive should comply with relevant existing pharmaceutical legislation, including the provisions on pharmacovigilance summarised above. The new directive provides for a transitional period of 7 years until 2011, by which time manufacturers should comply with the regulations.

Australia

In Australia, complementary medicines are regulated as medicines under the Therapeutics Goods Act 1989 (the Act).[35] The Therapeutic Goods Administration (TGA) is the authority responsible for administering the Act.

The Act defines a complementary medicine as a therapeutic good consisting wholly or principally of one or more designated active ingredients, each of which has a clearly established identity and a traditional use. Traditional use means use of the designated active ingredient that is well documented, or otherwise established, according to the accumulated experience of many traditional healthcare practitioners over an extended period; it should also accord with well-established procedures of preparation, application and dosage. Complementary medicines comprise medicinal products containing herbs, vitamins, minerals, nutritional supplements, homeopathic medicines and certain aromatherapy products; the category includes traditional medicines (including traditional Chinese medicines, ayurvedic medicines and Australian indigenous medicines). The Therapeutic Goods Regulations 1990 designate the types of active ingredients that may be used in such medicines.[36]

As with other medicines in Australia, complementary medicines are regulated under a two-tier regulatory framework based on risk, although all products must be manufactured according to good manufacturing practice (GMP) standards. Products are regulated as 'low-risk' Listed medicines (designated AUST L on the product label) or as higher-risk Registered medicines (AUST R).

Listed complementary medicines may contain only certain ingredients permitted by the TGA and are authorised only for claims relating to health maintenance, health enhancement or non-serious self-limiting conditions; serious diseases or conditions, or claims for treatment or prevention, are generally not permitted. Listed medicines are not assessed individually for efficacy: sponsors must certify to the TGA that they hold evidence to support all claims made for the product. Evidence, products and ingredients may be audited by the TGA as part of target or random auditing. Most complementary medicines authorised in Australia are Listed medicines.

Registered complementary medicines are assessed individually for quality, safety and efficacy before marketing. Efficacy is usually supported by data from controlled clinical trials, but in some circumstances bibliographic data may be used.

Sponsors of all authorised complementary medicines are obliged to report to the TGA any adverse reactions associated with their products.

In consultation with industry, the TGA has developed the Australian Regulatory Guidelines for Complementary Medicines (ARGCM)[37] to assist sponsors of complementary medicines to meet their legislative obligations.

New Zealand

The current regulatory framework for complementary medicines in New Zealand has strong similarities to that in the UK before the introduction of the European Union Traditional Herbal Medicinal Products Directive.

A herbal remedy is a special subcategory of medicine, defined in section 2 of the Medicines Act 1981.[38] A herbal remedy is a medicine that does not contain a prescription, restricted or pharmacy-only medicine, and consists of a substance derived from plant material that has been dried or crushed (or derived through any other similar process). It may also be an aqueous or alcoholic extract of the dried or crushed plant material, or a mixture of that material with another inert substance. Ministerial consent is not required for the distribution of a herbal remedy that is sold or supplied without any recommendation as to its use and the labelling complies with the requirements of section 28 of the Medicines Act, whereas ministerial consent is required for the distribution of a herbal remedy that is sold with a recommendation for use for a therapeutic purpose.

Homeopathic remedies are those prepared under the principle of homeopathy, in which the active ingredient to be administered is in a concentration not more than 20 p.p.m, and the remedy is labelled only with the name of the active ingredient, trade name (if any) and a statement that as it is a homeopathic remedy it does not normally require ministerial consent before distribution. The product label or associated advertising material must not contain therapeutic claims or indications for use. A homeopathic remedy that is labelled or advertised with claims as to its therapeutic purpose is a medicine and subject to the full control of the medicines legislation.

Sterile homeopathic preparations intended for injection or for administration to the eyes are regarded as medicines and are therefore subject to the full control of the medicines legislation.

Most products considered to be complementary medicines are currently regulated as 'dietary supplements' and are regulated under the Dietary Supplement Regulations 1985,[39] under the Food Act 1981.[40] The Dietary Supplement Regulations 1985 provide some restrictions on ingredients of dietary supplements, and no therapeutic claims are allowed; however, many manufacturers ignore these requirements.

Medsafe, the regulatory authority for medicines and medical devices in New Zealand, and the New Zealand Food Safety Authority (NZFSA), have recently written to manufacturers of dietary supplements to inform them of planned changes to the Dietary Supplements Regulations 1985. The changes are likely to include transfer of responsibility from the NZFSA to the Ministry of Health for 'therapeutic-type dietary supplements'.[41]

This follows the recent failure of the proposals for a joint Australia New Zealand Therapeutic Products Authority (ANZTPA) to achieve sufficient parliamentary support in New Zealand. The joint authority would have been responsible for regulating medicines, including complementary medicines, medical devices and blood products, across Australia and New Zealand. As Australia has existing regulations for complementary medicines, ANZTPA would have introduced similar regulations, including pharmacovigilance requirements, for complementary medicines in New Zealand.[42]

The United States of America

In the USA, most complementary medicines (termed 'dietary supplements') are regulated under the Dietary Supplements Health and Education Act 1994 (DSHEA).

Under the regulations, dietary supplements are defined as: vitamins, minerals, amino acids, herbs or other botanicals, dietary substance to supplement the diet by increasing the total dietary intake, or a concentrate, metabolite, constituent, extract or combination of any of the above ingredients.[43,44] Also, products must state 'dietary supplement' on the label, be intended for ingestion as a tablet, capsule or liquid, and not be represented for use as a conventional food or a sole item of a meal or the diet.

Product labels may include a 'claim' or statement that:

- describes the role of a nutrient or dietary ingredient intended to affect the structure or function in humans
- characterises the documented mechanism by which a nutrient or dietary ingredient acts to maintain such structure or function
- describes a general wellbeing that may arise from consumption of a nutrient or dietary ingredient.

The manufacturer of the dietary supplement should have substantiation that the statement is truthful and not misleading, and the label must include, prominently displayed and in boldface type, the following:[43]

> This statement has not been evaluated by the Food and Drug Administration. This product is not intended to diagnose, treat, cure, or prevent any disease.

In 2006, the Dietary Supplement and Nonprescription Drug Consumer Protection Act was passed, which requires manufacturers, packers or distributors whose names appear on the label of a non-prescription drug or dietary supplement marketed in the USA to: submit to the Secretary of Health and Human Services, within 15 business days, any report of a serious adverse event associated with use of such drug or supplement in the USA; submit within 15 business days any related medical information that is received within 1 year of the initial report; maintain records related to each report for 6 years; and permit inspection of such records.[45]

Also, on 22 June 2007, the Food and Drug Administration (FDA) published its final regulations for GMP for dietary supplements.[46]

Canada

Regulations for complementary medicines (termed 'natural health products' or NHPs) in Canada were introduced in 2004. The new regulatory framework has a 6-year transition period for sponsors to meet the requirements such that sale of all natural health products must comply with the Regulations by 1 January 2010.

Under the regulations, NHPs are considered to be herbal remedies, homeopathic remedies, traditional medicines (e.g. traditional Chinese herbal medicines), vitamins, minerals, probiotics, essential fatty acids or amino acids that are used to prevent, diagnose or treat disease, restore or correct function, or maintain or promote health, and are endorsed for self-care purposes.[47] Products authorised under the scheme must be for OTC use: the label and package insert must provide sufficient information for the consumer to use the product safely and effectively without the need to consult a healthcare provider.

Sponsors of NHPs must apply for, and be awarded, a product licence for their products. Product licence applications have several categories, including traditional and non-traditional claims. There are different requirements for licence applications in each category, e.g. traditional claims are those products that have been used within a cultural belief system or healing paradigm for at least 50 consecutive years.[48] To make a traditional use claim, the method of preparation should be considered to be traditional and a minimum of two traditional references should be submitted supporting the recommended conditions of use or one acceptable pharmacopoeia reference. For non-traditional claim applications, scientific evidence supporting the safety and efficacy of the product according to the recommended conditions of use must be submitted.

Under the NHP Regulations, product licence holders are responsible for providing Health Canada with information about adverse reactions to their products.[47] Serious and serious unexpected adverse reactions to *any dose* of an NHP must be reported within 15 days of becoming aware of them ('case report'), whereas an annual report should include only those adverse reactions occurring at the *labelled dose* ('summary report').

Information on safety and efficacy of complementary medicines

There is a general lack of objective information on the safety of many complementary medicines. This has arisen in part because, under the current regulatory framework, there is little incentive for manufacturers to carry out preclinical tests and clinical trials. Postmarketing surveillance studies involving certain HMPs have been conducted by some manufacturers (usually those based in Germany), but this is the exception. Generally speaking, there is a lack of information on the types and frequency of adverse effects, including interactions with other medicines, foods, alcohol, disease, etc. and other aspects relevant to safety for complementary medicines, such as their active constituents, pharmacokinetics, pharmacology, use in special patient groups (e.g. children, older people, individuals with renal or hepatic disease, pregnant or breast-feeding women), effects of long-term use.[4]

It is often argued that complementary medicines, particularly herbal medicines, have a long history of traditional use and that this provides evidence for their safety (and efficacy). However, although the 'test of time' may have identified inherently toxic plants, it cannot, for example, identify delayed adverse effects, effects that may arise from use in patients with 'modern' illnesses, such as HIV/AIDS, and safety issues arising from how herbal medicines are utilised today, e.g. together with conventional medicines.[49] Certainly, there are examples of type A reactions (those that typically are dose dependent and related to the pharmacological effects of the medicine), type B reactions (typically unrelated to dose, idiosyncratic) and other types of ADRs (e.g. delayed effects in the user or offspring remote from medicine use in the user) associated with the use of certain herbal medicines.[33]

In addition, the efficacy of many complementary medicines has not been evaluated in randomised clinical trials (RCTs). Even for well-tested herbal medicines, such as certain extracts of St John's wort herb that have been assessed in around 30 RCTs in depression, only a small number of participants in clinical trials have been exposed to a specific manufacturer's product. Furthermore, there are few long-term clinical trials of complementary medicines intended for long-term use. For comparison, conventional medicines have been tested on up to 5000 patients before they reach the market, and this is still considered to be a small number.[50] The lack of information on the safety and efficacy of complementary medicines makes it difficult to carry out benefit–risk assessments.

Methods for pharmacovigilance of complementary medicines

Some standard methods used in pharmacovigilance, particularly spontaneous reporting schemes, are used to monitor the safety of complementary medicines, although these methods are less well established than for conventional medicines. Other methods, such as prescription event monitoring, are now being considered for exploring the safety of herbal medicines. All available pharmacovigilance tools have important limitations with regard to their use in investigating the safety of complementary medicines, in addition to those already recognised, and it is likely that modified, even novel, methods are required.[5]

Spontaneous reporting schemes

Spontaneous reporting schemes typically comprise reporting (which is usually, but not always, voluntary) to a regional or central authority by healthcare professionals, and in some countries patients, of suspected adverse effects of medicines. The future of spontaneous reporting schemes in pharmacovigilance has been questioned,[3] although it is likely that this point was raised in relation to conventional medicines for which other well-established tools, such as computerised health-record databases, can be used for pharmacovigilance purposes. By contrast, spontaneous reporting for complementary medicines is in the early stages of its development; at present, in the absence of other tools and/or resources, it is the main method of generating and detecting signals of potential safety concerns associated with complementary medicines. Spontaneous reporting schemes appear to function reasonably effectively as a pharmacovigilance tool for herbal medicines, e.g. in countries such as Germany where HMPs have been regulated as medicines, frequently prescribed by doctors and are well known to other healthcare professionals, particularly pharmacists.[51] However, spontaneous reporting is likely to be far less effective in countries such as the UK, where herbal and complementary medicines have been marketed mainly as unlicensed products, with no obligation for manufacturers to report suspected ADRs to the competent authority, and complementary medicines are used mostly in self-treatment with no supervision from a healthcare professional. Similar problems arise in developing countries.[52–54]

International monitoring of suspected ADRs associated with herbal medicines

Adverse drug reaction reports, including herbal ADR reports, from the CSM/MHRA Yellow Card scheme, and (in January 2007) those from 81 other countries (plus 18 associate member countries) with national ADR monitoring schemes, are fed into the WHO/Uppsala Monitoring Centre (UMC).[55] The UMC recognises the problems inherent in ADR reporting for herbal medicines and has established a traditional medicines project to stimulate reporting in this area and to standardise information on herbal medicines, particularly with regard to nomenclature.[56] For example, a special set of herbal anatomical–therapeutic–chemical (ATC) codes has been developed that is fully compatible with the regular ATC classification system for conventional medicines,[57] and another initiative provides guidance on accepted scientific names for medicinal plants.[58]

The UMC database, established in 1968, holds over 3.5 million reports of suspected ADRs (2006), of which around 0.5% involve herbal medicines. For the period 1968–97, almost 9000 reports involving herbal medicines were received by the UMC. Most reports for herbal medicines originate from Australia, France, Germany, the UK and the USA.[56]

UK national spontaneous reporting scheme and complementary medicines

The MHRA's national spontaneous reporting scheme for suspected ADR reporting by healthcare professionals (also known as the Yellow Card scheme) has been applied to licensed medicines, including licensed complementary medicines, since its inception in 1964. However, the inclusion of licensed complementary medicines in the scheme was not well publicised until October 1996, over 30 years later, when the scheme was extended to include reporting for unlicensed herbal medicines.[59] This move followed a 5-year study of traditional remedies and food supplements, carried out by a British medical toxicology unit,[60] which identified suspected ADRs associated with these types of products. The extension allowed those with official reporter status – at the time, doctors, dentists and coroners only – to submit reports for unlicensed herbal medicines, but did not (and could not) place any statutory obligation on manufacturers to report suspected ADRs associated with their unlicensed herbal products.

In April 1997 and November 1999, the scheme underwent further extensions to allow reporting of suspected ADRs by all hospital and community pharmacists, respectively.[61] Further extensions to the reporter base for the Yellow Card scheme occurred in October 2002, when all nurses, midwives and health visitors became recognised reporters.[62] At the same time, electronic reporting of suspected ADRs over the internet was launched in an attempt to facilitate reporting,[63] and in April 2003 a pilot scheme was introduced to allow patient reporting of suspected ADRs via one of the NHS's 22 NHS Direct telephone call centres.[64] Subsequently, a pilot scheme for direct patient reporting of suspected ADRs via Yellow Cards in doctors' surgeries was initiated in January 2005. Direct patient reporting was introduced country wide in October 2005, and 2000 patient reports of suspected ADRs (associated with all types of medicines) were received during the first 6 months of the introduction of direct patient reporting.[65]

Despite these initiatives to stimulate reporting of suspected ADRs associated with both licensed and unlicensed complementary medicines, particularly herbal medicines, the numbers of herbal ADR reports submitted remain very low relative to numbers of reports submitted for conventional medicines. From 1964 until the end of 1995, 832 reports for herbal medicines were received.[66] For the period 1996 (when the Yellow Card scheme was extended to unlicensed herbal medicines and its inclusion of herbal medicines was first well publicised) to 2002 inclusive, 467 reports of suspected ADRs associated with herbal medicines were received (Figure 6.1). Most frequently, these reports related to products containing the herbal ingredients St John's wort (*Hypericum perforatum*), ginkgo (*Ginkgo biloba*), peppermint (*Mentha piperita*), *Echinacea* species, senna and valerian (*Valeriana officinalis*). It is not known whether the low numbers of reports of suspected ADRs associated with herbal medicines simply reflect a low frequency of adverse effects with herbal medicines, or whether there are other explanations, e.g. substantial under-reporting.

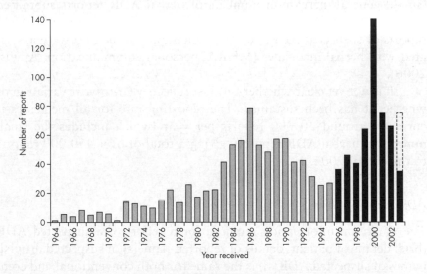

Figure 6.1 The number of reports of suspected adverse drug reactions associated with herbal medicines received by the UK Committee on Safety of Medicines/Medicines and Healthcare products Regulatory Agency's (CSM/MHRA) Yellow Card scheme for the period 1964 to 25 July 2003. (Source: Adverse Drug Reactions On-line Information Tracking.[66] This figure was first published in Barnes[5] and is reprinted here by kind permission of Adis International Ltd, Auckland, New Zealand.)

Figure 6.1 shows the numbers of reports of suspected adverse drug reactions associated with herbal medicines received by the UK CSM/MHRA's Yellow Card scheme for the period 1964 to 25 July 2003. Pale bars (i.e. pre-1996) represent licensed herbal medicines; dark bars (1996 onwards) represent reports for both licensed and unlicensed herbal medicines following extension of the scheme to unlicensed herbal medicines in October 1996; the dotted line above the 2003 bar represents an estimate of the total number of reports for the full year.

The number of herbal ADR reports received increased over the period 1999–2002, with a peak in the year 2000 around the time that reports emerged of suspected interactions between St John's wort and certain prescription medicines. In part, this simply reflected an increase in numbers of reports of suspected ADRs associated with St John's wort (60% [82/140] of herbal reports for the year 2000 [42% for 1999 and 13% for 1998] and 40% [138/345] of all herbal reports received during this period related to St John's wort, with around 40 reports in total describing drug interactions with St John's wort) but there was also a (small) general increase in numbers of herbal ADR reports submitted during this period.[66] In 2005, the MHRA received a total of 20 925 reports of suspected ADRs for all medicines, of which 80 were associated with herbal medicines (MHRA, personal communication, August 2006).

It is not yet clear whether this just reflects year-to-year variation or whether it has been sustained. The reporting rate for all medicines is currently around 20 000 reports per year (which includes the small number of herbal ADR reports), giving a total of over 450 000 reports to the end of 2002.

ADR reporting forms

The minimum information required for a report of a suspected ADR (brief details of patient, details of reporter, name[s] of suspected drug[s], names of suspected ADR[s]) is the same for both conventional and complementary medicines and, in most countries, a standard form (the Yellow Card in the UK) is used to collect data, regardless of the type of preparation implicated. It is not desirable to introduce different reporting forms for different types of preparations, but modifications to the existing reporting card could be made so that important details on herbal and complementary medicines can be requested. The WHO has produced a template of a modified spontaneous reporting form with specific data fields relating to HMPs.[1] A small number of countries have introduced a specific ADR reporting form for herbal medicines.[67]

Typically, existing ADR reporting forms have not been designed with complementary medicines in mind and, therefore, have several deficiencies with regard to prompting for and collecting information on complementary medicines implicated in ADR reports. The UK Yellow Card provides a convenient case study to illustrate this point (Box 6.1).

Box 6.1 Limitations of ADR reporting forms for collecting information on suspected adverse drug reactions (ADRs) associated with herbal and complementary medicines

In 2000, a modified Yellow Card was introduced which included in the section for 'Other drugs' the prompt '(including self-medication and herbal remedies)',[68] but there was otherwise no specific mention on the form of complementary medicines or any related terms. In addition, the section 'Suspected drug' presents several problems. First, the reporter is asked to provide the brand (proprietary) name of the suspected drug(s). Although licensed herbal medicinal products are likely to have brand names, unlicensed herbal products legally are not permitted to use them – only the vernacular and/or botanical name, such as St John's wort or *Hypericum perforatum*, should be used, although this is ignored by some manufacturers. For unlicensed herbal medicines it would be more appropriate to request the name of the herbal ingredient(s) and the name of the manufacturer/supplier. Identifying the manufacturer is particularly important for reasons mentioned earlier, namely because the composition of products containing the same herbal ingredient can vary both qualitatively and quantitatively between manufacturers. Also, there may be other problems with the pharmaceutical quality (e.g. contamination) of unlicensed herbal products, which should be considered when assessing ADR reports. Ideally, the form should also include space to indicate whether a sample of the suspected product(s) is available.

Other relevant information not specifically requested includes the method of processing the crude herbal material (e.g. type of extract), because this can also influence the precise chemical composition and, therefore, the potential toxicity of a herbal preparation,[51] the strength of the preparation (e.g. drug:extract ratio) and the formulation of the product (e.g. tablets, tincture). Also, many herbal medicinal products contain several herbal ingredients, some include non-herbal ingredients, such as vitamins and minerals, and herbal practitioners often prescribe several herbal tinctures supplied together as a mixture. With respect to these preparations, one or more herbal ingredient(s) may be the suspected agent(s), yet there is limited space on the current Yellow Card to provide this level of detail.

A critical point is that, to identify specifically the herbal ingredient(s) implicated, the binomial botanical name (genus and species) should be given, and recommendations for standardisation of botanical nomenclature used in pharmacovigilance have been made.[69] For example, 'echinacea' is insufficient, because three different *Echinacea* species (*E. purpurea*, *E. pallida* and *E. angustifolia*) are used medicinally, and these differ in their phytochemical composition. In addition, the specific plant part used should also be stated, because one or more plant parts may be used medicinally and, again, the phytochemical composition can vary. For example, both the root and the herb (aerial parts) of *E. purpurea* and nettle (*Urtica dioica*) are used medicinally. However, typically, ADR reporting forms do not include any prompts for these details.[5]

Signal detection and assessment

At present, because of the relatively small number of reports of suspected ADRs associated with complementary medicines held on databases of national pharmacovigilance centres (e.g. the MHRA's ADROIT [Adverse Drug Reaction On-line Information Tracking]), signals are usually detected simply by numbers of reports. For conventional medicines, statistical methods, such as proportional reporting ratios (PRRs), are used to identify suspected ADRs that occur more frequently in the database than expected. It may be possible to obtain PRRs for some suspected ADRs associated with certain herbal medicines, such as St John's wort products, for which there are substantial numbers of reports (e.g. in the UK, at least 150 reports for St John's wort have been received since 1996).[5]

The WHO/UMC process for signal detection involves the calculation of a measurement of association known as the 'information component'. For herbal medicines, the comparison is made against the rest of the database, rather than only against the subset of herbal ADR reports. The assumptions made in proportional analysis, and the importance of considering the effect of selected backgrounds, have been discussed in the context of conventional medicines.[70] As there are additional biases and other issues in pharmacovigilance of complementary medicines, choice of an appropriate comparator requires consideration and some preliminary work has explored this issue.[71]

After confirmation of a signal relating to a safety concern, the next stages in its evaluation are also difficult with respect to complementary medicines. In most cases, quantifying the risk is probably impossible because there is no reliable way of determining the number of individuals exposed to the complementary medicine of interest. Benefit–risk analysis is problematic because of the limited clinical data on safety and efficacy of complementary medicines, and identifying at-risk groups is also difficult because the user profile for complementary medicines is poorly defined. A particular problem is that a specific complementary medicine can have numerous uses and may be taken by healthy individuals for 'general wellbeing', as well as by patients with chronic disease. These problems are further compounded if, for example, the variation in different preparations containing the same herbal ingredient(s) is considered. The concerns regarding kava-kava (*Piper methysticum*) and hepatotoxicity illustrate the process of assessing and responding to safety issues relating to unlicensed herbal medicinal products (Box 6.2).

Box 6.2 Kava-kava (*Piper methysticum*) and hepatotoxicity: the UK regulatory response

A signal concerning kava-kava and liver toxicity was first raised in 2000 following a cluster of cases reported in Switzerland, and was strengthened a year or so later following further spontaneous reports from Switzerland and Germany.[72] The British Committee on Safety of Medicines (CSM) undertook an initial evaluation, including causality assessment, and found that the risks of kava-kava appeared to outweigh its benefits. No regulatory action was taken at that time, although the herbal sector instigated a voluntary withdrawal of products containing kava-kava while the safety concerns were investigated further.

The next stage involved further data collection and evaluation. The CSM set up a working group to assess the issue and requested additional data on benefits and risks of kava-kava from the herbal sector and regulatory authorities. When the CSM next considered the issue in July 2002, a total of 68 reports originating from several countries had been received, although only 3 originated in the UK.[72] The severity of the liver damage described in the reports varied from abnormal liver function test results to liver failure and death; six patients received liver transplants. Different preparations of kava-kava were available (e.g. different types of extracts) and consideration was given to whether only certain types of kava-kava preparation might be associated with liver toxicity. However, there appeared to be no relationship between the method of processing/type of extract, strength or dose, and the adverse reactions. Thus, on the basis of the data available, the CSM advised that the possible benefits of preparations containing kava-kava do not outweigh the risks, kava-kava had the potential to cause hepatotoxicity that could be serious in nature, and kava-kava should be prohibited in unlicensed medicines. On 13 January 2003, a statutory order came into effect in the UK prohibiting the sale, supply and import of unlicensed medicines containing kava-kava. Product licences for licensed kava-kava products were revoked.[73]

Some of the difficulties in assessing safety concerns with unlicensed herbal medicines were evident here, e.g. the number of unlicensed herbal products containing kava-kava available in the UK, their extent of use and the extent of use of kava-kava preparations by patients consulting medical herbalists were not known; reports involved different types of kava-kava preparations; only a very low number of reports was received in the UK; the quality and completeness of the reports were poor, and some reports were duplicated; there are few clinical trials of kava-kava products and a lack of clear evidence of efficacy; regulatory options in responding to the signal were limited, and alternatives, such as including warning information with products, would have required the voluntary cooperation of manufacturers of unlicensed kava-kava products and the MHRA would have had no means of enforcement.

In 2005, evidence relating to the hepatotoxicity associated with kava was reviewed in a public consultation and later that year by the Expert Working Group set up to consider the evidence. The Expert Working Group's report was published in July 2006 and concluded that there was insufficient new evidence to support a change in the regulatory position, hence the inclusion of kava in unlicensed medicines in the UK remains prohibited.[23] The report also identified several new questions and issues that may be important with respect to hepatotoxicity of kava, including the possibility that other alkaloid and/or amide constituents may be present, and their possible contribution to hepatotoxicity, and the need for a systematic evaluation of all marketed kava products and their source material, and of the variation in the phytochemistry of kava cultivars.[23]

Strengths and weaknesses of spontaneous reporting schemes

Spontaneous reporting schemes have recognised advantages and limitations, and several of these may be even more important with regard to complementary medicines (Box 6.3). In particular, under-reporting is a well-recognised, important and inevitable limitation of any spontaneous reporting scheme, but for several reasons it may be an even greater problem for complementary medicines.

Box 6.3   Summary of advantages and limitations of spontaneous adverse drug reaction (ADR) reporting schemes with respect to complementary medicines

Advantages
Monitor all drugs, including all complementary medicines, all the time and for all consumers and patients

Provide early warnings of undocumented drug safety concerns; important for complementary medicines as information on safety is limited

Relatively cheap to run; important as the complementary medicine sector may not have the resources to conduct large-scale post-marketing surveillance studies

Limitations

Under-reporting; likely to be substantial for complementary medicines

   Poor quality of data available to or provided by reporter; ADR reporting forms do not cater specifically for recording information on complementary medicines as suspected and/or concomitant drugs

Biases in reporting

Cannot estimate frequency of an ADR because do not provide accurate information on number of individuals exposed to the drug of interest; probably not possible to obtain denominators for complementary medicines, particularly unauthorised products

   Suspected ADRs may be identified/reported outside the formal system (e.g. to herbalists and other complementary medicine practitioners, health-food store staff)

Modified from Barnes[5] (Reprinted by kind permission of Adis International Ltd, Auckland, New Zealand).

Under-reporting of suspected ADRs associated with complementary medicines could occur at several levels. First, because of the perception that complementary medicines are 'safe', users of these preparations may not associate an adverse event with their use of a complementary medicine, particularly if they are taking other (conventional) medicines.[5] If the user does make an association between use of a complementary medicine and an adverse event, they may take steps to resolve the problem themselves (e.g. stop taking the preparation) and/or may not inform a healthcare professional.[9] Under-reporting can also occur at the level of the healthcare professional, because doctors, pharmacists and other recognised reporters could filter out reports of suspected ADRs described by patients.[74] Reasons for under-reporting among healthcare professionals are well documented, although studies exploring this area have been carried out in the context of conventional medicines, and it is not known if these same reasons apply to under-reporting for complementary medicines.

Pharmacist reporting of suspected ADRs associated with complementary medicines

When community pharmacists were recognised as official reporters to the 'Yellow Card' scheme, they were encouraged by the then CSM and MHRA to concentrate on areas of limited reporting by doctors, namely licensed and unlicensed herbal products, and other non-prescription medicines.[61] This extension followed a 1-year pilot scheme for community pharmacist ADR reporting, carried out in the four CSM regions during 1997–8 and involving around 3200 pharmacies; this showed that community pharmacists, compared with general practitioners (GPs), submitted a greater proportion of reports of suspected ADRs associated with herbal medicines (the numbers of herbal ADR reports as a proportion of the total number of reports submitted by pharmacists and GPs were 4/96 [4.2%] and 8/1975 [0.4%[, respectively; $p < 0.001$).[75] However, numbers of herbal ADR reports submitted by both groups of reporters were very low and represented an average of only one and two reports per CSM region for pharmacists and GPs, respectively. Evaluation of the pilot scheme indicated that the completeness of all reports submitted by community pharmacists and GPs was similar.[75]

Several studies involving community pharmacists indicate that many pharmacists are unaware that they should report suspected ADRs associated with herbal medicines. A cross-sectional survey carried out in 1998 of over 1300 community pharmacists (response rate: 67%) not involved in the CSM/MHRA pilot scheme for community pharmacist ADR reporting found that: 47% of respondents were not aware that the Yellow Card scheme applied to herbal medicines at all; 37% were aware that it applied to licensed herbal medicines; and only 16% knew that it applied to both licensed and unlicensed herbal medicines.[14] This finding is not so surprising because these pharmacists were not recognised reporters at the time of the study and would not have received training materials on ADR reporting. Of more concern are that studies conducted since all community pharmacists became recognised reporters and were encouraged to focus on reporting suspected ADRs associated with herbal and other non-prescription medicines, which have continued to find that many community pharmacists are unaware of the need to report suspected ADRs associated with herbal medicines,[76,77] particularly unlicensed herbal medicines.[76] There may also be biases favouring ADR reporting for complementary medicines. An audit of medicines information pharmacists working in a medicines information centre in Wales found that, although they encouraged only 41% of enquirers about ADRs to complete Yellow Cards, they were more likely to give encouragement when an 'alternative' medicine was involved rather than a conventional medicine.[78] In addition, all these studies revealed deficiencies in community pharmacists' knowledge on other aspects of ADR reporting, such as the level of certainty required about a causal relationship.

To date, there are very few studies that provide any information on the extent of under-reporting of suspected ADRs associated with complementary medicines. In one cross-sectional survey of community pharmacists who were not involved in the CSM/MHRA pilot scheme for community pharmacist ADR reporting (see earlier), respondents were asked to describe any reports of suspected ADRs associated with complementary medicines that they had received or identified over the previous 12 months.[13,14] In total, among 818 respondents, 44 reports of suspected ADRs associated with herbal medicines were described, an average of 1 report per 19 pharmacists. By contrast, the CSM/MHRA pilot scheme, which ran over approximately the same period covered by the survey, and involved around 3200 pharmacies, received only four reports.[75,79] Conclusions cannot be drawn from these crude comparisons, because these studies used different methodologies, involved pharmacists/pharmacies in different regions of the UK, etc. They do, however, raise the hypothesis that there is significant under-reporting by pharmacists of suspected ADRs associated with herbal medicines.

It is recognised that pharmacists can make an important contri-bution to ADR reporting for complementary medicines, but it is likely that greater vigilance on the part of the pharmacist and initiatives to encourage complementary medicine ADR reporting by pharmacists are required. Against this background, there have been several recent papers in a journal received by all UK pharmacists,[16,80,81] and a fact-sheet on ADR reporting by pharmacists has been produced by the Science Committee of The Royal Pharmaceutical Society of Great Britain (the professional and regulatory body for all pharmacists in the UK), which provides guidance and reminds pharmacists of their professional and ethical responsibilities in this regard.[82]

Complementary medicine practitioner reporting of suspected ADRs associated with complementary medicines

In many countries, complementary medicines are widely available from a range of outlets without the need for interaction with a conventional healthcare professional. Suspected ADRs associated with complemen-tary medicines may, therefore, be identified by or reported to an individ-ual (e.g. herbalist or other complementary medicine practitioner) who is outside the formal system for ADR reporting. Health-food stores are a major outlet for complementary medicines, but it is not known if staff in these outlets receive reports of suspected ADRs associated with such products and, if they do, what action, if any, they take.[5]

At present, in the UK herbal medicine and other complementary medicine practitioners are not recognised as reporters by the MHRA Yellow Card scheme. Several herbal medicine practitioners and other herbal sector organisations have initiated their own ADR reporting schemes for herbal medicines based on the MHRA scheme. Although this is a responsible and potentially useful step forward where these schemes have developed a link with the MHRA or WHO/UMC so that reports are eventually collated, ad hoc schemes are not encouraged because there is a risk that reports will be dispersed and signals may be not be detected as early as possible, or may be missed completely. As with any spontaneous reporting scheme, schemes initiated by the herbal sector are also likely to be prone to limitations such as under-reporting. It is not known whether reasons for under-reporting of suspected herbal ADRs by the herbal sector are different from those for herbal ADR reporting by conventional healthcare professionals.[5] It is possible that there may be concerns among the herbal sector that the availability of herbal medicines and their freedom to practise herbal medicine may be threatened if significant numbers of herbal ADR reports are submitted.

The National Institute of Medical Herbalists (NIMH), the major organisation for medical herbalists in the UK, requests reports from its members of suspected ADRs associated with herbal treatments. Reports are submitted on a modified Yellow Card form, which has some additional data fields relevant to herbalists' prescriptions. The NIMH sends an annual summary of reports received to MHRA. Since 1994, when the scheme was established, 42 reports have been received by the NIMH.[83] Most reports described reactions experienced by patients who had received a combination of several herbs, which is typical of medical herbalists' treatment approach. A similar scheme has been set up by the Register of Chinese Herbal Medicine (RCHM), which also uses a modified Yellow Card form to collect data from its practitioners of Chinese herbal medicine. The RCHM scheme also has a link with the MHRA; the RCHM had received reports from 3% (around 15) of its 500 or so members up to 2006.[84]

Other schemes have been established that are not restricted to herbal medicine practitioners. Phytonet is a password-protected, internet-based system for gathering reports of suspected ADRs associated with herbal medicines; it was set up by a UK university on behalf of the European Scientific Co-operative on Phytotherapy in 1996.[85] Phytonet uses an electronic form based on the CSM/MHRA Yellow Card, but differs from the schemes described above in that it accepts reports from healthcare professionals, herbal practitioners, patients and the public. Submitted reports are assessed by an expert panel and, where appropriate, fed into the WHO/UMC. Few reports have been received, however, and support is needed to revive the system. In the UK, as there is no obligation for manufacturers to report suspected ADRs associated with their unlicensed herbal products, the British Herbal Medicine Association (BHMA), members of which include many herbal medicine manufacturers, has addressed this in its voluntary code of practice for its members.[86] The code includes the requirement that manufacturers send reports of suspected ADRs associated with their unlicensed herbal products to the BHMA, which may, at its discretion, forward such reports to the MHRA. However, up to 2003, the BHMA had not received from its members any reports of suspected ADRs associated with unlicensed HMPs.

Prescription event monitoring

The methodology of prescription event monitoring (PEM) in monitoring the safety of newly marketed prescription drugs is well established.[87] In brief, PEM is a hypothesis-generating, non interventional, observational form of monitoring for newly marketed medicines carried out by the Drug Safety Research Unit, Southampton, UK. Current PEM methodology involves sending a 'green form' to GPs who have prescribed the medicine being studied; these data are obtained from the UK Prescription Pricing Authority. The green form comprises a simple questionnaire, which requests data on all health events that the patient who was prescribed the drug experienced during treatment. These forms are usually sent to the GPs around 6 months after the patient was first prescribed the medicine under study. The valuable contribution that PEM has made to pharmacovigilance of conventional medicines is clear, but the existing method is of little use at present for pharmacovigilance of complementary medicines because they are rarely prescribed.

A protocol for modified PEM methodology has been developed by the same unit in Southampton, in collaboration with the NIMH and other herbal medicine and pharmacovigilance specialists. This approach involves using herbalists to provide adverse event data on green forms for patients treated with a specific herbal medicine. Where patients give permission, a green form requesting adverse event data would also be sent to their GP. There are limitations to this method, such as whether sufficient patient numbers could be achieved and, particularly, that the herbal medicine of interest is not 'newly marketed' so there may be preconceptions about its safety profile. Nevertheless, the protocol represents a step forward in attempting to develop methods for pharma-covigilance of complementary medicines. Another potential approach, based on PEM concepts, is to use community pharmacists to recruit a cohort of purchasers (where consent is given) of a specific HMP, who would then be followed up over time and adverse event data collected. The feasibility of this approach has been demonstrated in a pilot study using a conventional non-prescription medicine.[88,89] Pilot work assessing the feasibility of these models has been undertaken.[90,91]

Other pharmacoepidemiological study designs

The methodology for case–control and cohort studies is well established and these study designs can be used to investigate safety concerns with complementary medicines, although few studies have been carried out to date. One study explored the relationship between colorectal cancer and use of preparations containing anthranoid laxatives[51] and a prospective, observational cohort study, involving 131 medical prac-tices in Germany and a total of 662 outpatients, assessed the type and frequency of adverse events associated with the use of anthroposophi-cal medicines.[92] Several other cohort and cross-sectional studies have examined the use of complementary medicines, particularly herbal medicines, during pregnancy.[93–97]

The strengths and limitations of case–control and cohort studies are well documented,[98] but, as with other study designs, some of the problems are compounded when these study designs are applied to complementary medicines. For example, it is particularly problematic to establish and verify exposure of both cases and controls to the comple-mentary medicine(s) of interest because, in many countries, complemen-tary medicines are rarely prescribed by conventional healthcare professionals; even where complementary medicines are purchased from pharmacies, pharmacists do not routinely record use of comple-mentary medicines and other non-prescription medicines on compu-terised patient medication records.[13,14] In addition, for reasons explained earlier, there are likely to be variations in different manufacturers' prod-ucts and, therefore, defining exposure precisely will be difficult at best.

Case–control and cohort studies involving conventional prescribed medicines can be carried out using computerised health-record databases such as the UK General Practice Research Database and the Medicines Monitoring Unit database, but such tools are currently of no use for studies involving complementary medicines for the reasons given above, namely that complementary medicines are rarely prescribed and information on non-prescription medicines, including complementary medicines, rarely recorded on GPs' patient records.

As with case–control and cohort studies, experimental studies can be applied to investigating the safety of complementary medicines. At present, notwithstanding recognised limitations, such as sample size and ethical considerations, well-designed and well-conducted RCTs overcome some of the difficulties that complementary medicines present for other pharmacoepidemiological studies, e.g. precisely establishing exposure is simpler because compliance checks can be carried out, and RCTs are less likely to use complementary medicines, e.g. HMPs (containing the same herbal ingredient) from different manufacturers, so the possibility of product variation and batch-to-batch variation in products is reduced.[5] However, clinical trial participants could take purchased complementary medicines in addition to the study medication.

Systematic reviews and meta-analyses of adverse event data from RCTs of specific complementary medicines have been carried out, but this introduces other problems. Many existing RCTs of complementary medicines are of poor or limited methodological quality, and/or published reports of studies do not follow Consolidated Standards of Reporting Trials (CONSORT) guidelines.[99] In addition, different clinical trials of a particular herbal ingredient will usually have been carried out using different manufacturers' products, but systematic reviews and meta-analyses often ignore variations between products. An elaboration of item 4 in the original CONSORT guidelines, aimed at improving the quality of reporting descriptions of herbal medicine interventions tested in RCTs, has been published.[100,101] The elaborated guideline is also applicable to other clinical study designs and preclinical experiments.

Communication of information on safety concerns associated with complementary medicines

The importance of the timing, content and method of delivery of messages about safety concerns has been discussed extensively, and the requirements for successful communication of safety concerns should apply equally to complementary medicines. However, communicating information on these products presents additional difficulties for several reasons. Standard forms of communication, such as 'Dear Doctor/ Pharmacist' letters, can be sent, but healthcare professionals are unlikely to know which of their patients are using complementary medicines and, therefore, will be unable to pass on safety messages to specific individuals. Complementary medicine practitioners may keep some records of their patients' treatment, but, as complementary medicine practitioners are typically unregulated at present, there are no uniform standards with regard to record-keeping. Importantly, lists of all individuals practising complementary medicine are not available.

Most users of complementary medicines obtain their medicines from outlets where there is no healthcare professional present and without seeking professional advice. Methods aimed at reaching the public directly (e.g. the internet) and the popular media are often the only ways of communicating information on safety concerns to such individuals.

There is also a lack of research on how complementary medicine users interpret information on risks associated with complementary medicines. It should not be assumed that users' understanding of risk associated with complementary medicines is the same as that for prescription medicines or conventional non-prescription medicines. It has been shown that individuals may overestimate the risks of adverse effects associated with prescription medicines and conventional non-prescription medicines,[102,103] but, given that complementary medicines are widely perceived to be safe, the hypothesis that users of complementary medicines may underestimate risks needs to be tested. In the EU, the new directive on traditional HMPs requires manufacturers of products registered under the new national scheme to provide systematic information with their products, including information on adverse events and special warnings. The impact of this on users' perceptions of the risks associated with herbal medicines will also require evaluation.[5]

The action taken by the MHRA in the UK to communicate information on interactions between St John's wort and certain prescription medicines provides an example of the process of communicating information on herbal safety concerns (Box 6.4).

Box 6.4 Communication of information on St John's wort (*Hypericum perforatum*) herb products and drug interactions in the UK

In the year 2000, evidence emerged relating to important interactions between products containing St John's wort and certain prescription medicines. Following its decision that manufacturers should include warning information on product packaging, the Medicines and Healthcare products Regulatory Agency (MHRA) used various ways of communicating the message. 'Dear Doctor/Pharmacist' letters were sent, and pharmacists in particular were asked to provide advice to consumers and patients on interactions between St John's wort and conventional medicines. A telephone helpline was set up, and information for patients was posted on the MHRA website. However, it is difficult to assess the effectiveness of these measures. Since February 2000 when the information was made public, the Committee on Safety of Medicines (CSM)/MHRA Yellow Card scheme has continued to receive reports of suspected interactions between St John's wort and conventional medicines (more than 30 from February 2000 to April 2003), e.g. reports of breakthrough bleeding and unintended pregnancy in women taking St John's wort products together with oral contraceptives.[66] Pharmacists also received several other tailored items of information describing this safety issue;[104,105] despite this, in a small pseudo-patient study, a quarter of pharmacists provided unsatisfactory information on the potential interaction between St John's wort products and oral contraceptive agents.[106]

It is also likely that there is scope for improving communication with healthcare professionals and patients/consumers on complementary medicine safety issues. In recognition of this, an area on the MHRA website has been set up that is dedicated to providing early information on herbal safety concerns.[22]

The future for pharmacovigilance of complementary medicines

The potential for complementary medicines to have a significant negative impact on public health needs to be kept in perspective. Nevertheless, a parallel can be drawn between the lack of a formal medicine regulatory system before the thalidomide disaster and the current situation in several countries where complementary medicines are unregulated. In such countries, complementary medicines, including imported herbs with which there is no experience of traditional use in the importing country, are sold without any requirement to demonstrate to the licensing authority evidence of quality, safety and efficacy.

Post-thalidomide, new initiatives in drug safety monitoring initially followed further high-profile drug safety problems.[107] Likewise, several recent high-profile herbal safety concerns, such as renal failure and urothelial cancer associated with exposure to *Aristolochia* species,[108] drug interactions with St John's wort[109] and hepatotoxicity associated with kava-kava,[23] have contributed to the increasing awareness of the need to monitor the safety of herbal and complementary medicines. Against a background of increasing use of complementary medicines, particularly by patients using conventional drugs concurrently and those with serious chronic illness, it is likely that new safety concerns will continue to emerge.

Improvements in the safety and pharmacovigilance of complementary medicines, particularly herbal medicines, can be expected in the EU following the introduction of a new Directive for traditional HMPs that requires manufacturers of traditional HMPs registered under national schemes established under the Directive to adhere to recognised standards for pharmaceutical quality, provide bibliographic evidence of the safety of their products and comply with regulatory provisions on pharmacovigilance. These improvements may not happen immediately across all manufacturers, because some may take advantage of the 7-year transition period.

Another effect of the Directive may be to shift the emphasis of research involving herbal medicines. At present, most research in the herbal medicine area is aimed at discovering the pharmacological activities of medicinal plants and providing evidence of clinical efficacy; rather less effort is focused on investigating safety. However, as the proposed traditional HMP Directive does not require manufacturers to demonstrate efficacy (other than by way of traditional use), there may be more interest among manufacturers and researchers to extend knowledge of the safety of herbal medicines. Although research into the safety of herbal medicines is to be welcomed, research into efficacy is also needed in order to develop HMPs with favourable benefit–harm profiles.

Statutory regulation of herbal medicine practitioners is expected to be implemented over the next few years in several countries; some states of Australia and provinces of Canada have already taken this step. Once this has been achieved, it seems reasonable to expect that spontaneous reporting schemes would recognise statutory regulated herbal medicine practitioners as reporters (where they are not already encouraged to report), who would be encouraged to report suspected ADRs associated with herbal medicines.

In the longer term, modified, even novel tools for monitoring the safety of complementary medicines may be introduced. Pharmacy–record linkage is used in the Netherlands for pharmacovigilance purposes, and this could be an invaluable tool for monitoring safety of complementary medicines purchased through pharmacies. In the UK, a Department of Health report[110] has discussed the possibility of community pharmacists being able to access a common electronic health record, which will be created for all patients. Although such a system would probably apply only to prescription medicines initially, with technological advances it might also be developed into a computerised record–linkage database that could be used to monitor the safety of herbal and other non-prescription medicines. A small number of countries have already taken steps to allow patients/consumers a greater role in pharmacovigilance by including them as recognised reporters in spontaneous reporting schemes; consideration could be given to further extending the direct contribution of patients to monitoring the safety of complementary medicines, e.g. by collecting data directly from patients in studies based on modified PEM methodology.

In the future, publications describing case reports of suspected ADRs associated with complementary medicines may improve if authors of such reports and journal editors adhere to guidelines resulting from a joint initiative between members of the International Society of Pharmacovigilance and the International Society of Pharmacoepidemiology.[111] The guidelines include reference to publications of case reports of ADRs associated with herbal medicines.

Ensuring the safety of complementary medicines may lie, at least in part, with pharmacogenetics and pharmacogenomics. The importance of genetic factors in determining an individual's susceptibility to ADRs is well documented,[112] and this applies to complementary medicines as well as to conventional drugs.[113] However, optimising treatment, including reducing the potential for ADRs, on the basis of a patient's genotype has barely been discussed in the context of complementary medicines.

References

1. World Health Organization. *WHO Guidelines on Safety Monitoring of Herbal Medicines in Pharmacovigilance Systems.* Geneva: WHO, 2004.
2. World Health Organization. *The Importance of Pharmacovigilance.* Geneva: WHO, 2002.
3. Waller PC, Evans SJW. A model for the future conduct of pharmacovigilance. *Pharmacoepidemiol Drug Safety* 2003;**12**:17–29.
4. European Commission. Directive 2004/27/EC. Brussels: European Commission, 2004.
5. Barnes J. Pharmacovigilance of herbal medicines. A UK perspective. *Drug Safety* 2003;**26**:829–51.
6. Thomas KJ, Nicholl JP, Coleman P. Use and expenditure on complementary medicine in England: a population based survey. *Compl Ther Med* 2001; **9**:2–11.
7. MacLennan AH, Wilson DH, Taylor AW. The escalating cost and prevalence of alternative medicine. *Prev Med* 2002;**35**:166–73.

8. Eisenberg DM, Davis RB, Ettner SL, et al. Trends in alternative medicine use in the United States, 1990–1997: results of a national follow-up survey. *JAMA* 1998;**280**:1569–75.
9. Barnes J, Mills SY, Abbot NC et al. Different standards for reporting ADRs to herbal remedies and conventional OTC medicines: face-to-face interviews with 515 users of herbal remedies. *Br J Clin Pharmacol* 1998;**45**:496–500.
10. Gulian C, Barnes J, Francis S-A. Types and preferred sources of information concerning herbal medicinal products: face-to-face interviews with users of herbal medicinal products [abstract]. *Int J Pharm Prac* 2002;**10**(suppl):R33.
11. Vickers AJ, Rees RW, Robin A. Advice given by health food stores: is it clinically safe? *J R Coll Physicians Lond* 1998;**32**:426–8.
12. Quinn CG, Waterman P. A comparison of the teaching of herbal medicine in the United Kingdom and Europe. Undergraduate dissertation, University of Strathclyde, Glasgow, 1997.
13. Barnes J, Abbot NC. Experiences with complementary medicines: a survey of community pharmacists [abstract]. *Pharm J* 1999;**263**:R37, R43.
14. Barnes J. An examination of the role of the pharmacist in the safe, effective and appropriate use of complementary medicines. PhD thesis, University of London, 2001.
15. Cockayne NL, Duguid M, Shenfield GM. Health professionals rarely record history of complementary and alternative medicines. *Br J Clin Pharmacol* 2004;**59**:254–8.
16. Barnes J. Herbal therapeutics (1): an introduction to herbal medicinal products. *Pharm J* 2002;**268**:804–6.
17. Barnes J, Anderson LA, Phillipson JD. *Herbal Medicines*, 3rd edn. London: Pharmaceutical Press, 2007.
18. De Los Reyes GC, Koda RT. Determining hyperforin and hypericin content in eight brands of St John's wort. *Am J Health Syst Pharm* 2002;**59**:545–7.
19. Kressman S, Muller WE, Blume HH. Pharmaceutical quality of different *Ginkgo biloba* brands. *J Pharm Pharmacol* 2002;**54**:661–9.
20. Loew D, Kaszkin M. Approaching the problem of bioequivalence of herbal medicinal products. *Phytother Res* 2002;**16**:705–11.
21. Woodfield R. Senecio species in unlicensed herbal remedies [letter]. London: Medicines Control Agency, 2002.
22. Medicines and Healthcare products Regulatory Agency. *Herbal safety news*. Available at: http://medicines.mhra.gov.uk (accessed 29 July 2003).
23. Committee on Safety of Medicines' Expert Working Group (Kava). Report of the CSM's expert working group on the safety of kava. Medicines and Healthcare products Regulatory Agency, July 2006. Available at: www.mhra. gov.uk (accessed 25 September 2006).
24. Medicines and Healthcare products Regulatory Agency. *Black Cohosh*. UK Public Assessment Report. MHRA, July 2006. Available at: www.mhra. gov.uk (accessed 25 September 2006).
25. Medicines Control Agency. *Traditional Ethnic Medicines: Public health and compliance with medicines law*. London: Medicines Control Agency, 2001.
26. Barnes J, Teng L, Shaw D. TCM: balancing choice and risk? *Pharm J* 2004; **273**:342.

27. Teng L, Shaw D, Barnes J. Traditional Chinese herbal medicine. *Pharm J* 2006;**276**:361–3.
28. Williamson EM. Ayurveda: introduction for pharmacists. *Pharm J* 2006; **276**:108–10.
29. World Health Organization. *National Policy on Traditional Medicine and Regulation of Herbal Medicines.* Report of a WHO global survey. Geneva: WHO, 2005.
30. Adcock H. Medicines Control Agency proposes ban for kava-containing products. *Pharm J* 2002;**269**:128.
31. De Smet PAGM, Hänsel R, Keller K et al., eds. Toxicological outlook on quality assurance of herbal remedies. In: *Adverse Effects of Herbal Drugs*, Vol 1. Berlin: Springer Verlag, 1992.
32. Busse W. The significance of quality for efficacy and safety of herbal medicinal products. *Drug Inf J* 2000;**34**:15–23.
33. De Smet PAGM. Health risks of herbal remedies. *Drug Safety* 1995;**13**:81–93.
34. Commission of the European Communities. Directive 2004/24/EC on Traditional Herbal Medicinal Products. Brussels: European Commission, 2004.
35. Therapeutics Goods Act 1989. Available at: www.comlaw.gov.au (accessed 3 June 2008).
36. Therapeutic Goods Regulations 1990. Available at: www.comlaw.gov.au (accessed 3 June 2008).
37. Australian Regulatory Guidelines for Complementary Medicines (ARGCM). Available at: www.tga.gov.au/docs/html/argcm.htm (accessed 3 June 2008).
38. Medicines Act 1981. Available at: www.legislation.govt.nz (accessed 11 December 2007).
39. Dietary Supplement Regulations 1985. SR 1985/208. Available at: www. legislation.govt.nz (accessed 11 December 2007).
40. Food Act 1981. Available at: www.legislation.govt.nz (accessed 11 December 2007).
41. Medsafe and New Zealand Food Safety Authority. Letter to organisations involved in the manufacture, distribution and advertising of dietary supplements in New Zealand, 2007. Available at: www.medsafe.govt.nz (accessed 11 December 2007).
42. Australia New Zealand Therapeutic Products Authority. Postponement of the ANZTPA establishment project. Available at: www.anztpa.org (accessed 11 December 2007).
43. Food and Drug Administration. Department of Health and Human Services. Dietary Supplement Health and Education Act of 1994, Public Law 103–417, 103rd Congress. Available at: www.fda.gov/opacom/laws/dshea.html#sec3 (accessed 11 December, 2007).
44. Office of Dietary Supplements, National Institutes of Health. *Dietary Supplements. Background information.* Available at: http://ods.od.nih.gov/factsheets/DietarySupplements.asp (accessed 11 December, 2007).
45. GovTrack.us. S. 3546–109th Congress (2006): Dietary Supplement and Nonprescription Drug Consumer Protection Act, *GovTrack.us (database of federal legislation).* Available at: www.govtrack.us/congress/bill. xpd?bill=s109–3546 (accessed 11 December 2007).

46. Food and Drug Administration. Department of Health and Human Services. *Current Good Manufacturing Practice in Manufacturing, Packaging, Labeling, or Holding Operations for Dietary Supplements; Final Rule.* Federal Register: June 25, 2007;**72**(121);34751–958. Available at: www. cfsan.fda.gov/~lrd/fr07625a.html (accessed 11 December 2007).

47. Natural Health Products Regulations. *Canada Gazette* 2003;**137**(13). Available at: http://canadagazette.gc.ca/partII/2003/20030618/html/sor196-e. html (accessed 11 December, 2007).

48. Natural Health Products Directorate. *Natural Health Products Directorate Guidance Document.* Available at: www.hc-sc.gc.ca/dhp-mps/prodnatur/ legislation/docs/license-licence_guide_tc-tm_e.html (accessed 11 December 2007).

49. Ernst E, De Smet PA, Shaw D et al. Traditional remedies and the 'test of time'. *Eur J Clin Pharmacol* 1998;**54**:99–100.

50. World Health Organization. *WHO Policy Perspectives on Medicines. Pharmacovigilance: ensuring the safe use of medicines.* Geneva: WHO, 2004.

51. De Smet PAGM. An introduction to herbal pharmacovigilance. In: De Smet PAGM, Keller K, Hänsel R et al. (eds), *Adverse Effects of Herbal Drugs,* Vol 3. Berlin: Springer-Verlag, 1997: 1–13.

52. Chen Y. Safety monitoring of Traditional Chinese medicines in China. *Drug Safety* 2006;**29**:352 (abstract).

53. Dodoo ANO, Appiah-Danquah A, Gysana-Lutterodt M, Duwiejua M. Safety monitoring of herbal medicines in Ghana: challenges and opportunities. *Drug Safety* 2006;**29**:352 (abstract).

54. Dodoo ANO, Appiah-Danquah A. Safety of herbal medicines: the practitioners' view. *Drug Safety* 2006;**29**:350 (abstract).

55. Uppsala Monitoring Centre. *Global Intelligence Network for Benefits ad Risks in Medicinal Products.* UMC. Available at: www.who-umc.org (accessed 20 January 2007).

56. Farah MH, Edwards R, Lindquist M et al. International monitoring of adverse health effects associated with herbal medicines. *Pharmacoepidemiol Drug Safety* 2000;**9**:105–12.

57. World Health Organization Collaborating Centre for International Drug Monitoring. *Guidelines for Herbal ATC Classification.* Uppsala: The Uppsala Monitoring Centre, 2004.

58. World Health Organization Collaborating Centre for International Drug Monitoring. *Accepted Scientific Names of Therapeutic Plants and Their Synonyms.* Uppsala: The Uppsala Monitoring Centre, 2005.

59. Anon. Extension of the yellow card scheme to unlicensed herbal remedies. *Curr Prob Pharmacovigilance* 1996;**22**:10.

60. Shaw D, Leon C, Kolev S et al. Traditional remedies and food supplements: a 5-year toxicological study (1991–1995). *Drug Safety* 1997;**17**: 42–56.

61. Extension of the yellow card scheme to pharmacists. *Curr Prob Pharmacovigilance* 1997;**23**:3.

62. Committee on Safety of Medicines and Medicines and Healthcare Products Regulatory Agency. The yellow card scheme: extension of the yellow card scheme to nurse reporters (online). Available at: http://medicines.mhra.gov.uk/ aboutagency/regframework/csm/csmhome.htm (accessed 25 July 2003).

63. News item. MCA launches web version of yellow card scheme. *Pharm J* 2002; **269**:631.
64. News item. Patients able to report ADRs via NHS Direct. *Pharm J* 2003; **270**:608.
65. Raine J. The new European regulatory framework: implications for safety and pharmacovigilance of herbal medicines. Lecture presentation at International conference on Pharmacovigilance of herbal medicines: current state and future directions. London, April 2006.
66. Medicines and Healthcare products Regulatory Agency. *Adverse Drug Reaction On-line Information Tracking (ADROIT)S.* London: MHRA, 2003.
67. Barnes J, Aggarwal AM. Spontaneous reporting of ADRs associated with herbal medicines: final results of a cross-sectional survey of national pharmacovigilance centres. *Drug Safety* 2006;**29**:359 (abstract).
68. Updated 'yellow card' launched. *Pharm J* 2000;**265**:387.
69. Farah MH, Olsson S, Bate J et al. Botanical nomenclature in pharmacovigilance and a recommendation for standardisation. *Drug Safety* 2006;**29**: 1023–9.
70. Gogolak VV. The effect of backgrounds in safety analysis: the impact of comparison cases on what you see. *Pharmacoepidemiol Drug Safety* 2003;**12**: 249–52.
71. Bate A, Ericsson J, Farah M. International data mining for signals of herbal ADRs. *Drug Safety* 2006;**29**:353 (abstract).
72. Medicines Control Agency. Consultation MLX 286: proposals to prohibit the herbal ingredient kava-kava (*Piper methysticum*) in unlicensed medicines. London: Medicines Control Agency, 2002.
73. The Medicines for Human Use (Kava-Kava) (Prohibition) Order 2002 (SI2002/3170). London: The Stationery Office, 2003.
74. Van Grootheest K, de Graaf L, de Jong-van den Gerg LTW. Consumer adverse drug reaction reporting: a new step in pharmacovigilance? *Drug Safety* 2003;**26**:211–17.
75. Davis S, Coulson R. Community pharmacist reporting of suspected ADRs: (1) the first year of the yellow card demonstration scheme. *Pharm J* 1999;**263**: 786–8.
76. Wingfield J, Walmsley J, Norman C. What do Boots pharmacists know about yellow card reporting of adverse drug reactions? *Pharm J* 2002;**269**:109–10.
77. Green CF, Mottram DR, Raval D et al. Community pharmacists' attitudes to adverse drug reaction reporting. *Int J Pharm Prac* 1999;**7**:92–9.
78. Biscoe R, Houghton JE, Woods FJ. An audit of the level of encouragement given by medicines information pharmacists to enquirers of suspected adverse drug reactions to complete a yellow card report: perspectives in patient safety (abstract). 28th UK Medicines Information Conference Proceedings, 19–21 September 2002, Chester, UK.
79. News item. Pharmacists' adverse drug reaction reporting to start on April 1. *Pharm J* 1997;**258**:330–1.
80. Major E. The yellow card scheme and the role of pharmacists as reporters. *Pharm J* 2002;**269**:25–6.
81. Cox A. Embracing ADR reporting could improve pharmacists' standing (letter). *Pharm J* 2002;**269**:14.

82. Moffat T. *Adverse Drug Reaction (ADR) Reporting by Pharmacists.* London: Royal Pharmaceutical Society of Great Britain, 2003.
83. Broughton AL. Adverse event reporting by herbal practitioners: the National Institute of Medical Herbalists yellow card reporting scheme. *Drug Safety* 2006;**29**:348 (abstract).
84. Booker T. The Register of Chinese Herbal Medicine 'yellow card scheme'. *Drug Safety* 2006;**29**:349 (abstract).
85. Mills S. The ESCOP perspective on ADRs and ADR reporting. *Drug Safety* 2006;**29**:350 (abstract).
86. British Herbal Medicine Association. *Code of Good Practice: Unlicensed herbal remedies.* Bournemouth: British Herbal Medicine Association, 1997.
87. Shakir SAW. PEM in the UK. In: Mann RD, Andrews EB (eds), *Pharmacovigilance.* Chichester: Wiley, 2002: 333–44.
88. Layton D, Sinclair HK, Bond CM et al. Pharmacovigilance of over-the-counter products based in community pharmacy: methodological issues from pilot work conducted in Hampshire and Grampian, UK. *Pharmacoepidemiol Drug Safety* 2002;**11**:503–13.
89. Sinclair HK, Bond CM, Hannaford PC. Pharmacovigilance of over-the-counter products based in community pharmacy: a feasible option? *Pharmacoepidemiol Drug Safety* 1999;**8**:479–91.
90. Layton D, Denham A, Whitelegg ME et al. Methodology of a feasibility study to assess the application of prescription event monitoring (PEM) to monitor the safety of herbal medicines. *Drug Safety* 2006;**29**:355 (abstract).
91. Aggarwal AM, Barnes J. A pilot study of community-pharmacy-based pharmacovigilance of an over-the-counter herbal medicine ginkgo (*Ginkgo biloba*): methodological issues from work in progress. *Drug Safety* 2006; **29**:358 (abstract).
92. Hamre HJ, Witt CM, Glockmann A, Tröger W, Willich SN, Kiene H. Use and safety of anthroposophic medications in chronic disease. A 2-year prospective analysis. *Drug Safety* 2006;**29**:1173–89.
93. Chuang CH, Doyle P, Wang JD, Chang PJ, Lai JN, Chen PC. Herbal medicines used during the first trimester and major congenital malformations. An analysis of data from a pregnancy cohort study. *Drug Safety* 2006;**29**: 537–48.
94. Nordeng H, Havnen GC. Use of herbal drugs in pregnancy: a survey among 400 Norwegian women. *Pharmacoepidemiol Drug Safety* 2004;**13**:371–80.
95. Tsui B, Dennehy CE, Tsourounis C. A survey of dietary supplement use during pregnancy at an academic medical center. *Am J Obstet Gynecol* 2001; **185**:433–7.
96. Gibson PS, Powrie R, Star J. Herbal and alternative medicine use during pregnancy: a cross-sectional survey. *Obstet Gynecol* 2001;**97**(suppl 1):S44–5.
97. Gallo M, Sarkar M, Au W et al. Pregnancy outcome following gestational exposure to Echinacea: a prospective controlled study. *Arch Intern Med* 2000;**160**:3141–3.
98. Strom BL. How should one perform pharmacoepidemiology studies? Choosing among the available alternatives. In: Strom BL (ed.), *Pharmacoepidemiology*, 3rd edn. Chichester: Wiley, 2000: 401–13.

99. Moher DG, Schulz KF, Altman DG. The CONSORT statement: revised recommendations for improving the quality of reports of parallel-group randomized trials. *Ann Intern Med* 2001;**134**:657–62.

100. Gagnier JJ, Boon H, Rochon P, Moher D, Barnes J, Bombardier C, for the CONSORT group. Reporting randomized, controlled trials of herbal interventions: an elaborated CONSORT statement. *Ann Intern Med* 2006;**144**: 364–7.

101. Gagnier JJ, Boon H, Rochon P, Moher D, Barnes J, Bombardier C, for the CONSORT Group. Recommendations for reporting randomized controlled trials of herbal interventions: explanation and elaboration. *J Clin Epidemiol* 2006;**59**:1134–49.

102. Berry DC, Knapp PR, Raynor DK. Is 15% very common: informing people about the risks of medication side effects. *Int J Pharm Prac* 2002;**10**:145–51.

103. Berry DC, Raynor DK, Knapp P et al. Patients' understanding of risk associated with medication use: impact of European Commission guidelines and other risk scales. *Drug Safety* 2003;**26**:1–11.

104. Barnes J, RPSGB Complementary Medicine Working Group. *Herb–medicine Interactions: St John's wort (*Hypericum perforatum*). Useful information for pharmacists.* London: RPSGB, 2002 (factsheet).

105. Barnes J, Anderson LA, Phillipson JD. Herbal therapeutics (10). Herbal interactions. *Pharm J* 2003;**270**:118–21.

106. Consumers' Association. Can your pharmacist cope? *Which?* 2004; February:10–13.

107. Edwards IR, Olsson S. WHO programme: global monitoring. In: Mann RD, Andrews EB (eds), *Pharmacovigilance*. Chichester: Wiley, 2002: 169–82.

108. Cosyns J-P. Aristolochic acid and 'Chinese herbs nephropathy': a review of the evidence to date. *Drug Safety* 2003;**26**:33–48.

109. Henderson L, Yue QY, Bergquist C et al. St John's wort (*Hypericum perforatum*): drug interactions and clinical outcomes. *Br J Clin Pharmacol* 2002;**54**:349–56.

110. Department of Health. *A Vision for Pharmacy in the New NHS*. London: Department of Health, 2003.

111. Kelly WN, Arellano FM, Barnes J et al. Guidelines for submitting adverse event reports for publication. *Drug Safety* 2007;**30**:367–73.

112. Pirmohamed M, Park BK. Genetic susceptibility to ADRs. *Trends Pharmacol Sci* 2001;**22**:298–305.

113. Pirmohamed M. Pharmacogenomics and herbal medicines. *Drug Safety* 2006;**29**:356 (abstract).

Part 2

Therapies involving
use of medicines

7

Homeopathy and anthroposophy

Steven B Kayne

Homeopathy, because of its availability under the National Health Service (NHS) in the UK since its inception in 1948, is often considered to be the most important of the complementary disciplines. In fact, it is not the UK's most popular therapy by total market value, and it is likely that herbal and perhaps also aromatherapy products will be fully reimbursable under the NHS in the foreseeable future.

Anthroposophical medicine is associated with homeopathy but has some important differences. These are discussed at the end of the chapter.

Homeopathy

Definition

Homeopathy is a complementary discipline based on the law of similars, which involves the administration of ultra-dilute medicines prepared according to methods specified in various homeopathic pharmacopoeias with the aim of stimulating a person's own capacity to heal.

The terms 'law of similars' and 'homeopathic pharmacopoeias' will be further defined in the text.

History

The development of modern homeopathy

The practice of homeopathy has changed little in the last 200 years or so in the way that its medicines have been used. In direct contrast to orthodox medicine (OM), only a handful of new medicines have joined the modern homeopath's armamentarium. For this reason, the founder of modern homeopathy, the German physician and apothecary Samuel Hahnemann, left a powerful legacy to successive generations. The medicines are largely prepared and administered as they were in the very early days of the discipline. Thus, the history of homeopathy, and especially that of its founder, occupies an important part in teachings on the subject.

Christian Friedrich Samuel Hahnemann was born just before midnight on 10 April 1755 in Meissen, the ancient town renowned for its porcelain and situated on the banks of the river Elbe, approximately 180 km south of Berlin.

His parents were Johanna Christiane and Christian Gottfried Hahnemann. To avoid confusion with the many other family members with the same first name, the infant was known throughout his long and eventful life as Samuel. He qualified as a physician at the Frederick Alexander University in Erlangen in 1779. At this time disease was viewed as an invader to the body, to be fought with whatever chemical or other method that was in favour at the time. Blood letting, purgatives, emetics and leeches were all used, as was the administration of large quantities of chemicals, including arsenic and mercury.

Increasing frustration with such methods of treatment caused Hahnemann to withdraw from medical practice and concentrate on writing. In 1790 he translated and annotated *Materia Medica* (Figure 7.1), written by the eminent Scottish physician William Cullen (1710–90), who practised in Edinburgh and was considered to be a medical guru by many of his European colleagues during the second half of the eighteenth century.

Cullen had devoted 20 pages in his book to Cinchona (Peruvian bark), a drug that was administered widely for the treatment of malaria, then known as the ague or marsh fever. Hahnemann disagreed with Cullen's suggested mechanism of action as an astringent, and he decided to test the drug by taking relatively large doses himself. He found that the resulting toxic effects were very similar to the symptoms suffered by patients with marsh fever. Similar effects were witnessed for the use of Belladonna to treat scarlet fever, a disease with similar symptoms to those shown by people suffering from Belladonna poisoning.

Hahnemann then tried a number of other active substances on himself, his family and volunteers to obtain evidence to substantiate his findings. In each case he found that the medicines could bring on the symptoms of the diseases for which they were being used as a treatment. Thus he systematically built up considerable circumstantial evidence for

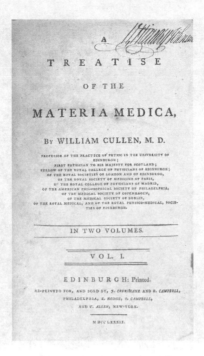

A

T R E A T I S E

OF THE

MATERIA MEDICA,

By WILLIAM CULLEN, M. D.

PROFESSOR OF THE PRACTICE OF PHYSIC IN THE UNIVERSITY OF
EDINBURGH;
FIRST PHYSICIAN TO HIS MAJESTY FOR SCOTLAND;
FELLOW OF THE ROYAL COLLEGE OF PHYSICIANS OF EDINBURGH;
OF THE ROYAL SOCIETIES OF LONDON AND OF EDINBURGH,
OF THE ROYAL SOCIETY OF MEDICINE OF PARIS,
OF THE ROYAL COLLEGE OF PHYSICIANS OF MADRID,
OF THE AMERICAN PHILOSOPHICAL SOCIETY OF PHILADELPHIA,
OF THE MEDICAL SOCIETY OF COPENHAGEN,
OF THE MEDICAL SOCIETY OF BERLIN,
OF THE ROYAL MEDICAL, AND OF THE ROYAL PHYSICO-MEDICAL, SOCIE-
TIES OF EDINBURGH.

IN TWO VOLUMES.

VOL. I.

EDINBURGH: Printed.
RE-PRINTED FOR, AND SOLD BY, J. CRUKSHANK AND E. CAMPBELL,
PHILADELPHIA, E. HODGE, T. CAMPBELL,
AND T. ALLEN, NEW-YORK.

M DCC LXXXIX.

Figure 7.1 Cullen's *Materia Medica* was Hahnemann's inspiration for his involvement in homeopathy while translating the book. (From the author's collection.)

the existence of a law of cure based on the concept of using 'like to treat like'. He called the systematic procedure of testing substances on healthy human beings in order to elucidate the symptoms reflecting the use of the medicine a *Prüfung*, which is translated into English as 'proving'.

Hahnemann returned to medicine in 1801, using his new homeopathic principles. Many colleagues viewed his methods with considerable scepticism despite a number of spectacular successes. In 1810 Hahnemann published his most famous work, the *Organon of the Rational Art of Healing*.[1] A total of five editions of this book appeared during Hahnemann's lifetime; the manuscript for a sixth edition was not published until many years after his death. The subject matter in the sixth edition was set out in 291 numbered sections or aphorisms, usually denoted in the literature by the symbol § and the relevant section number.

Following the death of his first wife Johanna in 1830, Hahnemann married the Marquise Melanie D'Hervilly-Gohier, a colourful and eccentric companion many years his junior. The couple moved to Paris, where he died in 1843.

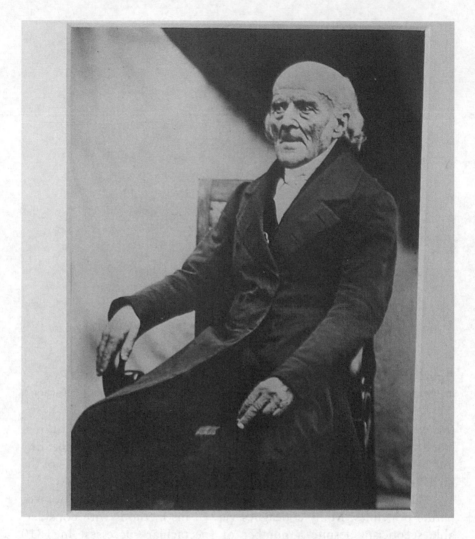

Figure 7.2 Photograph of Samuel Hahnemann taken on 30 September 1841 by H Foucault of Paris. (Courtesy of Faculty of Homeopathy Museum.)

Figure 7.2 shows a photograph of Hahnemann 2 years before his death. The photograph was originally the property of the Reverend T. Everest, who recorded:

> It was a dark rainy day, with violent gusts of wind, all which circum-stances by increasing the difficulty of taking the photograph, have given the countenance of Hahnemann an air of stiffness. Hahnemann was, moreover, rather unwell that day.

Theory

The mechanisms of action of homeopathy are not understood, although many possible explanations for them have been put forward. There are claims that the apparent success of homeopathy is due solely to a placebo effect. This may well be true to some extent (as in orthodox medicine), but is only part of the story.

The vital force

Homeopaths consider disease to be an expression of the vital force of each individual. As all individuals are quite different in their expression of the vital force, patients are treated according to their idiosyncratic, rather than their common, symptoms. The symptoms are important only in that they act as an indicator for the selection of an appropriate medicine.

Hahnemann introduced the word 'dynamis' to describe the vital force indicating that life was dynamic and took an active part in organising biological activity. He called the process of potentising medicines (see below) 'dynamisation', a term that is still widely used by French and German homeopaths. Vitalists believe that the body comprises a hierarchy of parts (cells, tissues, organs and systems) that are all fully interdependent in both ascending and descending order, and with an interrelationship that is controlled by a vital force. Under normal conditions, the vital force is thought to be responsible for the orderly and harmonious running of the body, and for coordinating the body's defences against disease. However, if the force becomes disturbed by factors such as emotional stress, poor diet, environmental conditions or certain inappropriate allopathic drugs, then illness results.

It is suggested that the vital force operates on three different vibratory levels:

1. Mental: changes in understanding and consciousness are recorded (e.g. confusion and lack of concentration)
2. Emotional: changes in emotional states are recorded (e.g. anxiety and irritability)
3. Physical: changes to the body's organs and systems are recorded (e.g. organ malfunction and disease).

Classic homeopaths consider the body's functions to be a *mélange* of all these levels when determining which homeopathic medicine is appropriate to restore the vital force to its normal levels. They consider the totality of symptoms rather than looking at individual planes in isolation. If only a partial image of the total symptom picture is acquired, they consider that the effect of the medicine will be limited to that vibrational level.

This comprehensive approach is not the only way homeopathic medicines can be used. It is possible to administer medicines chosen for their local effect in the physical plane alone. This approach is used especially for first aid and the treatment of many simple self-limiting situations.

The three principles of homeopathy

There are three important principles of homeopathy according to Hahnemann: like cures like, minimal dose and single medicine.

Like cures like

This principle first appeared in an article entitled 'Essay on a new principle for ascertaining the curative power of drugs'.[2] Hahnemann believed that, in order to cure disease, one must seek medicines that can excite similar symptoms in the healthy human body. This idea is summarised in the phrase *similia similibus curentur*, often translated as 'let like be treated with like'.

Examples of such treatment might be the homeopathic use of the following:

- Apis (from the bee) to treat histamine-type reactions resulting from a sting
- Coffea (from the green coffee bean) to treat insomnia
- Urtica (from the nettle) to treat an urticarial rash.

At first sight, this method is rather different to the orthodox approach, in which the use of a laxative to treat diarrhoea might be viewed rather strangely! However, there are examples of this practice in orthodox medicine where large doses of digoxin cause many of the cardiac arrhythmias for which it is a treatment and large doses of aspirin cause headaches.

It was this method of prescribing according to the matching of symptoms and drug pictures that prompted Hahnemann in 1807 to coin the term 'homeopathy' from the Greek words *homoios* (similar) and *pathos* (disease or suffering). He termed the more orthodox treatment by the law of contraries 'allopathy' from *alloios*, meaning contrary. This term is still widely used today.

Minimal dose

When Hahnemann carried out his original work he gave substantial doses of medicine to his patients, in keeping with contemporary practice. This often resulted in substantial toxic reactions; fatalities were not uncommon. He experimented to try to dilute out the unwanted toxicity while at the same time maintaining a therapeutic effect. There is much speculation as to how Hahnemann developed the method of serial dilution and agitation of his medicines, which achieved his aim better than he could have hoped. To his surprise Hahnemann found that, as the medicines became more dilute, they became more potent therapeutically. To reflect this effect he called his new process 'potentisation'. The potentisation process is described in detail below.

Single medicine

Hahnemann believed that one should use a single medicine to treat a condition. Provings in all materia medicas relate to single medicines and there is no way of knowing whether or how individual medicine drug pictures are modified by combination with other ingredients. Classic homeopaths observe this rule carefully. In later life Hahnemann did use mixtures of two or three medicines and there are a limited number of such mixtures still used today, including Arsen iod, Gelsemium and Eupatorium (AGE, for colds and flu) and Aconite (or sometimes Arsen alb), Belladonna and Chamomilla (ABC, for teething).

Holistic approach

In addition to the three principles stated above, Hahnemann believed that homeopathy should be practised according to the holistic principles that are common to all complementary disciplines (see Chapter 1). Each patient should be treated as a complete individual. This means that medicines (or procedures) appropriate for one patient might be totally inappropriate for another even though the symptoms may be similar. Conversely, the same medicine may be used to treat very different conditions in different patients. Both general practice and homeopathic consultations are organised around the key task of treating patients' health-related problems. Despite their different theories of healing, interactions between professionals and patients in both share many features, although there are also clear differences in the ways in which patients and professionals go about the process of problem-solving.[3]

Homeopathic laws of cure

There are three laws of cure that may be applied to the practice of homeopathy: Hering's law, Arndt's law and the law of minimum action.

Hering's law

This law is attributed to the American homeopath Dr Constantine Hering. It states that cure takes place:

- from the top to the bottom of the body
- from the inside to the outside
- from the most important organs to the least important
- in reverse order of the onset of symptoms.

Hence mental symptoms (emotions) might be expected to improve before physical symptoms are resolved, and recent symptoms will subside before long-standing chronic symptoms. A good example of this law in practice is the resolution of asthma, which is often associated with skin conditions. It is not uncommon to see the physical symptoms of asthma improving only to find an underlying skin condition becoming more pronounced.

Arndt's law

This is a general law that states that:

- weak stimuli encourage living systems (e.g. homeopathy)
- medium-strength stimuli impede living systems (e.g. biochemical pathway blockers)
- strong stimuli tend to destroy living systems (e.g. chemotherapy).

It is suggested that small quantities of homeopathic medicine administered to an individual stimulate the body's own defence mechanisms to deal with disease. In fact, the situation is probably much more complicated than this simplistic explanation suggests, and is not as yet understood (see below).

Law of minimum action

The third law is associated with the minute doses administered in homeopathy:

- A change in nature is effected by the least possible action.
- The decisive amount of action needed to produce change is always the minimum.

Clinical experience suggests that the minute amounts of active ingredients administered by homeopaths are still sufficient to produce a therapeutic effect. It is generally accepted that the frequency of administration is more significant than the size of the dose.

Proving homeopathic medicines

All homeopathic medicines have a 'drug picture', a written survey of the symptoms noted when the drug was given to healthy volunteers, a process known as 'proving the drug'. Hahnemann defined very precisely guidelines for carrying out provings.

Theoretically, the proving of a substance refers to all the symptoms induced by the substance in healthy people, according to Hahnemann's original instructions. However, drug pictures may also contain symptoms derived from the following sources:[4]

- Observations of toxological effects arising from therapeutic, deliberate or accidental administration
- Observations of pathological symptoms regularly cured by the medicine in clinical practice: this is the source of many seemingly strange symptoms that occur in some drug pictures.

In some instances the complete drug picture may be derived from toxicological or clinical observations and not from a true proving at all.

The drug pictures are collected together in materia medicas, many of which have been computerised. These are usually consulted when an appropriate medicine is being chosen to treat a patient (see below).

Nomenclature of homeopathic medicines

Homeopathic products are traditionally called remedies, although the term 'medicine' is preferred by many people. The existing nomenclature of homeopathic medicines and the connected abbreviation system by which medicines are identified have evolved over 200 years and are full of irregularities and mistakes. Traditionally medicines are described by an abbreviation of the Latin name together with an indication of the potency. There are so many synonyms, different spellings, different abbreviations and differences in the source material used for the medicine preparation that it is difficult to avoid confusion. However, within a particular country it is unlikely that any conflict will arise. Patients are well advised to take any prescribed medication with them when they travel because the medicine obtained abroad may be different to the medicine that they are used to buying in their own country.

Some examples that illustrate sources of potential confusion have been highlighted in a report prepared under the auspices of the European Committee for Homeopathy.[5] Most botanical names currently used in homeopathy are still similar to the current botanical nomenclature used for the source material. However, other medicines have other synonyms that do not correspond with either the pharmacopoeias or the current botanical names. For example, Belladonna (more correctly *Atropa belladonna*), Cactus grandiflorus (*Cercus grandiflorus*) and Chamomilla (*Matricaria chamomilla*) all have commonly used homeopathic names that are incorrect. Further, the botanical nomenclature used in homeopathy does not indicate the part of the plant that has been used. In some countries the whole plant is used; in other countries it can be the root, seeds, leaves, or flowers or fruits.

Most zoological names currently used in homeopathy are still similar to the current zoological nomenclature, such as *Apis mellifica* (bee), *Latrodectus mactans* (spider) and *Vespa cabro* (wasp). Some, however, are not. For example, the medicine known as Cantharis would be more correctly called *Lytta vesicatoria*. Medicines from chemical sources have their problems too. Compounds with fluorine, calcium, bromium, iodine, oxygen and sulphur ions are usually called fluoratums, bromatums, iodatums, sulphuratums, etc., but calcium fluoride is called Calcarea fluorica in some countries and Calcium fluoricum in others, which is inconsistent (Calcium fluoratum would be more logical).

Many of the nosode names (nosode is defined below) currently used in homeopathy are insufficiently specified names, e.g. Psorinum, Carcinosinum, Tuberculinum and Medorrhinum. The nosodes often show different starting materials and manufacturing methods in different communities.

Homeopathy needs a consistent international nomenclature system to ensure the accurate supply of currently available medicines and the logical incorporation of new medicines in the future. The European

Committee on Homeopathy has made proposals for the development of a more logical system of abbreviations that will ensure international standardisation.

Difficulties with nomenclature are not confined to naming medicines. A group of Latin American and European authors have pointed out that international confusion also exists as to the exact meaning of many words used routinely in homeopathy and they suggest that many inaccurate or imprecise terms should be replaced.[6]

The manufacture of homeopathic medicines

The homeopathic pharmacopoeias

Homeopathic medicines are prepared in accordance with the methods described in various national homeopathic pharmacopoeias. For many years British manufacturers have relied on a selection of foreign reference works, principally the *German Homeopathic Pharmacopoeia* (GHP, or HAB in the German abbreviation) with its various supplements, together with the *French Pharmacopoeia* and the *Homeopathic Pharmacopoeia of the US* (HPUS), for most of their information, particularly with regard to the analysis of starting materials. After an interval of almost 100 years a new edition of the *British Homeopathic Pharmacopoeia* (BHomP) was published by the British Association of Homeopathic Manufacturers (BAHM) in 1993[7] and this is used alongside the GHP, although the BHomP has not been formally adopted as a national pharmacopoeia by the Medicine and Healthcare products Regulatory Agency (MHRA) and has no status under European legislation (see the section on Regulatory affairs, below). A second edition of this text was published in 1999.[8]

The methods of preparing medicines differ between the various pharmacopoeias and this introduces an international variable, e.g. the German text states that to make a mother tincture the source material must be macerated for at least 10 days at a temperature not exceeding 30°C, whereas the French publication specifies a period of 3 weeks. Little research has been carried out to quantify the variance in active principles that may occur, although nuclear magnetic resonance techniques exist for testing different source materials.[9] These differences mean that medicines may well differ from country to country even though the potencies appear to be equivalent.

The source materials

Plant material

Well over half of all homeopathic medicines are prepared from extracts of plant materials and, because of this, homeopathy is often confused with herbalism. However, the ways of producing the two types of medicines are quite different. Herbal products are generally the result of an aqueous or alcoholic extraction alone, whereas in homeopathy an additional dilution process is involved. Either the whole plant may be used or only selected parts, as specified in the pharmacopoeia monographs. The specimens are collected in dry sunny weather and cleaned by careful shaking, brushing and rinsing with distilled water. They are then examined to ensure the absence of moulds and other imperfections. Fresh plant material is desirable, but for a variety of reasons dried specimens are sometimes used. Arnica, for example, grows best above 3000 metres and is often subject to conservation orders at certain times of the year, whereas Nux vomica is readily available in relatively large amounts, but is difficult to obtain in the very small quantities required by homeopathic pharmacists. Soil differences may mean that the most easily accessible plants are not the most suitable. Crataegus, the hawthorn, varies in quality from country to country. These difficulties may be appreciated if one considers the analogy of wines: grapes grown in different soil and climatic conditions, even if adjacent to each other, produce wines with different characteristics. Calendula, which is used for the treatment of superficial abrasions, is illustrated in Figure 7.3.

Animal and insect material

This material must be obtained from healthy specimens. The bee yields Apis, a medicine used to treat peripheral oedematous conditions and the effects of stings. Other examples are medicines made from snake and spider venoms, musk oil and the juice of the cuttlefish (Sepia). Musk is obtained from the African cevit, a fox-like animal kept in battery accommodation, mainly in Ethiopia. There have been calls recently for the practice of milking animals to be discontinued in favour of synthetic production.

Other biological material

Biological source material is used to prepare isopathic medicines (for definition of isopathy see below) that include:

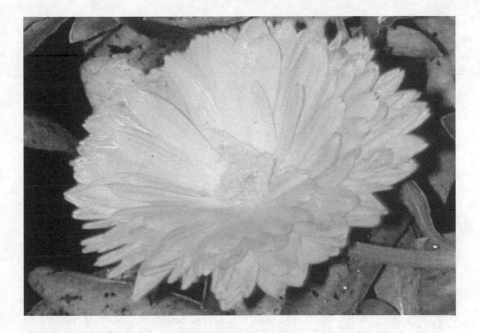

Figure 7.3 *Calendula officinalis* (marigold): the plant is used to make oral and topical products in both homeopathy and herbalism.

- allergodes (e.g. grass pollens, flowers, animal hair, feathers, foods)
- sarcodes (e.g. bacterial cultures or healthy secretions)
- nosodes (pathological samples).

Chemical material

Highly purified chemical material is rarely used in the preparation of medicine, e.g. Calcium carbonicum is obtained from the interspaces of oyster shells and is not prepared in the laboratory. Sulphur is obtained from a naturally occurring source (e.g. a geothermal area) and is not precipitated in the laboratory. Chemical material and drugs may also be used in the preparation of isopathic medicines known as tautodes (see below).

Imponderables

Homeopathy uses the word imponderables for all the medicines that are not material substances. Examples include:

- Magnetis poli ambo, magnetis polus arcticus, magnetis polus australis (medicines from magnetism)
- Sol (sunlight)
- Ultraviolet (UV) rays
- X-ray.

Preparation of medicines

The preparation of homeopathic medicines is graphically represented in Figure 7.4

Stage 1: extraction procedure

Mother tinctures are liquid preparations resulting from the extraction of suitable vegetable source material with, usually, alcohol/water mixtures. They form the starting point for the production of most homeopathic medicines, although some are used orally (e.g. Crataegus) or topically (e.g. Arnica). The resulting extract solutions contain on average one part drug to three parts mother tincture, although this strength can vary depending on the species and type of extraction process. The solutions are strained to remove any extraneous pieces of debris.

Insoluble chemicals such as Aurum (gold), Graphites (graphite or lead) and Sulphur (and most isopathic preparations) must be processed differently. The solid material is triturated with lactose in a pestle and mortar. The resulting triturate may be compressed directly into trituration tablets or administered as a powder. More usually, however, trituration continues until the particle size has been reduced sufficiently to facilitate the preparation of a solution, usually achieved after three to six serial dilutions depending on the scale being used. From this point the standard potentisation procedure described below can be followed.

In the case of soluble chemicals, solutions of known concentration in distilled water or alcohol can be prepared initially as the starting solution.

Stage 2: the potentisation ('dynamisation') process

With some medicines, e.g. Arnica or Calendula, the mother tincture may be applied directly to the skin, or it may be diluted and used as a gargle; Crataegus mother tincture is often administered as five drops in water. Most mother tinctures, however, are diluted in a special manner. As this dilution increases the homeopathic strength (although the

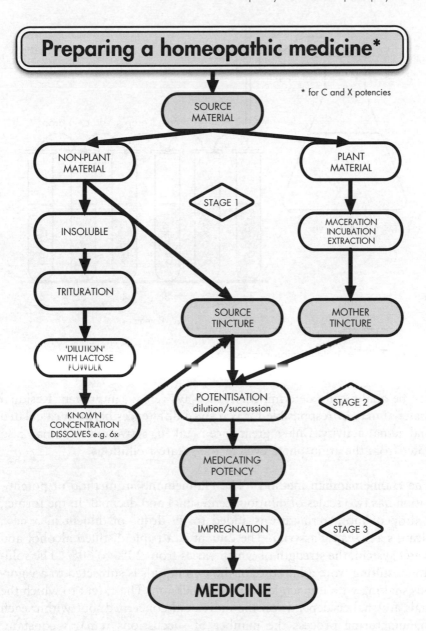

Preparing a homeopathic medicine*

* for C and X potencies

SOURCE MATERIAL

NON-PLANT MATERIAL

PLANT MATERIAL

STAGE 1

INSOLUBLE

MACERATION INCUBATION EXTRACTION

TRITURATION

SOURCE TINCTURE

MOTHER TINCTURE

'DILUTION' WITH LACTOSE POWDER

POTENTISATION dilution/succussion

STAGE 2

KNOWN CONCENTRATION DISSOLVES e.g. 6x

MEDICATING POTENCY

IMPREGNATION

STAGE 3

MEDICINE

Figure 7.4 Summary of preparation process.[10]

chemical concentration decreases), the process is known as potentisation (Figure 7.5). In homeopathy, as elsewhere, dilution is never perfect, particularly at low concentrations where surface absorption may well be a major factor, so that the real degree of dilution beyond the levels that

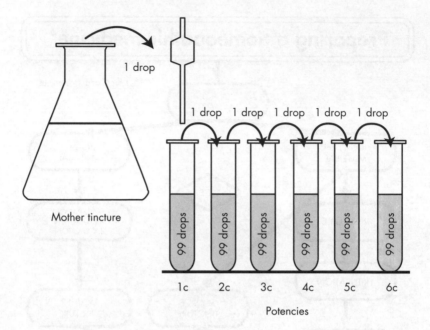

Figure 7.5 The potentisation process.

can be analytically determined will always remain unproven. Residual material may be responsible for perceived differences between calculated and actual activity. Unless great care is taken, active material may also enter from the atmosphere even at the greatest dilutions.

The Hahnemannian method The Hahnemannian method of potentisation has two scales of dilution: centesimal and decimal. In the former, 1 drop of mother tincture is added to 99 drops of diluent in a new, clean, screw-cap glass vial. The diluent is a triple-distilled alcohol and water system, the strength of which varies from 20% to 60%. The solution resulting from admixture of the two liquids is subjected to a vigorous shaking with impact, known as succussion. The extent to which the vials are shaken depends on the individual concerned, but within each manufacturing process the number of succussions remains constant. Hahnemann's ideas on how often to succuss the vial varied widely from once or twice right up to 100 times. After the initial process, successive serial dilutions are made, using fresh glass vials at each stage until the solution reaches 12c, 30c, 200c, etc. (the number refers to the number of successive 1 in 100 dilutions and 'c' indicates the centesimal method). The stages are summarised in Table 7.1. In the decimal scale, one drop

Table 7.1 Centesimal potencies

Centesimal potency	Concentration	Dilution
1 (1c or 1cH)	10^{-2}	1:100
6 (6c or 6cH)	10^{-12}	$1:10^{12}$
12 (12c or 12cH)	10^{-24}	$1:10^{24}$
30 (30c or 30cH)	10^{-60}	$1:10^{60}$
200 (200c or 200cH)	10^{-400}	$1:10^{400}$
M^a	10^{-2000}	$1:10^{2000}$
10M^a	$10^{-20\,000}$	$1:10^{20\,000}$

^{a}Korsakovian dilutions

Table 7.2 Decimal potencies

Decimal potency	Concentration	Dilution
1x (D1)	10^{-1}	1:10
6x (D6)	10^{-6}	$1:10^{6}$
12x (D12)	10^{-12}	$1:10^{12}$
00x (D00)	10^{-70}	1.10^{70}

of mother tincture is added to nine drops of diluent. This is indicated by a number and 'x' (e.g. 6x). At the higher centesimal dilutions, letters are normally used. The 1000 dilution level is therefore M and 100.000 is CM (Table 7.2).

Potencies up to 200c are often still made by hand by skilled operators agitating the container between each serial dilution stage by striking it on the heel of the hand. Most large manufacturers have small mechanical shakers that perform the task with rather less effort. At very high potencies medicines are usually made robotically using the Korsakovian method

The Korsakovian method There is some doubt concerning how M and 10M potencies are made. These are often described as being 1000 and 10 000 centesimal dilutions. Although it is still possible to prepare potencies of this magnitude according to Hahnemann's original instructions using special machinery, many of these medicines are prepared robotically using a method described in 1832 by the Russian homeopath Nicolaevich Korsakov, although they are seldom correctly labelled to show this.

A first dilution known as 1K or 1cK is prepared by adding a measured volume of mother tincture to an appropriate volume of diluent and the resulting solution succussed thoroughly. Liquid is then removed from the vial by suction or inversion, leaving droplets of solution adhering to the container wall. New solvent is then added, the vial agitated vigorously and the process repeated. Korsakovian potencies are usually denoted by a number denoting the number of serial dilutions followed by the letter 'K' (e.g. 1000K).

The LM method   In later life Hahnemann began using potencies based on serial dilutions of 1:50 000 at each level. These are called LM (or occasionally Q) potencies. Medicines are triturated to the third centesimal level with lactose before being diluted according to the scale described above. Homeopaths often instruct patients to succuss LM potencies before taking each dose to minimise the possibility of developing the symptoms of the medicine.

The effects of potentisation   One of the fundamental tenets of homeopathy is the concept of potentisation, and yet it continues to be one of the major stumbling blocks to its widespread acceptance, with many sceptics claiming that it is just a myth.[11] It is not known how Hahnemann came upon the procedure of potentisation; most probably it arose from his knowledge of chemistry and alchemy. Over the past three decades research into structure formation and structure conservation in water systems has created significant interest in the homeopathic community. Geometric and dynamic models have been constructed to try to explain how medicines can be therapeutically active at such extreme dilutions.[12]

It is possible to construct a mathematical model for the potentisation process, identifying an interrelationship of the dilution factor, the number of succussions and the oscillatory function, which is said to contribute to a biological effect. Among the simpler explanations are those based on molecular geometries or shapes, and a concept of hydration shells formed by the close association of water molecules with the ions of medicine molecules.

Succussion involves the effect of pressure changes due to the shock waves produced. The magnitude of this pressure has not been well examined but may be estimated, from conservation of energy equating kinetic energy with strain energy, to be about 5–100 MPa, dependent on the procedure[13]

The simplest explanation for succussion is that it may merely facilitate a complete mixing. Another possibility is that the structure of solvent molecules may be electrochemically changed by succussion, enabling it to acquire an ability to 'memorise' an imprint of the original medicine.

Stage 3: presentation – the dose forms

Solid dose forms   In allopathic medicine tablets and capsules are made in different forms to control the speed at which the active ingredient is delivered. In homeopathy one is not faced with this necessity, so the choice of carrier is governed by convenience rather than therapeutic efficiency. The main solid dose forms are shown in Figure 7.6.

Tablets (A) are similar to the classic biconvex plain white tablets used widely in conventional medicine. The size is about the same as a 75 mg dispersible aspirin tablet. The tablets are manufactured commercially from lactose and appropriate excipients. On an industrial scale blank lactose tablets and granules, or sucrose pills, can be surface inoculated by spraying on the liquid potency in alcoholic tincture or as a syrup in a revolving pan, rather like the old method of sugar coating.

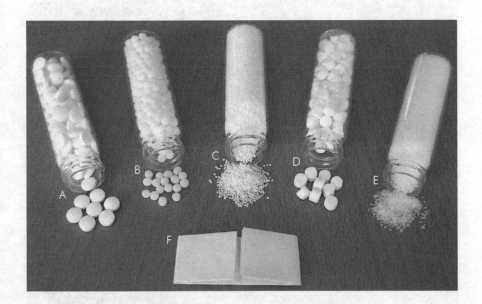

Figure 7.6 Solid dose forms.

The exact amount of medicine to be applied to ensure an even covering is determined using dyes. Pills are similarly prepared.

On a small scale in the pharmacy, the solid dose forms may be placed in glass vials and medicated by placing drops of liquid potency in strong alcohol on the surface; the number of drops used depends on the amount of solid dose form being medicated (Figure 7.7). The container is agitated in a manner similar to succussion to disperse the medicine throughout the dose form. On a large industrial scale tablets may be made by the pharmaceutical method of compressing medicated granules or applying the medicated potency as a spray to the tablets in a revolving pan.

Crystals (C) are made from sucrose and have the appearance of granulated sugar.

Soft tablets (D) are loosely compressed lactose tablets that melt quickly in the mouth.

Granules (E) are mainly made from lactose, and are about the size of the 'hundreds and thousands' used as cake decorations. They can be useful for infants and animals.

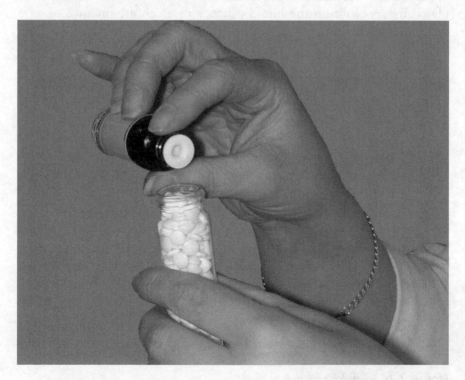

Figure 7.7 Medicating tablets by hand.

Individual powders (F) are made from lactose impregnated with liquid potency and are useful where small numbers of doses are required.

Liquid dose forms   Liquid potencies, prepared from the mother tinctures by serial dilution as described above, may be administered directly, in water or on a sugar cube.

Mother tinctures may also be taken orally (e.g. Crataegus), usually in water. They are more often applied topically, either singly (e.g. Arnica for bruising, Thuja for warts or Tamus for chilblains) or in mixtures (e.g. Hypericum and Calendula).

Topical dose forms   Ointments, creams, lotions and **liniments** (generic and patent) usually contain between 5% and 10% of mother tincture or, in a few cases where no mother tincture exists, liquid potency (e.g. Graphites or Sulphur) incorporated in a suitable vehicle. Absorption of homeopathic substances applied to the skin varies greatly depending on their physical and chemical properties. The skin's structure is especially suited to the absorption of lipophilic compounds into deeper-lying tissues. Using a flat-bed electrophoresis device and thin-layer chromatography it was shown that Hamamelis and Hypericum moved more quickly than Arnica and Calendula.[14]

Eyedrops have caused manufacturers licensing difficulties and at the time of writing are restricted in the UK to prescription on a named-patient basis. However, Calendula, Cineraria and particularly Euphrasia eyedrops are all extremely useful and are likely to prove very popular if and when they become more widely available.

Containers   There has been much discussion as to whether plastic or glass containers are appropriate for solid dose forms. The traditionalists still favour neutral glass containers, suggesting that there is a possibility of chemicals leeching out from the plastic. Little work has been done to investigate whether the fears of those eschewing plastic have a firm foundation.

There have also been suggestions that the glass may play some part in 'holding' the potency. Again, these have not been substantiated.

Liquids are packed in glass dropper bottles. The major suppliers use amber screw-cap bottles with a plug in the neck with a channel that facilitates the delivery of one measured drop (0.05 ml). Silicone rubber teat droppers are also used.

Legal classification of homeopathic medicines

Manufactured homeopathic medicines are subject to careful scrutiny to ensure that they are of the highest quality and safety. In the UK they have been treated as medicines since the inception of the National Health Service in 1948 and are available on medical prescription just as orthodox medicines are. As a result, they are subject to rules governing their manufacture and supply.

In Europe there are four routes by which homeopathic medicines can be registered.

1.   Products with limited claims of efficacy based on bibliographic evidence, and injections, may be registered under national rules (if the rules have been adopted by a member state). Several products have been registered under the UK national rules that came into force in 2006.
2.   Products that are 4x and above may be registered on the basis of quality and safety only (i.e. making no claims of efficacy) under an abbreviated European scheme.
3.   Products with claims of efficacy supported by clinical trials may be licensed under European legislation just like orthodox medicines. No homeopathic medicine has been licensed under this classification.
4.   Medicines for veterinary use may be registered under the Veterinary Regulations (see below).

Most registered homeopathic medicines for human use may be sold without restriction in a wide range of retail outlets. Exceptions include certain formulations such as eyedrops and injections that may contain unlicensed ingredients and are restricted to medical prescriptions on a named-patient basis.

At the time of writing the situation with regard to nosodes is uncertain. It is appropriate to exert some voluntary control when supplying certain nosodes for self-treatment in the over-the-counter (OTC) environment.

Some unlicensed medicines obtained from homeopathic manufacturers holding special manufacturing licences in the UK may be classified pharmacy only (P) and should not be placed on open shelves.

Homeopathic medicines may be prepared extemporaneously by pharmacists in a registered pharmacy if they have appropriate expertise.

In the USA homeopathic medicines are subject to the Food, Drug and Cosmetic Act of 1938 and regulations issued by the Food and Drug Administration (FDA).[15] Pre-market approval is by way of monograph approval by the Homeopathic Pharmacopoeia Convention of the United States (HPCUS).[16] Although homeopathic drugs are also subject to the FDA's non-prescription drug review, the FDA has not yet used this authority. However, manufacturing, labelling, marketing and sales of homeopathic medicines are subject to FDA compliance rules. These rules, with the exception of provisions for expiry dating, tablet imprinting and finished product testing, are functionally identical to the rules for their allopathic counterparts. Good manufacturing practice (GMP) standards for homeopathic and allopathic drugs are the same. Subject to the relevant FDA regulations homeopathic medicines indications may be given on the label and there are no limitations of where they can be sold.

The labelling requirements for human homeopathic medicinal products and the provisions for controlling the import, export and manufacture of homeopathic medicinal products are specified in the European Directive. The label must contain the words 'Homeopathic medicinal product without approved therapeutic indications' and 'Consult your doctor if symptoms persist'. Brand names, and names that indicate possible uses (sometimes called fantasy names), are officially banned, but there appear to be areas where the licensing authorities will allow some latitude in the regulations with respect to the naming of homeopathic products containing a number of different medicines. Following representations from some manufacturers on the basis of safety, some complex medicines containing several ingredients are being licensed with names of the type 'Medicine X Co' to obviate the necessity of attempting to remember a long list of ingredients when requesting an OTC medicine or writing a prescription. There is a potential source of confusion here, for some products that were on the market before the new legislation being adopted are still allowed to use brand names and even make limited claims of effectiveness. The authorities have not announced a date by which the products licensed under the old regulations have to be relicensed under the new EU regulations. Until this happens, the two types of medicine will exist side by side, although many manufacturers are beginning to register their products voluntarily.

A multidisciplinary expert committee, known as the Advisory Board on the Registration of Homeopathic Products, was established in the UK in 1993 to give advice to the MHRA, the government body responsible for assessing the safety and quality of homeopathic medicines before licensing. The Committee comprises a number of practising doctors, pharmacists and vets as well as academics. Similar bodies exist in other EU countries.

None of the above precludes experienced homeopathic practitioners and pharmacists from continuing to recommend and supply medicines compounded for individual needs.

The practice of homeopathy

Types of homeopathic medicine

Three subgroups of homeopathic medicines may be identified from the thousands that are available:

- Polychrests
- Isopathic medicines
- Constitutional medicines.

Polychrests

Over-the-counter prescribing in pharmacies is generally, but not exclusively, based on polychrests. Polychrests are medicines with drug pictures that show a very wide spectrum of activity and therefore have a broad range of applications. The term 'polychrest', meaning 'many uses', was taken from the Greek by Hahnemann and was first used by him in an 1817 article on Nux vomica. This group of 20–30 medicines forms the basis of most commercially available homeopathic ranges as they lend themselves to prescribing based on abbreviated drug pictures (Table 7.3) without protracted consultations. Although they are used mainly for first aid and acute situations, polychrests are also often indicated in chronic disease because they affect so many body tissues. Many polychrests are also constitutional medicines (see below).

Isopathic medicines

In general, modern isopathic medicines are administered on the basis of the principle *aequalia aequalibus curentur* (let same be treated by same) rather than the classic *similia similibus curentur* (let like be treated by like). Most have not been subjected to provings and therefore do not appear in the materia medica. Some of the older nosodes and sarcodes do have drug pictures, although their use is limited to rather specialised circumstances. Examples include Bacillinum, Medorrhinum and Psorinum (nosodes), and Lachesis (sarcodes).

Isopathic medicines are classified according to the origin of the source materials.

Table 7.3 List of common polychrest medicines

Polychrest	Main feature of drug picture
Aconite	Fear, first signs of cold
Allium cepa	Allergies and colds
Arnica	Mental and physical tiredness
Arsen alb	Diarrhoea (food)
Belladonna	Sudden-onset bursting headache
Bryonia	Productive cough, arthritic pain (better from cold, worse movement)
Calc carb	Abdominal pains, swelling of joints, sweating
Calc phos	Forgetful, restless, catarrh
Cantharis	Burns, frequent urination with burning sensation
Carbo veg	Wind; collapse accompanied by 'blueness'
Chamomilla	Teething and colic
Euphrasia	Allergies accompanied by eye symptoms; acid lacrimation
Gelsemium	Colds and flu; anxiety about failing
Hypericum	Painful injuries, especially of digits – blood and crush remedy
Ignatia	Effects of grief
Ipecac	Wheezing cough
Natrum mur	Sneezing, cold sores
Nux vom	Effects of over-eating, constipation
Pulsatilla	PMS; catarrh (bland, yellow or green in colour)
Rhus tox	Arthritic pain (better from heat, movement), strains
Ruta	Soft tissue injuries; sprains
Sepia	Premenstrual syndrome

Allergodes These are potentised allergens derived from many sources (e.g. grass and flower pollens, moulds, house-dust mites, animal hair, chocolate, milk, shellfish, wheat). Several companies produce OTC packs of allergodes, specifically mixed pollens and mixed grasses. These can be used effectively, provided that the patient knows that he or she is allergic to that substance. There are geographical variations that need to be considered. Allergodes have been shown to be effective in the treatment of a range of allergic reactions.[17]

Nosodes The Heads of European Medicines Agencies Homeopathic Medicinal Product Working Group (HMPWG) have defined nosodes as being homeopathic preparations made from products of human or animal disease processes, from pathogens or their metabolic products, from the decomposition products of animal organs, or from cultured microorganisms (see www.hma.eu/index.php?id=6). It is important to note that many nosodes are derived from pathological secretions taken from the host subject and they therefore contain not only the causative organism, but also the products of the immune system reactions of the host to it, i.e. they contain the overall, the specific and the unspecific immune response of the host organism to the pathogen.

Nosodes are prepared from diseased plant, animal or viral material (e.g. fluid from an arthritic joint, bowel tissue and vesicles). Autoisopathics are similar to nosodes but are prepared from an individual patient's own products (e.g. blood, pustules, urine, warts and verrucae,) or milk from a cow or sheep suffering from mastitis. There are various childhood illnesses represented among the nosodes, e.g. whooping cough (Pertussin) and German measles (Rubella). There are also tropical nosodes, such as cholera and malaria (Box 7.1).

Sarcodes These are generally obtained from bacterial cultures or healthy secretions, such as Lac can (dog's milk) or Moschus (musk oil). Among the sarcodes, Lachesis, from bushmaster snake venom, is a medicine that has a comprehensive drug picture.

Tautodes These are derived from drugs (e.g. chloramphenicol, diazepam, nitrazepam, penicillin), chemicals (e.g. pesticides, industrial fluids and biological washing powders) or synthetic products (e.g. nylon, plastics and rubber latex). One of the first tautopathic preparations was made during World War II from mustard gas. Most tautodes (or tautopathic medicines) are administered on the basis that they cause the condition for which they are being used therapeutically, but there are a few, mainly derived from allopathic drugs, that have a drug picture and can be used classically.[18] Attempts to use homeopathic dilutions of certain drugs of abuse to wean patients off their habit have met with partial success.

Box 7.1   Isopathic medicines as 'vaccines'

The word 'vaccine' is sometimes used erroneously by homeopaths to describe sarcodes, nosodes and tautodes when used to stimulate the autoimmune response. As a general rule sarcodes are used prophylactically, nosodes are used to treat the symptoms of a disease and tautopathics (made from orthodox vaccines) to treat adverse reactions resulting from immunisation. Unfortunately the exact source of the material used to manufacture the medicine is seldom stated on the label. There could conceivably be three variants of each so-called vaccine. It should be noted that none of these medicines are true vaccines and there is little scientific evidence as to whether or not they can confer any protection against a disease when given prophylactically. The UK Faculty of Homeopathy counsels against the use of any medicines by members of the public in such circumstances (see http://tinyurl.com/288oye).

An interesting randomised study has demonstrated that a nosode made from infected tissue could confer some protection on laboratory mice subjected to bacterial challenges.[19] High-potency medicines prepared from tissue infected with *Francisella tularensis* were administered to the test animals. It was found that 75% of the untreated controls died while only 53% of the isopathically treated group succumbed. Because of the implications for public health, pharmacists are normally best advised to refer requests for these so-called vaccines to a registered medical practitioner. In the case of the nosode Pertussin, specific instructions to this effect were circulated by the health authorities some years ago. It may be considered that a prescription, although not legally necessary, would provide appropriate evidence that this advice has been followed.

In the USA terminology differs from the above. The *Homeopathic Pharmacopoeia of the United States* (HPUS) provides the following definitions.

- **Isodes,** sometimes called **detoxodes**, are homeopathic dilutions of botanical, zoological, or chemical substances, including drugs and excipients, that have been ingested or otherwise absorbed by the body and are believed to have produced a disease or disorder.
- **Nosodes** are homeopathic attenuations of: pathological organs or tissues; causative agents such as bacteria, fungi, ova, parasites, virus particles and yeast; disease products; and excretions or secretions.
- **Sarcodes** are homeopathic attenuations of wholesome organs, tissues or metabolic factors obtained from healthy specimens.
- **Allersode** is the term used to describe homeopathic dilutions of antigens, i.e. substances that, under suitable conditions, can induce the formation of antibodies. Antigens include toxins, ferments, precipitinogens, agglutinogens, opsonogens, lysogens, venins, agglutinins, complements, opsonins, amboceptors, precipitins and most native proteins.

Constitutional medicines

In any given population the following may be observed:

- People react to homeopathic medicines with different levels of intensity.
- Some people respond especially well to a particular medicine; among people in this unique group, certain physical and mental characteristics appear to be common (skin texture, hair colour, height and weight). Further, these people also tend to have similar complaints; for example Pulsatilla and Sepia are both used for pre-menstrual tension. However, 'Pullsatilla ladies' tend to be weepy while 'Sepia ladies' tend to be tall and slim with a darker complexion.
- Parallels can often be drawn between certain characteristics shared by people in this group, and the physical or chemical properties of a medicine. Pulsatilla (the Windflower) is a slender flower that bends in the wind, a characteristic that may be considered analogous to having a changeable temperament.

The constitutional characteristics of the patient prevail in the absence of disease. They are also aspects of the individual that may intensify during illness to become symptoms. Particular physical characteristics, body functions and psychological traits may become exaggerated. If a person's constitutional medicine coincides with the symptom picture being presented there is a strong possibility of a favourable outcome.

The use of constitutional medicines is a skill that eludes most novice prescribers. A great deal needs to be known about the patient and the medicine and their use is not recommended unless appropriate knowledge and experience have been gained.

Homeopathic practitioners

In the UK, Ireland and many other English-speaking countries, most health professionals have responded reactively to a demand for homeopathy from clients, rather than encouraging its use proactively, although with improved access to training this position is changing. In these countries homeopathy may be practised not only by statutorily registered, qualified health professionals but, under common law, also by professional homeopaths (also known as non-medically qualified practitioners or NMQPs) and lay homeopaths with no formal training. Professional homeopaths are recognised by some NHS health boards in the UK. Common law permits freedom of choice of patients to choose the healthcare provision that they feel appropriate, and the freedom of people to practise homeopathy if they so wish. The main drawback of such a liberal system is that it allows a person to set up as a homeopath with little or no training.

Medical homeopathy, together with veterinary homeopathy, other professions allied to medicine and professional homeopaths, have quite separate educational facilities and governing bodies. Practice by the first is supervised by the Faculty of Homeopathy, which was founded in 1950 by an Act of Parliament. The Faculty accredits training courses for health professionals, awarding the qualification of Licentiate (LFHom with appropriate professional suffix) as a basic qualification for all health professionals and Membership (MFHom) and Fellowship (FFHom) for dental surgeons, medical doctors, nurses, pharmacists, podiatrists and veterinary practitioners. A pharmacy diploma is also available that covers dispensing, manufacture and counter prescribing. Currently more than 500 doctors hold the MFHom qualification. In addition there are 620 with the LFHom and an unspecified number of prescribers occasionally prescribing homeopathy, but who do not have a formal qualification. By contrast, in Germany 7000 medical doctors have homeopathic training and in France 5500.[20]

Dental and pharmacy diplomas are also available.

Training for professional homeopaths is offered by a number of colleges, each giving their own qualification. Homeopaths registered with the Society of Homoeopaths in Northampton may use the letters RSH (or FSH) after having followed a course of instruction and a period of clinical supervision. Another professional body is the UK Homeopathic Medical Association, the full members of which must complete similar requirements. These practitioners use the initials MHMA.

Despite their substantial training in well-established colleges, the professional homeopaths were formerly regarded with disdain by medical homeopaths, an opinion that continued into the 1980s. However, the two groups are moving together slowly with a number of joint working groups being formed. There are NHS homeopathic hospitals in Bristol, Glasgow and London. A hospital in Tunbridge Wells was forced to close down its NHS facilities in 2008 after funding was withdrawn. At the time of writing the future of The Royal London Homeopathic Hospital is in some doubt.

Germany also has two classes of practitioners: doctors (95% of whom practise some form of complementary medicine) and *Heilpraktikers*. The latter group, translated as 'health practitioners', developed in the 1930s, when doctors did not have a monopoly on the delivery of healthcare. At present the ratio of practising *Heilpraktikers* to physicians is about 1:4. *Heilpraktikers* are not obliged to undertake formal medical training, but are obliged to take a test administered by the local health authority. If a candidate fails, he or she may continue to resit until successful. The *Heilpraktiker's* activities are comparable to those of NMQPs in the UK, except that the former tend to use several different therapies concurrently and place more emphasis on diagnostic procedures.[21]

Approaches to the practice of homeopathy

There are many schools of thought around the world as to how homeopathy should be practised with respect to the choice of medicine, and the potency and frequency with which medicines should be administered. There is no established norm. Writers on homeopathy frequently refer to classic or European homeopathy, usually with the implication that this is the most complete and authoritative version of Hahnemann's views and most closely represents his methods. However, such claims do not correspond with the historical facts. The influence of the great American homeopaths has also been significant in shaping current practice. The notion that there is a standard or pure form of homeopathic practice has been criticised, with the argument that instead the so-called classic homeopathy is really a complex mixture of ideas drawn from a variety of sources.[22]

There are broadly three ways in which homeopathic medicines are administered in Europe and in other countries where European influence is strong:

1. *One medicine at a time* in a single dose or repeated doses is prescribed by those claiming to be classic or unicist homeopaths. This approach is generally favoured by homeopaths in the UK. However, Hahnemann changed his ideas several times, especially towards the end of his life, and so the term 'classic' could be applied to several different methods of using medicines and not just unicist prescribing.
2. *More than one medicine at a time*, given simultaneously in alternation or concurrently. This is called pluralist prescribing and claims to treat more than one aspect of a patient's condition. It is common in France, Germany and Italy, and where medicines from these countries are available.

3.   *Mixtures in one container* of different medicines and different
     potencies, selected and combined for their combined effect on par-
     ticular disease states. This method is known as complex prescri-
     bing and is very popular in France and Germany, where it is not
     uncommon to have 15–20 medicines ranging from very low to
     high potencies in the same preparation. It is likely that many of
     these complex mixtures will appear in the UK market within the
     foreseeable future. They do have some advantages for the OTC
     environment, as Table 7.4 shows. Classic homeopaths claim that
     this is not true homeopathy because there is no individual match-
     ing of the symptom and drug picture. Furthermore, no provings
     exist of the mixtures. Interestingly, this complex approach to
     prescribing is being adopted in modern orthodox medicine as an
     element of care plans involving the treatment of various diseases,
     including diabetes.

Supply of a named homeopathic medicine

Almost all human homeopathic medicines are classified as part of the
general sales list (GSL) in the UK and may be sold without restriction in
a wide range of retail outlets. Exceptions include very low potencies of
traditional poisons (e.g. Aconite and Belladonna), which have little if
any use in homeopathy, and certain formulations such as eyedrops and
injections that are presently unlicensed. It is appropriate to exert some
voluntary control when certain nosodes are being used as human or
veterinary vaccines (see previous section).

Table 7.4 Comparison of single (simplex) and combination (complex) remedies

Single-remedy prescribing	Combination-remedy prescribing
More difficult to pick remedy – needs time for repertories	Easier to prescribe – covers number of indications
Carefully targeted to patients' requirements – more precise	'Blunderbuss' approach
Provings available	No provings available for combination remedies
Outcome clearly attributable to remedy	Doubt as to which remedy is working
No problems with interactions	No knowledge of how remedies might interact with each other
Favoured by classic prescribers	Resistance among classic prescribers

Interpreting a written or verbal request for a homeopathic medicine

The request for supply may be by prescription signed by either a medical practitioner or an NMQP or by an OTC request from a client. Vets and dental surgeons may also issue private prescriptions. Thus, the stimulus prompting the purchase of a medicine may come from the practitioner, who may issue a formal prescription or give verbal instructions on what to buy. Other prospective purchasers are influenced by friends, family and the media. In order to comply with a request the following information is required:

- **Name of medicine**: care should be taken to ensure that the abbreviations used are correctly interpreted, e.g. *Staph*. could be *Staphylococcus* or *Staphisagria*. If in doubt, revert back to the practitioner.
- **Potency**: normally in the UK the potency will be on the centesimal scale (6c or 30c) or the decimal scale (6x). Very high potencies such as M and 10M may also be requested. Some pharmacists believe that high potencies should not be used to self-treat and may sell these medicines only in small quantities to ensure that they are not being misused.
- **Dose form**: ideally the dose form should be specified. Therapeutically the carrier is thought to be insignificant (although this has not been proven experimentally), but there may be other reasons why one or other form is preferred.
- **Quantity**: solid dose forms in the UK are often made available in 7, 14 or 25 g glass vials, indicating the capacity of the container. These correspond to approximately 55, 125 and 250 tablets, respectively, depending on the physical characteristics of the tablet. Tablets may also be available in quantities of 100 or 125. Liquid potencies and mother tinctures are supplied in 10, 20 and 50 ml dropper bottles that can deliver their contents dropwise.
- **Dose**: it is necessary to specify the dose required on prescriptions, rather than state 'as directed'. Some of the homeopathic dose regimens are complicated and easy to forget, especially by older patients.

Dispensing the medicine

Endorsing the prescription

To avoid contaminating the medicine, especially in the early days of dealing with homeopathic prescriptions, it is probably wise to issue an original pack as near as possible to the amount specified. Homeopathic medicines have been available under the UK NHS since its inception in 1948 and the prescription form (or, in Scotland, the doctor's stock order) should be endorsed with the amount supplied and the supplier's name if not given by the prescriber. Adding the trade price will be helpful to the pricing bureau. If in doubt, suppliers are usually very willing to give advice. If the bulk is broken solid dose forms should not be handled or tablets counted in a tablet counter, but instead transferred by first shaking them into the lid.

Increasingly, the costs of private homeopathic treatment are being met by health insurance schemes but, as the situation changes from month to month, patients should be advised to check with their own insurer before presenting their prescription.

Labelling

Dispensed medicines should be labelled in the normal way and a clear indication given of the name and potency. Occasionally it may be necessary to reinforce complicated instructions with a separate sheet of written instructions.

Counselling

Most patients will know that they are likely to receive a homeopathic prescription if they attend a suitably qualified practitioner, but some may not. There may be evidence of some anxieties about the validity of the therapy and it may be considered necessary to say a few words about the general features of homeopathy so that the patient is aware of the type of treatment being given. It can be said that it is safe, will not interfere with other medicines and is tailored to the patient's particular requirements. It is difficult to give exact guidelines because each individual situation is different. However, something appropriate should be said.

The other important information concerns taking the medicine. As the active ingredient is placed on the surface of the dose form and is absorbed through the oral mucous membranes, a number of precautions should be taken (shown in Box 7.2).

Box 7.2   Precautions in taking the medicine

The solid dose forms should not be handled to prevent deterioration due to bacterial or chemical contamination. They should be transferred to the mouth by way of the container cap. If dropped on the floor they should be discarded.

The solid dose forms should be allowed to dissolve in the mouth rather than being chewed and/or swallowed.

Liquid medicines should be held in the mouth for 20–30 s before swallowing.

Medicines should be taken half an hour before or after food, drink, tobacco or sweets. Aromatic flavours are thought to inactivate homeopathic medicines. Ideally, peppermint-flavoured toothpaste should be avoided, but if it is being used then at least 1 h should be allowed between cleaning the teeth and taking the medicine and the mouth should be rinsed out thoroughly with water before taking the medicine.

Medicines should be kept in the original container and stored in a cool dry place.

Existing allopathic medication should not be stopped without the permission of the original prescriber.

Safety

Potential sources of concern on safety issues include inappropriate treatment, toxicity, aggravation and interactions.

Inappropriate treatment

Most ranges of homeopathic medicines available for sale commercially over the counter are designed to be used for the treatment of simple self-limiting conditions. Some may also be used for ongoing conditions such as back pain or soft tissue injuries. Clients who request unusual medicines or who return repeatedly to purchase the same medicine on several occasions should be gently reminded that advice from a physician or registered homeopath might be appropriate to confirm that their condition lends itself to self-treatment.

It is vital that all practitioners offer advice and treatment only according to their levels of competency. Patients whose problems fall outwith these boundaries should be referred to suitably qualified colleagues.

Toxicity

Adverse reactions have been investigated using electronic databases, hand searching, searching reference lists, reviewing the bibliography of trials and other relevant articles, contacting homeopathic pharmaceutical companies and drug regulatory agencies in the UK and the USA, and by communicating with experts in homeopathy.[23] The authors, Dantas and Rampes, reported that the mean incidence of adverse effects of homeopathic medicines was approximately 2.5 times greater than for placebo in controlled clinical trials, but effects were minor and transient. There was a large incidence of pathogenic effects in healthy volunteers taking homeopathic medicines but the methodological quality of these studies was generally low. It was found that anecdotal reports of adverse effects in homeopathic publications were not well documented and mainly reported aggravation of current symptoms. Case reports in conventional medical journals pointed more to adverse effects of mislabelled homeopathic products than of true homeopathic medicines. It was concluded that homeopathic medicines in high dilutions, prescribed by trained professionals, were probably safe and unlikely to provoke severe adverse reactions. Once again it is difficult to draw definite conclusions because of the low methodological quality of reports claiming possible adverse effects of homeopathic medicines.

Some isolated cases of adverse reactions in the literature have also been highlighted.[24] Two dermatological problems were reported after the use of a medicine containing mercury in low potency.[25,26] However, another more recent paper concluded that the dosage of arsenic, mercury and lead in homeopathic medications manufactured under GMPs and following the US pharmacopoeia guidelines is generally below the detection level and not thought to be a risk to health.[27]

From time to time lactose sensitivity is encountered. This can be overcome by using a sucrose-based carrier or a liquid potency.

Aggravation

Grabia and Ernst[28] considered the frequency of homeopathic aggravations in placebo and verum groups of double-blind randomised trials. They identified 24 trials for evaluation, using 8 independent literature reviews. The average number of aggravations was low with a total of 50 aggravations being attributed to patients treated with placebo and 63 to patients treated with homeopathic medicines. The authors concluded that their review did not provide clear evidence that the phenomenon of homeopathic aggravations exists.

However, not withstanding these comments, clinical experience shows that in about 10% of chronic cases the patient's condition may be exacerbated within 2–5 days of taking a medicine. Typically, a skin condition may become worse after taking a low-potency medicine. Such a reaction usually occurs only the first time that the medicine is used. This reaction, known as an aggravation, has been described as an adverse drug reaction (ADR), and in the sense that it is unwanted by the patient it might be considered thus. When told of the possibility of aggravation many patients will say that they expect to get worse before they get better. Far from being upset by the apparent ADR they consider an aggravation as a sign that the medicine is working.

If an aggravation appears, the patient should be instructed to cease taking the medicine until the symptoms subside and then recommence taking the medicine at a lower frequency. If the symptoms continue to get worse when the medicine has been temporarily suspended, it is likely that the wrong medicine is being taken. Patients who are receiving prescribed medication should be advised to consult their practitioner for ways of dealing with aggravations.

Interactions

There is no evidence that homeopathic medicines interfere with any concurrent allopathic medicines, and indeed they are particularly useful for treating trivial conditions in people who are taking several orthodox medications. It is thought that steroids may inactivate homeopathic medicines to some extent and, although this potential interaction is certainly not dangerous, it could reduce their expected effectiveness. Some homeopathic medicines are considered to be an antidote to or to inactivate other medicines in some circumstances, e.g. Camphor, Aconite and Nux vom. Traditionally, homeopaths usually advise patients to refrain from taking coffee, tea, chocolate and spicy food when taking homeopathic medication, but there is little evidence that such abstinence is necessary.

It has been recommended that healthcare providers should ask their patients not only if they use homeopathic pharmaceuticals in general but to specify which products they are using, bearing in mind the possibility that they may contain mother tinctures or products at such low dilutions that they contain material doses and potentially interfere with conventional treatment.[29]

Prescribing homeopathic medicines

Prescribing a homeopathic medicine can be a long and complex process.[30] It is possible to prescribe for acute and self-limiting conditions by the following six steps:

1. Taking a decision on whether to treat or to refer
2. Obtaining the necessary information
3. Deciding on a particular medicine
4. Establishing a dose regimen
5. Providing the medicine
6. Follow-up.

Step 1: deciding whether to treat or refer

Working within the bounds of competency is implied in the codes of ethics of all healthcare providers. The decision, which with experience can be taken without an in-depth investigation, is based on the severity and type of symptoms being presented, the length of time during which symptoms have been experienced, etc. Having decided to treat, the next question is whether to treat with homeopathy or allopathy. Normally a healthcare provider using homeopathy as an adjunct to existing skills would not seek to widen his or her portfolio of conditions treated with homeopathy, but would rather endeavour to complement existing methods of responding to requests for advice. There are one or two exceptions to this. Requests for help with examination nerves can be effectively met with Arsenicum album or Gelsemium, and Cocculus may be suggested with confidence to women suffering from nausea during the first trimester of pregnancy. In neither case do suitable allopathic products exist. Homeopathy might also be indicated for patients with an existing extensive portfolio of medication where adding extra drugs might cause worries about interaction.

Step 2: obtaining the necessary information

Before choosing an appropriate medicine to prescribe, information is required from:

•   the patient: signs and symptoms, both observed and reported
•   the practitioner's observational and listening skills
•   the practitioner's own knowledge and limits of competency
•   sources of reference, including materia medicas and repertories.

A useful acronym to use when assessing a case is provided by the letters LOAD, standing for listen, observe, ask and decide:

Listen to what the patient tells you about his or her symptoms.
Observe the patient's general demeanour, appearance, temperament, etc.

Ask the patient appropriate questions to learn more about the condition. Decide what to do next after assessing the information provided.

Given the restrictions on resources in most pharmacies it is not possible to pursue the extended consultations felt necessary by most complementary practitioners. This means that the conditions being treated are likely to be restricted to simple self-limiting conditions using polychrests.

Step 3: deciding on a particular medicine

If all the preparatory work in step 2 has been carried out assiduously, the choice of medicine is not as daunting as it might appear. Another acronym may be useful: ACT, which stands for assess, confirm and talk.

Assess Having gathered all the requisite information, an appropriate medicine can be chosen. Most practitioners keep the drug pictures of 20–30 simple medicines in their memory and can often prescribe a polychrest quickly without reference to the repertory. For most of us it is necessary to use the repertory, a textbook that lists disease states and gives medicines with a drug picture in which the various symptoms appear. An appropriate medicine may be chosen by using a repertory to identify one or more medicines that might fit the symptom picture, and using the materia medica to see which drug picture fits best. There are several materia medicas and repertories available. Boericke's *Materia Medica and Repertory* has both texts in the same book and is probably the easiest for the beginner to use. It has the disadvantage that the language is rather old-fashioned and written in patient's terminology, hence the appearance of words such as 'brain-fag'. In some instances lateral thinking must be used to navigate through the index. The repertory gives medicines in normal type and italics: italic type indicates a higher importance of medicine than normal type.

Probably the most widely used text is the *Repertory of the Homeopathic Materia Medica* by Kent, the great American homeopath.[31] This text gives three grades of medicine, indicated by plain, italic and bold text. Other examples of repertory include texts by Murphy,[32] Phatak[33] and Schroyens.[34] In some cases the drug picture may be very extensive. Arnica, for example, extends over several pages and it would be impossible to identify a complete match. When used for acute conditions the polychrests can be prescribed on the basis of an abbreviated drug picture, picking out just a handful of the most important symptoms. These symptoms, known as keynotes, are considered to be important because they have been reported more often than have other symptoms by volunteers taking part in provings. Examples of keynotes are given for some common polychrests at the end of this chapter. When starting out it is perfectly possible to counter prescribe using keynotes, provided that only acute self-limiting conditions are prescribed for.

Computerised repertories are increasing in popularity but tend to be rather complicated for most beginners. RADAR and Cara are the programs most frequently used by professionals; other less extensive programs are available.

Confirm   Having chosen the medicines most likely to be of assistance, the final decision must be made. This can be achieved by checking the materia medica drug picture and asking a few confirmatory questions, particularly about modalities and what makes the condition better or worse.

Examples of modalities are that the condition is made better or worse by:

• the application of heat or cold to the affected part
• movement
• exposure to warm or wet weather.

For example, the medicines Rhus tox and Bryonia are both indicated for the treatment of rheumatic pain. Patients who find that they are stiff first thing in the morning but improve as the day proceeds, and for whom the application of heat is beneficial, respond well to Rhus tox. Patients who find any movement painful and for whom the application of cold is beneficial respond well to Bryonia.

Talk   It might also be appropriate to give the patient some general information on homeopathy, especially if the pharmacist is acting proactively rather than reactively to a request for homeopathic medicines from the client.

Step 4: establishing a dose regimen

• In first-aid situations the medicine is given frequently – up to every 10–15 min for 6–8 doses in some cases. Here the term 'first aid' refers to a suggested initial treatment for any condition being treated, not just for an injury, as in orthodox medicine.

- With acute prescribing the dose should be taken three times daily for 7–10 days.
- In chronic conditions frequencies of once or twice a day (or even once a month) are more appropriate.

By convention it is generally stated that the dose for a child under 12 years should be half that of an adult (i.e. one tablet instead of two).

Step 5: providing the medicine

Having chosen the medicine, the patient should be given information on how to take it.

Step 6: follow-up

After the dose regimen periods stated above the treatment should be reviewed. A number of responses are possible and are shown in Figure 7.8.[35] There are four main options:

1. The medicine has proved successful and may be discontinued.
2. The outcome is not satisfactory, but the client has not been taking the medication according to instructions – instructions should be given to restart the course of treatment.
3. The outcome is unsatisfactory, but the client has returned too soon – the course should be completed before further action is taken.
4. The client appears to have completed the treatment but the outcome is unsatisfactory – consider changing the medicine or referring.

Demand for homeopathic medicines

Size of market[36]

The last decade has seen an increase in the European market for homeopathic and anthroposophical medicines (see below) from €590m in 1995 to €775 in 2001 (15 EU states) and €930m in 2005 (25 EU states). In many markets the growth in sales has been less steady since 2001 than it was in the preceding 5 years. The 2005 figure of €930m represents €1771m at consumer prices or €4 per head of population.

Many European countries have a long-standing tradition in the use of homeopathic medicines. In most of the former socialist states

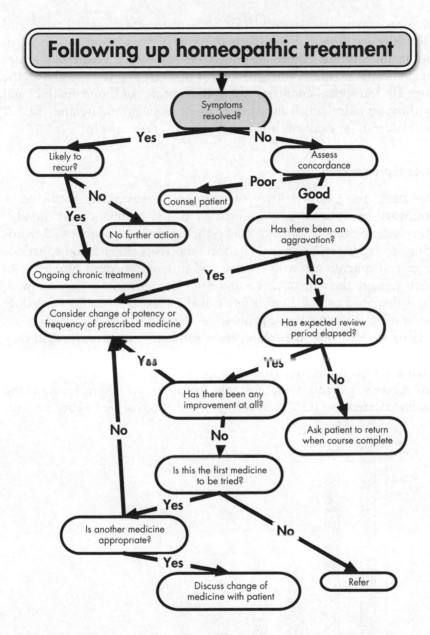

Following up homeopathic treatment

Symptoms resolved?

Yes → Likely to recur?

No → Assess concordance

Poor → Counsel patient

Good → Has there been an aggravation?

Likely to recur? — No → No further action

Likely to recur? — Yes → Ongoing chronic treatment

Has there been an aggravation? — Yes → Consider change of potency or frequency of prescribed medicine

Has there been an aggravation? — No → Has expected review period elapsed?

Has expected review period elapsed? — Yes → Has there been any improvement at all?

Has expected review period elapsed? — No → Ask patient to return when course complete

Has there been any improvement at all? — Yes → Consider change of potency or frequency of prescribed medicine

Has there been any improvement at all? — No → Is this the first medicine to be tried?

Is this the first medicine to be tried? — Yes → Is another medicine appropriate?

Is this the first medicine to be tried? — No → Refer

Is another medicine appropriate? — No → Consider change of potency or frequency of prescribed medicine

Is another medicine appropriate? — Yes → Discuss change of medicine with patient

Figure 7.8 Follow-up chart.

homeopathy was restricted by the government but is now expanding. Conversely, in some western European states a lack of robust evidence has resulted in decreased availability of homeopathic treatment. Eight member states are responsible for 90% of the total sales. France and Germany are both major markets in terms of population and are leading manufacturers. Figure 7.9 shows the top 10 EU countries for size of homeopathic and anthroposophical market. Figure 7.10 shows the top 10 European countries by consumption of homeopathic and anthroposophical medicines per head of population. Ireland (€1.17) and UK (€0.78) rank twelfth and thirteenth, respectively

User characteristics

To study the characteristics of users of homeopathic medicine, a four-part questionnaire was distributed by Furnham and Bond.[37] Respondents were required to read eight vignettes (each about 70 words long) describing a British male patient who visits either a homeopath or a general practitioner with specific and different medical problems. In each vignette the patient gets better after treatment or remains unwell; he is described as being either emotionally balanced (stable) or slightly neurotic in character. Participants were required to rate each vignette on criteria such as: Did they think the treatment was effective? Did they think the person would remain feeling better? A total of 165 people completed the questionnaire. Homeopathy was perceived as more effective for treating patients with unstable psychological characteristics and orthodox medicine (OM) was seen as more effective for treating patients

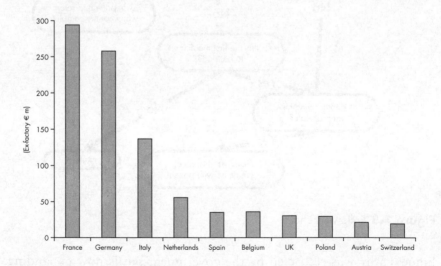

Figure 7.9 Top 10 EU countries for size of homeopathic and anthroposophical market.

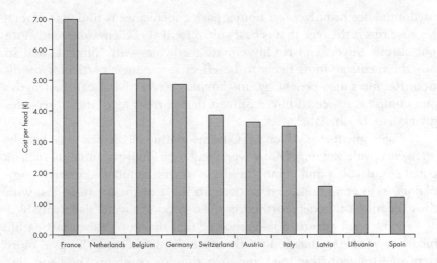

Figure 7.10 Top 10 European countries by consumption of homeopathic and anthroposophical medicines per head of population.

with stable psychological characteristics. Homeopathy was perceived as more effective by participants who themselves used complementary medicine. Participants who had visited a complementary therapist felt more strongly that psychological factors were important in illness than participants who had never consulted a complementary practitioner. Non-complementary medicine users perceived OM to be more effective than complementary medicine users.

As homeopathic medicines are readily available at a number of outlets (pharmacies, health stores, etc.), they provide consumers with an attractive option for self-treating. The buyer characteristics of the British homeopathic OTC market have been investigated.[38] In a questionnaire-based study of 407 purchasers in 109 pharmacies, it was found that very few people under the age of 25 bought OTC homeopathic medicines, and only 12% of buyers aged 25–35 years were male. Most respondents bought the medicine for themselves rather than for other members of their family, emphasising the individualistic nature of homeopathic medicines. As regards the main medicine grouping of the homeopathic medicines bought, the most popular were polychrests (medicines with a wide spectrum of activity, making them well suited to the OTC environment) and complex medicines (mixtures of medicines usually with specific uses). There were a small number of branded medicines. The most frequently purchased polychrests were Arnica (6.3% of all purchases), Pulsatilla (3.0%) and Rhus tox (2.3%). The predominance of polychrest homeopathic medicines is understandable, because this is the type that is best suited to the OTC environment. With polychrests buyers can readily equate medicines with ailments and so buy the medicine most likely to be effective for their particular condition. Retailers also benefit by not having to offer what can be lengthy and complex advice to buyers, given that current legislation precludes giving uses on the label.

The ailments for which OTC homeopathic medicines were bought were very wide ranging. Many were acute self-limiting ailments such as coughs and colds and minor injuries; others included digestive complaints, skin conditions and anxiety. In most of these categories, with the exception of anxiety, orthodox OTC products were also available.

Most respondents (60%) reported that they took the homeopathic medicine as sole medication for their problem; others (27%) used more than one homeopathic medicine at a time or combined homeopathic and allopathic medicines (13%).

Concern should be expressed at the excessive length of time for which some respondents take their medicines. Most homeopathic medicines offered for sale over the counter are designed for short-term administration. Long-term chronic conditions are best treated under the guidance of a practitioner; this should ensure the choice of appropriate therapy, as well as minimising the possibility of provings. Although taking homeopathic medicines for long periods should not cause any irreversible harm, because the medicines are not in themselves toxic, patients may suffer because they may not be receiving appropriate treatment for their condition.

A similar study in New Zealand produced comparable results.[39] There was a high degree of awareness of homeopathy in New Zealand, with 92% of a sample of 503 pharmacy clients claiming to have heard of homeopathy; 67% said that they had used the therapy.

Evidence

Homeopathy is enjoying increased consumer-led demand, even though objectively convincing data to support its claims tend to be conflicting[40] due to difficulties in obtaining consistent results with conventional medical trials.[41] To secure general acceptance for homeopathy it is crucial to secure an overall theory to explain its effects.

According to Walach 'we face the situation that homeopathy, as a medical theory, is only weakly supported by experimental facts, and highly endorsed by circumstantial and anecdotal evidence, which is unique in the history of medicine over such a long time'.[42]

Ernst has been particularly active in questioning the evidence produced for homeopathy (and indeed other complementary disciplines), asking whether the demise of homeopathy was imminent[43] and whether we should be using 'powerful placebos'.[44] His views were branded 'misleading'[45] and 'neither balanced nor penetrating'.[46]

It is beyond the scope of this chapter to look at the research carried out in homeopathy in great detail, particularly that associated with evidence on effectiveness. The reader is referred to specialist texts on this subject for such information.[47,48] The library at Hom-Inform (see below) is able to locate appropriate books and papers. In this section a flavour of the topics available is offered.

There is much circumstantial evidence from case studies that homeopathy is effective, from both patients and practitioners. Scientific evidence is rather sparse and much of what is available suffers from poor methodology.[49] The influence of indicators of methodological quality on study outcome in a set of 89 placebo-controlled clinical trials of homeopathy has been investigated.[50] It was concluded that, in the set studied, there was clear evidence that studies with better methodological quality tended to yield less positive results. Examples of poor methodology include dubious accuracy of test materials, inappropriate measurements and poor randomisation techniques.

This is unfortunate, to say the least, because, increasingly, decisions on whether or not to use or purchase homeopathic services require evidence of positive outcomes and value for money. The availability of funds for research is limited. Organisations such as the Homeopathic Trust (now merged with the British Homeopathic Association) and the Scottish Homeopathic Research and Education Trust have generously supported workers over many years, but the sums available are modest. The relatively small value of the market means that manufacturers have little to invest in research outwith their own commercial requirements.

Broadly, homeopathic research falls into five main categories:

1. Placebo studies designed to demonstrate that homeopathy is not merely a placebo response and satisfy criticism from sceptics
2. Clinical trials to establish efficacy
3. Physicochemical studies on mechanisms of action
4. Audit and case study collection to establish effectiveness and improve the use of homeopathy

5.   Attitudes and awareness studies and sociological research to determine why and how homeopathy is used.

Walach et al.[51] focused on reviews and other 'landmark' papers dealing with different strands of homeopathic research. The authors found that many plant and animal models have been studied during laboratory research and numerous effects and anomalies reported. However, no single model has been sufficiently widely replicated. Basic research, trying to elucidate a purported difference between homeopathic medicines and control solutions, has produced some encouraging results but again without independent replication. Clinical research included pathogenic trials (provings) and therapeutic trials. Reports on clinical trials for single conditions were limited and, in many cases, conflicting. By contrast, observational research into uncontrolled homeopathic practice consistently gave strong therapeutic benefits for patients.

Placebo studies

The placebo response

A reason that is widely held to be responsible for any success in homeopathy, is what is commonly called 'the placebo response'.

In 1651 the English scholar Robert Burton wrote:

An empiric oftentimes, and a silly chiurgeon, doth more strange cures than a rational physician – because the patient puts confidence in him.

Physicians have known for at least several centuries that patients often display marked improvement of symptoms when given a sugar pill or some other substance having no known medicinal properties, under the impression that it is an active drug. With the advent of large-scale clinical drug trials during the last 30–40 years placebos have become an important way of eliminating investigator bias in medical research. As a result we have learned much about the placebo and its effect in studying other therapies. Unfortunately researchers have not devoted much attention to rigorously defining what exactly is meant by the placebo effect, and to delineate the types of phenomena to which the terms should apply. What is known suggests that a patient's beliefs or expectations can influence the body state. This in turn appears to have implications for the mind and body.

The word 'placebo' is derived from the Latin, 'I shall please'. From an original religious use the word acquired a medical and negative connotation.

Definition

The term placebo may be defined as:[52]

An inactive substance administered to a patient usually to compare its effects with those of a real drug, but sometimes for the psychological benefit to the patient through his believing he is receiving treatment.

A more comprehensive definition is provided by Shapiro:[53]

- A placebo is any therapeutic procedure (or the component of any therapeutic procedure) that is given deliberately to have an effect, or unknowingly has an effect on a patient, symptoms or disease, but which is objectively without specific activity for the condition being treated.
- The therapeutic procedure may be given with or without conscious knowledge that the procedure is a placebo, may be an active (non-inert) or non-active (inert) procedure.
- The placebo must be differentiated from the placebo effect, which may or may not occur and which may be favourable or unfavourable.
- The placebo effect (or response) is defined as the changes produced by a placebo.

Placebo effects

Placebo interventions may have an effect on most organ systems in the body. Benefits have been reported in postoperative pain, angina, cough, headache, peptic ulcer, hypertension, anxiety and arthritis.[54]

Studies have also shown that symptoms can change even when an active therapy expected to be present has in fact been withdrawn. In 1988 Hashish et al. investigated the outcome resulting from the application of ultrasound after the extraction of wisdom teeth.[55] Unknown to the therapist the machine was switched on and off without his knowledge. Patients' symptoms improved in both cases. Sham surgery has also been used in investigating angina and improvements noted in both the patients who had received a surgical intervention and those who *thought* that they had been given an operation.[56,57]

There is no doubt that physiological and psychological changes, both beneficial and non-beneficial, can result from the administration of a technically inert therapy.

The placebo effect is most powerful under the following conditions:[58]

- When the patient expects the symptoms to improve
- When the practitioner expects the patient's symptoms to improve
- When treatment is administered by someone considered to be of high status and authoritative by the patient
- When the treatment appears to be effective and credible to the patient
- When a positive practitioner–patient interaction is established.

None of the above factors exists in isolation. It is likely that a placebo effect results from the interaction of all the foregoing. The placebo effect should be viewed as an interactive process, in which the patient, treatment characteristics and practitioner all play an important part.

A general characteristic of the placebo effect is its relatively short duration: from 2 to 6 weeks is often quoted in the literature. In a two-part trial of patients with chronic rheumatoid arthritis in which separate groups of patients were treated with homeopathic medicines, salicylates and placebo, 60% of the patients receiving placebo withdrew from the study in 3 weeks dissatisfied with their progress.[59] By 6 weeks all the placebo patients had withdrawn from the study, whereas after a year the homeopathic group still had 74% of its patients and the salicylate group 15% of its patients. Improvement in long-standing chronic conditions as a result of using homeopathy cannot therefore be due solely to a placebo effect.

Placebo studies in homeopathy

The first investigation of the placebo effect used the hypothesis that homeopathy was due to a placebo response rather than the converse.

Following a pilot trial in 1983 with 35 patients,[60] the hypothesis was tested in a double-blind, placebo-controlled trial, using a model based on the use of mixed grass pollens to treat 144 hayfever patients.[61] The authors concluded that homeopathy appeared to be effective in its own right, i.e. they disproved their original hypothesis. This result was reinforced by further work in this area.[62]

It has been suggested that the evidence supporting the hypothesis that homeopathy may be solely a placebo response can be considered under a number of headings:[63]

- Theoretical evidence: immunological-type responses to minute quantities of stimulant are well documented

- Practical evidence: outcome measures based on patient-oriented methods demonstrate an improvement in both overall wellbeing and clinical symptoms
- Laboratory research: difficult to replicate and apply to in vivo situations
- The self-healing response: in assembling the varying sources of evidence for the existence of a placebo response to homeopathy, the interesting idea is introduced of replacing the term 'placebo' with 'intention-modified self-healing response', which is affected by the circumstances of the healing encounter.

Reilly[63] suggested that the intention-modified self-healing response may exist alone or be combined with an intervention to give a therapeutic, intention-modified, self-healing response.

A meta-analysis on 89 randomised clinical trials (RCTs) assessed whether or not the clinical effect reported in RCTs of homeopathic medicines was equivalent to that reported for placebo.[64] The results of the meta-analysis were not compatible with this hypothesis, but insufficient evidence was found from these studies that homeopathy was clearly efficacious for any single clinical condition.

Three independent systematic reviews of placebo-controlled trials on homeopathy, assessed by Jonas et al.,[65] reported that the effects of homeopathy appear to be more than placebo, whereas one review found its effects to be consistent with placebo. The reviews comprehensively searched for all clinical trials and used standard methods for their quality evaluation and analysis. Only high-quality studies were selected for analysis (e.g. those with adequate randomisation, blinding, sample size and other methodological criteria that limit bias). There was evidence from several series of trials that homeopathy may be effective for the treatment of influenza, allergies, postoperative ileus and childhood diarrhoea, but ineffective for migraine, delayed-onset muscle soreness and prevention of influenza.

Randomised clinical trials: meta-analyses and reviews

It used to be said that constructing RCTs for homeopathic medicines was impossible because of the individualisation required in prescribing. Over the years various techniques have been developed for RCTs, and they have been carried out for a number of single medicines including Arnica,[66-69] Arsenicum album[70] and Rhus tox.[71] However, most RCTs set out to test homeopathy as an intervention versus placebo, rather than to test a specific medicine.

Homeopathic RCTs are always scrutinised very carefully by the scientific community, so their quality needs to be extremely high for the outcomes to be accepted. The objective of one of the most frequently cited papers on homeopathic clinical trials[72] was to establish whether or not there was any firm evidence of the effectiveness of homeopathy from all the many controlled trials that have been carried out in recent years. The methodological quality of 107 controlled trials published in 96 journals worldwide was assessed. The trials were scored using a list of predefined good criteria. A total of 81 positive trials were recorded. The 5 allergic trials included in the analysis were all positive: the next most successful therapeutic group, with 90% of its 20 trials positive, was trauma and pain. The authors acknowledge that the weight of presented evidence was probably not sufficient for most people to make a decision on whether homeopathy works or not, but that there would probably be enough evidence to support several common applications if it were an orthodox therapy.

A systematic review has been carried out of 32 trials (28 placebo-controlled, 2 comparing homeopathy and another treatment, and 2 comparing both, i.e. comparing outcomes from trials comparing homeopathy with a placebo with outcomes from trials comparing homeopathy with another non-homeopathic treatment) involving a total of 1778 patients.[73] The methodological quality of the trials was highly variable. In the 19 placebo-controlled trials providing sufficient data for meta-analysis, individualised homeopathy was significantly more effective than the placebo effect but, when the analysis was restricted to the methodologically best trials, no significant effect was seen. The results of the available randomised trials suggest that individualised homeopathy had a greater effect than placebo. The evidence was not convincing because of methodological shortcomings and inconsistencies.

Several individual trials have yielded negative results.[74-76] A high-quality, randomised, double-blind, placebo-controlled trial was conducted involving 63 patients on the homeopathic prophylaxis of migraine using a technique approved by the International Headache Society under good clinical practice.[77] The authors concluded that homeopathy could not be recommended for migraine prophylaxis.

The results from a German randomised, double-blind, placebo-controlled trial were presented at the Sixth Annual Symposium on Complementary Medicine at Exeter in December 1999. The clinical efficacy and tolerance of Caulophyllum D4 was investigated using 40 pregnant women with premature amnion rupture.[78] The effect of the medicine in D4–D18 on smooth muscle was also investigated in vitro.

Patients between gestational weeks 38 and 42 with premature amnion rupture, no regular contractions and cervix dilatation of < 3 cm were randomised. Appropriate tests were used to measure outcomes. In the second experiment the effect of the homeopathic medicines was measured on the spontaneous contraction activity of smooth muscle obtained from the uterus and stomach of guinea-pigs and rats. It was concluded that the medicine was tolerated without adverse reactions, and had no myogenic effects.

Mathie[79] examined all published clinical trials on human subjects that appeared in full papers from 1975 until December 2002, and that compared homeopathic treatment with placebo or with another medication, using a randomised and/or double-blind study design. Mathie identified a total of 93 original articles, of which 79 were placebo controlled and the remaining 14 compared homeopathy with a conventional treatment. He suggested that from the first group it appeared that the present weight of evidence favours homeopathic treatment effectiveness in childhood diarrhoea,[80,81] muscle soreness,[82] hayfever and allergic rhinitis,[83] influenza,[84] pain,[85] adverse effects of radio- and chemotherapy,[86] traumatic injury[87] and upper respiratory infection.[88] The weight of evidence did not favour the use of homeopathy in the treatment of headache,[74] stroke[89] or warts.[90] With regard to the studies comparing homeopathy with allopathy, there was insufficient evidence either to favour or to find no support for homeopathy in nine of the ten conditions investigated. For upper respiratory tract infection a weight of evidence suggested that homeopathy and conventional medicine (aspirin) were equally effective in treating the common cold. Mathie emphasises the need for much more and better directed research in homeopathy. He states that many homeopaths rely on their own successful clinical evidence. However, if homeopathy truly enables people to attain better health, it is vitally important that it achieves much wider respect within medicine at large. He calls for a fresh agenda of enquiry that goes beyond (but includes) the placebo-controlled trial. Each study should adopt research methods and outcome measurements linked to the clinical significance of homeopathy's effects.

A review of papers investigating the effectiveness, safety and cost-effectiveness in general practice was published by a group of Swiss workers.[91] They reported that many high-quality investigations of pre-clinical basic research proved that homeopathic high potencies can influence regulative and scientific changes in cells or living organisms. Of the 22 systematic reviews analysed by the authors 20 detected at least a trend in favour of homeopathy. In their estimation five studies yielded results indicating clear evidence for homeopathic therapy. The evaluation of 29 studies involving upper respiratory tract infections/allergic reactions showed a positive overall reaction in favour of homeopathy. Eight of 16 placebo-controlled studies were significantly in favour of homeopathy. A general health economic statement about homeopathy could not be made from the available data.

Bias in the conduct and reporting of trials is a possible explanation for positive findings of placebo-controlled trials. In both conventional and homeopathic trials it has been shown that smaller studies and those of lower quality tend to show greater numbers of positive effects. Shang et al.[92] compared the findings from 110 homeopathic trials with those from 110 matched conventional medicine trials. In both groups, smaller trials and those of lower quality showed more beneficial treatment effects than larger and higher-quality trials. The researchers concluded that there were biases in both homeopathy and conventional trials. The evidence for a specific effect of homeopathic medicines was weak but the evidence for specific effects of conventional medicine was strong. The finding was claimed to be compatible with the notion that the clinical outcomes of homeopathy were the result of a placebo effect. Although the review claimed to be based on over 100 homeopathy studies, in fact the conclusion was based on only 8 trials, many being excluded for unclear reasons.

Mathie[79] stated at the end of a substantial review that, given the wide-ranging clinical benefits that homeopathy brings, there might be many more medical conditions – not presently listed in *any* category of evidence – that can become included in a future list of those confirmed by research to be effectively treated by homeopathy.

Studies on mechanisms of action of homeopathic medicines

Usually patients are not worried about – or in many cases are not even interested in – how a medicine works. Their main concern is safety and a positive outcome. The emphasis on proving that homeopathy works has been overtaken by a wish to improve its use. However, there is no doubt that homeopathy would benefit from a plausible explanation of its mechanisms of action.

Where there are material doses of medicine present, generally below the 12c potency, it is easier to accept a pharmacological response, albeit not one that can necessarily be explained in standard pharmacological terms. It has been proposed that there is an active therapeutic ingredient in homeopathic medicines and it acts pharmacologically in the body's vomeronasal system.[93] The vomeronasal organ (Jacobson's organ) is the receptor site for the detection of non-odorant molecules, e.g. pheromones, in reptiles, amphibians and mammals.

Once the medicine has been diluted beyond Avogadro's number, theoretically there are no molecules of the drug present, so how can the potentisation process possibly give a therapeutic result? How, indeed! It has to be said that we are not even close to finding out. There has not been much progress since George Vithoulkas wrote in 1985 'as far as is yet known, there is no available explanation in modern physics or chemistry for the phenomenon of potentisation' (page 106).[94] The literature contains numerous hypotheses that seek to explain how homeopathic medicines might work – some are so plausible that they are as difficult to disprove as to prove!

There are three main diluents used during the potentisation process: water, alcohol and, in the case of non-soluble source materials, lactose. All of these are thought to play an important part in the mode of action.[95]

One of the most controversial ideas on the mechanisms of action of homeopathy was suggested in the 1980s. The 'memory of water', a concept by which the properties of an aqueous preparation are held to depend on the previous history of the sample, will be forever linked to the name of the late Jacques Benveniste. The term first appeared in the French newspaper Le Monde, commenting on a fierce controversy that blew up in the pages of the leading scientific journal Nature in 1988. In June of that year, Nature published a paper by a large international group led by Benveniste, which made the sensational claim that the antibody anti-IgE, in dilutions far into the 'ultramolecular' range, triggers degranulation of human basophils in vitro.[96] Nature had resisted publishing the paper, and the then editor, John Maddox, agreed to do so only on the condition that Benveniste allowed an inspection team, nominated by Maddox, to visit his laboratory after publication. The team duly visited and, a month later, published its report denouncing Benveniste's work as 'pseudoscience', but nevertheless justifying its decision to publish.[97] Two subsequent attempts to reproduce Benveniste's results failed,[98,99] although he remained defiant until his death in October 2004.

Teixeira[100] has claimed that the memory of water idea is not compatible with our knowledge of pure water. If an explanation on physical grounds is to be found, research must focus on other aspects of the preparation, such as the presence of other molecules and dissolved gases. There is significant debate on the nature of the active therapeutic ingredient in homeopathic medicines and whether the effect of homeopathic medicines is exerted locally. Texeira's paper accepts that there is an active therapeutic ingredient in homeopathic medicines that acts pharmacologically in the body and proposes a possible receptor site. As mentioned above, the vomeronasal organ (Jacobson's organ) is the receptor site for the detection of non-odorant molecules. The organ forms the main part of a chemoreceptor system known as the vomeronasal system. This paper proposes that it is this system that constitutes the receptor for homeopathic medicines in both animals and humans.

In 2001 a team in South Korea discovered a whole new dimension to what happens when a substance is dissolved in water and the resulting solution is further diluted.[101] Conventional wisdom says that the dissolved molecules simply spread further and further apart as a solution is diluted. But two chemists have found that some do the opposite: they clump together, first as clusters of molecules, then as bigger aggregates of those clusters. Far from drifting apart from their neighbours, they got closer together. The discovery could provide the first scientific insight into how some homeopathic medicines work.

In the last few years, the most radical challenge in the entire history of homeopathy has emerged with the emergence of a non-local causality hypothesis, based on 'entanglement theory'.[102,103] This combines two theories based on complexity theory and quantum mechanics.

Following consideration of various new models, Milgrom[104] has suggested that conventional medicine could be considered to be a special case of a broader therapeutic paradigm also containing homeopathy.

The HomBRex database indexes basic research on homeopathy (www.carstens-stiftung.de/hombrex).[105] It includes research on effects of homeopathic preparations in bioassays and physicochemical effects of the homeopathic preparation process (potentisation). At the end of 2006 it contained more than 1100 experiments in more than 900 original articles, including 1014 biological studies.

Audit, perception of benefit studies and case study collection

Audit

In the current climate of audit collection it is not surprising that homeopathy has begun to get its act together with respect to gathering data on outcomes. Proposals have been presented for Europe-wide data collection.[106] Data-gathering schemes have also been suggested in Germany.[107]

Thompson et al.[108] explored motivation for and expectation of hospital attendance from a patient perspective by administering a questionnaire to 110 consecutive patients attending Bristol Homeopathic Hospital outpatients and 20 parents of children with asthma and eczema. They found encouragement from doctors, self-motivation and word of mouth most motivated patients to come to the hospital

The Society of Homeopaths has also been involved in an audit of patients treated by practitioners registered by the Society.[109]

Mathie and Farrar[110] conducted a pilot data collection study, in which 14 homeopathic dentists collected clinical and outcome data over a 6-month period in their practice setting. The multi-practitioner pilot study indicated that systematic recording of practice data in dental homeopathy was both feasible and capable of informing future research.

Perception of benefit

A typical perception outcome study has been reported.[111] It involved patients being treated by homeopathic medicine at the Tunbridge Wells Homeopathic Hospital in England during 1997. The study aimed to assess, first, the range of diagnoses presented by patients and, second, patients' own impressions of benefit. A total of 1372 questionnaires were completed by patients, after their consultations, to record their impressions of the effects of homeopathic treatment. Patients were asked to score their responses on a +3 to −3 scale. The three main diagnostic groups were dermatology, musculoskeletal disorders and malignant disease, especially carcinoma of the breast. Overall, 74% of patients recorded positive benefits, with 55% recording scores of 3 or 2.

Case study collection

Detailed anecdotal information is usually called 'a case report'. To be acceptable these reports must be rigorously structured and not subject to journalistic enhancement.[112] There is a requirement for information on the disease and its extent, and information about any other patients who did not recover after being administered similar treatment. From an orthodox point of view such observations are interesting but do not necessarily mean that the next patient will respond in the same manner. Despite this several orthodox medicines, especially in the field of psychiatry, are administered on the basis of case studies, although the acceptability of such justification is often challenged by more orthodox colleagues. The case report is one of the chief sources of clinical knowledge for the homeopath. In teaching seminars the world over, most established teachers will present only cases that fulfil stringent quality criteria.[113] A good case brings the different parts together into a coherent narrative whereas in materia medicas and provings the information can feel jumbled and unconnected. Cases demonstrate the practical application of the principles of homeopathy direction of cure, prescribing strategies, potency choices, etc. By supplying cases, without details of medicines given, teachers of homeopathy have the perfect tool for modern 'problem-based learning'. There is a growing momentum in conventional medicine to recognise the value of patients' narratives.[114]

A Japanese study to investigate the effect of homeopathic treatment on 60 patients with chronic skin disease found that it provoked a good response, suggesting that it might be a useful strategy alongside conventional therapies.[115]

The collection of case studies has always been an important aspect of homeopathic practice. Several publications accept these, including the Faculty of Homeopathy Newsletter *Simile.*

Attitude and awareness studies

These studies provide important information on topics such as why people turn to homeopathy and how they obtain the necessary guidance on which medicines to purchase. The attitudes of providers of homeopathy are also important. Examples of such studies in the pharmacy environment have been provided.[116,117]

Materia medica

Examples of common medicines

In this abbreviated materia medica section some useful medicines are given with indications. The details given are not comprehensive.

Aconite Anxiety, distress, fear – almost terror – before and after receiving bad news. Aconite is also given at the first sign of a sneeze. It may be combined with other medicines in mixtures like ABC (Aconite, Belladonna and Chamomilla).

Arnica Mental and physical fatigue. Bruises, sprains and after accidents. Pre- and postoperatively. Pre- and post-childbirth.

Argent nit Feelings of fear and nervousness (but not terror), especially of an anticipatory nature. Exam nerves with gastrointestinal symptoms (often diarrhoea) and insomnia.

Arsen alb Effective for simultaneous diarrhoea and vomiting; when patient is chilly and restless.

Belladonna Burning, hot, flushed appearance. Tonsillitis, sore throat, earache. Generalised effects of sunstroke. Bursting headache. Sudden onset of symptoms.

Bryonia Joint pains that are worse on movement and with warmth (compare Rhus tox), better for pressure. Dry hacking cough.

Cantharis Burns, scalds, sunburn. Cystitis with burning feeling and frequent desire to urinate, hot, scalding urine. Gnat bites.

Chamomilla Teething in infants and for exceedingly irritable children who are quiet when carried.

Colocynth Colic (especially in infants), abdominal pain and other gastric upsets.

Euphrasia Allergic symptoms, especially red weepy eyes.

Ferrum phos First stage of head cold, croup, stiff neck.

Gelsemium Useful for influenza. Pre-exam nerves, when the mind goes blank.

Hamamelis Blood and crush injuries, especially those involving digits.

Ignatia Stress, especially following bereavement, nervous headaches.

Ipecacuanha Constant nausea not relieved by vomiting. Unproductive cough, with loose chesty rattle. Infantile diarrhoea with green-coloured stools.

Ledum Used to treat puncture wounds.

Nux vomica Effects of overeating and drinking. Indigestion, nausea constipation.

Pulsatilla Non-corrosive, thick, coloured catarrh that is better in the open air.

Rhus tox Rheumatic and arthritic conditions where symptoms are made worse by initial movement but improved with gentle continuing movement and the application of heat.

Ruta Soft-tissue injuries. May be combined with Rhus tox or Arnica.

Specialities In addition to the complexes for internal use, there are medicines on the market that might be called specialities – products that are usually produced by one manufacturer alone. Examples are Weleda UK's Combudoron gel for burns, scalds, sunburn, bites and skin rashes, and Nelson's insomnia medicine, Noctura. With the implementation of UK National Rules allowing homeopathic medicines to be registered with limited claims of effectiveness (based on bibliographic evidence of use), the range of these products in the UK is likely to expand.

Symphytum Assists in repair of bone injuries.

Repertory

In this section the process of counter prescribing has been greatly simplified: this will upset purists who resist the shortening of drug pictures in this way. However, this pragmatic approach, using polychrests, enables a relatively quick response to a request for treatment. Using a repertory style of presentation, appropriate choices can be made from Tables 7.5–7.14. Homeopathy has applications in the following:

- The initial treatment for simple self-limiting conditions (coughs, colds and flu) and for injuries (abrasions and soft-tissue injuries) and allergies (Tables 7.5–7.10)
- Allergies (Table 7.11)
- Dental surgery[118] – before and after treatment (Arnica) and for anxiety (Aconite or Argent nit: Table 7.12)
- Conditions associated with women (Table 7.13)
- Sports care – treating simple conditions and injuries in athletes (Arnica, Ruta: Table 7.14)
- First aid and travel (Table 7.15)
- Veterinary medicine (pets and farm animals) notwithstanding the limits on counter prescribing afforded by the Veterinary Surgeons Act 1961, which restricts diagnosis and treatment to veterinarians and owners (as there are no provings on animals, despite anatomical variances veterinary uses generally mirror human applications).

Tables 7.5–7.15 offer guidance on how to respond to requests for assistance in treating a number of common conditions. They are not meant to be comprehensive – there are many excellent repertories and prescribing guides[119] available – but will serve to illustrate what can be treated. The indications represent a highly abbreviated drug picture that highlights the most common uses for each of the medicines.

Table 7.5 Medicines used for colds and flu

Nasal symptoms	Other symptoms	Modalities	Comments	Medicine
Sneezing, congestion	Thirst	Worse in stuffy atmosphere	Initial stages of colds and flu	Aconite
Runny nose, sore nostrils	Streaming eyes – lacrimation bland	Better wrapped up	Treatment of colds	AGE[a]
Streaming coryza, sneezing	Streaming eyes, hot, thirsty, sore throat	Better for fresh air		Allium cepa
Sore red nostrils	Sore eyes 'aching bones'	Better for warmth	Treatment of flu	Gelsemium
Right nostril congested	Yellow nasal discharge, neuralgia	Better in open air	Pulsatilla	

[a]AGE is a combination of three remedies – Arsen iod, Gelsemium and Eupatorium.

Table 7.6 Medicines used for gastrointestinal problems

Condition	Symptoms	Modalities	Comments	Medicine
Colic	Severe abdominal cramps	Better from drawing up knees or bending double	May be associated with diarrhoea Infant colic	Colocynth
Colic	Abdominal pain, distension, wind		Infant colic and discomfort from teething	Chamomilla
Constipation	Stools hard, dry, thick and brown, nausea and thirst	Worse in the morning		Bryonia
Constipation	Frequent ineffectual straining; patient cold and irritable	Worse in the morning		Nux vomica
Diarrhoea	Colic, watery stool, flatulence, trembling	Better from warmth	Anxiety related ('exam nerves') Worried about failing exam	Argent Nit Gelsemium

Table 7.6 *Continued*

Condition	Symptoms	Modalities	Comments	Medicine
Diarrhoea	Rectal pain, small dark stools	Worse from cold	Food related	Arsen alb
Diarrhoea	'Explosive' frequent diarrhoea with flatulence	Better with gentle rubbing over hepatic region	With indigestion; common in children	Podophyllum
Indigestion	Belching and flatulence; cold sweat; nausea in morning	Worse in evening and from cold air	May be combined with Belladonna for irritable bowel syndrome	Carbo veg
Nausea	Accompanied by abdominal pain; retching	Better after stool passed	Associated with over-eating	Nux vomica
Nausea	Accompanied by vomiting		Morning sickness in pregnancy; also for motion sickness	Cocculus (Tabacum specific for sea sickness)

Table 7.7 Medicines used for coughs

Speed of onset	Symptoms	Modalities	Comments	Medicine
Slow	Hacking productive cough	Worse with change of atmosphere and after food	Best as cough mixture sipped slowly in warm water	Bryonia
Slow	Dry; long lasting	Worse at night and with exertion	Often after flu	Phosphorus
Steady	Spasmodic, dry and irritating	Worse at night in bed	Said to be associated with whooping cough	Drosera
Sudden	Wheezing cough with shortness of breath, nasal coryza	Worse at night especially when lying down		Ipecac
Sudden	Dry 'bark', headache	Worse with excitement and cold air Better from lying down		Spongia

Table 7.8 Medicines used for headaches

Speed of onset	Symptoms	Modalities	Comments	Medicine
Sudden	Bursting pain with flushed appearance	Better for lying down in dark room	May be caused by exposing head to cold	Belladonna
Gradual	'Blinding' headache	Better in open air	May follow eyestrain and emotional stress – students?	Natrum mur
Gradual	Splitting or crushing pain in occiput	Worse with warmth and motion	Patient irritable	Bryonia
Occasional	Throbbing pain	Worse when standing	May result from lack of food	Sulphur

Table 7.9 Medicines used for mental states

Condition	Symptoms	Modalities	Comments	Medicine
Fear terror	Bursting sensation in head	Worse in warm room	Will not go to the dentist; will not fly	Aconite
Anticipatory anxiety of event to come	Headache	Better for fresh air	Will do both of above but extremely unhappy	Argent nit
Worry about not performing well; failure of exams	Dry mouth, tremble	Worse when weather wet	Desire to be left alone	Gelsemium (also for agitated pets)
Grief	Crying; mood swings, headache	Worse from open air	Used for recent bereavement	Ignatia
Grief	Irritable, depressed, Headache	Better from open air	Ongoing effects of grief	Natrum mur

Table 7.10 Medicines used for skin conditions

Condition	Symptoms	Modalities	Comments	Medicine
Abrasions – superficial	Cuts, grazes, nappy rash Cold sores		Topical application Painful abrasions especially on fingers or toes	Calendula Hypercal[a] Hypericum
Acne, eczema	Rough dry skin, oozing sores Abscesses, suppurating and unhealthy skin Dry, scaly, itching and burning	Worse with warmth and at night Worse from exposure to cold winds Worse with scratching and washing with warm water	Topical or oral if skin broken	Graphites Hepar sulph Sulphur
Allergic response	Urticarial type skin rash	Worse from touch and scratching		Urtica
Boils	Abscesses, boils, cracks at end of fingers; coldness in extremities	Worse from washing	Has 'drawing' effect: expels foreign bodies from wounds	Silica
Burns	Burns and scalds Throbbing red rash	Better with rubbing Worse with touch	Sun burn	Cantharis Belladonna
Chilblains			Topical (ointment, cream or mother tincture) if skin unbroken; if skin broken oral as tablets, etc.	Tamus
Insect bites	Puncture wound – cold to the touch	Better with cold	Also rheumatism in feet	Ledum

Table 7.10 *Continued*

Condition	Symptoms	Modalities	Comments	Medicine
Insect stings	Histamine reaction	Worse with heat and touch	Also for oedema in extremities	Apis
Warts			As with Tamus above	Thuja

ª Hypercal is a mixture of the remedies Hypericum and Calendula.

Table 7.11 Medicines used for allergiesª

Symptoms	Symptoms	Modalities	Medicine
Bland lacrimation	Watery bland coryza	Worse in cold air – causes cough	Allium cepa
Acid burning lacrimation	Fluid watery coryza	Worse indoors and at night	Euphrasia
Heavy swollen eyes	Sneezing, watery coryza, sore throat	Worse in damp weather and with excitement	Gelsemium
Urticarial rash on skin	Profuse discharge	Worse from touch	Urtica

ª Isopathic remedies – allergodes and tautodes – may also be considered for the treatment of allergies and contact dermatitis.

Table 7.12 Medicines used in dentistry

Condition	Medicines to be considered
Anxiety, fear of dentist	Aconite, Argent nit
Preoperative	Arnica
Postoperative	Arnica, Calendula, Hypercal
Gum disorders	Merc sol
Mouth ulcers	Borax orally or Calendula mouthwash

Table 7.13 Medicines used for treating women

Condition	Symptoms	Modalities	Comments	Medicine to consider
Cystitis	Burning pains, frequent urge to urinate Constant involuntary 'dribble' especially when coughing or sneezing	Worse in the morning Worse in cool dry weather		Cantharis Causticum
Premenstrual syndrome	Breasts painful, irregular scanty periods, weepy Abdominal pain, cystitis, flatulence	Worse from heat and after eating Better by going to bed	Best in short and stoutish fair-skinned women who are affectionate Best for tall slim women with waxy skin who are lacking in affection	Pulsatilla Sepia
Heartburn	Indigestion and wind			Carbo veg
Insomnia	Difficulty in getting to sleep	Worse from cold and excitement	May be associated with toothache	Coffea
Morning sickness	Nausea with fainting and vomiting Nausea, heartburn and sore breasts	Worse with food or smoking Worse lying down		Cocculus Conium
Pregnancy: Before delivery After delivery	Anxiety To help recovery To help delivery To reduce bruising		Commence at around 35 weeks	Argent nit Arnica Caulophyllum Arnica

Table 7.14 Medicines or remedies useful for sportspeople

Condition	Symptoms	Modalities	Comments	Medicine to consider
Anxiety before competition	Worry, diarrhoea, sweating, dry mouth			Argent nit
Diarrhoea			From anxiety From excess or rich food	Argent nit Arsen alb
Muscle tiredness	Delayed onset muscle soreness		May be combined with Rhus tox	Arnica
Sprain	Ligament damage causing impaired movement	Better for warmth Better for cold		Rhus tox Bryonia
Strain	Soft tissue injury, pain		May be combined with Rhus tox and/or Arnica	Ruta
Tennis elbow	Painful elbow; detachment of muscular and tendinous fibres			Argent met

Table 7.15 Examples of medicines used in first aid and travel

Condition	Medicine	Form	Comments
Abrasions (superficial), scratches Antiseptic use	Calendula	Mother tincture Cream, ointment	Dilute with water Should not to be used topically for deep cuts
Allergies	Euphrasia Mixed pollens/grasses	Tablets, pills, granules Eyedrops (prescription only) Tablets, pills, granules	Particularly where red itchy watery eyes Use twice daily Depends on area visited *Other remedies available*
Anxiety (about travelling)	Argent nit (worry) Aconite (terror) Rescue Remedy	Tablets, pills, granules Tablets, pills, granules Liquid and spray	Start taking night before travel Start taking 2 days before travel Flower remedy

Table 7.15 *Continued*

Condition	Medicine	Form	Comments
Blood and crush injuries	Hypericum	Tablets, pills, granules Mother tincture diluted with water	Take every 10–15 min Do not use topically where severe injury
Bruising	Arnica	Mother tincture Cream, ointment and gel Tablets, pills, granules	May be diluted with water Apply topically When associated with general trauma, tiredness
Diarrhoea and vomiting	Arsen alb	Tablets, pills, granules	May need concurrent rehydation therapy Seek advice if lasts more than 2–3 days (especially in tropical climates)
Heat effects, headache and flushing with sudden onset	Belladonna	Tablets, pills and granules	Seek advice if persists
Indigestion, effects of over-eating and drinking	Nux vomica	Tablets, pills, granules	
Insect bites	Apis mel Ledum	Tablets, pills, granules Tablets, pills, granules Mother tincture diluted with water	Stings; surrounding area warm/hot Puncture wounds; cold to touch Apply topically
Insomnia	Coffea Passiflora	Tablets, pills, granules Tablets, pills, granules	Take before retiring; repeat if necessary
Jetlag	Arnica	Tablets, pills and granules	Take before, during and after flight as necessary
Motion sickness	Cocculus Petroleum Tabacum	Tablets, pills, granules Tablets, pills, granules Tablets, pills, granules	Air or car travel Associated with nausea and headache, Sea travel
Sore throat, mouthwash/gargle	Calendula	Mother tincture	Dilute with water
Sun burn	Belladonna Cantharis Urtica	Tablets, pills, granules Tablets, pills, granules Cream, ointment Tablets, pills, granules	Hot, flushed with headache; rash Hot burning skin Use topically to soothe skin Take orally if skin broken in place of topical

Veterinary use of homeopathy

There is an increasing demand from the public for homeopathic medicines to treat animals. Under the Veterinary Surgeons Act 1966, diagnosis and treatment of animals are restricted to veterinarians and owners. Pharmacists are able to advise on the availability of different items, but the final choice of medicine must always rest with the owner. If in doubt, the case should be referred to a veterinary practitioner.

Potential problems

Potential problems include the supply of nosodes that are used by homeopathic veterinarians against a variety of conditions, including kennel cough, leptospirosis and parvo. Owners who seek to protect their animals from disease by using homeopathic nosodes should not do so without obtaining professional advice from a suitably qualified veterinary surgeon. They should be reminded that insurance policies may be invalidated by not using orthodox immunisation programmes.

Registered homeopathic veterinary products

Under the Veterinary Regulations (renewed annually) provision was made for the registration of homeopathic veterinary products in the category. Authorised Veterinary Medicine – General Sales List (AVM-GSL) for non-food-producing animals. The use of registered homeopathic medicines was extended to food-producing animals as well as pets under the 2007 Regulations. A small range of products has been registered by a Scottish manufacturer.

As a result of the limited number of veterinary products available the common practice of owners using human homeopathic medicines to treat animals continues. Under a grandfather clause in the 2006 Veterinary Regulations products that were on the market before 1994 may be registered with the Veterinary Medicines Directorate (VMD) and placed on the market without further action. Details of all homeopathic veterinary medicines registered by the VMD may be found at http://tinyurl.com/23qmqa

If a fully registered homeopathic veterinary product exists then it must be supplied if prescribed, even if it is requested generically.

Unregistered products

A vet may use medicines 'off-label' under the 'prescribing cascade' subject to a strict hierarchy. These provisions apply to both orthodox and homeopathic practice:

• If there is no licensed veterinary medicine available for a particular condition or for use in a particular species similar veterinary products may be used.
• If there are no suitable veterinary products a human medicine may be prescribed.
• If no suitable human product is available a pharmacist or a vet may prepare the required medicine extemporaneously provided that they have the necessary expertise.

The biochemic tissue salts

The tissue salts are often included under the homeopathic umbrella, although their inventor insisted that they were quite separate from homeopathy.

Dr Wilhelm Heinrich Schüssler, a German homeopathic physician from Oldenburg, introduced a number of inorganic substances in low potency to his practice in 1872, and developed the idea of biochemic tissue salts. Proponents cite unhealthy eating practices that could lead to deficiencies of various salts considered to be vital for the healthy functioning of the body. It is argued that this situation may be corrected by taking tissue salts.

There are 12 single biochemic tissue salt medicines, together with some 18 different combinations. They are made by a process of trituration, each salt being ground down with lactose sequentially up to the sixth decimal potency (6x) level. The resulting triturate is then compressed directly into a soft tablet. Although most of the salts are soluble, there is no intermediate liquid stage, and surface inoculation is not used as it is thought to render the tissue salts ineffective. The tablet readily dissolves in the mouth, releasing fine particles of mineral material that can be absorbed into the bloodstream through the mucosa. The salts are often referred to by a number, from 1 to 12 in order of their names. They are listed in Table 7.16.

Table 7.16 Tissue salts and examples of their indications for use

Number	Tissue salt	Indication
1	Calc fluor	Maintain elasticity of tissues, for impaired circulation
2	Calc phos	Impaired digestion and teething
3	Calc sulph	Acne, pimples, sore lips
4	Ferr phos	Coughs, colds, chills
5	Kali mur	Respiratory ailments, children's fevers
6	Kali phos	Nervous exhaustion
7	Kali sulph	Catarrh, skin eruptions
8	Mag phos	Antispasmodic, neuralgia, flatulence
9	Nat mur	Watery colds, flow of tears, loss of smell or taste
10	Nat phos	Gastric disorders, heartburn
11	Nat sulph	Bilious attacks, flu. 'The liver salt'
12	Silica	Boils, brittle nails

For many ailments, more than one tissue salt is required. In order to simplify treatment there are a number of combination medicines containing three, four or five different salts, usually referred to by the letters A–S and given specific indications. For example, combination A contains Ferr phos, Kali phos and Mag phos, and is used for sciatica and neuralgia, and combination S contains Kali mur, Nat phos and Nat sulph, and is used for stomach upsets.

Homotoxicology

The brain child of German doctor Hans-Heinrich Reckeweg (1905–85) is also based on homeopathy. Drawing on a vast knowledge of herbal lore and medicines, Dr Reckeweg compounded a store of medicines that trod a line between folk medicine and basic plant pharmacology. Homotoxicologists endeavour to identify and treat the underlying toxic causes of ill health, rather than merely to suppress symptoms. The therapy is used widely in Germany but is less well known in the rest of the world.

Anthroposophy

Echoing the ancient Greek axiom 'Man, know thyself', Rudolf Steiner, the founder of anthroposophy, described it as 'awareness of one's humanity'. The Austrian-born Steiner (1861–1925) was the head of the German Theosophical Society from 1902 until 1912, at which time he broke away and formed his Anthroposophical Society. One of his main motives for leaving the theosophists was that they did not consider Christian teachings as special.[120]

Steiner's most lasting and significant influence has been in the field of education. In 1913 at Dornach, near Basel, Switzerland, Steiner built his *Goetheanum*, a 'school of spiritual science'.

Steiner designed the curriculum of his schools around his spiritual ideas and ascribed the following qualities to the living body:

- A life force that maintains the physical body functions
- An etheric body of non-physical formative forces, particularly active in growth and nutrition
- An astral body, particularly active in the nervous system
- A spiritual core or ego, reflected in a person's ability to change him- or herself inwardly.

Anthroposophical practitioners seek to understand illness in terms of the way in which these four elements interact. Anthroposophy embraces a spiritual view of the human being and the cosmos, but its emphasis is on knowing, not purely on faith.

Steiner's early experiments in Switzerland finally led to the founding of the Waldorf School Movement, which by 1969 had 80 schools attended by more than 25 000 children in the USA and Europe. Many other projects grew out of Steiner's work, including centres for handicapped children, schools of art, sculpture and drama, and research centres.

People who follow an anthroposophical way of life use antibiotics restrictively and have few immunisations, and their diet usually contains live lactobacilli, which may affect the intestinal microflora. In a cross-sectional study, 295 children aged 5–13 years at two anthroposophical (Steiner) schools near Stockholm, Sweden, were compared with 380 children of the same age at two neighbouring schools in terms of history of atopic and infectious diseases, use of antibiotics and immunisations, and social and environmental variables.[121] Prevalence of atopy was found to be lower in children from anthroposophical families than in children from other families. It was concluded that lifestyle factors associated with anthroposophy may lessen the risk of atopy in childhood. Rhythmical massage therapy is an important element of anthroposophic practice (Chapter 17).

Anthroposophical medicines

Great care is taken in collecting raw materials for preparing anthroposophical medicines.[122] Vegetable material is grown using methods of biodynamic farming, a development of organic practice in which the soil is fed to improve its structure and fertility. Soil additives are restricted to homeopathic medicines; all other hormones and chemicals are excluded. Due cognisance is taken of the natural cycles of the moon, sun and seasons. The first growth of plants is harvested and composted, and a second crop grown on the composted material. The process is repeated, and the third generation of plants is used to prepare the medicine. Manufacturers prefer to produce their own source material whenever possible. Weleda of Ilkeston, Debyshire, one of 26 Weleda companies worldwide, grows many medicinal plants in its extensive herb gardens. Anthroposophical pharmacy uses different temperatures during the manufacturing process according to the particular medicine involved. Aconite, said to exhibit the properties of coolness, is prepared at a lower temperature than Crataegus, a medicine acting on heart muscle and therefore active at body temperature. Anthroposophical practitioners believe that there is a link between warmth and the ego. Paying attention to temperature during preparation can be seen as helping to relate the medicines to human use. The medicines are extracted, diluted and used without potentisation, or prepared using the homeopathic process of serial dilution and succussion. Iscador, marketed by Weleda in the UK, is a mistletoe preparation used for cancer care. Its complex method of extraction involves mixing winter and summer sap. Drops of winter sap are added to a fine film of summer sap on a rapidly spinning disc; there is also a controlled fermentation process.

Although an anthroposophical prescription is often highly individualised, taking into account the physical and spiritual features of a patient, there are specifics, usually mixtures of several potentised medicines, that can be used in all patients to alleviate certain symptoms. There are treatments for bruises and sprains, burns, chilblains, constipation, indigestion and many other common ailments. Two examples are:

1.   Formica (red ant juice) and Bambusa (bamboo nodes), combined with either silver or tin, is indicated for a variety of acute or chronic back pain problems.
2.   Silicea comp. contains potencies of Silica (quartz), Belladonna (deadly nightshade) and Argent nit (silver nitrate) and is used to treat sinusitis.

Availability of anthroposophical medicine[123]

There are anthroposophical medical associations in at least 15 EU member states (Austria, Belgium, Czech Republic, Denmark, Estonia, Finland, Germany, Italy, Latvia, Netherlands, Poland, Romania, Spain, Sweden, the UK) as well as in other European countries. These account for more than 2000 trained medical practitioners. In addition anthroposophical medicines are prescribed by approximately 30 000 general medical practitioners and specialists.

Evidence

Evidence of successful outcome of treatment for anthroposophical medicine is sparse, although there are considerable anecdotal data. In a German study 18 unselected patients with chronic inflammatory rheumatic conditions, including 10 with confirmed rheumatoid arthritis, were treated according to anthroposophical principles in an open prospective uncontrolled pilot study with a mean follow-up period of 12 months.[124] Main outcome targets were local and systematic inflammation, subjective status and functional capacity. Treatment comprised a combination of Bryonia, Rhus tox, Apis, Formica and Vespa, individualised to each patient's requirements. There appeared to be a definite reduction in local and systemic inflammatory activity and an improvement in mental symptoms. These results must be considered to be of limited validity because the patients were self-selected, in that they asked to be treated using anthroposophical medicine, the numbers of patients were low and there was no double-blinding.

Anthroposophical physicians have prolonged consultations with their patients, taking an extended history, addressing constitutional, psychosocial and biographic aspects of patients' illness, and selecting optimal therapy. In Germany, health benefit programmes have included the reimbursement of this additional physician time. Patients treated by anthroposophical physicians after an initial prolonged consultation have been shown to enjoy a long-term reduction of chronic disease symptoms and improvement of quality of life.[125]

Further, in patients starting anthroposophical therapies for chronic disease, total health costs did not increase in the first year and were reduced in the second year.[126] This reduction was largely explained by a decrease of inpatient hospitalisation. Within the limits of a pre-post design, study findings suggest that anthroposophical therapies are not associated with a relevant increase in total health costs.

More information

Homeopathy

Faculty of Homeopathy & British Homeopathic Association (Administration)
15 Clerkenwell Close, London EC1R 0AA
Tel: 020 7566 7810
Fax: 020 7566 7815
Email: info@trusthomeopathy.org/faculty
Website: www.trusthomeopathy.org/faculty

Society of Homoeopaths
2 Artizan Road, Northampton NN1 4HU
Tel: + 44 1604 621400
Fax: + 44 1604 622622
Email: info@homeopathy-soh.org
Website: www.homeopathy-soh.org

Hom-Inform, British Homeopathic Library
Glasgow Homeopathic Hospital
1053 Great Western Road, Glasgow G12 0XQ
Tel: + 44 141 211 1617
Fax: + 44 141 211 1610
Email: hom-inform@dial.pipex.com
Website: www.hom-inform.org

Academic Department (AdHom) and Faculty of Homeopathy in
  Scotland
Glasgow Homeopathic Hospital, 1053 Great Western Road
Glasgow G12 0XQ
Tel: + 44 141 337 1824
Fax: + 44 141 211 1610
Email: carolanderson@dial.pipex.com
Website: www.adhom.org

Anthroposophy

Anthroposophical Society of America
1923 Geddes Ave, Ann Arbor, MI 48104–1797, USA
Tel: + 1 734 662 9355
Fax: + 1 734 662 1727
Email: Information@anthroposophy.org
Website: www.anthroposophy.org

Allgemeine Anthroposophische Gesellschaft
Goetheanum Postfach 134, CH-4143 Dornach, Switzerland
Tel: + 61 706 4242
Fax: + 61 706 4314
Email: wochenschrift@goetheanum.ch
Website: www.goetheanum.ch

Rudolf Steiner Library
65 Fern Hill Rd, Ghent NY 12075, USA
Tel: + 1 518 672 7690
Fax: + 1518 672 5827
Email: rsteinerlibrary@taconic.net
Website: http://rslibrary.elib.com

Further reading

Edmunds F. *An Introduction to Anthroposophy: Rudolf Steiner's world view*,
    updated edn. London: Rudolph Steiner Press, 2005.
Kayne SB. *Homeopathic Pharmacy*, 2nd edn. Edinburgh: Elsevier Churchill
    Livingstone, 2005.
Kayne SB, Kayne LR. *Homeopathic Prescribing*. London: Pharmaceutical Press,
    2007.
Kayne SB, ed. *Homeopathic Practice*. London: Pharmaceutical Press: 2008.

National Library for Health, CAM Specialist Library. *Homeopathy Annual Evidence Update*. Available at: http://tinyurl.com/6pttk7.
The Annual Evidence Update on Homeopathy aims to identify, organise and present the most up-to-date evidence on this topic. Searches in a large number of databases are carried out. The searches aim to identify all relevant systematic reviews and randomised controlled trials published during the previous year.
Owen D, ed. *Principles and Practice of Homoeopathy: The therapeutic and healing process*. Edinburgh: Elsevier Health Sciences, 2007.

References

1. Hahnemann CS. *Organon of the Rational Art of Healing*. Dresden: Arnold, 1810.
2. Hahnemann CS. Versuch uber ein neues Prinzip zur Auffindung der Heilkerafte der Arzneisubstanzen. *Hufland's J* 1796;**2**:2, 3 (translated into English by RE Dudgeon) London: Lesser Writings, 1852: 295–352.
3. Ruusuvuori J. Comparing homeopathic and general practice consultations: the case of problem presentation. *Commun Med* 2005:123–35. PubMed
4. Belon P. Provings. Concept and methodology. *Br Homeopath J* 1995; **84**:213–17.
5. Dellmour F, Jansen J, Nicolai T et al. *The Proposal for a Revised International Nomenclature System of Homeopathic Medicines and their Abbreviations*. Brussels: European Committee for Homeopathy, 1999.
6. Guajardo G, Bellavite P, Wynn S et al. Homeopathic terminology: a consensus quest. *Br Homeopath J* 1999;**88**:135–41.
7. BAHM. *British Homeopathic Pharmacopoeia* (BHomP), vol. 1. Ilkeston, Derbyshire: BAHM, 1993.
8. BAHM. *British Homeopathic Pharmacopoeia* (BHomP), vol. 1, 2nd edn. Ilkeston, Derbyshire: BAHM, 1999.
9. Kayne SB. *Homeopathic Pharmacy – An introduction and handbook*. Edinburgh: Churchill Livingstone, 1997: 57.
10. Kayne SB, Kayne LR. *Homeopathic Prescribing*. London: Pharmaceutical Press, 2007: 14.
11. Isbell W, Kayne SB. Potentization – just a myth? *Br Homeopath J* 1997; **86**:156–60.
12. Schulte J. Effects of potentisation in aqueous solutions. *Br Homeopath J* 1999;**88**:155–60.
13. Chaplin MF. The memory of water: an overview. *Homeopathy* 2007; **96**:43–150
14. Schmolz M. Thin-layer chromatography in electrophoresis of homeopathic single medicines. *Biomed Ther* 2000;**18**:202–3.
15. Bourneman JP, Field RL. Regulation of homeopathic products. *Am J Health-Syst Pharm* 2006;**63**:86–91.
16. Food, Drug, and Cosmetic Act of 1938, Pub. L. 103–417, 52 Sta. 1041 (1938), as amended and codified in 21 U.S.C. §321(g)(1) (1938).
17. Beattie N, Kayne SB. The treatment of allergies with isopathy. *Br Homeopath J* 2008;in press.

18. Julian O. *Materia Medica of New Homoeopathic Medicines*. Beaconsfield: Beaconsfield Publishers, 1979.
19. Jonas WB. Do homeopathic nosodes protect against infection? An experimental test. *Altern Ther Health Med* 1999;**5**:36–40.
20. European Coalition on Homeopathic and Anthroposophic Medicinal Products. *Homeopathic and Anthroposophic Medicines in Europe – Facts and figures*. Brussels: ECHAMP, 2007: 91.
21. Ernst E. Towards quality in complementary health care: is the German 'Heilpraktiker' a model for complementary practitioners? *Int J Qual Hlth Care* 1996;**8**:187–90.
22. Campbell A. The origins of classical homeopathy? *Compl Ther Med* 1999;**7**:76–82.
23. Dantas F, Rampes H. Do homeopathic medicines provoke adverse effects? A systematic review. *Br Homeopath J* 2000;**89**(suppl 1):S35–8.
24. Barnes J. Complementary medicine: homoeopathy. *Pharm J* 1998;**260**:492–7.
25. Montoya-Cabrera MA, Rubio-Rodriguez S, Velazquez-Gonzalez E, Montoya SA. Intoxicacion mercurial causada por un medicamento homeopatico. *Gac Med Mex* 1991;**127**:267–70.
26. Wehner-Caroli J, Scherwitz C, Schweinsberg F, Fierbleck G. Exazerbation einer Psoriasis pustulosa bei Quecksilber-intoxikation. (Pustular psoriasis with exacerbation from mercury toxicity.) *Hautarzt* 1994;**45**:708–10.
27. Clement RT. Lead, mercury, and arsenic in complex homeopathic medicines and child safety. *Townsend Lett* 1998;**176**:102–3.
28. Grabia S, Ernst E. Homeopathic aggravations; a systematic review of randomised, placebo controlled trials. *Homeopathy* 2003;**92**:92–8.
29. Cuesta Laso LR, Alfonso Galán MT. Possible dangers for patients using homeopathy: may a homeopathic medicinal product contain active substances that are not homeopathic dilutions? *Med Law* 2007;**26**:375–86. PubMed
30. Whitmarsh T. The complexities of homeopathic prescribing or how do we decide to do what we do? *Homeopathy* 2007;**96**:71.
31. Kent JT. *Repertory of the Homeopathic Materia Medica*, 2nd edn. London: Homeopathic Book Service, 1986.
32. Murphy R. *Homeopathic Medical Repertory*, 2nd edn. Pagosa Springs, CO: Hahnemann Academy of North America, 1998.
33. Phatak SR. *Concise Repertory of Homeopathic Medicines*, 2nd edn. Bombay: Homeopathic Medical Publishers, 1977.
34. Schroyens F. *Synthesis*, 7th edn. London: Homeopathic Book Publishers, 1998.
35. Kayne SB, Kayne LR. *Homeopathic Prescribing*. London: Pharmaceutical Press, 2007: 38.
36. ECHAMP. *Homeopathic and Anthroposophic Medicines in Europe – Facts and Figures*. Brussels ECHAMP, 2007: 11–13.
37. Furnham A, Bond C. The perceived efficacy of homeopathy and orthodox medicine: a vignette-based study. *Compl Ther Med* 2000;**8**:193–201.
38. Kayne SB, Beattie N, Reeves A. Self-treatment using homeopathic medicines bought over-the-counter (OTC) in a sample of British pharmacies. *Br Homeopath J* 2000;**89**(suppl 1):S50.

39. Kayne SB, Usher W. Homeopathy – attitudes and awareness amongst pharmacy clients and staff in New Zealand. *NZ Pharm* 1999;**19**:32–3.

40. Walach H, Magic of signs a non-local interpretation of homeopathy. *Br Homeopath J* 2000;**89**:127–40.

41. Stevinson C, Dearer VS, Fountain-Barber A, Hawkins S, Ernst E. Homeopathic arnica for prevention of pain and bruising: randomized placebo-controlled trial in hand surgery. *J R Soc Med* 2003;**96**:60–5.

42. Walach H. Entanglement model of homeopathy as an example of generalised entanglement predicted by weak quantum theory. *Forsch Komp Klass Natur* 2003;**10**:192–200.

43. Ernst E. The demise of homoeopathy? *Pharm J* 2000;**264**:66.

44. Ernst E. Should we use 'powerful placebos?' *Pharm J* 2004;**273**:795.

45. Kayne SB, Kayne LR. Misleading. (Letter) *Pharm J* 2000;**264L**:94.

46. Mathie RT, Kayne LR. Unbalanced opinion. (Letter) *Pharm J* 2004;**273**:815.

47. Bellavite P, Signorini A. Is homeopathy effective? In: *Homeopathy. A frontier in medical science*. Berkeley, CA: North Atlantic Books, 1995: 37–55.

48. Ernst E, Hahn EG, eds. *Homeopathy. A critical approach*. Oxford: Butterworth-Heinemann, 1998.

49. Kayne SB. *Homeopathic Pharmacy – An introduction and handbook*. Edinburgh: Churchill Livingstone, 1997: 164–7.

50. Linde K, Scholz M, Ramirez G et al. Impact of study quality on outcome in placebo-controlled trials of homeopathy. *J Clin Epidemiol* 1999;**52**:631–6.

51. Walach H, Jonas WJ, Ives J, van Wijk R. Weingärtner O. Research on homeopathy: State of the art. *J Altern Compl Med* 2005;**11**:813–29.

52. *Chambers Dictionary*. Edinburgh: Chambers Harrap, 2000.

53. Shapiro AK. A contribution to a history of the placebo effect. *Behav Sci* 1960;**5**:109–35.

54. Turner JA, Richard AD, Loeser JD et al. The importance of placebo effects in pain treatment and research. *JAMA* 1994;**271**:1609–14.

55. Hashish I, Feinman C, Harvey W. Reduction of post operative pain and swelling by ultrasound: a placebo effect. *Pain* 1988;**83**:303–11.

56. Benson H, McCallie DP. Angina pectoris and the placebo effect. *N Engl J Med* 1979;**300**:1424–8.

57. Diamond EG, Kittle CF, Crockett JF. Comparison of internal mammary artery ligation and sham operation for angina pectoris. *Am J Cardiol* 1960;**5**:483–6.

58. Mitchell A, Cormack M. *The Therapeutic Relationship in Complementary Health Care*. Edinburgh: Churchill Livingstone, 1998:80.

59. Gibson RG, Gibson SI, MacNeill AD, Watson-Buchanan W. The place for non pharmaceutical therapy in chronic rheumatoid arthritis: a critical study of homoeopathy. *Br Homeopath J* 1980;**69**:121–33.

60. Reilly DT, Taylor MA. Potent placebo or potency? A proposed study model with initial findings using homeopathically prepared pollens in hayfever. *Br Homeopath J* 1985;**74**:65–75.

61. Reilly DT, Taylor MA, McSharrry C, Aitchison TC. Is homeopathy a placebo response? Controlled trial of homeopathic potency with pollen in hayfever as model. *Lancet* 1986;**ii**:881–8.

62.   Taylor MA, Reilly D, Llewellyn-Jones RH et al. Randomised controlled trial of homoeopathy versus placebo in perennial allergic rhinitis with overview of four trial series. *BMJ* 2000;**321**:471–6.

63.   Reilly D. Is homeopathy a placebo response? What if it is? What if it is not? In: Ernst E, Hahn E G (eds), *Homeopathy – A critical approach*. Oxford: Butterworth-Heinemann, 1998: Chapter 8.

64.   Linde K, Clausius N, Ramirez G et al. Are the clinical effects of homoeopathy placebo effects? A meta-analysis of placebo-controlled trials. *Lancet* 1997;**350**:834–43.

65.   Jonas W, Kaptchuk TJ, Linde KA. Critical review of homeopathy. *Ann Intern Med* 2003;**138**:393–9.

66.   Ernst E, Pitler MH. Efficacy of homeopathic arnica: A systematic review of placebo and controlled clinical trials. *Arch Surg* 1998;**133**:1187–90.

67.   O'Meara S, Wilson P, Bridle C, Wright K, Kleijnen J. Homoeopathy. *Qual Safety Hlth Care* 2002;**11**:189–94.

68.   Stevinson C, Devaraj VS, Fountain-Barber A, Hawkins S, Ernst E. Homeopathic arnica for prevention of pain and bruising: randomized placebo-controlled trial in hand surgery. *J R Soc Med* 2003;**96**:60–5.

69.   Brinkhaus B, Wilkens JM, Lüdtke R, Hunger J, Witt CM, Willich SN. Homeopathic arnica therapy in patients receiving knee surgery: results of three randomised double-blind trials. *Compl Ther Med* 2006;**14**:237–46.

70.   Datta S, Mallick P, Khuda Bukhsh AR. Efficacy of a potentized homoeopathic drug (Arsenicum Album-30) in reducing genotoxic effects produced by arsenic trioxide in mice: Comparative studies of pre-, post- and combined pre- and post-oral administration and comparative efficacy of two microdoses. *Compl Ther Med* 1999;**62**:75.

71.   Fisher P, Greenwood A, Huskisson EC, Turner P, Belon P. Effect of homeopathic treatment on fibrositis. *BMJ* 1989;**299**:365–6.

72.   Kleijnen J, Knipschild J, ter Riet G. Clinical trials of homoeopathy. *BMJ* 1991;**302**:316–23.

73.   Linde K, Melchart D. Randomized controlled trials of individualized homeopathy: a state-of-the-art review. *J Altern Compl Med* 1998;**4**:371–88.

74.   Walach H, Haeusler W, Lowes T et al. Classical homeopathic treatment of chronic headaches. *Cephalalgia* 1997;**17**:119–26.

75.   Hart O, Mullee MA, Lewith G, Miller J. Double blind placebo-controlled randomised clinical trial of homeopathic arnica C30 for pain and infection after total abdominal hysterectomy. *J R Soc Med* 1997;**90**:73–8.

76.   Ernst E, Barnes J. Are homeopathic medicines effective for delayed-onset muscle soreness? A systematic review of placebo-controlled trials. *Perfusion* 1998;1 4–8.

77.   Whitmarsh T, Coleston-Shields DM, Steiner TJ. Double blind randomised placebo-controlled trial of homeopathic prophylaxis of migraine. *Cephalalgia* 1997;**17**:600–4.

78.   Beer A-M, Heiliger F, Lukanov J. Caulophyllum D4 to introduction of labour in premature rupture of membranes – a double blind study confirmed by an investigation into the contraction activity of smooth muscles. *FACT* 2000;**5**:84–5.

79. Mathie RT. The research evidence base for homeopathy: a fresh assessment of the literature. *Homeopathy* 2003;**92**:84–91

80. Jacobs J, Jiminez LM, Gloyd SS et al. Treatment of acute childhood diarrhea with homeopathic medicine: a randomized clinical trial in Nicaragua. *Pediatrics* 1994;**93**:719–25.

81. Jacobs J, Jimenez LM, Malthouse S, *et al.* Homeopathic treatment of acute childhood diarrhea: results from a clinical trial in Nepal. *J Altern Compl Med* 2000;**6**:131–9.

82. Tveiten D, Bruseth S, Borchgrevink CF, Norseth J. Effects of the homoeopathic medicine Arnica D30 on marathon runners: a randomized, double-blind study during the 1995 Oslo Marathon. *Compl Ther Med* 1998;**6**:71–4.

83. Taylor MA, Reilly D, Llewellyn-Jones RH et al. Randomised controlled trial of homoeopathy versus placebo in perennial allergic rhinitis with overview of four trial series. *BMJ* 2000;**321**:471–6.

84. Papp R, Schuback G, Beck E et al. Oscillococcinum in patients with influenza-like syndromes: a placebo-controlled double-blind evaluation. *Br Homeopath J* 1998;**87**:69–76.

85. Stam C, Bonnet MS, van Haselen RA. The efficacy and safety of a homeopathic gel in the treatment of acute low back pain: a multi-centre, randomised, double-blind comparative clinical trial. *Br Homeopath J* 2001;**90**:21–8.

86. Balzarini A, Felisi E, Martini A, De Conno F. Efficacy of homeopathic treatment of skin reactions during radiotherapy for breast cancer: a randomised, double-blind clinical trial. *Br Homeopath J* 2000;**89**:8–12.

87. Chapman EH, Weintraub RJ, Milburn MA et al. Homeopathic treatment of mild traumatic brain injury: A randomized, double-blind, placebo-controlled clinical trial. *J Head Trauma Rehabil* 1999;**14**:521–42.

88. de Lange de Klerk ES, Blommers J, Kuik DJ et al. Effect of homoeopathic medicines on daily burden of symptoms in children with recurrent upper respiratory tract infections. *BMJ* 1994;**309**:1329–32.

89. Savage RH, Roe PF. A double blind trial to assess the benefit of *Arnica montana* in acute stroke illness. *Br Homeopath J* 1977;**66**:207–20.

90. Kainz JT, Kozel G, Haidvogl M, Smolle J. Homoeopathic versus placebo therapy of children with warts on the hands: a randomized, double-blind clinical trial. *Dermatology* 1996;**193**:318–20.

91. Bornhoft G, Wolf U, von Ammon K et al. Effectiveness, safety and cost-effectiveness of homeopathy in general practice. *Forsch Komplementärmed* 2006;**13**(suppl 2):19–29.

92. Shang A, Huwiler-Müntener K, Nartey L, Jum P et al Are the clinical effects of homeopathy placebo effects? Comparative study of placebo-controlled trials of homeopathy and allopathy. *Lancet* 2005;**366**:726–32.

93. McGuigan M. Hypothesis: do homeopathic medicines exert their action in humans and animals via the vomeronasal system? *Homeopathy* 2007;**96**:113–19.

94. Vithoulkas G. Homeopathic experimentation: the problem of double blind trials and some suggestions. *J Complement Med* 1985;**1**:10–15.

95. Singh PPP, Chabra HL. Topological investigation of the ethanol/water system and its implications for the mode of action of homeopathic medicines. *Br Homeopath J* 1993;**82**:164–71.

96. Davenas EE, Beauvais F, Amara J et al. Human basophil degranulation triggered by very dilute antiserum against IgE. *Nature* 1988;**333**:816–18.

97. Maddox J, Randi J, Stewart WW. 'High-dilution' experiments a delusion. *Nature* 1988;**334**:287–90.

98. Ovelgönne JH, Bol AW, Hop WC, van Wisk R. Mechanical agitation of very dilute antiserum against IgE has no effect on basophil staining properties, *Experientia* 1992;**48**:504–8.

99. Hirst SJ, Hayes NA, Burridge J, Pearce FL Foreman JC. Human basophil degranulation is not triggered by very dilute antiserum against human IgE. *Nature* 1993;**366**:525–7.

100. Teixeira J. Can water possibly have a memory? A sceptical view. *Homeopathy* 2007;**96**:158–62.

101. Coughlan A. Bizarre chemical discovery gives homeopathic hint. *Chemical Communications*, 2001: 2224. Available at: http://tinyurl.com/cdbjf (accessed April 2008).

102. Fisher P. Entangled, or tied in knots? (Editorial) *Homeopathy* 2004; **93**:171–2.

103. Milgrom LR. Journeys in the country of the blind: entanglement theory and the effects of blinding on trials of homeopathy and homeopathic provings. *Evid Based Compl Altern Med* 2007;**4**:7–16.

104. Milgrom LR. Toward a unified theory of homeopathy and conventional medicine. *J Altern Compl Med* 2007;**13**:759–69.

105. Van Wijk R, Albrecht H. Classification of systems and methods used in biological basic research on homeopathy. *Homeopathy* 2007;**96**:247–51.

106. Haselen van R, Fisher P. Describing and improving homeopathy. *Br Homeopath J* 1994;**83**:135–41.

107. Heger M. Prospective documentation in homoeopathic practice – an essential contribution to quality assurance. *Hom Int Res Dev News Lett* 1998;**2**:3–18.

108. Thompson E, Dahr J, Susan M, Barron S. Setting standards in homeopathic practice – A pre-audit exploring motivation and expectation for patients attending the Bristol Homeopathic Hospital. *Homeopathy* 2007;**96**:243–6.

109. Relton C, Chatfield K, Partington H, Foulkes L. Patients treated by homeopaths registered with the Society of Homeopaths: a pilot study. *Homeopathy* 2007;**96**:87–9.

110. Mathie RT, Farrer S. Outcomes from homeopathic prescribing in dental practice: a prospective, research-targeted, pilot study. *Homeopathy* 2007;**96**:74–81.

111. Clover A. Patient benefit survey: Tunbridge Wells Homoeopathic Hospital. *Br Homeopath J* 2000;**89**:68–72.

112. Ernst E Anecdotal obsessions? A comment on the use of anecdotes by the general media to support claims in CAM. *Compl Ther Nurs Midwifery* 2004;**10**:254–5.

113. Dr Massimo Mangialavori's website, Cases and articles. Available at http://tinyurl.com/288owf (accessed 8 November 2007).

114. Greenhalgh T, Hurwitz B. Why study narrative? *BMJ* 1999;**318**:48–50.

115. Itamura R. Effect of homeopathic treatment of 60 Japanese patients with chronic skin disease. *Compl Ther Med* 2007;**15**:115–20.

116. Alton S, Kayne SB. A pilot study of the attitudes and awareness of homeopathy shown by patients in three Manchester pharmacies. *Br Homeopath J* 1992;**81**:189–93.

117. Davies M, Kayne SB. Homeopathy – a pilot study of the attitudes and awareness of pharmacy staff in the Stoke-on-Trent area. *Br Homeopath J* 1992;**81**:194–8.

118. Varley P. What do homeopathic dentists do? *Homeopathy* 2007;**96**:72–3.

119. Kayne SB, Kayne LR. *Homeopathic Prescribing*. London: Pharmaceutical Press, 2007.

120. *The Skeptics Dictionary*. Available at: http://skepdic.com/steiner.html (accessed 3 June 2008).

121. Alm JS, Swartz J, Lilja G et al. Atopy in children of families with an anthroposophic lifestyle. *Lancet* 1999;**353**:1485–8.

122. Evans M, Rodger I. *Anthroposophical Medicines*. London: Thorson, 1992.

123. ECHAMP. *Homeopathic and Anthroposophic Medicines in Europe – Facts and figures*. Brussels: ECHAMP, 2007: 92.

124. Simon L, Schietzel T, Artner CG et al. An anthroposophical treatment design for inflammatory rheumatic conditions. *J Anthroposoph Med* 1997; **14**:22–40.

125. Hamre HH, Witt CM, Glockmnan A, Ziegler R, Willich SN, Kiene H. Anthroposophic medical therapy in chronic disease: a four-year prospective cohort study. *BMC Compl Altern Med* 2007;**7**:10. Available at: http://tinyurl.com/ynkx67 (accessed 8 November 2007).

126. Hamre HH, Witt CM, Glockmnan A, Ziegler R, Willich SN, Kiene H. Health costs in anthroposophic therapy users: a two-year prospective cohort study. *BMC Health Serv Res* 2006;**6**:65. Available at: http://tinyurl.com/277ubw (accessed November 2007).

8

Medical herbalism

Steven B Kayne

Introduction

Only the medical aspects of herbalism are considered in this chapter, leaving aside the cosmetic applications – creams, bath additives and hair care products, to name just a few examples. Some authorities would say that the inherent 'feel good factor' associated with the use of such products could be considered to be a positive activity that promotes a significant health benefit and there may be some merit in this argument. Another psychological benefit may accrue from the process of growing herbs, as well as taking them medicinally or using them to make food more interesting and palatable. In his book entitled *The Therapeutic Garden*, Donald Norfolk,[1] an osteopath, suggests that gardening is the oldest of the healing arts and says that the 'high-tech' medical profession recognises that the sick and despairing respond to gardens. The fact that postoperative patients recover sooner if they are given a view of grass and trees has led to demands to revive the old tradition of hospital gardens.

The body of knowledge about plants, herbs and spices, and their respective and collective roles in promoting human health, is modest.[2] Dietary compounds and their roles in maintaining human health and interactions with established nutrients require much investigation.

Herbal medicines are becoming increasingly popular with the public:

- They are readily available from health stores and pharmacies, as well as from other specialist outlets.
- They are often highly effective.
- They provide clients with the means to self-treat a range of conditions for which orthodox over-the-counter (OTC) medicines are limited or unavailable.
- As they are 'naturally occurring', herbal medicines are perceived as being free of side effects, and in some cases complementary to

western or orthodox medicines. Unfortunately these latter two beliefs are not entirely true because there is evidence to the contrary in a number of well-researched circumstances, necessitating the observance of caution, particularly when self-treating.

Definition

Quite simply medical herbalism may be defined as the practice of using products in which all active ingredients are of herbal origin to treat the sick.[1] In practice rather more detail is required. According to the World Health Organization (WHO) Guidelines, herbal medicines are considered to be:[3]

> Plant-derived materials or products with therapeutic or other human health benefits which contain either raw or processed ingredients from one or more plants. In some traditions materials of inorganic or animal origin may also be present. (page 6)

The European Directive defines a herbal medicine thus:[4]

> A substance or combination of substances of herbal origin presented for treating or preventing disease or with a view to making a medical diagnosis or to restoring, correcting or modifying physiological functions.

Yet another definition is provided by the UK Medicines Act 1968, (Section 132), much of which has now been superseded by pan-European Union legislation:

> A 'herbal medicine' is a medicinal product consisting of a substance produced by subjecting a plant or plants to drying, crushing or any other process, or of a mixture whose sole ingredients are two or more substances so produced, or of a mixture whose sole ingredients are one or more substances so produced and water or some other inert substances.

This definition underlines the belief that products comprising both herbal and non-herbal ingredients (e.g. minerals) are generally not considered to be herbal medicines in the West.

The term 'phytotherapy' was suggested by Henri Leclerc (1870–1955) who published numerous essays on the use of medicinal plants in the French journal *La Presse Médicale*.

History

The exact origins of herbalism are unknown. Probably it was several different groups of prehistoric peoples who discovered that some herbs were good to eat, whereas others had curative powers. Humans also discovered plants with peculiar, reality altering, stimulating and inebriating effects. In ancient cultures these were considered to be 'plants of the gods'. Ingesting them could lead to contact with the realms of the gods and demons, their ancestors or various other forces of nature not normally visible. Some of these plants had interesting side effects – many were considered to be aphrodisiacs, awakening sexual desire and increasing pleasure.[5] But we must turn our attentions to more mundane matters!

The opium poppy, *Papaver somniferum*, is perhaps the earliest medicinal plant, being well known in ancient Greece.[6] Hippocrates mentions the use of poppy juice as a cantharic, hypnotic, narcotic and styptic. Pliny the Elder indicates the use of the seed as hypnotic and the latex as an effective treatment for headaches, arthritis and curing wounds. The smoking of opium was not noted until much later; it was extensive in China and other countries in the Far East in the latter part of the eighteenth century.

The mechanism of action of herbs remained a mystery for centuries – and in some cases still remains a mystery. Only the development of sophisticated techniques of chemical analysis in the last century has begun to provide some of the answers. Those who took a special interest in the healing powers of herbs, acquiring a special knowledge and skill, came to enjoy an honoured place in society.

The earliest medicine men assumed a link with religion, believing that their powers were divinely granted. The first medical records date from ancient Assyria, China, Egypt and India.

William Turner was the first person to study plants scientifically in the sixteenth century. He travelled widely throughout Europe and grew plants in his gardens in south-west London (later the Royal Botanical Gardens, Kew). At this time the Doctrine of Similars determined how plants were used. It was promoted by Paracelsus (1493–1541). According to this paradigm every plant acted in effect as its own definition of its medical application, resembling either the part of the body afflicted or the cause of the affliction. Nicholas Culpepper (1616–54) was an influential proponent of the Doctrine of Signatures as well as various astrological theories, by which herbs were set under the domination of the sun, moon or one of the five planets then known. His herbal, published in 1652, was extremely successful, being reprinted many times.

Subsequently, the apothecaries, who had acquired healing skills in addition to merely selling herbs, took over. A number of physic gardens were set up to produce important medicinal herbs under controlled conditions to ensure an uninterrupted supply.

By the end of the eighteenth century the heyday of herbalism was passing, but an interest was still maintained. Plants were classified and studied carefully. Expeditions were mounted to uncharted territories to collect new species that could be used medicinally. Several important discoveries were made including digoxin from the foxglove and quinine from cinchona bark.

In America the name of Samuel Thomson (1769–1843) deserves attention.[7] Samuel is usually referred to as being a medical doctor in the literature. This does considerable credit to the man who enjoyed but one month's schooling in his life. Thomson's practice involved using simple herbs for bodily correction. He was so successful that opposition from the medical profession was strong and uncompromising. They succeeded in prosecuting him, but his name was cleared and he became universally recognised as an outstanding figure in the medical world. His fame spread to England where, thanks to the promotion by a Mr George Lees, the Thomsonian system (Figure 8.1) was embraced by

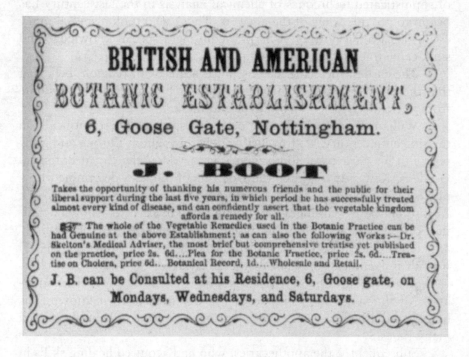

Figure 8.1 Advertisement.

Mr Jesse Boot when he opened the first of what was to become the UK's biggest multiple pharmacy chain, in Goose Gate, Nottingham in 1872.

Renewed interest in 'natural' medicines has led to a resurgence of demand for herbal medicines in the last 20 years.

Theory[8]

Traditionally, the herbalist has recognised four clear stages when offering treatment for any particular condition, individualising the prescription according to holistic methodology to take account of their patients' particular needs:

1. Cleansing the body: removal of toxins and other noxious influences – real or imagined – that might cause a physical or mental barrier to treatment. Diuretics, expectorants and laxatives are involved here.
2. Mobilising the circulation: traditionally disease was seen as a 'cold' influence on the body and before any other treatment the body should be comforted by 'heating agents'. Hot spices and pungent medicines (e.g. ginger) and more gentle warming medicines are available for this purpose. Hot spicy food prompts gastric defence against enteric infections in the tropics.
3. Stimulating digestion: inappropriate or too much heat in the body manifests itself as fevers and inflammatory conditions. Thus, the so-called 'cooling medicines' are those used to treat these circumstances, leading to improved digestion. Anti-inflammatories, anti-allergics and sedatives are examples of therapeutic classes of drugs that fall into this category.
4. Nourishment and repair: in this phase the herbalist deals with the debility arising from disease in the body. The term 'tonic' covers a wide range of medicines used to support the body. Examples include hawthorn (*Crataegus oxycanthoides*), milk thistle (*Silybum marianus*) and St John's wort (*Hypericum perforatum*).

There is a tendency in modern herbalism (as in homeopathy) to skip this measured approach and seek a medicine that deals with local problems rather than the body as a whole. This has been called, perhaps unkindly, a 'fire-fighting' approach. In part this has been fuelled by the growing OTC market, which has produced a number of medicines labelled for use in specific conditions, making it easy for the seller and buyer alike. Therapists claim that this approach goes against the principles of complementary practice. On the other hand, the public seem to be satisfied that the medicines that they buy work in many situations, otherwise they would have voted with their feet – in the opposite direction – long ago. There is no doubt that long-term chronic conditions do need the considered approach offered by qualified practitioners.

Sources of reference

Having carried out an extended consultation common to all complementary disciplines, the following texts are used routinely by herbal practitioners to facilitate the choice of medicine (see Further reading):

- Materia medica: a comprehensive list detailing the main characteristics and uses of medicines, e.g. *Potter's Cyclopaedia of Botanic Drugs*
- Repertory: a comprehensive list of medical conditions with suggested medicines for treatment, e.g. *Herbal Medicine* by Miller and Murray
- The *British Herbal Pharmacopoeia* gives identification and usage information as well as providing instructions on how medicines should be prepared and the *British Herbal Compendium* provides up-to-date summaries of the available scientific knowledge on medicinal plants (http://tinyurl.com/2cy66z)
- The *American Herbal Pharmacopeia* (www.herbal-ahp.org) began developing qualitative and therapeutic monographs in 1994, and intends to produce 300 monographs on botanicals, including many of the ayurvedic, Chinese and western herbs most frequently used in the USA. Once completed, these monographs represent the most comprehensive and critically reviewed body of information on herbal medicines in the English language, and will serve as a primary reference for academicians, healthcare providers, manufacturers and regulators.

Herbal medicines

The use of herbals as a source for drugs

Many of the plants used in modern herbal preparations contain active ingredients the effects of which can be pharmacologically demonstrated. For some OTC products in particular the situation is complicated by the frequent use of drugs in 'polypharmaceutical' combinations. In these circumstances prescriptions are often empirical, resulting from clinical observation and experience rather than scientific deduction.

The main reasons for the attraction of using herbal source material are:

- the long periods of experience with traditional medicines
- the many isolated constituents found in modern drugs
- the large pool of plant material available, particularly important in developing countries
- profit for pharmaceutical companies – a wish for 'part of the action' in many cases in response to customer demand.

Differences between herbal and orthodox medicine

- Use of whole plant: herbalists believe that giving an extract from a whole plant rather than using active principles in isolation (when known) allows them to take advantage of a synergism that is believed to exist between the various constituents. There are some cases where the synergistic effect of the herb might be more helpful than giving an isolated agent. There is also some evidence that the active ingredients in certain whole herbs (e.g. glycyrrhizic acid from liquorice) are absorbed differently from when extracted in pure form, and thus the whole herb might be less dangerous than a particular extract.
- Combination of medicinal herbs: herbalists tend to use mixtures of herbs to treat different aspects of a disease in order to exhibit the individualistic therapy demanded by using a holistic approach to medicine. It is true to say that in orthodox medicine it is usual for patients to be given extra drugs during the progression of their disease (e.g. patients with diabetes may be given antihypertensives and diuretics in addition to hypoglycaemic drugs), but initially 'polypharmacy' is not viewed sympathetically. This practice also disagrees with Hahnemann's view of a single medicine in homeopathy.
- Although orthodox drugs are synthetic, homogeneous and standardised, herbals are naturally occurring and extracted, heterogeneous and, in many cases, non-standardised.
- Diagnosis: herbal treatments are often symptomatic in their approach, whereas most orthodox practitioners tend to seek a diagnosis on the basis that if one can treat the cause of a disease the symptoms will resolve naturally.

General types of medicinal herbs used

Practitioners use medicinal plants with:

- powerful actions, e.g. liquid extracts of foxglove and belladonna, with substantial toxic risk
- intermediate actions, e.g. tinctures of arnica and khella, with some adverse drug reactions (ADRs)
- gentle actions, e.g. infusions of German camomile and peppermint with less risk of ADRs.

In many instances conditions can be treated by drugs in each of the three groups, e.g. cardiac disease responds to foxglove in the powerful group, arnica in the intermediate group and hawthorn in the gentle group. Herbal medicines for nervous diseases include opium in the powerful group, St John's wort in the intermediate group and valerian in the gentle group. Examples of the main therapeutic groups of herbal medicines are summarised in Table 8.1. Some medicines (including garlic and ginger) have wide spectra of activity and may be considered as being equivalent in some respects to the homeopathic polychrests.

Active constituents in herbal medicines[9,10]

Herbal medicines contain a bewildering array of chemicals. In this section the most frequently occurring types to be found in common herbs are mentioned.

Table 8.1 Examples of the therapeutic use of herbal remedies

Therapeutic group	Example of herbal remedy
Anticoagulants	Alfalfa, arnica, fucus, garlic, ginger
Coagulant	Mistletoe
Cardioactive	Coltsfoot, devil's claw, ginger, ginseng, parsley, wild carrot
Diuretic	Burdock, dandelion, elder, juniper, pokeroot, squill
Hyperglycaemic	Devil's claw, ginseng, liquorice
Hypoglycaemic	Alfalfa, garlic, ginger, juniper, marshmallow, myrrh
Hypolipidaemic	Alfalfa, garlic, ginger
Hypertensive	Blue cohosh, coltsfoot, gentian, ginger, liquorice
Hypotensive	Celery, devil's claw, fucus, garlic, ginger, St John's wort
Sedative	Camomile, hops, passionflower, St John's wort, valerian

General classes of constituents

Bitters Traditionally these were used extensively to stimulate appetite (i.e. in the final fourth stage of the healing process outlined above). It is now thought that they will be effective only if a malnourished state exists. The bitter constituents simulate the bitter receptors in the taste buds at the back of the mouth and give rise to an increase in the psychic secretion of gastric juice. The most effective chemicals are the monoterpene secoiridoid glycosides of gentian. Other extracts that have been used as bitters include quassia, quinine (Cinchona) and strychnine (Nux vomica).

The 'hot' medicines The three most commonly used 'hot' medicines include black pepper (*Piper nigrum*), cayenne pepper (*Capsicum*) and ginger (*Zingiber*). They are used as metabolic stimulants, more specifically as a 'facilitating agent' to accompany other herbs whose stimulatory activity may be augmented.

Resins The term 'resin' is applied to the sticky water-insoluble substance of complex chemical nature often exuded by the plant, soon hardening to protect an injury. The constituents include resin acids, resinols, resin tannols, esters and chemically inert compounds known as resenes. On heating resins soften and eventually melt. Resins are usually produced by the plant in ducts or cavities, but may also be found in special cells elsewhere, e.g. in elements of the heartwood of guaiacum and the internal cells of the male fern. The term may also be applied to that part of a plant that is soluble in ether or alcohol (e.g. guaiacum resin and kava resin).

Resins are used as astringents and antiseptics of the mouth and throat and have also been applied to inflammatory conditions of the upper digestive tract.

Propolis, a product collected by bees from resinous plants, is used in herbal medicine, although it is not strictly herbal in nature. The product is also used in homeopathy.

A 'balsam' (e.g. balsam of Peru and balsam of Tolu) is an oleoresin containing a high proportion of aromatic balsamic acid.

Saponins Saponins are glycosides that produce frothy aqueous solutions. Plants containing these compounds (e.g. *Quillaia saponaria*) have been used for centuries as gentle detergents. Decoctions of soapwort (*Saponaria*) have been used to wash and restore ancient fabrics. They also have haemolytic properties and when injected into the bloodstream are highly toxic. When taken by mouth saponins appear to be comparatively harmless. Sarsaparilla is rich in saponins but is widely used in the preparation of non-alcoholic drinks.

Two distinct types of saponins may be recognised. The steroidal saponins are of great pharmaceutical importance because of their relationship to compounds such as the sex hormones, cortisone and the cardiac glycosides. Some species of the yam (*Dioscorea* spp.) and potato (*Solanum* spp.) contain steroidal saponins.

The second group of saponins is known as the pentacyclic triterpenoid saponins. This includes quillaia bark and liquorice root (*Glycyrrhiza*). The former is used as an emulsifying agent, the latter as a flavouring agent, demulcent and mild expectorant.

Tannins   This is not a specific phytochemical group but a name for a group of chemicals that have a particular characteristic. The term 'tannin' was first applied by Seguin in 1796 to denote substances present in plant extracts that were able to combine with animal proteins in the hides, preventing putrefaction and converting them to leather. Most tannins have molecular masses (Mr) of about 1000–5000 and many are glycosides.

Tannin-producing drugs will precipitate protein and have been used traditionally externally as styptics, and for burns and weeping eczema, and internally for the protection of inflamed surfaces of the mouth and throat. They are also claimed to be antioxidants. Witch-hazel (*Hamamelis virginiana*) is a tannin-containing drug used principally for its astringent properties.

Volatile oils   Volatile oils are dealt with in greater detail in Chapter 9 which explains the medical use of aromatherapy.

As the name suggests volatile oils are volatile in steam. They differ widely in both chemical and physical properties from fixed oils. They are secreted in oil cells, in secretion ducts or cavities, or in glandular hairs, and are frequently associated with gums and resins.

With the exception of oils derived from glycosides (e.g. bitter almonds and mustard oil), volatile oils are generally mixtures of hydrocarbons and oxygenated derivatives mainly responsible for odour and taste. In some oils (e.g. oil of turpentine) the hydrocarbon portion dominates whereas in others (e.g. oil of cloves) the opposite is true.

Volatile oils are used in perfumery and cosmetics (e.g. oil of rose, oil of bergamot), in food flavourings (e.g. oil of lemon) as well as in medicine.

Many oils with a high phenolic content (e.g. clove and thyme) have antiseptic properties, whereas others are used as carminatives. Oils showing antispasmodic activity include peppermint (*Mentha piperita*) and camomile (*Matricaria chamomilla*).

Phytochemical groups of constituents

Alkaloids   Alkaloids show great variation in their botanical and bio-chemical origin, chemical structure and pharmacological action. Consequently a precise definition is difficult. Typical alkaloids are basic, contain one or more nitrogen atoms, and have a marked physiological action on humans and animals.

Coumarins   Coumarins are benzo-α-pyrones generally with a hydroxyl or methoxy group in position 7. They are often associated with glyco-sides. Simple coumarins have a pleasant odour, variously described as being like 'new-mown hay' or vanilla. The widespread nature of coumarins – they have been found in about 150 different species – means that they are consumed by humans, being present in carrots, celery and parsnip. Simple substituted coumarins are used as pigments in sunscreens.

Flavonoids   Flavonoids consist of a single benzene ring joined to a benzo-γ-pyrone structure. They are widespread in herbal material functioning as plant pigments and being responsible for the colours of flowers and fruit. Although the name is derived from 'flavus', meaning yellow, many of the pigments are in fact blue, purple, red and white.

About three-quarters of the 2000 types are known as glycosides, the balance being aglycones. According to the state of oxygenation derivatives include flavones, flavonols and flavonones.

Glycosides   Glycoside is a term that covers many different combina-tions comprising a monosaccharide part (e.g. fructose or glucose) and a non-sugar part, which may be a simple phenol, flavonoid, anthraquinone, triterpenoid or other structure, known as 'aglycone'. It is this last part that determines the therapeutic characteristics.

Some glycosides may occur as anthraquinones, reduced derivatives, anthranols and anthrones; the last occur either free or combined as glycosides.

Cardiac glycosides contain deoxysugars (e.g. cyamarose) as the sugar part of their molecules. Cardiac glycosides from the foxglove (*Digitalis purpurea*) and lily of the valley (*Covalleria majalis*) both act on the heart, increasing the contractile force and speed of the cardiac muscle.

Polysaccharides   Polysaccharides are polymers based on sugars and uronic acid. They are found in all plants, especially as a component of the cell wall. Some plants accumulate polysaccharides (e.g. *Aloe vera*).

Polysaccharides are thought to have an important role as immunoenhancing agents (e.g. Echinacea)

The preparation and presentation of herbal medicines

The medicines are made according to standards quoted in the appropriate pharmacopoeias, e.g. *British Herbal Pharmacopoeia*. Herbal medicines may be administered as crude drugs or extracts. The latter include infusions, decoctions and cold aqueous macerates that can be freshly prepared by the consumer. There are also liquid extracts, tinctures and solid and dry extracts that are industrially produced.

Solid dose forms and topical preparations in which herbal ingredients have been incorporated are also available.

Crude drugs

Crude drugs are still widely available both commercially and from professional medical herbalists. They are extracted by the consumer as an infusion if the herbs are of a light fleshy nature or as a decoction if fibrous and woody (roots and barks). The extraction process is outlined below. The advantages are that the extraction is freshly prepared and is particularly appropriate for herbs with active constituents that need to be given hot.

Infusions and decoctions

Infusions   This is the preferred method of extracting fresh active ingredients from light leafy herbs. The drug may be extracted alone or in the form of a herbal tea, of which there are simple (e.g. camomile, peppermint) and more complex varieties with more than one active principle and a number of excipients. They are convenient when the active constituents are water soluble.

The extraction process for infusions

- Plants containing aromatic oils, e.g. anise, fennel and juniper fruit, should be crushed or 'bruised'; other plants should be finely chopped or minced.
- Pour 150–200 ml boiling water over the herbal material and allow to stand for 10–30 min; if the material contains volatile oils it should not be boiled; infusions made from drug material that does not include volatile oils (e.g. hawthorn) may be simmered on a low flame for an additional 5 min or so.
- Strain and take in divided doses during day of preparation.

The herbal tea

Commercially available medicinal teas are ready formulated for the consumer and are usually prepared freshly as an infusion before taking. They contain the following constituents:[11]

- The remedium cardinale: one or more basic medicinal agents, e.g. a laxative tea may contain senna leaves and frangula bark.
- The adjuvans: one or more auxiliary medicines that enhance the action of the basic medicine or reduce undesirable side effects. Thus, drugs with carminative (anise, caraway or fennel) and/or spasmolytic properties (camomile flowers, silverweed) may reduce unwanted side effects of senna.
- The constituens, corrigens and colorants: fillers and aesthetic agents to improve aroma, appearance, colour or texture. Up to 20% of the tea may be a filler (e.g. raspberry leaves) which prevents it from separating into its components. To ensure concordance, herbal teas must be reasonably palatable; this is especially important for children. Widely used excipients include bitter orange peel, orange blossom, hibiscus flowers and peppermint leaves. Colorants such as cornflower, mallow and marigold are also used.

Decoctions Roots and barks may be extracted using a decoction method:

- Pour about 200 ml cold water over the prescribed amount of finely divided botanical material and allow to simmer at around 30°C for about 30 min.
- Cool, strain and take on day of preparation.

Liquid extracts

Strengths Traditionally practitioners have used liquid extracts as the preferred method of administering herbal medicines, despite their unpalatable bitter taste in many instances. The strength of a liquid is usually expressed as a ratio. Thus a 1:5 ratio means that 5 ml of the final liquid preparation is equivalent to 1 g of original dried herb. Liquid preparations weaker than 1:2 are usually called 'tinctures', whereas 1:1 and 1:2 preparations are called 'extracts'. Tinctures are usually made by maceration and extracts by percolation.

Use of liquids Although liquid extracts are still used widely and are relatively easy to make, because of worries over inconsistent quality there has been a move towards 1:5 tinctures, with doses of 2.5–5 ml three times daily. In other countries herbalists use much smaller doses – 15–20 drops of a diluted tincture is not uncommon in the USA. The manufacturing process for tinctures and liquid extracts does differ, principally in that no heat and stronger alcohol are involved in the preparation of the former. Calculating an equivalent dose may be difficult because it is likely that there could be some variance in the active constituents.

The extraction processes

Cold water extracts

Macerates

Occasionally extracts are made at room temperature because of a high starch content (e.g. marshmallow root) or to improve tolerance (e.g. bearberry leaves).

- Place minced material in cold water and leave to stand for 8 hours with occasional stirring.
- Strain and bring to the boil briefly to kill any bacterial contamination before allowing to cool and taking.

Extraction with solvent under vacuum

- Percolate or macerate chopped-up drug using appropriate solvent
- Evaporate under vacuum.

More permanent preparation

Alcoholic tinctures

Used for resins and volatile oils:

- Made by extracting material with varying strengths of alcohol solvent
- Strained and strength adjusted
- Elegant and long-lasting preparation.

The strength of alcohol used for the extraction process is important. An investigation into the extraction of volatile oil from camomile plants found that 55% alcohol (ethanol) was the optimum strength.[12] Another worker has found that 40–60% alcohol provided the best range for extracting a range of different herbs.[13]

Other extracts   The following extracts are occasionally seen:

- Solid extracts are pastes made by evaporating expressed juice or liquid extract.
- Dry extracts are solid extract dried under vacuum.

The practice of medical herbalism

Supply of herbal medicines

The UK law relating to the sale and supply of OTC herbal medicines (section 12.2 of the Medicines Act 1968) has now been replaced by the European Directive on Traditional Herbal Medicinal Products of the European Parliament (2004/24/EC) and of the Council of 31 March 2004 amending (available at http://tinyurl.com/2w9nfw). This establishes a registration scheme for industrially produced OTC herbal medicines, under which manufacturers have to demonstrate safety and quality, but not efficacy. The first five products were registered under the scheme in October 2007. A further 13 products including Echinacea, St John's Wort and Valerian were registered in the next ten months.

The European Directive allows an exemption for herbal medicines made up by practitioners after a personal consultation. Further advice on the Traditional Herbal Medicines Registration Scheme is available at the UK Medicines and Healthcare products Regulatory Agency (MHRA) site at http://tinyurl.com/26yhf6. The rules also apply to Chinese herbal medicines (see Chapter 12).

The herbal practitioner

The herbal practitioners' activities are covered by Part III of the Supply of Herbal Medicines Order 1977, which lists medicines that may be used in the surgery during a consultation. There are special exemptions through the terms of the Medicines Act 1968 (Sections 12(1) and 56(2)). Conditions that need to be satisfied include the following:

- The practitioner must supply medicines from premises (apart from a shop) in private practice 'so as to exclude the public'.
- The maximum permitted dose must not be exceeded for a list of certain medicines.
- The practitioner must exercise his personal judgement in the physical presence of the patient before prescribing treatment.
- For systemic treatment medicines are subject to a maximum dose restriction. All labelling on internal medicines must clearly show the date, correct dosage and instructions for use.
- Proper clinical records must be kept.
- Herbal practitioners often prepare their own tinctures, using ethanol for which registration with Customs and Excise is required.

It has been recommended in a report by a Department of Health steering group that there is an urgent need to proceed with the statutory regulation of practitioners of herbal medicine and other traditional medicine systems.[14] The primary reasons for this recommendation are to safeguard the public by allowing removal of failing practitioners from the statutory register and to enable informed choice by those who wish to access these forms of treatment. The group also recommended that the supply of herbal medicines to individual patients, without the need for a marketing authorisation, should be limited to those on the statutory register.

Training of herbalists

Prospective members of the National Institute for Medical Herbalists (NIMH), a professional body that accredits training courses, are expected to follow a programme of academic study (normally 3–5 years' duration) and to complete a minimum of 500 hours of clinical training.

Schools and universities offering courses in herbal medicine must apply to the board and pass through the accreditation procedure to enable their graduates to become practising members of the NIMH. Each course must reach the minimum standards as set out in the accreditation board's guidelines. Core subjects studied include: anatomy, physiology, pathology, diagnosis, pharmacology, pharmacognosy, botany, materia medica, communication skills and complementary medicine, as well as nutritional and herbal therapeutics. Critical skills and research methodology are also required. Clinical practice is supervised by experienced practitioners.

Applications of herbalism

A wide range of conditions respond to treatment and/or management with herbal medicines. They may be used alone or to complement other orthodox or non-orthodox treatments. Some of the most common conditions are listed below. The list is not meant to be exhaustive. It is designed to give some idea of the scope of what may be achieved. For further detailed information the reader is referred to the excellent text by Mills and Bone from which the following is adapted:[15]

Generalised conditions
Autoimmune conditions
Acute inflammation of muscles, joints and connective tissues
Psoriasis and other skin conditions

Debility
Chronic fatigue syndrome
Fatigue and debility after illness
Fatigue linked to depression
Support during terminal illness

Fevers
Fevers resulting from infectious causes
Febrile symptoms of non-infectious origin

Infectious disease
Unlike homeopathy, i.e. not directly effective on body invaders, herbalism may be used in these circumstances. The following conditions respond:
Acute gastrointestinal, respiratory, and urinary infections

Topical bacterial infections
Minor-to-moderate febrile infections
Minor-to-moderate chronic bacterial, fungal and viral infections

Malignant diseases
Cancers of varying types
Symptoms resulting from cancer
Problems with body systems

Cardiovascular system
Hypertension
Angina
Ongoing symptoms of cardiac disease
Patients with heart disease are reported to benefit from treatment with herbal medicine with fewer side effects[16]

Gastrointestinal (GI) system
Dyspepsia, GI reflux
Food intolerance and allergies
Constipation and diarrhoea
Genitourinary system
Urinary tract infections
Benign prostate hypertrophy
Impaired lactation

Menopausal problems
Premenopausal syndrome (PMS)

Nervous system
Anxiety states
Insomnia
Nervous exhaustion
Pain control
Stress symptoms

Respiratory system
Upper respiratory tract infections
Allergic rhinitis
Bronchitis
Asthma

Skin diseases
Acne
Allergic reactions
Eczema.

Herbalism and pharmacy

Most pharmacists are likely to become involved with herbalism through the sale of OTC products that are pre-packaged and labelled with indications and instructions. The Royal Pharmaceutical Society of Great Britain (RPSGB) has produced a factsheet on herbal products that gives useful information. It notes that pharmacists supplying herbal products have a professional responsibility not to recommend any product where they have any reason to doubt its safety or quality, and only to offer advice on herbal products if they have appropriate knowledge. Whenever possible only licensed products should be offered for sale.

It is possible to dispense herbal preparations extemporaneously in response to requests for assistance similar to homeopathic counter prescribing. There is a small, but growing, market for dispensing herbal prescriptions. Figures 8.2 and 8.3 show an orthodox and herbal practice in Dunedin, New Zealand

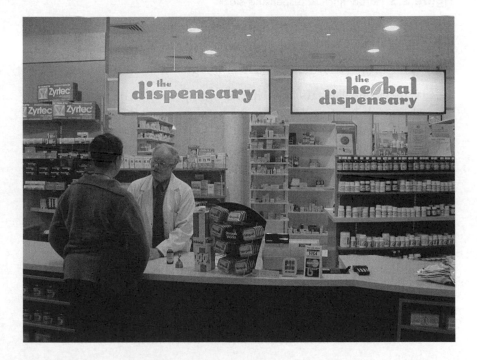

Figure 8.2 Integrating orthodox and herbal pharmacy at the Meridian Pharmacy, Dunedin, New Zealand.

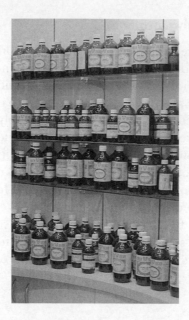

Figure 8.3 Herbal tincture dispensing stock.

When to consider herbalism

Herbal medicine is particularly useful in two situations:

1. Where a well-established herbal compound is being used for a short, self-limiting condition such as a cold or the flu; when other OTC medicines would normally be appropriate, the course of treatment is no more than a couple of weeks, and no serious adverse effects have been reported in the scientific literature. An example of this would be the use of Echinacea to ward off or reduce the effects of a cold or ginger to prevent motion sickness.
2. In the case of a more serious or ongoing illness, where no effective orthodox treatment exists and where there is some evidence from the scientific literature that a particular herbal compound may help. In this kind of situation, it is extremely important that the person be under the close supervision of a physician well versed in the disease in question and who has reviewed the available studies on the herb to be used. An example of this latter situation would be the use of milk thistle extract in the treatment of cirrhosis of the liver.

As a result of all of the problems with dosage, testing and the presence of toxins in herbs, there is an understandable temptation to rely on conventional pharmaceuticals in the OTC environment. However, herbs remain one of the few inexpensive sources of treatment for a number of conditions. *Ginkgo biloba* appears to be one of the only compounds that is claimed to improve memory (as opposed to stimulants, which improve concentration only). It may even slow the progression of Alzheimer's disease. Milk thistle is one of only a handful of compounds that may actually reverse liver damage. Herbs remain the primary medicinal agents for most people in developing countries – most of the world's population.

Presentation of OTC products

Oral dose forms

The availability of herbal specialities in elegant OTC pharmaceutical presentations as tablets or capsules (Figure 8.4) provides a quick and easy way of self-treating. An important advantage is that palatability is greatly improved. However, they do not allow the same flexibility to change the dose regimen as liquid or crude drug formulations. Furthermore, it has been suggested that the substantial amount of processing required in making tablets and capsules may cause some denaturation of the active herbal principles. In addition, as they usually contain purified ingredients, the synergistic effect will be lost.

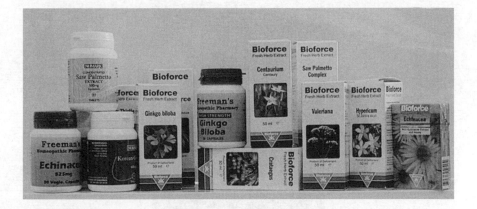

Figure 8.4 Examples of common branded and generic over-the-counter herbal products.

Powdered drugs have a substantial therapeutic advantage in that all the active constituents are included in the dose form rather than just those obtained during the extraction process (Figure 8.5). Drugs containing tannins are best given as a powder because tannins are only slowly dissolved from the herb matrix and are therefore still being released in an active form when the powdered herb reaches the colon.[17] It is important to give instructions to consume water along with or after ingestion, depending on the nature of the medicine being taken.

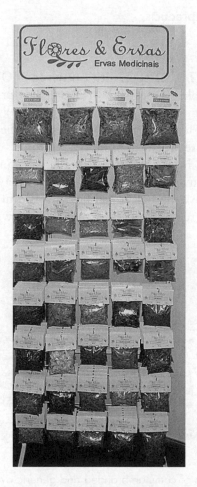

Figure 8.5 Display of powdered drugs for over-the-counter supply (Brazil).

Topical products

A wide range of topical products is available over the counter. These include creams, gels, lotions and ointments. There have been some problems with adulteration of Chinese herbal ointments (see 'Safety issues').

Applications for topical formulations   Conditions that may be treated with topical herbal preparations include the following:

• Burns
• Infestations
• Minor wounds and skin abrasions
• Oral inflammatory conditions
• Rheumatic conditions
• Skin eruptions
• Soft tissue injuries – muscular sprains and strains.

Examples of the therapeutic classes of topical medicines

Demulcents

These are herbs with a soothing effect to the skin. Aloe vera, marshmallow (*Althaea*) and slippery elm bark (*Ulmus fulva*) are examples of mucilages that form the basis of creams and poultices.

Anti-inflammatories

Marigold (*Calendula officinalis*) and camomile (*Matricaria chamomilla*) both possess anti-inflammatory properties and are used to treat skin inflammations. Echinacea is another example (Figure 8.6). Knitbone (*Symphytum officinale)* is also claimed to be effective. In an open, uncontrolled study, 105 patients with locomotor system symptoms were treated twice daily with an ointment containing a Symphytum active substance complex.[18] A clear therapeutic effect was noted on chronic and subacute symptoms that were accompanied mainly by functional disturbances and pain in the musculature. The preparation was effective against muscle pain, swelling and overstrain. Activity was weaker against degenerative conditions, for which the ointment may have an adjuvant role with the aim of improving muscular dysfunction and alleviating pain.

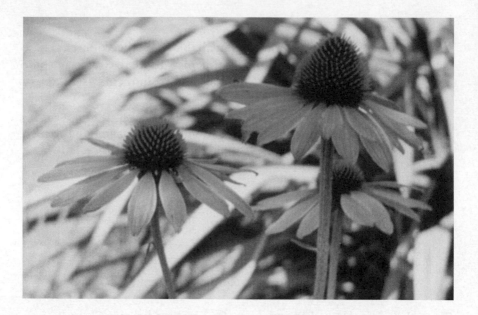

Figure 8.6 *Echinacea purpurea*, often called the 'herbal antibiotic'.

Antiseptics and disinfectants[19]

This section has been expanded to give the reader an example of just how many herbal medicines may be available for a given application. Furthermore, most of the chapter has been with reference to European herbs; in this section some examples of the plethora of traditional herbs from the native Antipodean communities are included.

Antiseptic literally means 'against putrefaction' or 'prevention of sepsis' but the term is usually used to describe agents applied to living tissues in order to destroy or inhibit the growth of infectious microorganisms. Disinfectants kill pathogenic agents and usually involve inanimate surfaces. Some naturally occurring medicines possess antimicrobial effects, and are effective in topical formulations as antiseptics and disinfectants.

Although the bacterial origin of infection was unknown before Pasteur's work in Paris, and Lister's work in the 1860s at Glasgow Royal Infirmary, antiseptics and disinfectants have been used empirically since the ancient Egyptians started embalming bodies.

What follows is a review of the most common 'natural' (i.e. non-synthetic) antiseptics and disinfectants that have been traditionally used in some communities of the northern and southern hemispheres. Many have no apparent scientific explanation for their action, but are nevertheless still in use, relying on the users' cultural traditions for maintaining a belief in efficacy.

- Bilberry (*Vaccinium myrtilus*): also known as huckleberry, the bilberry is related to the blueberry and cranberry. The fruit contains 7% tannic acid and a blue pigment, and is used, occasionally with the leaves, in an antiseptic mouthwash, together with the roots of the anti-inflammatory herb Tormentilla (*Potentilla* spp.). The latter contains 15–20% tannic acid and a red pigment and is used as an infusion on cuts, wounds, abrasions and sunburn.
- Blackcurrant (*Ribes nigrum*): this aromatic perennial shrub was formerly used in folk medicine as an infusion or gargle to treat sore throats. It is not considered to be of great medical importance now.
- Burnet saxifrage (*Pimpinelia saxifraga*): this herb is native to Europe, but has been introduced and naturalised in New Zealand and the USA. It may be used as a gargle or, externally, as a poultice or bath to treat wounds.
- Herb bennet (*Geum urbanum*): it can be applied to wounds to reduce inflammation and used as a gargle for sore gums and halitosis. It is rarely used now, except in folk medicine.
- Horsetail (*Equisetum arvense*): horsetail or 'bottlebrush' is native to Europe and thrives on moist waste ground. It contains silicic acid and a number of water-soluble silicic compounds, and is used in poultices to aid wound healing. A mild antiseptic. It is useful for eczemas.
- Hops *(Humulus lupulus)*: native to northern temperature zones, hops are best known for their involvement in brewing. A weak antibiotic, they have been used for urinary infections, and also occasionally as an application for skin conditions.
- Juniper (*Juniper communis*): juniper is applied externally to wounds and, with garlic, rosemary and Echinacea, it is used in poultices. Also used internally as a urinary antiseptic, especially in cystitis.
- Marjoram, wild (*Organum vulgare*): native to Europe, although now cultivated elsewhere, the herb grows on hillsides and in dry woodland; it has an aromatic scent. May be used externally in baths, inhalants or poultices where an antiseptic action is required.
- Nettle, stinging (*Urtica dioica*): a major ingredient of the oil is formic acid, with varying amounts of histamine, chlorophyll, iron,

plant enzymes and minerals. In the stinging hairs there is a nettle poison. Popular as an external application.

- Peppermint (*Mentha piperita*): one of the oldest and best-known European medicinal herbs, peppermint is said to produce a 'gentle disinfectant effect' (preventing fermentation) when there are abnormal decomposition processes in the stomach. Both the herb and its oil may be used externally in baths to treat cuts and skin rashes. The oil contains about 50% menthol.
- Savory, summer (*Satureja hotyrndid*): most commonly used as a culinary herb, but also possesses medicinal properties, and is an effective antiseptic gargle. Winter savory (*Satureja montana*) has similar properties.
- Sage, common (*Salvia officinalis*): it has been used as the constituent of a gargle, together with acriflavine and benzocaine. Another effective mixture is to bring equal parts of camomile flowers and sage leaves to the boil with milk, leaving the mixture to infuse, covered; it can then be used as an antiseptic mouthwash.
- Silver birch (*Betula pendula*): this deciduous tree can grow up to 20 m in height, and is common throughout central and northern Europe. The infusion is said to be a diuretic, whereas the buds and leaves may be added to bathwater to obtain a mild antiseptic action.
- Speedwell, common (*Veronica officinalis*): speedwell is still listed in the herbal materia medica, but its efficacy is uncertain; it was included in cough mixtures as a weak expectorant with some antiseptic properties.
- Tea tree oil (*Melaleuca alternifolia*): tea tree leaves contain about 2% of a pale, lemon-coloured, volatile oil with a strong nutmeg odour. The oil comprises about 60% terpenes and has germicidal activity. A study has found the oil to be effective in vitro against *Staphylococcus aureus*.[20] Tea tree oil should not be confused with tea oil, the sweet seasoning and cooking oil from pressed seeds of the tea plant.
- Thyme, garden (*Thymus vulgaris*): garden thyme is widely used as a culinary herb, being cultivated since the sixteenth century. The German apothecary Neuman first isolated the plant's essential oil in 1725 and this powerfully antiseptic substance is still used in pharmaceutical preparations. The oil contains up to 40% thymol. It also has rubefacient properties.
- Thyme, wild (*Thymus serpyllum*): herb baths and pillows. Used as poultice with onion, myrrh and melilot.

- Wormwood (*Artemesia absinthium*): also known as 'absinthe' or 'green ginger', wormwood is one of the most bitter herbs, but despite this has been a major ingredient of aperitifs and herb wines. 'Vermouth' is a French variation of the original German name 'Wemut'. It is thought to have antiseptic properties and may be used externally as a liniment.
- Wintergreen and myrrh are also used with other herbs in poultices and decoctions. Other herbs said to have antiseptic properties include species of fennel, hyssop and nasturtium.

The Antipodean pharmacy

The unique character of flora in the Antipodes is a result of the past history of the land and climate, and particularly of the long period in which the plants have been isolated from other flora. For example, despite the small area of New Zealand, it is a distinct botanical region, with 1796 species of plants having been identified. Examples of native herbal antiseptics are given below. There are numerous medicines for the treatment of cuts and abrasions; only those that are thought to have antiseptic properties are included.

Astringents

Decoctions of high tannin-containing drugs suspended in gum tragacanth are used to treat wounds. Examples are witch-hazel (*Hamamelis*) and tormentil root (*Potentilla*).

Other formulations

These include bath additives, inhalations (e.g. *Chamomilla*), mucilages (e.g. slippery elm), plasters (e.g. belladonna and cayenne), poultices (e.g. comfrey and marshmallow) and suppositories. Mullein oil (*Verbascum*) is used as eardrops for deafness associated with earwax, and eyebright (*Euphrasia*) for the eyes. Ideally both preparations should be sterile and extreme caution should be exercised in preparing them extemporaneously to minimise the chances of bacterial contamination. Eyebright, in liquid form, is often bought by clients to use as an eyewash. It should always be diluted with freshly boiled and cooled water before use.

Responding to requests for advice

Information to help colleagues respond to requests for advice is provided at the end of this chapter.

Counselling patients

Pharmacists should discourage the use of herbal products by patients when the source, active ingredients and composition are uncertain. Also, consumption of herbs and herbal preparations by patients on certain medications should be controlled, monitored or best avoided when the active ingredient is known to act either antagonistically or synergistically with the prescribed medication. Such safety issues are addressed in detail below.

It is prudent to counsel self-treating clients to observe the following 'rules':

• Try to choose a medicine that is specific for the condition being treated; if in doubt seek advice from the pharmacist or health shop assistant.
• If you are taking orthodox medicines seek advice from the pharmacist as to the likelihood of interactions.
• Do not take several medicines concurrently unless specifically directed to do so by a qualified medical herbalist.
• Use the lowest dose appropriate for the symptoms being treated; if a little works a lot more will not necessarily work better and may be dangerous.
• Make sure that you understand the dosage instructions.
• If symptoms do not improve significantly within 7 days seek advice from your family doctor.
• Do not self-treat for lengthy periods without seeking professional help to ensure that appropriate medication is being used.

Pregnant and nursing mothers

An American study has investigated the frequency of use of herbal and alternative medicine by women during pregnancy.[21] Two hundred and fifty pregnant women attending antenatal clinics were prospectively enrolled in a cross-sectional survey about use of herbal and alternative medical therapies; 244 women completed surveys (97%). Of the respondents, 9.1% reported use of herbal supplements during the current pregnancy, with 7.5% using these agents at least weekly. The most commonly used herbs during pregnancy were garlic, aloe, camomile, peppermint, ginger, Echinacea, pumpkin seeds and ginseng. There are no comparative statistics for the UK but it is likely that the use is rather less due to the fact that in the USA these products are considered to be food supplements whereas in the UK they are medicines.

A Swedish study during the period 1 July 1995 to end of 2004 investigated the characteristics of women using herbal drugs and the possible impact of use in early pregnancy on pregnancy outcome.[22] Women who reported use of herbal drugs were compared with all women giving birth during the period. Outcome variables included prematurity, birth weight, number of infants in delivery and congenital malformations. The most commonly reported herbal drugs used during pregnancy were iron-rich herbs, ginseng and valerian. No signs of unfavourable effect on pregnancy outcome were seen. The number of exposures was, however, low and so the effects on rare outcomes (e.g. specific malformations) could not be excluded. For this reason pregnant and lactating women should be as careful about medicinal herbs as they are about conventional medicines.[23]

Some compounds in herbs can cross the placenta and may be linked to birth defects or other problems in newborns. Some herbs may be passed to babies via breast milk. The use of black and blue cohosh, feverfew, garlic, ginseng and St John's wort during pregnancy is not recommended. Valerian is not recommended for lactating women (see 'Materia medica' below). The medicine Caulophyllum is also said to be contraindicated.[24] In homeopathy this medicine is actually recommended for administration immediately before and during childbirth. Lavender (*Lavendula angustifolia*) is one herbal medicine that is recommended for administration during pregnancy and for postpartum support. Dandelion (*Taraxacum officinales*), red raspberry leaf (*Rubus idaeus*) and nettle (*Urtica dioica*) are also used for this purpose.

An Australian trial that examined the safety and efficacy of raspberry leaf products consumed by a group of 51 mothers during their pregnancy, by comparison with a group of 57 mothers who did not, found that the herb can be consumed by women during their pregnancy to shorten labour with no identified side effects for the women or their babies.[25] The findings also suggested that women who ingest raspberry leaf might be less likely to develop an artificial rupture of their membranes, or require a caesarean section, forceps or vacuum birth than the women in the control group.

Paediatric use

Although most medicines have similar action in people of all age groups, the required dosage and potential adverse reactions tend to vary. This must be taken into consideration when prescribing for children, particularly infants. Children and infants are much more sensitive than adults to the effects of all medicines and so herbs should be given to these patients with great care. Doses should be carefully calculated. The following formulae may be used to calculate the appropriate amounts of herbs to be administered to children:

Clark's rule:

(Weight in lb/150) × Adult dose = Child's dose

Young's rule (for children 2 years and older):

(Age in years/[Age in years + 12]) × Adult dose = Child's dose.

Body surface area (BSA):

(BSA of child/1.73) × Adult dose = Child's dose.

where 1.73 = average adult BSA.

There are three main advantages in using herbal medicines for children:[26]

1. Many phytomedicines have a relatively good benefit–risk ratio.
2. Many herbal medicines for use in children fall into the 'gentle' classification, with actions that are perfectly adequate for children.
3. The methods of administration (e.g. inhalation, baths, ointments, syrups) commonly used in phytotherapy are particularly acceptable to children. This, together with the cooperation of parents who are often in favour of this therapy, provides for good concordance.

There is also a potential risk to children resulting from unintended access to medication. The accidental ingestion of a diuretic herbal medicine by a 2 year old, requiring admission and electrolyte monitoring, has prompted one physician to call for the mandatory use of child-resistant closures on containers bought over the counter in the UK.[27] The degree of control demanded of prescribable drugs does not extend to those of the herbal type. In view of the increasing use of such medicines, there is likely to be an increased risk of accidental ingestion. Childproof containers should be a legal requirement for herbal medicines. Parents should be cautioned to store such medicines out of the reach of children.

Liquid preparations are extremely useful for children, although the taste may be rather unpalatable, because the dose can be easily and accurately adjusted down to very small amounts with the aid of an oral syringe.

Caution should be exercised in applying camomile products to the gums of teething children. Valerian should not be given to children under the age of 3 years (see below 'Materia medica').

Elderly people

Interactions between medicinal herbs is a major concern especially for older patients, who may well be taking a substantial portfolio of prescription drugs. It may not be possible to obtain satisfactory answers to questions about the names of these drugs, partly because the patient may have forgotten them ('You know the ones – those little white tablets – what are they called?') or even that they have been taking the medicines for so long that they do not consider them to be worthy of mention.

It may be better to recommend that such patients take homeopathic medicines instead of herbal medicines in view of the lack of toxic effects with the former.

Sportscare

In the quest to find energy for that extra hundredth of a second and the medal that it may bring, sportspeople are constantly seeking products to enhance performance. Word is passed about some new discovery and it is taken without too much thought for safety or even legality. Ginseng is one such example. Unfortunately these drugs are often obtained in developing countries where control is non-existent and adulterants, the names of which do not appear on the label, may be on the International Olympic Committee list of banned substances.

As a general rule athletes should be instructed not to take herbal medicines unless they can be certain of purity.

Evidence

Many orthodox treatments were originally taken from herbal use, and most conventional drug prescriptions are still said to have a plant-derived component, but the renewed interest has focused on the traditional use of whole plant products. Western mainstream research has lagged behind the public shift in usage and this style of evidence is in its early stages of development: for all complementary and alternative medicine (CAM), the Cochrane Collaboration on Complementary Medicine, as of March 2000, noted 4700 randomised controlled trials (RCTs) and 204 systematic reviews, of which 1561 trials related to herbalism met the required criteria.[28]

Linde et al. have stated that systematic reviews are available on a range of herbal preparations prescribed for defined conditions.[29] However, there is a sparsity of evidence regarding the effectiveness of individualised herbal medicine and according to Guo et al. no convincing evidence to support the use of individualised herbal medicine in any indication.[30]

The range of investigations that has been carried out on herbal medicines varies widely, e.g. St John's wort has been extensively studied using both in vivo (animal and human) and in vitro studies. Echinacea has been widely studied, sometimes with contradictory results. A carefully controlled and double-blinded experiment has suggested that Echinacea does not work.[31] Some 399 volunteers agreed to be inoculated with rhinovirus type 39. For 7 days before the inoculation and 5 days afterwards, the young adult volunteers took one of three well-defined formulations of Echinacea or a placebo. Treatment was randomly allocated. Altogether 349 of the volunteers caught a cold. Compared with placebo, none of the formulations prevented infection, relieved symptoms or speeded up recovery. By contrast, a widely reported[32] meta-analysis involving 1630 participants from 14 trials reached a positive conclusion.[33] RCTs that compared Echinacea-containing products with placebo and that reported on cold incidence or duration were included. Where reported, the Echinacea species included were E. angustifolia, E. purpurea and E. pallida. Most studies included 'natural' virus exposure; three studies included inoculation with rhinovirus. Four studies included concomitant treatment with a variety of additional supplements: vitamin C, propolis, thyme, citric acid, peppermint, lemon grass leaf, spearmint, rosemary leaf, eucalyptus or fennel seed. Dosages and study duration varied between studies. Two studies evaluated the effect of Echinacea in children. Echinacea was found to reduce the incidence of catching a cold by 58% and reduce the duration of a cold by an average of 1.4 days; both reductions were statistically significant. Significant statistical heterogeneity was found.

Other medicines have been much less studied and rely on folkloric evidence for continued use.

For a thorough evaluation of herbal products the following procedures should ideally be performed:

• The active principle should be isolated and investigated.
• An extract from the entire plant from which the active principle was isolated should be investigated.
• A comparison of the herbal preparation with a similar synthetic pharmaceutical product should be carried out in a randomised double-blind trial.

Such a rigorous investigation is well beyond the resources of most manufacturers. For now most of the evidence base remains traditional knowledge and experience based on centuries of use, centred on clinical effectiveness. The principal sources are:

• Bibliographical: compiled from literature; meta-analysis of research studies
• Observational studies: audit
• Clinical experience: anecdotal
• Scientific analysis to identify active ingredients
• RCT where possible (still limited, partly from resource constraints).

This has formed the basis of most current herbal pharmacopoeias, e.g. the *German Commission E Monographs*[34] have reviewed existing data and the traditional knowledge, and then applied the principle of 'reasonable certainty'. These monographs have been criticised in recent months since they are actually expert opinion, rather than reviews. Other reference texts include the *American Herbal Pharmacopoeia*, the *Therapeutic Compendium* and the monographs of the European Scientific Cooperative on Phytotherapy (ESCOP).[35]

Evidence for applications, where it exists, is quoted in the 'Material medica'/'Repertory' sections at the end of this chapter.

Reasons for negative outcomes

There are a number of reasons why clients do not observe a positive outcome after taking herbal medicines. The most obvious is that an inappropriate treatment has been chosen or they are taking quantities of active ingredients that are below the therapeutic threshold.

302 Complementary and Alternative Medicine

- They may be using old herbs (herbs lose potency with age and the herbs on some health food store shelves are literally 'years' old).
- They may be using powdered herbs in capsules when really an extract is the only way to get a concentrated enough dose for physiological effect (gingko biloba is an example of an herb best used in concentrate form). Even using fresh herbs, many people do not brew medicinal teas correctly. Such a tea should be 'quite' concentrated and the technique for making it is more elaborate than just dumping a tea bag in water and letting it sit for a couple of minutes.
- The person may also not be using the herb in a manner that delivers the active agent. In many herbs (e.g. valerian), the active ingredient is an oil and so is not soluble in water. Hence, steeping it in water and brewing a tea is not going to get you very much of the compound. In these cases, extracts in oil or glycerine (or sometimes in alcohol) or directly consuming the powdered herb are the best way to deliver the agent. Inappropriate dose regimens may also be responsible for a negative result (see 'Incorrect dosage or instructions' below).

Safety issues

Herbal medicines are complex mixtures of chemicals, many of which have not been subjected to rigorous testing. Unlike homeopathy, material doses are being administered and, given the non-standardisation of many of the medicines, it is quite likely that instances of adverse drug reactions will occur, particularly as the numbers of people using herbalism are rising at a substantial rate.

In this section the major potential sources of problems are discussed.

Lack of appropriate treatment

Incomplete practitioner education, leading to individuals prescribing outwith their limits of competence, and inappropriate self-treatment have implications for safety issues. Conditions that are not treated correctly by misdiagnosis or because they were missed altogether may become more acute or lead to the lengthening of incapacitation.

Toxic effects and interactions

Many people who use herbal preparations believe that they are totally safe in all respects because they are naturally occurring, i.e. that the active ingredients all fall in the 'gentle group' mentioned above. In fact this is far from the truth and some herbal preparations can be potentially dangerous, even in therapeutic doses. Comfrey (Symphytum) was found to contain pyrrolizidine alkaloids in quantities that could be hepatotoxic[36] and it was withdrawn from sale in its crude form some years ago. Other herbal species containing the drug (e.g. coltsfoot, echinacea and senecio) also contain pyrrolizidines but remain available.

An initial surveillance of case enquiries between 1983 and 1988 and in 1981 by the National Poisons Unit identified 5563 enquiries related to traditional herbal medicines and food supplements. After a detailed assessment, a link was found between exposure and reported clinical effects in 49 cases, indicating a need for continuous surveillance of such exposures.[37] The patient's age, genetic constitution, nutritional state, concomitant diseases and concurrent medication may affect the risk and severity of adverse events, as can consumption of large amounts or a wide variety of herbal preparations or long-term use.[38] However, a number of other factors make an assessment of adverse effects associated with herbal products more complex than for pharmaceuticals. A classification has been reported for adverse reactions from herbal products.[39]

The potential for interactions between herbal and conventional medicines has been recognised for some time, although wider awareness has been recognised more recently.[40,41] An example is the incidence or severity of interactions between herbal products and anticoagulant therapy. These interactions are said to be difficult to predict,[42] but awareness of these potential interactions is necessary to achieve optimal anticoagulation therapy. In particular pharmacists can play a crucial role in identifying such interactions; clinicians should be informed to monitor the therapy closely, particularly when such products are started or discontinued. In a study carried out in Scotland in 2006 4% of patients prescribed a herbal medicine by GPs were, at the same time, prescribed conventional medication that has been documented to interact with herbal treatments.[43]

Intrinsic effects[44]

These adverse effects that result from the herb itself may be either predictable and dose dependent, or unpredictable.[45] Yohimbine, an alkaloid found in the bark of the tree *Pausinystalia yohimbe*, has α_2-adrenoceptor antagonistic activity; it is taken for male impotence, and can cause hypertension and anxiety in a predictable dose-related manner. The drug has also been found to have an unpredictable reaction and is known to cause serious bronchospasm in some patients.[46] Comfrey has already been mentioned above; another example of a drug causing concern is Aristolochia.[47]

Four popular herbal supplements are currently being subjected to safety checks under the US National Toxicology Program.[48] The programme, a coalition of agencies that includes the Food and Drug Administration (FDA), the National Institutes of Health and the Centers for Disease Control and Prevention, is testing aloe vera, which is commonly used to soothe burned skin, but it is increasingly turning up as a beverage, with claims that it can fight disease by 'cleansing' the digestive tract. It can cause skin irritation.[49] Researchers have noted some similarities between aloe vera and croton oil, a known carcinogen. The other herbs being investigated are ginseng, kava and milk thistle. More than 30 substances are tested by the programme each year through rodent and in vitro studies. No humans are involved.

Intrinsic effects also include the effects resulting from misuse, accidental overdose or interactions with orthodox pharmaceuticals. Excessive doses of ginseng, considered to be abuse of the medicine, have been reported to cause agitation, insomnia and raised blood pressure. Similar abuse of liquorice may cause oedema and hypertension. An Australian patient who overdosed on a herbal laxative taken as a weight control medicine suffered neuropathy and coma.[50] The medicine contained podophyllin.

Fraunfelder[51] carried out a review of the more significant herbal and nutritional agents of clinical importance to ophthalmologists. Cases were collected from spontaneous reports submitted to the WHO, the FDA and the National Registry of Drug-Induced Ocular Side Effects. Additional cases were collected from the literature. It was concluded that camomile, datura, *Echinacea purpurea*, *Ginkgo biloba* and liquorice are all associated with clinically significant ocular side effects.

In Canada herbal or other non-vitamin, non-mineral (NVNM) supplements are used widely, and concern has been expressed over public health implications associated with interactions with conventional medications.[52] This is a major concern for the clinical herbalist.[53] Herbal preparations may be inducers of various drug metabolising enzymes.[54] This may result in a reduction in blood levels and therapeutic effect of some medicines metabolised by these enzymes. As the level of active ingredients may vary from one preparation to another, and patients may switch between preparations, the degree of induction is likely to vary. Concurrent use of herbs may mimic, magnify or oppose the effect of drugs. The following examples serve to illustrate the problem:

- In 2000 the UK Committee on the Safety of Medicine (now replaced by the Commission on Human Medicines) recommended that St John's wort should not be used with ciclosporin, digoxin, indinavir, oral contraceptives, theophylline or warfarin. It is thought that St John's wort affects neurotransmitters in the brain and may interact with psychotropic medicines including selective serotonin reuptake inhibitors (SSRIs).

- Kava-kava (*Piper methysticum*) has gained recent popularity – and notoriety (see 'Materia medica' below) – due to its relaxing effects, both as a recreational herb and as a treatment for anxiety.[55] A case report suggests caution before using kava along with benzo-diazepine drugs. A patient apparently lapsed into a 'semicomatous state' as a result of an interaction between kava and the drug alprazolam (Xanax).[56] The benzodiazepines generally lose effect within 8–12 hours, but secondary metabolites capable of interact-ing with other substances linger in the blood for 24 or more hours afterwards. Interactions between alcohol and the benzodiazepine drugs are well known – alcohol potentiates their effects – but herbal interactions have not been studied or previously recorded.

- Another example is the concurrent use of *Ginkgo biloba* and the so-called 'blood thinning' agents.[57] This provides a significant risk. The potentiation of action caused by using a herb with a similar pharmacological effect[58] could provoke a serious bleeding disor-der. The risk is probably greatest with concurrent use of heparin, warfarin and coumarin derivatives, but recent anecdotes indicate that interactions may also occur with aspirin. Another report describes a case of spontaneous bleeding into the eye from the iris within a week of onset of daily treatment in a patient who had been taking *Ginkgo biloba* and aspirin.[59]

- Potentiation of oral and topical corticosteroids by liquorice has been reported.[60]

For a comprehensive list of the large number of potential inter-actions between orthodox drugs and herbal medicines the reader is referred to the excellent book *Herbal Medicines* edited by Joanne Barnes and colleagues.[61] An abbreviated list is provided in Table 8.2.

Table 8.2 Examples of potential interactions between orthodox medicines and herbal remedies

Orthodox drug type	Example of interacting herbal remedy	Potential outcome
Gastrointestinal		
Antacids	Comfrey	Exacerbation of symptoms
Antidiarrhoeals	Senna	Antagonist effect
Laxatives	Senna	Potentiation
Cardiovascular		
Antihypertensives	Garlic, hawthorn	Potentiation
	Blue cohosh, ginger	Antagonist effect
Beta blockers	Coltsfoot	Antagonist effect
	Alfalfa	Hypertension
Diuretics	Garlic, ginger, St John's wort	Difficulty in controlling diuresis, hypertension
Respiratory		
Antiallergics	St John's wort, valerian	Potentiation of drowsiness associated with antihistamines
Central nervous system		
Analgesics	Dandelion, elder	Increased risk of toxicity with NSAIDs
	Liquorice	Decreased plasma concentration of drug
Antidepressants	Comfrey, ginseng	Hypotension with MAOI
	St John's wort	Antagonist effect
Antiepileptics	Borage, evening primrose, sage	May enhance risk of seizure
Anxiolytics, hypnotics	Hops, valerian, St John's wort	Potentiation
Endocrine		
Anti-diabetic	Alfalfa, damiana	Potentiation
	Devil's claw, ginseng	Antagonist effect
Hypo- and hyperthyroidism drugs	Fucus, horseradish, myrrh	Interfere with orthodox therapy
Corticosteroids	Dandelion, elder	Increased potassium loss
	Liquorice	Increased water and sodium retention
Oral contraceptives	Alfalfa, ginseng	Reduction in effectiveness
	St John's wort	

Adapted from Barnes J, Anderson L, Phillipson DJ. *Herbal Medicines*, 3rd edn. London: The Pharmaceutical Press, 2007.
MAOI, monoamine oxidase inhibitor; NSAIDs, non-steroidal anti-inflammatory drugs.

It would be appropriate for pharmacists whose advice is sought on potential interactions to check that the medicines concerned do not fall into the same therapeutic group, when potentiation could occur, or into opposite therapeutic groups, when antagonism would be possible.

During the early part of this century there was much discussion about the availability of St John's wort and the drug was restricted to private prescription in Ireland in 2000. However, the regulations banning the open sale of the herb did not cover importation. Therefore, despite the fact that people are unable to buy St John's wort in the Irish Republic, they can import it for personal use. Concerns included possible interactions with a number of common medicines such as anticoagulant drugs and oral contraceptives, and an assertion that people should not really be self-treating anxiety and depression albeit of the mild variety.

Some culinary herbs also contain potentially toxic constituents. The safe use of these herbs is ensured by limiting the level of constituent allowed in a particular food product to a level not considered to represent a health hazard. The irritant principle present in the volatile oil of parsley, apiole, is said to be both an abortifacient and hepatotoxic.[62]

Examples of adverse effects that may occur with herbal ingredients are summarised in Table 8.3. They include allergic, cardiac, hepatic, hormonal irritant, purgative and toxic effects.

Extrinsic effects

Other sources of potential danger are associated with a number of extrinsic effects that are related to problems in commercial manufacture or extemporaneous compounding. This leads to a variability in the quality of the product (see Chapter 6).

Failure of good manufacturing practice Some manufacturers use inadequate standards of quality during the manufacturing process, leading to batch-to-batch variability.

Adulteration Herbal products should be free not only from toxic botanical adulterants but also from other contaminants such as substantial residues, pesticides (e.g. organic phosphates), toxic metals[59] (e.g. arsenic, cadmium lead or mercury) and even conventional pharmaceuticals (e.g. corticosteroids or non-steroidal anti-inflammatory drugs).[64] This could lead to potential toxicity in overdose, the signs and symptoms of which are often recognised late.[65]

Table 8.3 Examples of adverse drug reactions (ADRs) caused by certain herbal ingredients

Potential ADR caused by active ingredient	Active ingredient thought to cause ADR (if known)	Examples of herbs that could be implicated
Allergic		
Hypersensitivity	Sesquiterpene lactones	Arnica, feverfew
Phototoxicity	Furanocoumarins	Celery, wild carrot
Immunity problems	Canavanine	Alfalfa
Cardiac	Cardiac glycosides	Squill
Endocrine		
Hypoglycaemic		Alfalfa, ginseng
Hyperthyroid	Iodine	Fucus
Hormonal	Triterpenoids	Liquorice
	Isoflavonoids	Alfalfa
	Saponins	Ginseng
	Anti-androgenic agents	Saw palmetto
Irritant		
Gastrointestinal	Pyrrolizidine alkaloids	Comfrey
Renal	Aescin	Horse chestnut
Toxic		
Hepatotoxic	Pyrrolizidine alkaloids	Comfrey
Mitogenic	Proteins	Mistletoe
Convulsant	Volatile oil constituents	Camphor

Adapted from Barnes J, Anderson L, Phillipson DJ. *Herbal Medicines*, 3rd edn. London: The Pharmaceutical Press, 2007.

In the USA it was reputed that one case of arsenic poisoning resulting from the ingestion of herbal tea has occurred, and in another case small amounts of cocaine were said to have been found in two herbal teas. Topical presentations can also be a source of problems. A study found that 8 of the 11 herbal creams being used by patients attending their medical practice (at a cost of up to £35 [€44; $65] per week) contained the controlled steroid dexamethasone. Concentrations of the drug varied from 64 to 1500 µg/g,[66] with the highest concentration being prescribed for the face of a 4-month-old baby with eczema. Worryingly, the concentration of dexamethasone in creams prescribed for children was 5.2 times higher than that in those prescribed for adults. The risk of adverse reactions with such potent steroids is increased by their inappropriate use and application to areas of thin skin such as flexures and the face. Furthermore, many of the preparations were supplied in unlabelled containers without clear instructions. The authors called for closer regulation of herbal medicines to ensure adequate labelling and to prevent dispensing of unlicensed products in the guise of herbal treatments.

A total of 100 herbal products containing *Smilax myosotiflora* were purchased in a market by the Malaysian Drug Control Authority and analysed for mercury content using cold vapour atomic absorption spectrophotometry.[67] It was found that 89% of the above products did not exceed 0.5 p.p.m. of mercury. Heavy metal poisoning such as mercury has been associated with traditional medicines.

Accidental contaminants may also include allergens, pollen, insect parts, moulds and mould spores.[68]

Mycotoxins are contaminants in a wide variety of natural products.[69] The UN Food and Agriculture Organization (FAO) estimates contamination of 25% of the world production of foodstuffs and 20% of the EU cereal harvest There are three main genera involved: *Aspergillus* (aflatoxins B1, B2, G1, G2 and ochratoxin A), *Penicillium* (ochratoxin A and patulin) and *Fusarium* (fumonisins, zearalenon and trichothecenes). Relatively few data were available on herbs that are susceptible to contamination and screening is necessary to identify those herbs that may be involved, e.g. aflatoxins have been detected in many samples of senna fruit, nux vomica seed, figs, nutmeg, ginger root, cayenne pepper and Agnus castus fruit.

Some plants come from nature with a microbial burden that needs to be reduced during processing.[70] The *European Pharmacopoeia* (see Further reading) sets limits for bacterial and fungal microbial contamination for herbal medicines.

Misidentification The problem of nomenclature exists in herbalism as well as in homeopathy with at least four different methods of naming plants – the common English name, the transliterated name from another language (often Chinese or Indian), the Latinised pharmaceutical name and the scientific name.[71] It is important that physical and microscopic identification methods are used. This will ensure that the correct species of plant (and, later, the correct part of the plant) according to the appropriate herbal pharmacopoeia is used to make the medicine.

Substitution Many herbal medicines do not have both the common and the Latin names of the herb on the label. The suspicion exists that some companies do not give the Latin name because the common name is shared by several different herbs, only one or two of which are medicinal (and therefore usually more expensive). There are several different species of ginseng with different properties and a wide variation in cost. By using only the common name, companies are able to substitute a less effective or even completely non-medicinal herb for the medicinal variety without making untruthful declarations on the label.

Lack of standardisation The amount of pharmacologically active ingredient available in a herbal medicine may vary widely from plant to plant, so accurately regulating dosage can be difficult, e.g. glycyrrhizic acid, one of the primary pharmacological agents in liquorice root, occurs naturally in concentrations ranging, on average, from 2% to 7%, with some rare plants as high as 27%. A plant with a 7% glycyrrhizic acid concentration is delivering a dose more than twice that of a plant with a 2% concentration. It is therefore important to use a standardised herbal preparation whenever possible. Extracts of many herbs have been analysed for the percentage of active ingredient and adjusted so that every bottle contains the same amount. There are extracts of ginkgo biloba that are standardised to 24% ginkgolides and in the USA a brand of echinacea standardised to 4% echinacosides. Some branded extracts refer to the percentage concentration of the raw herb present, rather than the amount of active principle, still leaving the problem of varying dosages, e.g. the UK's leading brand of tincture states on the label simply that 'the product has been prepared from '*Echinacea purpurea* herb and root' and that '15 drops contains the equivalent of 285 mg of whole fresh plant or 64.5 mg of whole dried plant'.

Another British supplier offers far more comprehensive information for its ginkgo biloba. The label states 'each tablet provides on average *Ginkgo biloba* extract 60 mg (equivalent to 300 mg of ginkgo biloba leaf) which has been standardised to contain 24% ginkgo flavine-glycosides giving flavone-glycosides 1.4 mg ginkgolides and bilobalides 3.6 mg'. It should be acknowledged that standardisation is not possible in all cases. For many herbal medicines the active ingredients have not been isolated and in other cases no reliable quantitative test exists. Another difficulty may be that the wrong active ingredient is being used to standardise the herb. Hypericin is no longer thought to be the main active constituent of St John's wort, because one may change the concentration of this product without an apparent change in antidepressant activity.[72]

Incomplete labelling There have been numerous incidents of herbal products, mainly obtained in or from developing countries, that do not declare all constituents on the label. Thus, a mixture may contain herbs in addition to those declared as adulterants or substitutions. This could lead to adverse reactions or, in the case of a sportsperson, a positive drug test for a banned substance of which the unfortunate athlete had no knowledge.

Substitution A report of nine cases of nephritis in young women taking a Belgian slimming treatment[73] led to the discovery that *Aristolochia fangchi* containing the nephrotoxic component aristolochic acid had been introduced in place of *Stephania tetrandra*. Eighty cases have now been identified, many developing terminal renal failure.

Incorrect dosage or instructions In general terms herbal medicines are safe if used according to instructions and within a safe dosage range. There are so many different pharmaceutical forms in which medicines can be taken – some may be standardised and some may not be – that calculating the correct dose is difficult, in some cases impossible, for the client. It is important that guidance is given on the label. Dose suggestions given in texts often reflect a consensus opinion among herbal practitioners using different methods and philosophies so there is no definitive answer to the question 'What is the recommended dose for this medicine?' The activity of crude plant material may differ from that of the purified constituents, because some constituents may modify the toxicity of others. Clear instructions are vital. A case reported in a Sydney newspaper in 1994 concerned a herbalist's patient who suffered a heart attack after misinterpreting instructions on how to take aconite.

Monitoring adverse effects (see Chapter 6)

The complexities of processing herbal medicine data compared with orthodox medicines have been highlighted.[74] Areas of concern with respect to the safety of herbal medicines were also highlighted after the recent introduction of a classification system for herbal medicines

Between 1968 and 1997, 8985 individual case reports received by the WHO adverse reactions Monitoring Centre in Uppsala, Sweden involved herbal medicines. Germany submitted the most reports (1796) followed by France (1479), the USA (1073) and the UK (993). Most reports concerned 'non-critical' reactions. In 21 of the 2487 critical cases a fatality was involved. The number of reports for specific medicines was small although it was possible to determine trends in some cases, e.g. echinacea appeared to be responsible for acute hypersensitivity and anaphylaxis. The authors concluded that the adverse effects of herbal products were inadequately documented.

The RPSGB recommends that any suspected adverse reactions in the UK should be reported to the MHRA using the 'Yellow Card' system.

Conclusion

The information available on safety issues, whether from the comparatively small amount of scientific investigations or from anecdotal data collected by both medically and non-medically qualified practitioners, forms the basis of advice that can be given to potential patients. Used judiciously herbal medicines are as safe as orthodox medicines, but, like the latter, the potential for non-beneficial outcomes if the medicines are used inappropriately is a real possibility.

The treatment of herbal poisoning[75]

- If contact dermatitis is caused by direct exposure to plants such as poison ivy it should be treated by cleaning the area and offering symptomatic treatment, which may or may not include antihistamines. If a caustic plant such as rue comes into contact with the oral mucosa, milk may be given and the patient observed to make sure that airway closure does not occur.
- Gastrointestinal distress is a common symptom of plant poisoning and may require ongoing fluid replacement.
- Renal toxicity and primary renal failure from plants such as rhubarb leaves and autumn crocus may require urinary alkalinisation and correction of calcium balance to treat oxalate ingestion; rhubarb leaves are a good source of soluble oxalate salts.
- Herbal teas prepared from oleander, foxglove or lily of the valley may cause hyperkalaemia and heart block. Treatment may include use of muscarinic cholinergic blockers such as atropine or phenytoin, cardiac pacing and potassium-removal techniques.
- Ingestion of ergot alkaloids may cause arterial vasospasm; therapy may include close medical observation, nitroprusside or adrenergic blocking agents.
- Atropine-like symptoms produced by plants such as jimsonweed may require simple observation or judicious use of physostigmine.

- Nicotine found in both domestic and wild tobaccos may produce sequential peripheral ganglionic stimulation, then blockade, and may result in seizures, paralysis and death. Treatment includes control of seizures and provision of ventilatory support.
- Ingestion of volatile oils such as pennyroyal or eucalyptus, which are irritants and central nervous system (CNS) depressants, may cause seizures and aspiration. Medical personnel should provide close observation of the patient, and be ready to treat aspiration; the risk of aspiration may contraindicate induction of emesis. Non-oily cathartics may be used, because oily cathartics may increase absorption of the toxins.
- Plant resins, such as those found in American ipecacuanha, may cause severe vomiting and catharsis, CNS effects and muscle weakness. There are no known antidotes; treatment includes reduction of gastrointestinal effects and maintenance of hydration.
- Plant alkaloids, such as those found in senecio, may produce jaundice and mimic alcoholism, hepatitis or Reye's syndrome. Treatment is supportive and will depend upon the degree of hepatic failure. Plants such as pokeberries or pokeweed which contain certain mitogens may cause severe gastroenteritis, respiratory stress or plasmacytosis. Treatment is symptomatic

The Royal Pharmaceutical Society herbaria

The Royal Pharmaceutical Society's herbaria of dried plant specimens, plant extracts and plant parts of medicinal value were established in 1842,[76] to assist detailed investigations into crude drugs and the establishment of standards.[77] Before this date drugs, foods and spices had for many years been subject to gross adulteration, simply because there were no standards by which they could be identified or their quality controlled. The herbaria (or 'museum' as they are jointly called in the literature) were originally housed 'in a front room without a vestige of furniture' on the ground floor at the Society's headquarters in 17 Bloomsbury Square, London.

A succession of professors from the School of Pharmacy took charge of the collection on a part-time basis until 1872 when Mr Edward Morrell Holmes was appointed full-time curator at a salary of £150 per annum. Holmes is credited with setting up an active centre of study alongside the herbaria. He remained in charge for 50 years, after which the position became part-time again. One of Holmes's successors was Dr T. Wallis who took over in 1925, researching, maintaining and extending the collection until Professor Jack Rowson was appointed full-time curator in 1948. Rowson developed the research potential of the museum until his departure in 1957. Dr Wallis then took control again with a technical assistant until 1969 when the collection was transferred to Bradford School of Pharmacy for 13 years,[78] a move that did not meet with universal approval within the profession,[79] but which nevertheless prompted the unveiling of a plaque to commemorate the occasion.[80] When the university informed the Society that it no longer wished to maintain the collection, Council decided that it should be gifted to The Royal Botanic Gardens Kew[81] where it became integrated with the Economic Botany Collections in 1983. This proved to be a more popular arrangement.[82] The collections were subsequently moved to their present site in the Sir Joseph Banks Building in 1989.[83]

The Economic Botany Collections (see www.rbgkew.org.uk/ ecbot.html) were founded by the first official Director of the Gardens, Sir William Hooker. Sir William's rationale for the Economic Botany Collections is as relevant today as it was in 1847:

> ... to render great service, not only to the scientific botanist, but to the merchant, the manufacturer, the physician, the chemist, the druggist, the dyer, the carpenter and the cabinet-maker and artisans of every description, who might here find the raw materials employed in their several professions correctly named.[84] (page 2)

The 9000 specimens in the Society's three herbaria and drug collection range from South American strychnos, European mandrake root and African rauwolfia to Chinese rhubarb and arrow poisons from Borneo. There is a large and important selection of quinine barks, resins (e.g. frankincense and myrrh), specimens of aloes, cinnamon and opium poppy, and a large seed collection. Associated documentation and correspondence concerning collection of the material make fascinating reading.

The collection is available for inspection by prior arrangement with the Curator of the Economic Botany Collections, The Royal Botanic Gardens, Kew, Richmond, Surrey TW9 3AB.

Future directions for herbalism

It seems likely in the foreseeable future that the two streams of plant use will continue side by side: whole plant use developing traditional herbal approaches, and using that experience with traditional medicines to increase the already large numbers of isolated constituents used as modern drugs. For both practices a large pool of plant material is available. This is diminishing fast, however; for example, in Madagascar, 90% of forests have gone in 15 years.

It seems critical to preserve and study the richness of this fauna, as well as the knowledge and experience of traditional healers and healing systems – especially for those peoples of the world who do not have access to, or cannot afford, pharmaceuticals. Even as western medicine extends to these people, models of integrated local clinics are appearing with most of the medicines from villagers' local forests, with local herbalists cooperating with a doctor. Indeed when there is a choice people are pluralistic. Just as in Asia they use orthodox medicine for symptomatic relief of acute conditions and traditional medicine for chronic problems, here the so-called underdeveloped world has given a lead that the industrial world is starting to follow.

Spagyric medicine

Spagyric, sometimes called herbal alchemy, is the production of herbal medicine by alchemical procedures. Before work is started on the herb, Spagyrists must prepare themselves. This is done in solitude with a 24-hour fast with meditation and prayer. No words are spoken. The only things that are allowed to pass the lips are clean water and the breath (see http://tinyurl.com/g52er).

Spagyric processing was created by the sixteenth-century healer Paracelsus. He coined the word Spagyric from two Greek words, meaning 'separate' and 'recombine'. Spagyrics have been used as source material for homeopathic medicines or combined with homeopathic medicines, but this is not the norm. These procedures involve fermentation, distillation and the extraction of mineral components from the ash of the marc.

Repertory

An abbreviated materia medica of common medicines

The list below contains the most popular herbs that form the basis of many self-treatment 'kits'.

Alfalfa (Lucerne)[85]

Source: the leaves and flowering tops of *Medicago sativa*.

Active ingredients: alkaloids, coumarin derivatives flavones, isoflavones, proteins and amino acids, sterols, sugars.

Uses: aperient, bactericidal, cardiotonic, diuretic, emetic, stimulant.

Common applications: urinary and bowel problems; peptic ulcer. Skin inflammation. Often used to treat arthritis and diabetes, but no firm clinical evidence of effectiveness exists.

Presentation: infusions for internal and external use. Tablets also available.

Daily dose: 10–15 g of the drug.[86]

Adverse drug reaction (ADR): alfalfa use in humans has been associated with systemic lupus erythematosus, an inflammatory connective tissue disease, other skin reactions, gastrointestinal disturbances and raised serum urate levels, Saponins interfere with the utilisation of vitamin E. Eating large quantities of alfalfa seeds over extended periods can cause reversible blood abnormalities.[87]

Aloe vera[88]

Source: prepared from the clear jelly-like mucilage obtained from the parenchymal tissue making up the inner portion of the leaves of *Aloe vera* (syn. *A. barbadensis, A vulgaris*).[89]

Active ingredients: mono- and polysaccharides, lipids, saponins, vitamins and minerals.[90]

Uses: cathartic. Assists healing of wounds and burns, although evidence of latter confused.[91] Anti-inflammatory. Fibromyalgia.[92]

Common applications: constituent of topical pharmaceutical and sunburn preparations. Included in various cosmetics, including hair care products and bath additives.

Presentation: gel, lotions, ointments and creams.

Daily dose: none documented.[66]

ADR: often confused with aloes (dried leaf juice) which has a potent laxative action. Ingestion of gel adulterated with leaf juice may cause diarrhoea.

Camomile, German[93]

Source: flowers of *Matricaria recutita* (or *M. chamomilla*). *Chamaemelum nobile* (Roman camomile) is also used, but less widely.

Constituents:[94] a major component responsible for most of the plant's medicinal qualities is known as α-bisabolol. Other constituents include a complex mixture of flavonoids (of which apigenin is an important element) and coumarins, sesquiterpenoids and spiroethers.

Uses: antiemetic, anti-spasmodic, mild sedative, anti-inflammatory and wound healing.

Common applications: digestive upset and indigestion, inflammation of gastrointestinal tract, teething, inflammation of mucous membranes, mild insomnia and anxiety.

Presentation: dried flower heads, liquid extract, tincture, tea. Oral preparations for infant colic and teething; external preparations – ointments/creams for cracked nipples, nappy rash. Constituent of cosmetics and hair care products. Essential oil is also used.

Daily dose: 1.5–3.0 g camomile flowers, infusion, liquid extract and tincture taken orally three times daily.

ADR: individuals with a known allergy to ragweed, asters, chrysanthemums and other botanical species related to *Matricaria recutita* should be cautious in taking products containing German camomile.[95] Individuals with existing asthma, urticaria or other allergic conditions should also use camomile products with caution because of a chance of exacerbation of their symptoms. The application of camomile products to the gums of teething children is also cautioned.[89] Although no reason is given, it is assumed that this warning relates to the potential induction of an allergenic response. In my experience this is often done and I have not been advised of any such reaction by a client. Concentrated tea may have an emetic effect; the infusion should not be allowed in contact with the eyes.[96]

Cohosh, black[97]

Source: rhizome and roots of *Cimicifuga racemosa*.

Constituents: alkaloids, tannins, terpenoids, various acids and volatile oils.

Uses: some oestrogenic activity.

Common applications:[98] stimulation of menstruation, treatment of menopausal symptoms (black cohosh is a main constituent of Lydia Pinkham's Vegetable Compound – www.mum.org/MrsPink1.htm). A trial investigating efficacy of a combination of black cohosh and St John's wort over 16 weeks found menopausal and psychological symptoms significantly improved compared with placebo.[99]

Presentation: dried rhizome, liquid extract and tincture.

Daily dose: dried rhizome 0.3–2 g or by decoction three times daily, 0.3–2 ml liquid extract (BP 1898), 2–4 ml tincture (BPC 1934).

ADR: black cohosh can cause headaches and stomach discomfort. In clinical trials comparing the effects of the herb and those of oestrogens, a low number of side effects were reported, such as headaches, gastric complaints, heaviness in the legs and weight problems.[100] The herb may have an additive antiproliferative effect when taken together with tamoxifen.[101] It is contraindicated in pregnancy; an overdose may cause premature birth.[102]

Cohosh, blue[103]

Source: roots and rhizomes of *Caulophyllum thalictroides*.

Constituents: alkaloids, saponins with a number of other compounds including gum, resins and phosphoric acid.

Uses: anti-spasmodic, anti-rheumatic; might have some efficacy in inducing labour.[104]

Common applications: amenorrhoea, threatened abortion and conditions associated with uterine atony.

Presentation: dried rhizome or root and liquid extract.

Daily dose: rhizome/root – 0.3–1 g or by decoction three times daily. Liquid extract (1:1 in 70% alcohol) 0.5–1 ml three times daily.

ADR: reputed to be abortifacient and should be taken if required only after labour has started, not during pregnancy. Self-treatment with this drug is generally considered inappropriate because of the nature of its action.

Echinacea[105]

Source: the rhizome and root of *Echinacea pallida* and *E. angustifolia* (the USA) and whole plant of *E. purpurea* (Europe).

Constituents: polysaccharides, glycoproteins, alkylamides and caffeic acid derivatives. Exact constituents vary with species.

Uses: thought to be immunostimulant, increasing body's healing powers. Increases activity of phagocytes (not act directly on invader)? Stimulates cell-mediated immune system. Anti-inflammatory.

Common applications: common cold, fevers, upper respiratory tract infections,[106,107] oral inflammation, minor skin abrasions and wounds.

Presentation: liquid extract and tincture used to increase immunity – colds and flu. Capsules and external preparations used for boils, burns, inflammatory conditions, wounds.

Daily dose:[108] 6–9 ml of expressed juice (concentration = 2.5:1); tincture 30–60 drops three times daily.

ADR: nausea. Maximum duration of use 8 weeks.[109] Individuals with allergies to the sunflower family (Asteraceae or Compositae) may experience mild allergic symptoms when ingesting echinacea.[27]

Feverfew[110]

Source: aerial parts, especially leaves, of *Tanacetum parthenium* (syn. *Chrysanthemum parthenium*).

Constituents: sesquiterpene lactones (parthenolide), flavonoids, melatonin.

Uses: treatment and prevention of migraine.[111] Anti-inflammatory,[110] possible anti-arthritic.[112] Suggested that it may inhibit prostaglandin production and serotonin.

Common applications: migraine, arthritis.

Presentation: people may chew fresh leaves. Also available as air-dried or freeze-dried herb and as capsules or tablets containing dried herb. Also liquid extract.

Daily dose:[113] 50 mg–1.2 g of powdered leaf; 3 cups of infusion daily; 125 mg of dried feverfew leaf preparation standardised to 0.2% parthenolide daily.[114]

ADR: mouth ulceration or gastric disturbance[115] and inflammation of lips and tongue.[96] May be contraindicated in pregnancy.

Garlic

Source: the fresh bulb of *Allium sativum*, cultivated worldwide.

Constituents: sulphur-containing compounds (including allicin, ajoenes, alliin), enzymes (including alliinase), flavonoids.

Uses: antihypertensive,[116] anti-thrombotic,[117] lipid-lowering agent,[118,119] antimicrobial. Protective effect against cancer.[120]

Common applications: common cold, hypertension, gastrointestinal ailments, possibly including side effects of paracetamol (acetaminophen),[121] cholesterol-lowering agent.[122]

Garlic was called 'the great panacea' by Galen. The antiseptic action is said to be effective against bacteria acid fungi, and the cloves that are used in India and China to treat amoebic dysentery.

Presentation: available as dried powder, 'odourless' extracts, capsules. Sometimes eaten raw against colds and influenza.

Daily dose:[123] one to two fresh garlic cloves (about 4 g) or 8 mg essential oil.

ADR: garlic should be avoided before undergoing surgical procedures because of possible post-surgical bleeding,[124] although the potential to impair platelet function is in some doubt.[125] Heartburn, flatulence and gastrointestinal upset have been reported, usually at doses equivalent to five or more cloves daily.[126] Contact dermatitis (caused by direct skin contact with raw garlic) is also possible. A possible interaction with warfarin has been reported.[127]

Garlic may be contraindicated in pregnancy and breastfeeding.[128] The odour of garlic is noticeable in the milk of lactating women who take the herb. This has been reported to cause colic in infants.

Ginger[129]

Source: usually powdered dried root of *Zingiberis officinalis*; may also be from whole fresh root when it is known as 'green ginger'.

Constituents: oleoresins (gingerols and shogaols), essential oil (zingiberene).

Uses: antiemetic, anti-nauseant, anti-inflammatory, antimicrobial. Possible gastroprotective and haematological properties.[130]

Common applications: loss of appetite, motion sickness,[131] inflammatory conditions.

Presentation: dried herb, capsules, tea. For topical use: liniment.

Daily dose:[132] 2–4 g. The antiemetic dose is 2 g of freshly powdered drug. May also be used as 10–20 drops of tincture in water with meals.[133]

ADR: occasional dyspepsia, but no significant risk when consumed at stated dose levels. Large overdose may cause depression and cardiac arrhythmias.[77] Some publications discourage large doses of ginger during pregnancy because of concerns about mutations or abortion.[111] However, according to the Mayo Clinic (http://tinyurl.com/3reyle) preliminary studies suggest that ginger may be safe and effective for nausea and vomiting of pregnancy when used at recommended doses for short periods of time (< 5 days). Additional research is needed to determine the safety and effectiveness of ginger during pregnancy before it can be recommended for longer periods of time. Possible risk of increased bleeding after surgery.[134]

Ginkgo biloba[135,136]

Source: concentrated extract of the leaves of the tree *Ginkgo biloba*; prepared by extraction of dried green leaves with acetone/water solvent.

Constituents:[137] flavonoids (flavone glycosides), diterpenes (ginkgolides), sesquiterpenes (bilobalides).

Uses: claimed to be effective in treating ailments associated with ageing and cerebral insufficiency;[138] increases blood flow.[139] Claimed to enhance cognitive function and memory.[140,141] Antioxidant. Tinnitus.[142] Effects of poor circulation.

Common applications: tinnitus, vertigo, Symptoms of the early stages of Alzheimer's disease, Raynaud's syndrome, intermittent claudication.

Presentation: tea capsules, tablets.

Daily dose:[16] the equivalent of 300 mg dried leaf, 40 mg extract, standardised to 24% flavone glycosides and 6% terpenoids, three times daily.[116]

ADR: occasional gastrointestinal disturbances, headache and allergic skin reactions (especially from handling ginkgo fruit). The herb has also been reported to cause spontaneous bleeding and may interact with anticoagulants and antiplatelet agents.[143]

Ginseng[144]

Source: main and lateral root parts of several species of *Panax*, including *P. ginseng* (Chinese or 'Asian'), *P. japonicus* (Korean), *P. quinquefolium* (American/Canadian) and *Eleutherococcus senticosus* (Siberian). The last is not a member of the *Panax* genus and is therefore not a true ginseng.

Active ingredients: contains a complex mixture at least 13 saponins known as ginsenosides, and a small amount of volatile oil. Siberian ginseng contains no appreciable amount of saponins but instead lignans, coumarins and polysaccharides.

Uses:[145] *pan* = all, *akos* = cure. Thus 'panacea'. *Gin* = man, *seng* = essence. Chinese people believe that ginseng represents a crystallisation of the essence of the Earth in the form of man. Immunomodulatory activity.

Applications: promoted as tonic, stimulant, improving stamina and sexual performance. Believed to improve performance and recovery in athletes.

Common application: stress, fatigue, strengthen immune function, increase endurance. General 'tonic'.[146] Anti-ageing.[147] Folkloric use in diabetes.

Presentation: dried herb. Decoction.

Daily dose: 1–2 g root or equivalent. The decoction is taken three to four times daily over 3–4 weeks.

ADR: mild irritability and excitation, insomnia, diarrhoea. Not recommended during pregnancy.[148] Ginseng is thought to have an additive effect when used together with monoamine oxidase inhibitors (MAOIs).[149] Clients should be advised against taking ginseng at night because it may cause insomnia.

Hawthorn[150]

Source: extract from berries, flowers and leaves of several species of *Crataegus* including *Crataegus oxycanthoides* (*C. laevigata*) and *C. monogyna*.

Constituents:[151] flavonoids (including quercetin glycosides and flavone-C-glycosides) and oligomeric procyanidins.

Uses: beneficial effects on coronary blood flow, blood pressure and heart rate;[152] decreases cardiac output. Slow acting – long-term use

Common application:[153,154] hypotensive; treatment of angina. In sport to facilitate maximum effort.

Presentation: decoction, liquid extract, tea, capsules/tablets.

Daily dose: 5 g drug (in five to six divided doses) or 900 mg extract for minimum 6 weeks' duration.

ADR: none found. Possible interaction with orthodox hypotensive drugs.

Kava-kava[155,156]

Note: the sale and import of foods and herbal medicine products containing kava-kava was originally banned in the UK in 2002 after data given to the MHRA the year before by the CSM's Expert Working Group (EWG) and the Medicines Commission, which agreed that, in rare cases, the use of unlicensed medicinal products containing the herb could lead to possible liver damage. The Food Standards Authority (FSA) reviewed this evidence and, after consulting with the Committee on Toxicology (COT), agreed that the risk was also evident for food uses. The ban was reviewed in 2006 and upheld.

Source: the rootstock derived from *Piper methysticum*.

Constituents: kavalactones including the pyrones: kavain (kawain), dihydrokavain, methysticin, dihydromethysticin and yangonin.

Alkaloids: cepharadione A (an isoquinoline), pipmethystine (a pyridone, in the leaf only). Miscellaneous flavonoids and benzylketones.[157]

Uses: treatment of anxiety[158,159] and as a muscle relaxant. Antimicrobial, antiseptic, mild analgesic, antispasmodic, diuretic, stimulant, 'tonic'.

Common applications: genitourinary infections, vaginitis, pruritis, geriatric incontinence. Powerful soporific. Used as liquid to cause mood elevation and feeling of relaxation (especially in the Pacific Islands). Treatment of stress-related headaches and muscle spasm; possible alternative to benzodiazepines.[160,161]

Presentation: powder, liquid extract, lotion.

Daily dose: 2–4 g three times daily herb, decoction (30 g–5000 ml) and take half a cup three times daily. Lotion (30 g to 250 ml glycerine) as necessary for itching.

ADR: excessive consumption can result in disturbances of vision (photophobia, diplopia and oculomotor paralysis), yellowing of the skin, problems with equilibrium, dizziness and ultimately stupor.[141] A possible interaction between kava and alprazolam has been noted.[162]

Milk thistle (St Mary's thistle)[163]

Source: extract from fruit (seeds) of *Silybum marianus* (syn. *Carduus marianus*).

Constituents: flavanolignans (especially silymarin and its derivative silybin), fixed oil, flavonoids and sterols.

Uses: free radical scavenger; hepatoprotective activity.[164–166] Said to facilitate lactation in nursing mothers.

Common application: loss of appetite. Liver and gallbladder complaints,[167,168] dyspepsia. Occasional reports of use in psoriasis.[169]

Presentation: capsules, liquid extract and tincture. Injection claimed to be most effective, tea the least effective.[170]

Daily dose: (1) 12–15 g drug or 200–300 mg silymarin calculated as silybin;[171] (2) 200 mg standardised extract (70% silymarin) three times daily;[137] (3) 20 drops tincture three times daily.

ADR: occasional diarrhoea.

St John's wort[172]

Source: extract from the fresh or dried leaves and the golden yellow flowering tops of *Hypericum perforatum*.

Constituents: anthracene derivatives (including hypericin and pseudo-hypericin), flavonoids, phenolics (including hyperforin), procyanidins and volatile oil.

Uses: antidepressant. Also used as anxiolytic, sedative and antiviral.

Common applications: mild antidepressant. In a meta-analysis of 23 randomised trials including a total of 1757 outpatients with mild or moderate depressive disorders *Hypericum* was found to be significantly superior to placebo.[173] St John's wort is said to be as effective as imipramine.[174,175] Menopausal symptoms of psychological origin.[176] Crush injuries orally and topically. Topical application also for neuralgias and myalgias.

Presentation: capsules, tablets liquid extract, infusion, tincture; topical oil or cream/ointment.

Daily dose: 2–4 g of dried drug as infusion three times daily[177] or equivalent of 1.0–2.7 mg of total hypericin.

ADR: stated to be 'minor' but headache, nausea, dizziness, dry mouth and photosensitivity have been reported.[178] Slight in vitro uterotonic activity has been reported[155] as well as the ADR mentioned above, so probably wise to avoid use during pregnancy. St John's wort may represent a potential and possibly an overlooked cause of drug interactions in transplant recipients.[179]

The following drugs should not be used in combination with St John's wort or preparations containing derivatives of *Hypericum*:[51,180]

- MAOIs: phenelzine, tranylcypromine, isocarboxazid
- SSRIs: fluoxetine
- Dibenzazepine derivatives: amitriptyline, protriptyline, nortriptyline, desipramine, amoxapine, imipramine, doxepine, perphenazine, carbamazepine, cyclobenzapine, clomipramine, maprotiline, trimipramine
- Sympathomimetics: amphetamines, ephedrine (found in many cold and hayfever medicines), methyldopa, dopamine, levodopa, tryptophan
- Others: ciclosporin and oral contraceptives.

In view of the current interest in this herb the clinically important interactions of St John's wort are summarised in Table 8.4.

American physicians have been advised not to encourage the use of St John's wort, valerian or passionflower for the treatment of anxiety based on small or inconsistent effects in small studies.[181]

Table 8.4 Examples of clinically important interactions of St John's wort

Orthodox drug	Effect of interaction
Anticonvulsants	Reduced blood levels; possible risk of seizures
Ciclosporin	Reduced blood levels with risk of transplant rejection
Digoxin	Reduced blood levels and loss of control of heart rhythm or heart failure
HIV protease inhibitors	Reduced blood levels with possible loss of HIV suppression
Oral contraceptives	Reduced blood levels with risk of conception and break-through bleeding
SSRIs	Increased serotoninergic effects with increased incidence of adverse reactions
Theophylline	Reduced blood levels and loss of control of asthma or chronic airflow limitation
Triptans	Increased serotoninergic effects with increased incidence of adverse reactions
Warfarin	Reduced anticoagulant effect and resultant need for increased dose

From *Fact Sheet for Healthcare Professionals*. CSM, 29 February 2000.
SSRIs, selective serotonin reuptake inhibitors.

Saw palmetto[182]

Source: powdered, partially dried and fresh ripe fruit of the North American tree *Sabal serrulata* (syn. *Serenoa repens*). Seeds are nutty with vanilla aroma; characteristic 'soapy' taste.

Constituents: rich in fatty acids and phytosterols (notably β-sitosterol). Also contains flavonoids and polysaccharides.

Uses: as a phyto-oestrogenic effect.

Common applications: claimed treatment for benign prostatic hypertrophy.[183,184] Also promoted as 'urinary tonic', diuretic and for cystitis and irritable bladder, and as a 'male reproductive tonic'.

Presentation: liquid extract, capsules/tablets.

Daily dose: 2–4 g of dried herb or equivalent.

ADR: occasional gastric problems have been reported.[185] As a result of its anti-androgen and oestrogenic activity, saw palmetto may interact with orthodox hormonal therapy including hormone replacement therapy and oral contraceptives.[186]

Valerian[187]

Source: dried root and rhizome of *Valeriana officianalis* dried at temperatures below 40°C.

Constituents: valepotriates, volatile oil, sesquiterpenes, pyridine alkaloids, caffeic acid derivatives.

Uses:[188] sedative, hypnotic. May also treat exhaustion and excitability.

Common applications: used for insomnia.[189,190] Valerian is reputed to have muscle-relaxing properties and is used alone, or in combination with other herbs, in the management of musculoskeletal conditions.[191]

Presentation: available in number of 'official' and OTC preparations, teabags and mixtures. Extracts, powders, tinctures. Unpleasant nauseous odour.

Daily dose:[192] 3–9 g drug in divided doses; 2–6 ml liquid extract.

ADR: occasionally headaches, excitability and insomnia.[193] Valerian may potentiate the effects of CNS depressant drugs, including alcohol. The herb should be used with caution in children under 3 years of age, and in pregnant or lactating women.[131]

An abbreviated repertory of common conditions

This list is not designed to be exhaustive, merely an indication of herbal medicines that may be used to treat a range of conditions. Not all the medicines listed will be found in 'Material medica' above. The cited references are examples of articles that refer to recorded uses of each herb. They may not provide robust evidence for the quoted application.

Anxiety, depression[194]

Anxiety: Asian ginseng (*Panax ginseng*)

Depression: ginkgo (*Ginkgo biloba*), St John's wort (*Hypericum perforatum*)

Sedatives: lemon balm (*Melissa officinalis*), valerian (*Valeriana officinalis*), skullcap (*Scutellaria lateriflora*)

Stress: kava (*Piper methysticum*)

Benign prostatic hyperplasia[195]

Saw palmetto (*Serenoa serrulata*), nettle (*Urtica dioica*), African prune tree (*Pygeum africanum*)

Coughs

Coltsfoot, ephedra (*Ephedra* spp.), horehound (*Marrubium vulgare*), liquorice, mullein (*Verbascum thapsus*), thyme (*Thymus vulgaris*), wild cherry bark (*Prunus serotina*)

Ear and eye

Ear infections: echinacea (*E. purpurea*)

Ear wax: mullein (*Verbascum thapsus*)

Eye: eyebright (*Euphrasia officinalis*)

Gastrointestinal

Colic: camomile (*Matricaria chamomilla*)

Constipation: aloe (*A. barbadensis*), senna (*Cassia senna*), rhubarb (*Rheum palmatum*), cascara (*C. sagrada*)

Dandelion (*Taraxacum officinalis*)

Diarrhoea: barberry (*Berberis vulgaris*), bilberry (*Vaccinium myrtillus*)

Flatulence and dyspepsia:[196] angelica (*Angelica archangelica*), aniseed (*Pimpinella anisum*), clove (*Syzygium aromaticum*), ginger (*Zingiber officinalis*), lemon balm (*Melissa officinalis*), parsley (*Petroselenium crispum*), rosemary (*Rosinarinus officinalis*), sage (*Salvia officinalis*), thyme (*Thymus vulgaris*)

Haemorrhoids: horse chestnut (*Aesculus hippocastanumn*)

Motion sickness: ginger (*Zingiber officinalis*)

Nausea and vomiting: ginger (*Zingiber officinalis*)

Heartburn and indigestion: devil's claw (*Harpagophytum procumbens*), gentian (*Gentiana lutea*), liquorice (*Glycyrrhiza* spp.), peppermint (*Mentha piperita*)

Hyperlipidaemia[197]

Garlic (*Allium sativum*), globe artichoke (*Cymara scolymus*)
Ispaghula (*Plantago ovata*)

Influenza and colds,[198] *sore throat*

Echinacea (*E. angustifolia, E. pallida, E. purpurea*), elder (*Sambucus nigra*), ephedra (*Ephedra sinica* and other species), garlic (*Allium sativum*), golden seal (*Hydrastis*), nettle (*Urtica dioica*), usnea (*Usnea barbata*)

Insomnia[199]

Valerian (*Valeriana officinalis*), hops (*Humulus lupulus*), passionflower (*Passiflora incarnata*), lemon balm (*Melissa officinalis*), lavender (*Lavandula angustifolia*)

Rheumatics

Devil's claw (*Harpagophytum procumbens*), turmeric (*Curcuma longa*), yucca (*Yucca* spp.)

Skin conditions

Athlete's foot: myrrh (*Commiphora molmol*), tea tree (*Melaleuca alternifolia*)

Abrasions, superficial: marigold (*Calendula officinalis*)

Acne: burdock (*Arctium lappa*), tea tree (*Melaleuca alternifolia*)

Eczema: borage (*Borago officinalis*), sarsaparilla (*Smilax* spp.)

Psoriasis: cayenne (*Capsicum* spp.)

Wound healing: comfrey (*Symphytum*)

Urinary

Urinary tract infection (UTI): cranberrry (*Vaccinium macrocarpen*), uva ursi (*Arctostaphylos uva-ursi*)

Women's health[200]

Menopause: alfalfa (*Medicago sativa*), black cohosh (*Cimicifuga racemosa*), sage (*Salvia officinalis*)

Morning sickness: ginger (*Zingiber officinalis*), horehound (*Marrubium vulgare*)

Painful menstruation: black cohosh (*Cimicifuga racemosa*), blue cohosh (*Caulophyllum thalictroides*), cramp bark (*Viburnum opulus*)

PMS: agnus castus (*Vitex agnus castus*), St John's wort (*Hypericum perforatum*)

More information

National Institute of Medical Herbalists (NIMH): www.nimh.org.uk
British Herbal Medicine Association (BHMA): www.bhma.info
The Scottish School of Herbal Medicine : http://tinyurl.com/36mzws
American Botanical Council: http://tinyurl.com/33z6am
Herbal Medicine: Internet Resources: http://tinyurl.com/33w75r

Further reading

American Herbal Pharmacopeia. Available at: www.herbal-ahp.org.
Barnes J, Anderson L, Phillipson DJ. *Herbal Medicines A guide for health care professionals*, 3rd edn. London: The Pharmaceutical Press, 2007.
BHMA Scientific Committee, *British Herbal Pharmacopoeia.* Bournemouth: BHMA, 1996.
Boon H, Smith M. The *Botanical Pharmacy.* Kingston: Quarry Press, 1999.
British Herbal Compendium. Available at: http://tinyurl.com/2cy66z.
European Directorate for the Quality of Medicines (EDQM). *European Pharmacopoeia*, 6th edn. Strasbourg: Council of Europe, 2007.
Foster S, Tyler VE. *Tyler's Honest Herbal*, 4th edn. Binghamton, NY: The Haworth Health Press, 1999.
Liniger SW Jr, Gaby AR, Austin S et al. *The Natural Pharmacy.* Rocklin, CA: Prima Publishing, 1999.
Medical Economics Co. *PDR for Herbal Medicines.* Montvale, NJ: Medical Economics Co., 1998.
Meletis CD, Jacobs T. *Interactions between Drugs and Natural Medicines.* Sandy, OR: Eclectic Medical Publishers, 1999.
Miller L, Murray WJ, eds. *Herbal Medicinals – A clinician's guide.* Binghamton, NY: Pharmaceutical Products Press (The Haworth Press), 1998.
Mills S, Bone K. *Principles and Practice of Phytotherapy.* Edinburgh: Churchill Livingstone, 2000.

Ottariano SG. *Medicinal Herbal Therapy. A Pharmacist's viewpoint.* Portsmouth, NH: Nicolin Fields Publishing, 1999.
Williamson EM. *Potter's Cyclopaedia of Botanic Drugs.* Saffron Walden: CW Daniel CO. 2003.

References

1. Norfolk D. *The Therapeutic Garden.* London: Bantam Press, 1999.
2. Balentine DA, Albano MC, Nair MG. Role of medicinal plants, herbs and spices in protecting human life. *Nutr Rev* 1999;**57**:s41–5.
3. World Health Organization. *Guidelines for Appropriate Use of Herbal Medicines.* Western Pacific Series 22. Manila: WHO Regional Publications, 1998.
4. European Union. Directive EC 65/65. Brussels: EU Secretariat.
5. Ratsch C. *Plants of Love.* Berkeley, CA: Ten Speed Press, 1997.
6. Kapoor LD. *Opium Poppy.* New York: Food Products Press, 1997: xiii.
7. Hutchens AR. *Indian Herbology of North America.* Boston, MA: Shambhala, 1991: xxix.
8. Mills S, Bone K. *Principles and Practices of Phytotherapy.* London: Churchill Livingstone, 1999: 80–6.
9. Evans WC. *Trease and Evans Pharmacognosy*, 14th edn. London: WB Saunders, 1996.
10. Mills S, Bone K. *Principles and Practices of Phytotherapy.* London: Churchill Livingstone, 1999: 23–79.
11. Schilcher H. *Phytotherapy in Paediatrics*, 2nd edn. Stuttgart: Medpharm, 1992: 16–18.
12. Munzel K, Huber K. Extraction procedures in the preparation of chamomile fluid extract. *Pharma Acta Helv* 1961;**36**:194–204.
13. Meier B. The extraction strength of ethanol/water mixtures commonly used for the processing of herbal drugs. *Planta Medica* 1991;**57**(suppl 2):A26.
14. Report to ministers from The Department of Health Steering Group on the Statutory Regulation of Practitioners of Acupuncture, Herbal Medicine, Traditional Chinese Medicine and Other Traditional Medicine Systems Practised in the UK ('The Pittilo Report'). London: Department of Health, 2008. Available at http://hdl.handle.net/10059/176 (accessed 20 July 2008).
15. Mills S, Bone K. *Principles and Practices of Phytotherapy.* London: Churchill Livingstone, 1999: 132–255.
16. Ho JW, Jie M. Pharmacological activity of cardiovascular agents from herbal medicine. *Cardiovasc Hematol Agents Med Chem* 2007;**5**:273–7. PubMed
17. Mills S, Bone K. *Principles and Practices of Phytotherapy.* London: Churchill Livingstone, 1999: 121.
18. Kucera M, Kalal J, Polesna Z. Effects of Symphytum ointment on muscular symptoms and functional locomotor disturbances. *Adv Ther* 2000;**17**: 204–10. PubMed
19. Kayne S, Hayes P. Natural antiseptics and disinfectants. *New Zealand Pharmacy* 1996;**16**:23–6.

20.   Carson CF, Cookson BD, Farrelly HD, Riley TV. Susceptibility of methicillin-resistant *Staphylococcus aureus* to the essential oil of *Melaleuca alternifolia*. *J Antimicrob Chemother* 1995;**35**:421–4.

21.   Gibson PS, Powrie R, Star J. Herbal and alternative medicine use during pregnancy: a cross-sectional survey. *Obstet Gynecol* 2001;**97**(suppl 1):S44–5. PubMed

22.   Holst L, Nordeng H, Haavik S. Use of herbal drugs during early pregnancy in relation to maternal characteristics and pregnancy outcome. *Pharmacoepidemiol Drug Safety* 2007;151–9. PubMed

23.   Brinker F. *Herb Contraindications and Drug Interactions*, 2nd edn. Sandy, OR: Electric Medical Publications, 1998: 173–85.

24.   Mills S, Bone K. *Principles and Practices of Phytotherapy*. London: Churchill Livingstone, 1999: 99.

25.   Parsons M, Simpson M, Ponton T. Raspberry leaf and its effect on labour: safety and efficacy. *J Aust Coll Midwives* 1999;**12**:20–5. PubMed

26.   Schilcher H. *Phytotherapy in Paediatrics*. Stuttgart: Medpharm Scientific Publishers, 1997: 15–16.

27.   Houlder A-M. Letter. *BMJ* 1995;**310**:1473.

28.   Cochrane Collaboration. Complementary Medicine Field. *Newsletter* March 2000;**6**:2.

29.   Linde K, ter Riet G, Hondras M, Vickers A, et al. Systematic reviews of complementary therapies – an annotated bibliography. Part 2: Herbal medicine BMC. *Compl Altern Med* 2001;**1**:5. Available at: http://tinyurl.com/5f3aol (accessed 25 July 2008).

30.   Guo R, Canter PH, Ernst E. A systematic review of randomised clinical trials of individualised herbal medicine in any indication. *Postgrad Med J* 2007; **83**:633–7. Available at: http://tinyurl.com/63ghem (accessed 20 July 2008).

31.   Turner RB, Bauer R, Woelkart K, Hulsey TC, Gangemi JD. An evaluation of *Echinacea angustifolia* in experimental rhinovirus infection. *N Engl J Med* 2005;**353**:341–8 .

32.   Hawkes N. Herbal medicine really does cure a cold. *The Times*, 25 June 2007:11. Available at http://tinyurl.com/2tsrjg (accessed 12 November 2007).

33.   Shah SA, Sander S, White CM, Rinaldi M, Coleman CI. Evaluation of echinacea for the prevention and treatment of the common cold: meta-analysis. *Lancet Infectious Diseases* 2007;**7**:473–80.

34.   Blumenthal M, Busse W, Goldberg A et al. *The Complete German Commission E Monographs: Therapeutic guide to herbal medicine*. Austin, TX: American Botanical Council, 1998: 685.

35.   European Scientific Cooperative on Phytotherapy (ESCOP) Secretariat. *Uitwaardenstraat* 13, NL-8081. The Netherlands: HJ Elburg,

36.   Weston CFM, Cooper JD, Davies JD, Levine DF. Veno-occlusive disease of the liver secondary to the ingestion of comfrey. *BMJ* 1987;**295**:183.

37.   Perharic L, Shaw D, Murray V. Toxic effects of herbal medicines and food supplements. (letter) *Lancet* 1993;**342**:180–1.

38.   De Smet P. Health risks of herbal medicines. *Drug Safety* 1995;**13**:81–93.

39.   Drew AK, Myers SP. Safety issues in herbal medicine: implications for the health professions. *Med J Austr* 1997;**166**:538–41.

40. Barnes J, Anderson L, Phillipson JD. Herbal interactions. *Pharm J* 2003;**270**: 118–21.
41. Stargrove MB, Treasure J, Dwight AHG, McKee L. *Herb, Nutrient and Drug Interactions: Clinical implications and therapeutic strategies.* St. Louis, Mo: Mosby Elsevier, 2008.
42. Bourget S, Baudrant M, Allenet B, Calop J. Oral anticoagulants: a literature review of herb-drug interactions or food-drug interactions. *J Pharm Belg* 2007;**62**:69–75. PubMed
43. Ross S, Simpson CR, McLay JS. Homeopathic and herbal prescribing in general practice in Scotland. *Br J Clin Pharmacol* 2006;**62**:647–52.
44. Barnes J, Anderson L, Phillipson DJ. *Herbal Medicines*, 3rd edn. London: The Pharmaceutical Press, 2007: 7–9.
45. Winterhoff H. Toxicological aspects of phytomedicine. *Eur Phytotelegram* 1994;**6**:17–20.
46. De Smet PAGM, Smeets OSNM. Potential risk of health food products containing yohimbe extract. *BMJ* 1994;**309**:958.
47. Breckenridge, Prof. Letter from CSM. Renal failure associated with aristolochia in some Chinese herbal medicines. CEM/CMO/99/8 27 July 1999.
48. Gottlieb S. News. *BMJ* 1999;**319**:336.
49. Goldfrank L, Lewin N, Flomenbaum N, Howland MA. The pernicious panacea – herbal medicine. *Hosp Phys* 1982;**18**:64–7.
50. Dobb GJ, Edis RH. Coma and neuropathy after ingestion of herbal laxative containing podophyllin. *Med J Austr* 1984;**140**:496–6.
51. Fraunfelder FW. Ocular side effects from herbal medicines and nutritional supplements. *Am J Ophthalmol* 2004;**138**:639–47.
52. Pakzad K, Boucher BA, Kreiger N, Cotterchio M. The use of herbal and other non-vitamin, non-mineral supplements among pre- and post-menopausal women in Ontario. *Can J Public Hlth* 2007;**98**:383–8. PubMed
53. Brinker F. *Herb Contraindications and Drug Interactions*, 2nd edn. Sandy, OR: Electric Medical Publications, 1998.
54. Breckenridge A. Message from Chairman, CSM, concerning important interactions between St John's Wort (*Hypericum perforatum*) preparations and prescription medicines. London: MHR. 29 February 2000.
55. Bergner P. Herb-drug interaction. *Medical Herbalism* 1997;**9**:1.
56. Almeida JC, Grimsley EW. Coma from the health food store: interaction between kava and alprazolam. *Ann Intern Med* 1996;**125**:940–1.
57. Kleijnen J, Knipschild P. Ginkgo biloba. *Lancet* 1992;**340**:1136–9.
58. Rowin J, Lewis SL. Spontaneous bilateral subdural hematomas associated with chronic Ginkgo biloba ingestion. *Neurology* 1996;**46**:1775–6.
59. Rosenblatt M, Mindel J. Spontaneous hyphema associated with ingestion of ginkgo biloba extract. *N Engl J Med* 1997;**336**:1108.
60. Fugh-Berman A. Herb-drug interactions. *Lancet* 2000;**355**:134–8.
61. Barnes J, Anderson L, Phillipson DJ. *Herbal Medicines*, 3rd edn. London: The Pharmaceutical Press, 2007: 612–15.
62. Tisserand R, Balacs T. *Essential Oil Safety*. Edinburgh: Churchill Livingstone, 1995.
63. Ko RJ. Adulterants in Asian patent medicines. (Letter) *N Engl J Med* 1998; **339**:847.

64. De Smet PAGM. The safety of herbal products. In: Jonas WB, Levi JS (eds), *Essentials of Complementary Alternative Medicine*. Baltimore, MA: Lippincott, Williams & Wilkins, 1999: 108.

65. Perchant L, Shaw D, Murray V. Toxic effects of herbal medicines and food supplements. *Lancet* 1993;**342**:180–1.

66. Keane FM, Munn SE, du Vivier AWP, Taylor NF, Higgins EM. Analysis of Chinese herbal creams prescribed for dermatological conditions. *BMJ* 1999; **318**:563–4.

67. Ang HH, Lee KL. Evaluation of mercury contamination in *Smilax myosotiflora* herbal preparations. *Int J Toxicol* 2007;**26**:433–9. PubMed

68. Cooper CR. Herbal medicines. *Hosp Forum* 1982;**17**:1387–92.

69. Ascher S. *Mycotoxins in Herbal Medicinal Drugs*. Report of Pharmacovigilance of herbal medicines – current state and future directions at the Royal College of Obstetrics and Gynaecology London from 26 to 28 April 2006. *Pharm J* 2006;**276**:543–5.

70. Mills S, Bone K. *Principles and Practices of Phytotherapy*. London: Churchill Livingstone, 1999: 109.

71. But P. Need the correct identification of herbs in herbal poisoning (letter). *Lancet* 1993;**341**:637.

72. Lenoir S, Degenring F, Saller R. A double blind randomized trial to investigate three different concentrations of a standardized fresh plant extract obtained from the shoot tips of *Hypericum perforatum* L. *Phytomedicine*, 1999;**6**: 141–6.

73. Vanhaelen J-L, Depierreux M, Tielemans C et al. Rapidly progressing interstitial renal fibrosis in young women: association with slimming regimen including Chinese herbs. *Lancet* 1993;**341**:387–91.

74. Farah MH, Edwards R, Lindquist M, Leon C, Shaw D. International monitoring of adverse health effects associated with herbal medicines. *Pharmacoepidemiol Drug Safety* 200;**9**:105–12.

75. Kunkel DB, Spoerke DG. Evaluating exposures to plants. *Emerg Med Clin N Am* 1984;**2**:133–44.

76. Anon. History of the collection. *Pharm J* 1989;**243**:545.

77. Shellard EJ. Materia medica museum and herbaria. *Pharm J.* 1972;**208**:244–6.

78. Anon. Herbarium moves to Bradford. *Pharm J* 1969;**203**:117.

79. Editorial. Future of the Society's herbaria. *Pharm J* 1967;**202**:275.

80. Anon. Unveiling plaque marking transfer of Society's Herbaria to Bradford. *Pharm J* 1970;**204**:154.

81. Anon. Monthly meeting of Council – Report. *Pharm J* 1982;**229**:545.

82. Trease GE. Reminiscences of the Society's herbaria. (Letter) *Pharm J* 1982; **229**:655.

83. Anon. The Society's drug collection 'back to life' at Kew. *Pharm J* 1989;**243**: 544–5.

84. Hooker WJ. *Museum of Economic Botany. A popular guide to the useful and remarkable vegetable products in the two museum buildings of the Royal Gardens of Kew*. London: Longman, Brown, Green and Longmans & Roberts, 1958.

85. Berry M. Alfalfa. *Pharm J* 1995;**255**:353–4.

86. Medical Economics Co. *PDR for Herbal Medicines*. Montvale, NJ: Medical Economics Co., 1999: 962.
87. Malinow MR, Bardana Jr, Goodnight Jr SH. Pancytopenia during ingestion of alfalfa seed. (Letter) *Lancet* 1981;i:615.
88. Vogler BK, Ernst E. Aloe vera: a systematic review of its clinical effectiveness. *Br J Gen Practice* 1999;**49**:823–8.
89. Tyler VE. *Tyler's Honest Herbal*. New York: The Haworth Herbal Press, 1998: 27.
90. Barnes J, Anderson L, Phillipson DJ. *Herbal Medicines: A guide for health care professionals*, 3rd edn. London: The Pharmaceutical Press, 2007: 25–6.
91. Marshall JM. Aloe vera gel. What is the evidence? *Pharm J* 1990;**244**: 360–2.
92. Dykman KD, Tone C, Ford C, Dykman RA. The effects of nutritional supplements on the symptoms of fibromyalgia and chronic fatigue syndrome. *Intergr Physiol Behav Sci* 1998;**33**:61–71.
93. Berry M. The chamomiles. *Pharm J* 1995;**254**:191–3.
94. Craker LE, Simon JE, eds. *Herbs, Spices and Medicinal Plants*, Vol 1. Arizona: Onyx Press, 1986: 235–80.
95. Barnes J, Anderson L, Phillipson DJ. *Herbal Medicines*, 3rd edn. London: The Pharmaceutical Press, 2007: 296.
96. McGuffin M, Hobbs C, Upton R, Goldberg A. *Botanical Safety Handbook*. Boca Raton, FL: CRC Press, 1997: 74.
97. Barnes J, Anderson L, Phillipson DJ. *Herbal Medicines*, 3rd edn. London: The Pharmaceutical Press, 2007: 80–1.
98. Tyler VE. *Tyler's Honest Herbal*. New York. The Haworth Herbal Press. 1998: 51–2.
99. Uebelhack R, Blohmer JU, Graubaum HJ et al. Black cohosh and St John's wort for climacteric complaints. *Obstet Gynecol* 2006;**107**:247–55.
100. National Center for Complementary and Alternative Medicine. *Herbs at a Glance. Black Cohosh*. Available at: http://nccam.nih.gov/health/blackcohosh (accessed 12 November 2007).
101. Jacobson JS, Troxel AB, Evans J et al. Randomized trial of black cohosh for the treatment of hot flashes among women with a history of breast cancer. *J Clin Oncol* 2001;**19**:2739–45.
102. Phillipson JD, Anderson LA. Counterprescribing of herbal medicines – Part Two. *Pharm J* 1984;**233**:272–4.
103. Barnes J, Anderson L, Phillipson DJ. *Herbal Medicines*, 3rd edn. London: The Pharmaceutical Press, 2007: 82–3.
104. Selim L. *Professional Review – Blue Cohosh*. Available at: http://tinyurl.com/2qfgty (accessed 12 November 2007).
105. Hobbs C. Echinacea – a literature review. *Herbalgram* 1993;**30**:33–49.
106. Lindenmuth GE, Lindenmuth EB. The efficacy of Echinacea compound herbal tea preparation on the severity and duration of upper respiratory and flu symptoms: a randomized double-blind placebo-controlled study. *J Altern Compl Med* 2000;**6**:327–34.
107. Barrett B, Vohmann M, Calabrese C. Echinacea for upper respiratory infection. *J Family Practice* 1999;**48**:628–35.

108.   Medical Economics Co. *PDR for Herbal Medicines*. Montvale, NJ: Medical Economics Co., 1999: 819.
109.   McGuffin M, Hobbs C, Upton R, Goldberg A. *Botanical Safety Handbook*. Boca Raton, FL: CRC Press, 1997: 44.
110.   Berry M. Feverfew. *Pharm J* 1994;**253**:806–8.
111.   Vogler BK, Pittler MH, Ernst E. Feverfew as a preventative treatment for migraine: a systematic review. *Cephalagia* 1998;**18**:704–8.
112.   Pattrick M, Hepinstall S, Doherty M. Feverfew in rheumatoid arthritis: A double blind, placebo controlled study. *Ann Rheum Dis* 1989;**48**:547–9.
113.   Medical Economics Co. *PDR for Herbal Medicines*. Montvale, NJ: Medical Economics Co., 1999: 1172.
114.   Awang D. Feverfew fever – a headache for the consumer. *Herbalgram* 1993;**29**:34–26, 66.
115.   McGuffin M, Hobbs C, Upton R, Goldberg A. *Botanical Safety Handbook*. Boca Raton, FL: CRC Press, 1997: 113.
116.   Silagy CA, Neil HAW. A meta-analysis of the effect of garlic on blood pressure. *J Hypertension* 1994;**12**:463–8.
117.   Kiesewetter H, Jung F, Jung EM et al. Effect of garlic on platelet aggregation in patients with increased risk of juvenile ischaemic attack. *Eur J Clin Pharmacol* 1993;**45**:333–6.
118.   Silagy CA, Neil HAW. Garlic as a lipid lowering agent – a meta-analysis. *J R Coll Physicians Lond* 1994;**28**:39–45.
119.   Thomson M, Al-Qattan KK, Bordia T, Ali M. Including garlic in the diet may help lower blood glucose, cholesterol, and triglycerides. *J Nutr* 2006; **136**:800S–2S.
120.   Fleischauer AT, Poole C, Arab L. Garlic consumption and cancer prevention: meta-analyses of colorectal and stomach cancers. *Am J Clin Nutr* 2000; **72**:1047–52.
121.   Miller LG, Murray WJ, eds. *Herbal Medicinals. A clinical guide*. Bingha, NY: Pharmaceutical Products Press, 1998: 40.
122.   Warshafsky S, Kamer RS, Sivak SL. Effect of garlic on total serum cholesterol. *Ann Intern Med* 1993;**119**:599–605.
123.   Medical Economics Co. *PDR for Herbal Medicines*. Montvale, NJ: Medical Economics Co., 1999: 627.
124.   Petry JJ. Garlic and postoperative bleeding. [Letter, comment] *Plastic Reconstruct Surg* 1995;**96**:483–4.
125.   Scharbert G, Kalb ML. Duris M, Marschalek C, Kozek-Langenecker SA. Garlic at dietary doses does not impair platelet function. *Anesth Analg* 2007;**105**:1214–18.
126.   Tyler VE. *Herbs of Choice. The therapeutic use of phytomedicinals*. Binghamton, NY: Pharmaceutical Products Press, 1994: 209.
127.   Sunter W. Warfarin and garlic. *Pharm J* 1991;**246**:72.
128.   McGuffin M, Hobbs C, Upton R, Goldberg A. *Botanical Safety Handbook*. Boca Raton, FL: CRC Press, 1997: 6–7.
129.   University of Maryland Medical Center. *Medical Reference – Complementary Medicine – Ginger*. Available at: http://tinyurl.com/2y9kcd (accessed 12 November 2007).

130. Boon H, Smith M. *The Botanical Pharmacy*. Kingston: Quarry Press, 1999: 155–63.
131. Tyler VE. *Tyler's Honest Herbal*. New York: The Haworth Herbal Press, 1998: 181–2.
132. Medical Economics Co. *PDR for Herbal Medicines*. Montvale, NJ: Medical Economics Co., 1999: 1230.
133. Weiss RF. *Herbal Medicine*. Beaconsfield: Beaconsfield Publishers, 1988: 48.
134. Backon J. Ginger as an antiemetic: Possible side effects due to its thromboxane synthetase activity. (Letter) *Anaesthesia* 1991;**46**:669–71.
135. Kleijnen J, Knipschild P. Ginkgo biloba. *Lancet* 1992;**340**:1136–9.
136. Houghton P. Gingko. *Pharm J* 1994;**253**:122–3.
137. Pang Z. Ginkgo biloba: History, current status and future prospects. *J Altern Compl Med* 1996;**2**:359–63.
138. Vorberg G. *Ginkgo biloba* extract (GBE): A long term study of cerebral insufficiency in geriatric patients. *Clin Trials J* 1985;**22**:149–57.
139. Jung F, Mrowietz C, Kiesewetter H, Wenzel E. Effect of *Ginkgo biloba* on fluidity of blood and peripheral microcirculation in volunteers. *Arzneimittelforschung* 1990;**40**:589–93.
140. Ernst E, Pittler MH. Ginkgo biloba for dementia: a systematic review of double blind placebo controlled trials. *Clin Drug Invest* 1999;**17**:301–8.
141. Kennedy DO, Scholey AB, Wesnes KA. The dose-dependent cognitive effect of acute administration of *Ginkgo biloba* to healthy young volunteers. *Psychopharmacology* 2000;**151**:416–23.
142. Ernst E, Stevinson C. Ginkgo biloba for tinnitus: a review. *Clin Otolaryngol* 1999;**24**:164–7.
143. Fessenden JM, Wittenhorn W, Clarke L. Gingko biloba: a case report of herbal medicine and bleeding postoperatively from a laparoscopic cholecystectomy. *Am Surg* 2001;**67**:33–5. PubMed
144. Raman A. Ginseng. *Pharm J* 1995;**254**:150–2.
145. Vogler BK, Pittler MH, Ernst E. The efficacy of ginseng. A systematic review of randomized clinical trials. *Eur J Clin Pharmacol* 1999;**55**:567–75.
146. Schulz V, Hänsel R, Tyler VE. *Rational Phytotherapy: A physicians' guide to herbal medicine*. Berlin: Springer, 1998: 270–2.
147. Xiao PG, Xing ST, Wang LW. Immunological aspects of Chinese medicinal plants as anti-ageing drugs. *J Ethnopharmacol* 1993;**38**:167–75.
148. McGuffin M, Hobbs C, Upton R, Goldberg A. *Botanical Safety Handbook*. Boca Raton, FL: CRC Press, 1997: 81.
149. Stockley I. *Drug Interactions. A sourcebook of adverse interactions, their mechanisms, clinical importance, and management*, 3rd edn. Oxford: Blackwell Scientific Press, 1994.
150. Weiss RF. *Herbal Medicine*. Beaconsfield: Beaconsfield Publishers, 1988: 162–9.
151. Mills S, Bone K. *Principles and Practices of Phytotherapy*. London: Churchill Livingstone, 1999: 439–47.
152. Rodale JI. *The Hawthorn Berry for the Heart*. Wmmaus, PA: Rodale Books, 1971.

153. Barnes J, Anderson L, Phillipson DJ. *Herbal Medicines*, 3rd edn. London: The Pharmaceutical Press, 2007: 157–8.
154. Tyler VE. *Tyler's Honest Herbal*. New York: The Haworth Herbal Press, 1998: 206.
155. Bartram T. *Encyclopedia of Herbal Medicine*. Christchurch: Grace Publishers, 1885: 259.
156. Singh YD, Blumenthal M. Kava: an overview. *HerbalGram* 1997;**39**:34–55.
157. Boon H, Smith M. *The Botanical Pharmacy*. Kingston: Quarry Press, 1999: 133.
158. Woelk H. The treatment of patients with anxiety. A double blind study: kava extract WS1490 vs. benzodiazepine. *Z Allgemeine Med* 1993;**69**:271–7.
159. Lehmann E, Kinzler E, Friedemann J. Efficacy of a special kava extract (*Piper methysticum*) in patients with states of anxiety, tension, and excitedness of non-mental origin – a double-blind, placebo-controlled study of four weeks' treatment. *Phytomedicine* 1996;**3**:113–19.
160. Tyler VE. *Tyler's Honest Herbal*. New York: The Haworth Herbal Press, 1998: 230.
161. Bone K. Kava – A safe herbal treatment for anxiety. *Br J Phytother* 1993;**3**:147–53.
162. Almeida J, Grimsley E. Coma from the health food store: Interaction between kava and alprazolam. *Ann Intern Med* 1996;**125**:940–1.
163. National Center for Complementary and Alternative Medicine. *Herbs at a Glance – Milk Thistle*. Available at: http://nccam.nih.gov/health/milkthistle (accessed 12 November 2007).
164. Hobbs C. *Milk Thistle: The liver herb*, 2nd edn. Santa Cruz, CA: Botanica Press, 1992: 14–24.
165. Plomteux G, Albert A, Heusghem C. Hepatoprotector action of silymarin, in human acute viral hepatitis. *Int Res Commun Syst* 1977;**5**:259.
166. Blumenthal M, Brusse WR, Goldberg A et al. *The Complete German Commission E Monographs*. Austin, TX: American Botanical Council, 1998: 685.
167. Flora K, Hahn M, Rosen H, Benner K. Milk Thistle (*Silybum marianum*) for the therapy of liver disease. *Am J Gastroenterol* 1998;**93**:139–43.
168. Weiss RF. *Herbal Medicine*. Beaconsfield: Beaconsfield Publishers, 1988: 83.
169. Boon H, Smith M. *The Botanical Pharmacy*. Kingston: Quarry Press, 1999: 250–4.
170. Tyler VE. *Tyler's Honest Herbal*. New York: The Haworth Herbal Press, 1998: 254.
171. Medical Economics Co. *PDR for Herbal Medicines*. Montvale, NJ: Medical Economics Co., 1999: 1139.
172. Mills S, Bone K. *Principles and Practice of Phytotherapy*. Edinburgh: Churchill Livingstone, 2000: 542–52.
173. Linde K, Ramirez G, Mulrow C, Pauls A, Weidenhammer W, Melchart D. St John's wort for depression – an overview and meta-analysis of randomised clinical trials. *BMJ* 1996;**313**:253–8.

174. Vorbach EU, Arnoldt KH, Hubner W-D. Efficacy and tolerability of St. John's wort extract LI 160 versus imipramine in patients with severe depressive episodes according to ICD-10. *Pharmacopsychiatry* 1997;**30** (suppl 2):81–5.

175. Woelk H. Comparison of St John's wort and imipramine for treating depression: randomized controlled trial. *BMJ* 2000;**321**:536–9.

176. Grube B, Walper A, Wheatley MD. St John's wort extract: efficacy for menopausal symptoms of psychological origin. *Adv Ther* 1999;**16**:177–86.

177. Barnes J, Anderson L, Phillipson DJ. *Herbal Medicines*, 3rd edn. London: The Pharmaceutical Press, 2007: 250–1.

178. Ernst E, Rand JI, Barnes J, Stevinson C. Adverse effects profile of the herbal antidepressant St John's wort (*Hypericum perforatum*). *Eur J Clin Pharmacol* 1998;**54**:589–94.

179. Barone GW, Gurley BJ, Ketel BL, Abul-Ezz SR. Herbal supplements: a potential for drug interactions in transplant recipients. *Transplantation* 2001;**71**:239–41. PubMed

180. Boon H, Smith M. *The Botanical Pharmacy*. Kingston: Quarry Press, 1999: 283–90.

181. Saeed SA, Bloch RM, Antonacci DJ. Herbal and dietary supplements for treatment of anxiety disorders. *Am Fam Physician* 2007;**76**:549–56.

182. Mills S, Bone K. *Principles and Practice of Phytotherapy*. Edinburgh: Churchill Livingstone, 2000: 523–33.

183. Champault G, Patel JC, Bonnard AM et al. A double-blind trial of an extract of the plant *Serenoa repens* in benign prostatic hyperplasia. *Br J Clin Pharmacol* 1984;**19**:461–2.

184. Braeckman J. The extract of *Serenoa repens* in the treatment of benign pro-static hyperplasia: a multicentre open study. *Cur Ther Res* 1994;**55**:776–85.

185. McGuffin M, Hobbs C, Upton R, Goldberg A. *Botanical Safety Handbook*. Boca Raton, FL: CRC Press, 1997: 107.

186. Barnes J, Anderson L, Phillipson DJ. *Herbal Medicines*, 3rd edn. London: The Pharmaceutical Press, 2007: 238.

187. Houghton P. Valerian. *Pharm J* 1994;**253**:95–6.

188. Hobbs C. Valerian – a literature review. *Herbalgram* 1989;**21**:19–35.

189. Stevinson C, Ernst E. Valerian for insomnia? A systematic review. 1999 In print. (Cited in Ernst E. Herbal medicines as a treatment of some frequent symptoms during menopause. *J Br Menopause Soc* 1999;117–20.)

190. Oxman AD, Flottorp S, Håvelsrud K et al. A televised, web-based ran-domised trial of an herbal medicine (valerian) for insomnia. *PLoS ONE* 2007;**2**:e1040.

191. Boon H, Smith M. *The Botanical Pharmacy*. Kingston: Quarry Press, 1999: 308–13.

192. Mills S, Bone K. *Principles and Practice of Phytotherapy*. Edinburgh: Churchill Livingstone, 2000: 542–81.

193. McGuffin M, Hobbs C, Upton R, Goldberg A. *Botanical Safety Handbook*. Boca Raton, FL: CRC Press, 1997: 120.

194. Barnes J. Depression. *Pharm J* 2002;**268**:908–10.
195. Barnes J. Benign prostatic hyperplasia. *Pharm J* 2002;**268**:250–2.
196. Barnes J. Gastrointestinal system and liver disorders. *Pharm J* 2002:**268**: 848–50.
197. Barnes J. Hyperlipidaemia. *Pharm J* 2002;**269**:193–5.
198. Barnes J. Colds. *Pharm J* 2002;**269**:716–18.
199. Barnes J. Insomnia. *Pharm J* 2002;**269**:219–21.
200. Barnes J. Women's health. *Pharm J* 2003;**270**:16–18.

9

Aromatherapy

Steven B Kayne

Medicinal and cosmetic uses of aromatherapy are sometimes difficult to separate and there is often confusion in consumers' minds as to the different qualities of oils available for purchase.

Definition

The word 'aromatherapy' entered the English language in the early 1980s to describe the use of fragrant essential oils to affect or alter a person's mood or behaviour.[1] A broader definition that makes provision for massage with oils and transdermal absorption in addition to inhalation has been provided by Price and Price:[2]

> Aromatherapy is the use of essential fragrant oils (the pure volatile portion of aromatic plant products normally extracted by distillation) for therapeutic or medical purposes.

Strictly speaking the substances used in aromatherapy are not fragrances or aromatic mixtures (as used in the perfume industry) but pure essential oils (also known as volatile oils), volatile substances extracted from diverse parts of plants which have curative property.[3] Therefore, not everything that emits a pleasant smell is necessarily an essential oil. Frequently used as a synonym for essential oil is the term 'essence', which means a natural aromatic substance that a plant secretes from its reproductive organs; an essential oil is in fact an extract obtained by distilling an essence. Despite its name, an essential oil may or may not necessarily be oily in consistency.

History

The practice of using oils to treat illnesses is reputed to be at least 6000 years old and to have followed the westward course of civilisation, beginning in the oriental cultures of China, India, Persia and Egypt. The earliest Hindu scriptures mention several hundred perfumes and aromatic products, classifying their use for both liturgical and therapeutic applications.[4]

The Egyptians are known to have used plant products for many reasons, including medicine, massage therapy, preservation and mummification. Aromatic oils were made by soaking plant materials in base oils or fats. There is some evidence that later Egyptians experimented with crude methods of distillation.[1] The Greeks used aromatics and essential oils in warfare to stimulate aggression and heal battle wounds. Dioscorides, a first-century Greek surgeon in Nero's Roman army, included a chapter on oils in his medical encyclopaedia, which remained a standard medical text for more than 1000 years.

Modern aromatherapy owes its emergence to numerous European pharmacists and apothecaries, chiefly in France and Germany, whose improved methods of distillation and investigations on the nature and value of essential oils during the seventeenth and early eighteenth centuries contributed much to its wider acceptance. However, although by the end of the eighteenth century almost every herbalist and many physicians used essential oils to varying degrees, the practice received a major setback with the advent of chemistry. Using newly discovered techniques, alchemists began to extract what they believed to be active principles rather than using the plant and later even synthesised simple chemical drugs. The enthusiasm for naturally occurring treatments within the medically oriented professions receded until there was a revival in the 1920s.

The term *aromathérapie* is attributed to the French chemist René-Maurice Gattefossé, who published a book on the subject in 1937 and is generally considered to be the founder of modern aromatherapy.[5] It was not until this point in time that essential oil therapy was separated from mainstream phytotherapy by name. The first English translation of this book was published in 1993.[6] Gattefossé is said to have become interested in the study of essential oils in 1910 following a laboratory explosion in which he burnt his hand severely while working in his family perfumery. He is said to have plunged his hand into a conveniently placed bath of lavender oil. The hand not only healed within a few hours, but did so without scarring. This experience led him to investigate many essential oils and record the chemical constituents of each. During World War I Gattefossé used essential oils successfully to treat burns and prevent gangrene. With the advent of powerful modern drugs and in common with other complementary disciplines, aromatherapy fell into decline during the middle years of the twentieth century. In the 1960s a French doctor, Jean Valnet, who as an army surgeon had treated wounded soldiers with aromatherapy, followed up the work of Gattefossé. Together with one of his students, Margaret Maury, a biochemist, Valnet developed a method of applying the oils using massage. Maury introduced aromatherapy to the UK in the 1950s. Since then aromatherapy has enjoyed a considerable resurgence, with about 5000 trained aromatherapists now practising in the UK. It is now the fastest-growing complementary discipline in this country.

Theory

The basis for the action of aromatherapy is similar to modern pharmacology, with active principles entering the biochemical pathways, albeit in much smaller doses. Aromatherapy is thought to work at psychological, physiological and cellular levels.

Two mechanisms of action have been identified:

1.   Olfactory stimulation
2.   Dermal action.

The olfactory system

Aromatherapists believe that olfactory stimulation plays an important role in their treatment, the sense of smell being the most immediate of our senses.

Most mammals and reptiles have two distinct parts to their olfactory system: a main olfactory system and an accessory olfactory system.

Main olfactory system

The main olfactory system detects volatile, airborne substances that are inhaled through the nose, where they contact the main olfactory epithelium. Figure 9.1 is a diagram of the human olfactory system.

In the roof of each nostril is a region called the nasal mucosa. This region contains the olfactory epithelium covered by mucus. Odours are detected by the olfactory receptor neurons of the olfactory epithelium. These specialised cells possess a terminal enlargement (or dendritic

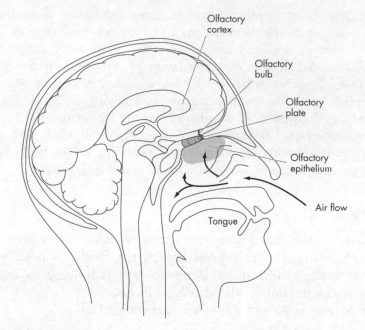

Figure 9.1 Diagram of the human olfactory system, showing the location of the olfactory epithelium. (The vomeronasal organ or accessory olfactory bulb [AOB] is located on the dorsal–posterior region of the main olfactory bulb.)

knob) that projects above the epithelial surface, from which extend about 8–20 non-motile olfactory cilia (Figure 9.2).

The receptors for odorants are located on these cilia. Olfactory receptor neurons in the olfactory epithelium transduce molecular features of the olfactory stimulants (or 'odorants') into electrical signals, which then travel along the olfactory nerve into the olfactory bulb. This is a highly organised structure, composed of several distinct layers, that passes on stimuli to the olfactory cortex in the brain. The cribriform plate of the ethmoid bone, separated at the midline by the crista galli, contains multiple small foramina through which the olfactory nerve fibres, or fila olfactoria, pass. These carry stimuli to the olfactory cortex located within the medial temporal lobes of the brain and responsible for the conscious awareness and identification of odours.

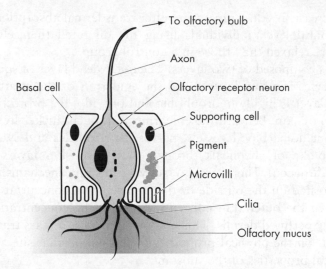

Figure 9.2 Olfactory receptor neuron.

Accessory olfactory system

The accessory olfactory system senses chemical stimuli in fluid phase primarily through the accessory olfactory bulb, also called the vomeronasal organ, which is located in the vomer bone between the nose and the mouth on the dorsal–posterior region of the main olfactory bulb. Known as pheromones, these chemicals trigger a natural behavioural response in another member of the same species. Examples include alarm pheromones, food trail pheromones, sex pheromones and many others that affect behaviour or physiology. From an accessory olfactory bulb located on the dorsal–posterior portion of the main olfactory bulb, stimuli pass to the amygdala and the hippocampus areas of the brain associated with emotional and learning processes. Learning processes are thought to be responsible for the memories evoked by various different odours (see below).

Dermal action

Traditional aromatherapists believe that volatile aromatic oils are effective only when their molecules come into contact with the nasal mucosa through inhalation (as detailed above).[7] However, application to the skin with or without massage has produced positive results, e.g. ylang ylang oil was found to cause a significant decrease in blood pressure and a significant increase in skin temperature after transdermal absorption.[8] At the behavioural level, individuals using the oil rated themselves calmer and more relaxed than those in a control group.

The skin is composed of two layers. The outer dead layer of squamous keratinocytes is a thin layer called the epidermis or the stratum corneum. This layer is highly hydrophobic and provides the protective barrier function of skin. Beneath the epidermis is a much thicker living layer of cells, including blood vessels, nerves, hair follicles and sweat glands. The uptake of chemicals through these two skin layers is controlled by diffusion. There are no active transport mechanisms. Chemicals deposited on the outside of the skin set up a concentration gradient between the outer skin concentration and the concentration within the richly perfused dermis. This gradient produces a mass transfer that depends on the physical properties of the skin at that site and also the chemical properties of the substance.

There are three types of chemical–skin interactions:[9]

1. The chemical may pass through the skin and contribute to the systemic load.
2. The chemical can induce local effects ranging from irritation through to burns or degradation of the barrier properties of the skin.
3. The chemical can evoke allergic skin reactions through complex immune system responses that can subsequently trigger responses in the skin at both the point of contact and skin sites remote to the contact.

The rate of essential oil absorption through the skin varies with a number of factors:

•   **Skin barrier**: the passage of a chemical through the skin barrier is dependent on many factors. The skin is not uniform in terms of thickness, epidermis:dermis ratio, density of hair follicles and many other parameters that affect permeability. The amount of material that may be absorbed will, as a consequence, vary depending on the anatomical site of the exposure.[10]
•   **Temperature**: a modest rise in the temperature of the skin is likely to cause enhanced blood flow and therefore lead to increased absorption of the essential oil. Many years ago the absorption of methyl salicylate was investigated and found to be enhanced by a rise in skin temperature consistent with taking a bath.[11] If the

temperature is too high, the volatile oils will evaporate, reducing the amount of essential oil available for absorption.

- **Water**: the presence of water influences the rate of absorption; it is thus beneficial to have a shower or bath before applying essential oils.
- **Skin occlusion**: covering the skin with a non-permeable dressing causes a change in the local environment: both temperature and hydration increase. As stated above, this will facilitate a more rapid absorption of essential oil. An American study with perfumes showed that almost 20 times as much fragrance was absorbed through the skin when it was covered than when it was left uncovered.[12] The application of a greasy ointment will have a partially occlusive effect in that it retards evaporation of water away from the skin. However, this also retards the passage of the essential oil and ointment bases are useful only for local effects.
- **Presence of detergent**: detergents and soaps increase skin permeability, so a good wash before aromatherapy is likely to be beneficial. The fat solubility of oil-based liniments and other oily topical applications (e.g. oily creams) helps the penetration of essential oils.

Unlike psychological mechanisms, the pharmacological mechanism for aromatherapy is not thought to involve any perception of the odour. Here the effects are thought to result from the compounds entering the body and acting directly on the brain, i.e. via the bloodstream by absorption through the lungs or olfactory mucosa.

Production of aromatherapy oils

Essential oils – composition and production

Essential oils are used in:[13]

- foods, as flavourings (e.g. orange or lemon oil)
- orthodox medicines (e.g. clove oil for toothache, peppermint oil for indigestion and eucalyptus as an inhalation, and are the constituents of many over-the-counter [OTC] patented products)
- complementary medicine (aromatherapy).

Extraction

The starting materials for true essential oils are 'essences'. These are generated by photosynthesis in highly specialised secretory cells that may be in the leaf, bark or other parts of the plant.[14] They may be stored within the same cell in which they are made or pass into a storage cell or duct. These cells are often just below the surface of the leaf and the essence may be released if the leaf is crushed, giving off a characteristic aroma. In other plants, storage ducts are in minute hairs on the leaf. These plants are highly aromatic and release their fragrance when simply brushed against. The proportion of essence in the plant varies with species and this accounts in part for the varying prices of essential oils. The particular plant used, and the part of that plant used, can have a significant effect on the final product.[15]

The best-quality essential oils are obtained from essences derived from a whole plant or plant parts (Table 9.1) by vapour or steam distillation. Ideally, a copper or stainless steel still that separates the plant material and steam is used. The separate chamber ensures that hot water will not break down or dilute the essential oils. The application of heat during the distillation process initiates certain chemical changes. The oil is slowly liberated from the plant material.

Other methods involving the passage of steam through the plant material, extraction with volatile solvents and cold pressing (mainly for citrus oils) are also available. Some plants may produce several oils as different sections of the plant are processed, e.g. from the leaves, flowers and fruit.

Table 9.1 Source of extracted essential oils

Part used for oil	Example
Bark	Cinnamon
Blossom	Orange (Neroli)
Bulbs	Garlic
Dried flower buds	Clove
Flowers	Jasmine, lavender, rose
Fruits	Lemon, mandarin
Grass	Lemongrass
Leaves	Eucalyptus, geranium, peppermint
Root tuber	Ginger
Seeds	Fennel
Wood	Sandalwood

Varying amounts of essential oil can be extracted from a particular plant. Over 100 kg of rose petals are required to obtain about 50 ml of essential oil, whereas lavender and lemon plants yield far greater quantities. The active principle of the citrus fruit is found in the outer coloured layer of the rind and the pulp, and the white pith must be removed before extraction can proceed. The peel is then squeezed and the resulting juice left to stand until the aromatic oil can be separated off. Other oils (jasmine, neroli and rose) are obtained by enfleurage or solvent extraction without any distillation. These are neither essential oils nor essences and are classified as 'absolutes'. All these variations are usually included in the aromatherapist's armamentarium under the general heading 'essential oils'.

It should be noted that some widely used oils are non-volatile (e.g. sunflower oil) and these are usually obtained by a simple crushing pressure known as expression.

Composition

Essential oils are highly complex chemicals containing perhaps as many as 100 or more constituents, many of which may be present in concentrations as low as 1%. Examples of typical chemical constituents in essential oils and their therapeutic properties are indicated in Table 9.2. Aromatherapists believe that the many constituents of essential oils combine synergistically, making the final therapeutic effect better than could be predicted from the sum of individual chemical group activities.

Table 9.2 Constituents of essential oils

Constituents	Therapeutic properties
Acids	Anti-inflammatory, hypothermic
Alcohols	Astringent
Aldehydes	Anti-inflammatory, astringent, bactericidal, hypothermic
Coumarins	Sedative, calming action
Dienes	Anticoagulant, anti-spasmodic
Esters	Anti-spasmodic, sedative
Ethers	Sedative, anti-spasmodic
Ketones	Anticoagulant, sedative, mucinolytic
Oxides	Mucinolytic, decongestant, expectorant
Phenols	Anthelmintic, bactericidal, fungicidal
Sesquiterpenes	Anti-inflammatory properties
Terpenes	Bactericidal, fungicidal; 'tonic'

This synergy works both to enhance outcomes directly and to reduce the possibility of side effects, by some constituents cancelling out the potentially damaging effects of others. This is known as 'quenching'.

An oil usually contains between three and five chemical groups. As a result of the synergistic effects it is not possible to determine the therapeutic properties by simply listing the properties associated with each constituent. The influence of one chemical group on another results in specific therapeutic properties, e.g. studies have shown that using whole essential oil is more effective than its isolated components (http://tinyurl.com/4v2kym).

Knowledge of environmental effects on essential oil content and the composition of aromatic crops is essential to determine the level of success that can be obtained in therapeutic use. Significant differences among essential oil contents can be observed between plants grown under field conditions and those grown in greenhouses.[16]

Chemotypes

Oils derived from the same source but with different characteristics are known as 'chemotypes'. There may be more than one chemotype for a given essential oil. For example:

- Most oils on the market derived from thyme (*Thymus vulgaris*) are rich in thymol, a compound with irritant properties. If the plant is cut in the spring the essential oil contains 30% thymol plus the monoterpene hydrocarbon *p*-cymene. If the same plant is cut in the autumn the essential oil may be found to contain 60–70% thymol and less *p*-cymene, changing its therapeutic potential.[17] There are several other chemotypes of thyme essential oils.
- There are three commercial types of camomile oil – German (*Matricaria recutita*), Roman or English (*Chamaemelum nobile*) and Moroccan (*Ormenis multicaulis*), all differing in genus and composition.
- At least three species of lavender may be identified: *Lavandula angustifolia* contains mainly alcohols and esters; *Lavandula latifolia* contains 1.8-cineole and camphor and fewer alcohols and esters; and *Lavandula stoechas* contains mainly ketones.[15]
- Eucalyptus oil can be extracted from 120 different species and at least 3 entirely different commercial oils are available.

Care should be taken to read the labels of such products to ascertain whether the ingredients are as expected. The selling price of an oil may reflect its composition. The chemical constituents of an essential oil represent a mixture of many organic compounds that have related, but distinct, types of chemical structure, giving the oil its odour, therapeutic properties and, in some cases, its toxicity.[18]

These constituents can vary with a number of different factors.

Growing conditions Conditions in which the plants have been grown can affect the composition of the oil. In drought or other extreme climatic circumstances, or if there are nutritional deficiencies in the soil, the plant's essential oils help to facilitate survival. The amount of essential oil in a plant is inversely proportional to the amount of water present. As the plant dries out it produces essential oils to compensate for the loss of water. Thus, the aroma from dried flowers is often more intense than that from fresh leafy material. Furthermore, the aroma from specimens of certain cultivated species may differ from that of similar wild species.[19] The wild variety of *Rosmarinus officinalis* (rosemary), which grows in various parts of Europe, contains an ester and ketone as its main active ingredients. The same variety cultivated in a greenhouse contains an oxide as the main chemical group. Geographical location may also affect the nature of the essential oil. The Mediterranean version of rosemary has a ketone as the main constituent and smells quite different to the wild or greenhouse varieties. The effect of various combinations of day and night temperatures and day lengths have been studied using dill plants in environmentally controlled chambers.[20] The concentration of essential oil was found to be highest during high-temperature periods; exposure to light was also important.

Plant maturity Different stages of a plant's development may affect the oil's characteristics, e.g. when *Verbena officinalis* is in bloom it gives off a pleasant perfume. However, soon after blooming this is replaced by a bitter odour. Hence plants destined for oil extraction must be harvested at specific times of the year.

Environmental conditions In many cases the time of day and environmental conditions at the time of harvesting are also important in determining the chemical and therapeutic nature of the essential oil. The period of time that elapses between collection of raw plant material and distillation must be as short as possible because chemical changes are initiated immediately after cutting. Significant differences in the essential oil content have been observed in camomile during protracted storage of harvested plants. After 31 months' storage at 16°C approximately 50% of the initial oil content was maintained.[21]

Production procedures Differences in production techniques and manufacturing equipment will result in differences in the quality and composition of the resultant oil.[6]

Storage Degradation from incorrect storage conditions can occur. The main degrading factor is atmospheric oxygen, which causes the oxidation of active principles, especially terpenes, and this process is enhanced by heat and light. Chemical change can result in the appearance of toxic chemicals. Terpene degradation in certain oils leads to the formation of compounds that can act as skin sensitisers.[22]

Quality of oils

Apart from the intrinsic nature of the oil and the possibility that its chemotypes may be confused, oils are liable to adulteration and contamination, possibilities that are said to be widespread.[23] Possible adulterants include other essential oils, and synthetic chemicals. Contaminants may include herbicides and pesticides. It is possible to detect these foreign materials using gas chromatography, mass spectroscopy, high-performance liquid chromatography and nuclear magnetic resonance: for consumers, it is important that aromatherapy products are purchased from a reputable source.

Some oils may not represent a naturally occurring state, but are changed for commercial reasons. White camphor oil is only a fraction of true camphor oil, whereas cornmint oil almost always has its menthol content halved.

Other oils may be fabricated by combining the same components as are found in the naturally occurring oil. There are probably no particular dangers associated with using these fabricated oils other than the possibility of allergic skin reactions. Examples of commonly fabricated oils include melissa and verbena. Other oils may be totally synthetic, e.g. wintergreen oil is almost always made from the chemical methyl salicylate.

The significant price difference between the different qualities of oils can be confusing to consumers who do not appreciate the difference between the variants.

Storage

It is recommended that essential oils should be used within 1 year of opening the container. As a result of the potential increase in the rate of degradation caused by heat and light, oils should be packed in amber bottles and kept in a cool place, preferably a refrigerator. Under these circumstances the lifespan of the oil may be doubled. Some oils become viscous if stored in a refrigerator, making them rather difficult to pour if they are not allowed to reach room temperature before use.

Incorrect storage may lead to the production of impurities that can cause dermatological problems.

Aromatherapy in practice

The term 'aromatherapy' is commonly applied both to treating ill health (i.e. therapy) and to cosmetic use, which relies on 'fragrancing'. Making a distinction between the two is not always possible: the use of aromatherapy in epilepsy, for example, is clearly designed to be therapeutic,[24] but where largely psychological factors might be involved a clear distinction is not easy.

Four basic types of use may be identified:[25]

1. **Cosmetic**: aromas are of a pleasurable type (bath essences, soaps)
2. **Holistic aromatherapy** for general stress
3. **Environmental fragrancing**: essential oils may be diffused into the atmosphere to enhance general wellbeing, for disinfectant purposes[26] or to mask unpleasant odours
4. **Medicinal or clinical aromatherapy**: used in the treatment of various conditions and where outcomes are measurable.

Fragrancing

Aromatherapy practitioners claim to be able to help a range of conditions, including eczema, digestive problems, muscular aches and pains, premenstrual syndrome (PMS), asthma, insomnia and headaches. As aromatherapy encourages relaxation, it is thought that patients suffering from stress-related conditions can also benefit.[27] Another aspect of aromatherapy is an enhanced feel-good factor, which may improve self-esteem, after a massage or a bath with essential oils. The current interpretation of the word 'perfume' illustrates the divergent course taken by modern fragrancing away from traditional aromatics.[28] As recently as the nineteenth century, 'to perfume' still meant 'to disinfect', i.e. to fumigate by using scent or, more literally, through smoke (i.e. per fume). When our ancestors scented themselves and their possessions or took a nosegay or scented handkerchief it was with a dual mood-enhancing and germicidal objective. Only in the past century or so has the purpose of fragrancing been divided between the aesthetic objectives of the modern perfume industry and the therapeutic objectives of aromatherapy. Aromas have also been used as a marketing tool, e.g. supermarkets are known to release aromas of newly baked bread or percolating coffee to enhance sales. Odours and taste are an important part of our everyday lives and are considered to be more than just a biological response.[29]

Olfactory remediation

As a way of including both medical and non-medical practice, the term 'olfactory remediation' has been suggested to describe the umbrella beneath which aromatherapy may coexist with a more scientific practice that also employs essential oils.[30] In this model aromatherapy is considered to be a largely experience-oriented discipline with a reliance on healing rather than scientific principles. It is usually practised by non-health professionals, who aim to treat a wide range of physical, mental and emotional symptoms, as well as being prescribed for general wellbeing.

The second area of olfactory remediation is not called aromatherapy formally, although its results may affect its practice. In this area olfactory stimulation is used therapeutically in a more specific manner to alleviate particular medical conditions only where appropriate. Studies on clinical outcomes have been published. Health professionals, especially nurses, are often involved in this variant. Although it is conceivable that pharmacists may be involved in both methods of using essential oils it is olfactory stimulation to which this chapter refers.

Aromatherapy massage

Aromatherapy massage is the combination of massage therapy and the utilisation of essential fragrant oils. Massage also provides the means for establishing a positive patient–practitioner healing relationship,[31] and can bring on the physiological benefits not only through the therapist's hands, which physically manipulate human tissue, but also by bringing about a psychological component of relaxation by using the sense of smell to strengthen the whole curative effect.[32] It is claimed that abdominal massage using essential oils with rosemary, lemon and peppermint can help relieve constipation in elderly people.[33]

Aromatherapy massage is a mixture of Swedish (soft tissue massage), shiatsu (massage at acupuncture points) and neuromuscular massage. Gentle rubbing movements may be used in some cases (see Chapter 13).

Gedney et al.[34] have identified 11 advantages of aromatherapy massage:

1. Promotes deep relaxation and relieves the physical and psychological weariness
2. Improves the function of the inherent internal organs indirectly or directly
3. Releases tense muscular pressure and decreases muscle pain
4. Promotes the blood circulation of the musculature and relieves the symptoms of inflammation and pain
5. Increases body elasticity and energy
6. Decreases the symptoms of arthritis and rheumatism
7. Restores and speeds up tissue healing of sprains and fractures
8. Promotes the function of the digestive system
9. Promotes the kidney and lymphatic systems to accelerate the suppression of toxins and waste
10. Relieves various kinds of headache symptoms
11. Promotes relaxation to increase mood and decreases psychological stress.

Route of administration

Essential oils may be administered by one or more of the following routes:

*   by inhalation
*   by topical application
*   by mouth
*   by rectal or vaginal administration.

Inhalation

Many conditions respond extremely well to essential oil inhalation. There are several commercially available inhalation products that include essential oils in their formulation (Karvol, Vick) as well as the standard inhalation of camphor and menthol BP. The oils can be inhaled using the old-fashioned bowl of hot water and towel over the head method or simply from one to two drops on a handkerchief or tissue. A few drops on the pillow may help a restless client sleep, but direct contact with the skin should be avoided. A variety of steam inhalers and fan-assisted apparatus is available. Used as a room fragrance, essential oils create a pleasant atmosphere, enhancing the mood and even creating a suitable ambience for meditation (Figure 9.3).

Topical application

Topical application is used during aromatherapy massage (see above). Essential oils are included in several patented products, including Vicks rub and Tiger Balm, where the ointment base serves as a carrier for both transdermal absorption and inhalation. Normally the oils are used in liquid form, although various gel and cream formulations exist. Compresses may also be used for skin conditions.

As the oils are highly concentrated they should not generally be applied to the skin undiluted, except under supervision. The use of aromatherapy oils contained in a vegetable carrier oil by skin massage is the most frequent route of administration. Aromatherapists dilute essential oils (0.5 ml:10 ml) with carrier oils, such as sweet almond, walnut, wheatgerm and hazelnut, which contain active vitamins and

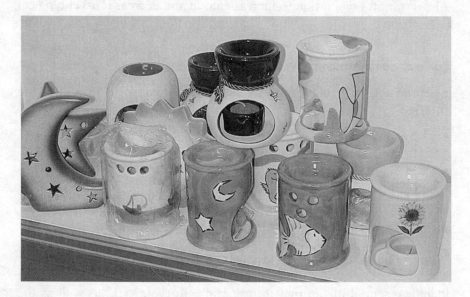

Figure 9.3 A selection of aromatherapy burners.

fatty acids. Other possible carrier oils are rapeseed, sunflower and soya bean.[35]

When contained in a suitable carrier oil dermal absorption is rapid, e.g. lavender oil enters the circulation within 5–10 min, with maximal blood concentrations being achieved after approximately 20 min.

Ready blended oils, comprising several essential oils mixed in a carrier, are available for specific purposes, e.g. rheumatics or insomnia. Essential oils can also be added to bath water. Here the cosmetic and medical applications become entwined. Clients often find it helpful to relax in a pleasantly scented bath for 20–30 min and this can also be used to relieve muscular strains and sprains. About six to eight drops of oil are suggested. The oil is normally eliminated from the body within about 90 min.

Oral administration

Some essential oils are used as orthodox medicines and are given orally. The oral use of peppermint oil[36] and some components of essential oils, such as pinene, limonene, camphene and borneol, is documented.[37,38] Various oils of the Umbelliferae family, e.g. caraway, dill and fennel, are used in medicines for indigestion, flatulence and dyspepsia in adults and infants. In general the oral administration of essential oils is not recommended, except under medical supervision, because it may carry a risk of an adverse reaction occurring. Significant levels of active ingredients in the bloodstream are achieved. Oral administration is not routinely used in the UK, although some practitioners do recommend the use of a weak aqueous solution as a mouthwash. Rinsing the mouth four times a day with 15 ml of a 5% solution of tea tree oil has been shown to be effective in treating a oral thrush.[39] Gargles and mouthwashes made from essential oils should not be swallowed.

Aromatherapy in France and Germany, in direct contrast to that in the UK and the USA, involves medically qualified doctors using essential oils as conventional internal medicines.

Other routes of administration

Vaginal administration (pessaries or tampons dipped in essential oils or douches) can be useful for localised symptoms. Tea tree oil has been used to treat candidiasis.[40] Suppositories may also be dipped in essential oils and used rectally. Being lined with mucous membranes, the rectum and vagina are both extremely sensitive to irritation.

Metabolism[41]

Essential oil components are metabolised differently according to the route of administration. After external application most essential oil components are likely to pass through the skin and enter the bloodstream.[42] Inhaled volatile essential oils are taken into the nose as vapour, dissolving in the mucosal layer. Orally administered essential oils are absorbed through the large and small intestine, and act directly on the brain via the circulation.[43] Possible neurochemical effects include the following:

- Inhibition of binding of glutamate, an excitatory neurotransmitter[44]
- Augmentation of γ-aminobutyric acid (usually abbreviated to GABA), an inhibitory neurotransmitter[45,46]
- Acetylcholine receptor binding.[47]

Most essential oils are fat soluble but, as they pass to the liver, enzymatic action will change them to more water-soluble structures, facilitating urinary excretion. Fat-soluble substances usually pass readily into the central nervous system and liver, more slowly into muscle and finally into adipose tissue, where a store of essential oil components may be built up slowly because of low blood flow. Once lodged in fat, most substances are inactive.

Essential oils are often electrically charged at body pH and can adhere easily to electrically charged molecules such as proteins. Ketones, esters, aldehydes and carboxylic acids, all of which are found in essential oils, tend to bind to plasma albumin, a soluble protein that is present in the blood in very high concentrations. Although it is not known whether this mechanism, which is found in drug distribution, applies to essential oils, these two facts make it a likely hypothesis.

The absorption pathways of essential oils are summarised in Figure 9.4

Choice of oil

A number of psychological responses to fragrant odours are possible, e.g. the individual's perception of the pleasantness of an odour and the individual's past association with an odour.[48] These variable individual psychological effects of odours are important because they are likely to influence treatment outcomes. In most circumstances a high concentration of most odours can be considered unpleasant; even when in small quantities they may be considered unpleasant. Individual experience of

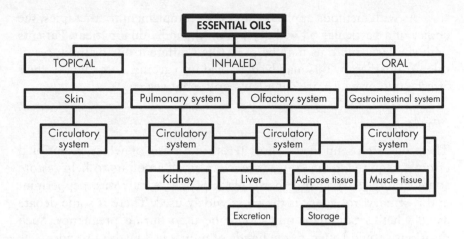

Figure 9.4 Absorption pathways of essential oils

an odour may also affect response. Consequently, patients for whom a particular odour has strong negative (or positive) associations may be expected to introduce interindividual variability in outcomes. It has been shown that individuals may even exhibit positive and negative attitudes to odour 'words'.[49]

Howard and Hughes[50] sought to establish whether lavender aroma and/or expectancies affect post-stress relaxation. They suggest that the previous associations of lavender aroma with assisted relaxation may have been influenced by expectancy biases, and that the relevant expectancies are easily manipulable.[50]

It is possible that aromatherapy might have its effects in the absence of any psychological perception of the smell. This is important, because many people with dementia may have little or no sense of smell due to the early loss of olfactory neurons[51] (see below).

Aromatherapy is frequently recommended for children but children's preferences for specific essential oils are not well documented. Fitzgerald et al.[52] studied the preferences of school-aged children for essential oils based on gender and ethnicity. Participants evaluated each scent's effect on mood and energy, stated their preferences, indicated if scents evoked particular thoughts and selected a favourite essential oil. Girls were more likely to feel happy when smelling sweet orange and more energetic with spearmint; all boys felt more energetic when smelling ginger. The results indicate that children have specific essential oil scent preferences. There is a trend towards differences based on gender and ethnicity.[52]

As with methods applicable to other complementary therapies, the choice of a particular oil will depend on the individual patient. Patients with similar symptoms may be prescribed different oils or mixtures of oils. Aromatherapy oils may be classified into groups according to their effects, two of which are stimulants and sedatives.

Stimulants

These oils are useful in the short term, in a crisis or when exceptional effort is required, or in convalescence in small amounts to help restore some vitality. They include basil, black pepper, eucalyptus, peppermint and rosemary; rosemary is the most widely used. There is some debate as to whether stimulant oils should be used during pregnancy. Such decisions should be left in the hands of a qualified health provider.

Sedatives

A number of essential oils are considered to be primarily calming or sedative. These include bergamot, camomile, lavender, marjoram, melissa and sandalwood. The most effective ways of using these oils are in massage and in baths, especially before going to bed.

Some oils have been shown to have both sedative and stimulant properties depending on the way in which they are used. These include geranium, neroli (orange flower) and rosewood.

Blends of oils for treating a variety of conditions are available. Most textbooks will give an indication of oils that can be mixed in a suitable carrier.

Conditions treated

Although the provision of evidence for the benefits of aromatherapy is slowly improving, the quality of many published trials is low and the range of conditions treated diverse. Aromatherapy is often misunderstood and consequently somewhat marginalised. As a result of a basic misinterpretation, the integration of aromatherapy into British hospitals is not moving forward as quickly as it might. Aromatherapy in the UK is primarily aimed at enhancing patient care or improving patient satisfaction, and it is frequently mixed with massage.[53] Little focus is given to the real clinical potential, except for a few pockets such as the Micap plc/Manchester Metropolitan University initiative, which led to a phase I clinical trial into the effects of aromatherapy on infection carried out in the Burns Unit of Wythenshawe Hospital.[54]

Examples of aromatherapy oils that are frequently used for self-treatment, together with appropriate routes of administration, are summarised in Table 9.3.

Evidence

Cooke and Ernst[55] make the point that trials of aromatherapy meet formidable methodological problems, e.g. the smell of the oils is difficult to mask and patient blinding can therefore be difficult.[55] Many studies use animal or tissue culture models.[56] There follows some examples of published research in a number of different applications. Primary sources of evidence should be carefully assessed for quality.

Table 9.3 Examples of essential oils and their uses

Condition to treat	Essential oil	Route of administration
Arthritis	Camomile, juniper, rosemary	Massage, bath additive
Athlete's foot	Lavender, tea tree	Footbath
Blisters	Lavender	Topical application
Burns	Lavender, camomile, eucalyptus, tea tree	Topical application, bath
Chilblains	Juniper, lavender, marjoram, rosemary	Topical application
Colds	Eucalyptus, orange, tea tree	Inhalation, massage/rub throat and chest
Coughs	Eucalyptus, lavender	Inhalation, massage/rub throat and chest
Flu	Eucalyptus, juniper, lavender, tea tree	Inhalation, massage/rub throat and chest
Insect bites	Camomile, lavender, tea tree	Topical application, bath, compress
Irritable bowel syndrome	Camomile	Massage abdomen, bath
Migraine	Lavender, marjoram, rosemary	Inhalation, massage head and neck
Muscle injuries	Eucalyptus, marjoram, rosemary, tangerine	Massage/rub affected area
Nausea	Lavender, mint	Inhalation
Sore throat	Lavender, sandalwood, tea tree	Massage/rub throat and upper chest

Review

The randomised controlled trial (RCT) literature on aromatherapy has been evaluated in order to define whether or not any clinical indication is backed up by evidence.[57] Studies on the local effects of oils and those involving healthy volunteers were excluded. Six RCTs were located, one each for the common cold, prophylaxis of bronchitis, smoking with-drawal symptoms, perineal discomfort after childbirth, anxiety and alopecia. With one exception these were all positive. A further six trials were found concerning the use of aromatherapy for anxiety and well-being in a variety of patient types in the hospital environment. Positive results were recorded in five of these studies, suggesting that aromather-apy may have an anxiolytic effect but that the evidence for other appli-cations was not 'compelling' for relaxation; the effects of aromatherapy are probably not strong enough for it to be considered for the treatment of anxiety. The hypothesis that it is effective for any other indication is not supported by the findings of rigorous clinical trials.

Anxiety

Aromatherapy is often promoted for the management of anxiety; how-ever, there is little evidence to support this. The systemic review by Cooke and Ernst[55] concluded that aromatherapy appears to have a transient effect in the reduction of anxiety but that there is no evidence of a lasting benefit from its use.

A randomised trial assessing the effectiveness of aromatherapy in reducing preoperative anxiety in women undergoing abortions has been carried out. Aromatherapy appeared to be no more effective than having patients sniff other pleasant odours in reducing pre-procedure anxiety.[57] A controlled, prospective study to evaluate the use of aro-matherapy to reduce anxiety before a scheduled colonoscopy or oesophagogastro-duodenoscopy did not show aromatherapy to be effective based on statistical analysis. However, patients did generally report the lavender oil as being pleasant.[58]

On a more positive note, aromatherapy massage with music reduced 'significantly' the anxiety and stress of emergency nurses.[59]

Menopausal symptoms

A Japanese research team have reported that aromatherapy could be effective as a CAM method for menopausal symptoms in the setting of a hospital obstetrics and gynaecology department.[60]

Research has suggested that aromatherapy massage can be used as an effective intervention to reduce abdominal subcutaneous fat and waist circumference, and to improve body image in postmenopausal women.[60,61]

Pain control

Evidence for the use of aromatherapy in pain control is patchy. An investigation into the use of aromatherapy in the management of acute postoperative pain concluded that further research was necessary before a firm conclusion could be reached.[62] Another rather more positive study concluded that lavender oil could be used to reduce the demand for opioids in an immediate postoperative period.[63] However, the authors said that further studies were required to assess the effect of this therapy on clinically meaningful outcomes, such as the incidence of respiratory complications, delayed gastric emptying, length of hospital stay or whether this therapy is applicable to other operations.

Kim et al.[64] compared the analgesic efficacy of postoperative lavender oil aromatherapy in 50 patients undergoing breast biopsy surgery; 25 patients received supplemental oxygen through a facemask with two drops of 2% lavender oil postoperatively. The remainder of the patients received supplemental oxygen through a facemask with no lavender oil. Outcome variables included pain scores (a numeric rating scale from 0 to 10) at 5, 30 and 60 minutes postoperatively, opioid requirements in the postanaesthesia care unit (PACU), patient satisfaction with pain control, as well as time to discharge from the PACU. There were no significant differences in opioid requirements and recovery room discharge times between the two groups. Postoperative lavender oil aromatherapy did not significantly affect pain scores. However, patients in the lavender group reported a higher satisfaction rate with pain control than patients in the control group.

A pilot study carried out by Kane et al.[65] presented eight patients with two odour therapies, lavender and lemon, two music therapies, relaxing and preferred music and a control condition, during vascular wound dressing changes. Although the therapies did not reduce the pain intensity during the dressing change, there was a significant reduction in pain intensity for the lavender therapy and a reduction in pain intensity for the relaxing music therapy after the dressing change.

Dementia

Aromatherapy is reported to be of benefit to people with dementia for whom verbal interaction may be difficult. It may provide an alternative option to neuroleptic drugs that are associated with side effects including sedation and falls.[66] It has been used to reduce disturbed behaviour,[67] promote sleep[68] and stimulate motivational behaviour.[69]

A placebo-controlled study, in which 72 patients with severe dementia were treated with lemon balm (*Melissa officinalis*) essential oil, demonstrated improvements in behavioural symptoms comparable with those seen with neuroleptic agents in patients with less severe dementia, but it also indicated secondary improvements in quality of life and activities.[70]

In a study using heated lavender oil (*Lavandula officinalis*) dispersed into the atmosphere by a small fan, observers detected improvement in 9 patients (60%) with a further 5 (33%) showing no change and only 1 (7%) showing a worsening of agitated behaviour.[71]

An RCT of the relaxing effects lavender oil massage on disordered behaviour in dementia was conducted by Smallwood et al.;[72] 21 patients were randomly allocated into one of 3 conditions: aromatherapy and massage, conversation and aromatherapy, and massage only. The aromatherapy and massage group showed the greatest reduction in the frequency of excessive motor behaviour of all three conditions. Almost all participants in the studies completed the course of treatment. This emphasises the excellent tolerability of aromatherapy, which is in contrast to many of the pharmacological treatments in this group of patients. It is common for 30% or more of the participants to be unable to complete a trial.[73]

Lavender has also been found to be as effective as an adjunctive therapy in alleviating agitated behaviours in Chinese patients with dementia.[74]

Bowles et al.[75] conducted a cross-over study of aromatherapy massage in 56 patients with moderate-to-severe dementia. Cream containing one of four essential oils (lavender, sweet marjoram, patchouli or vetiver) or cream alone was massaged into the skin five times daily for 8 weeks. The study showed a significant decrease in behavioural problems and resistance to care in the patients who received the cream with essentials oils compared with those who received the cream alone.

A note of caution on the use of aromatherapy oils to treat behavioural and psychological symptoms in dementia (BPSD) has been expressed by Nguyen and Paton.[76] They identified 11 prospective randomised studies in the literature with positive and negative consequences for both people with dementia and their carers. The authors concluded that, although a potentially useful treatment for BPSD, the expectations of clinicians and patients with respect to the efficacy and tolerability of conventional medicines should apply equally to aromatherapy. They also expressed concern that the side-effect profile of commonly used oils is virtually unexplored.

Childbirth

The use of aromatherapy during childbirth is becoming an increasingly popular care option with mothers and midwives. Burns et al.[77] investigated the feasibility of conducting an RCT on the use of aromatherapy during labour as a care option that could improve maternal and neonatal outcomes. They compared aromatherapy with standard care during labour: 251 women randomised to aromatherapy and 262 controls. Participants were randomly assigned to administration of selected essential oils during labour by midwives specifically trained in their use and modes of application. Unfortunately the study was underpowered so the results were of limited significance; however, the researchers demonstrated that it is possible to undertake an RCT using aromatherapy as an intervention to examine a range of intrapartum outcomes.[77] With this in mind it is to be hoped that more trials will be undertaken in the future.

An evaluation of a midwifery aromatherapy service for mothers in labour has been reported.[78] This study, of 8058 mothers in childbirth, is the largest research initiative so far undertaken in the use of aromatherapy within a healthcare setting. The study took place over a period of 8 years and a total of 10 essential oils were used plus a carrier oil, administered to the participants via skin absorption and inhalation. The study found little direct evidence that the practice of aromatherapy reduced the need for pain relief during labour or the incidence of operative delivery. However, a key finding of this study suggests that two essential oils – clary sage and camomile – are effective in alleviating pain. The evidence from this study suggests that aromatherapy can be effective in reducing maternal anxiety, fear and/or pain during labour. The use of aromatherapy appeared to facilitate a further reduction in the use of systemic opioids in the study centre, from 6% in 1990 to

0.4% in 1997 (per woman). A paper by Mousley[79] reported the results of the audit of a maternity aromatherapy service at a small maternity unit in the English Midlands. The service was introduced in May 2000 and the principal aims of the audit, conducted in October 2002 were to investigate clinical effectiveness, maternal satisfaction and staff training needs. The service has been shown to be effective in normalising childbirth and increasing satisfaction of mothers in respect of their labour experiences. A concurrent audit of staff demonstrated interest and enthusiasm of the service and identified areas for further development.

Cancer care

Aromatherapy and massage have gained wide popularity among nurses in clinical practice. An RCT has shown that a statistically significant psychological benefit was derived from giving foot massage to patients after cardiac surgery.[80] Evidence from an audit into the effects of aromatherapy massage in palliative and terminal care suggested that most patients derived some benefit.[81] The effect of massage with 1% Roman camomile in carrier oil has been investigated in patients receiving palliative care.[82] The control group was given massage alone. Anxiety scores improved in both groups but the aromatherapy group showed significant improvement in physical symptoms and quality of life. Other workers have not found significant improvements when using aromatherapy and massage over massage alone.[83] A number of other studies have demonstrated positive effects from massage.[84] However, aromatherapy massage may not confer benefit on cancer patients' anxiety and/or depression in the long term, although it seems to be associated with clinically important benefit up to 2 weeks after the intervention.[85]

Kyle evaluated the effectiveness of aromatherapy massage with 1% *Santalum album* (sandalwood) (group A) when compared with massage with sweet almond carrier oil (group B) or sandalwood oil (group C), in reducing levels of anxiety in palliative care.[86] The primary end-points of the research were to report a statistically significant difference in anxiety scores between experimental group B and comparison groups A and C, and to influence the integration of aromatherapy into all aspects of palliative care. The results were not substantial enough to generate coherent statistics, so no assumptions could be drawn from these results due to the inconsistencies that were bound to occur in such a small sample. However, the results seemed to support the notion that sandalwood oil is effective in reducing anxiety.

Epilepsy

Aromatherapy has been used by some patients suffering from epilepsy as a means of controlling their seizures. Certain oils, notably rosemary, can cause an increase in seizure frequency, so the appropriate oil must be carefully selected.

Common cold

Statistically significant differences have been noted between groups of patients suffering from a common cold who inhaled a mixture of camphor (35%), menthol (56%) and eucalyptus (9%), compared with those using a hot-water vapour control. Only 24 adults were involved in the trial.[87]

Cardiovascular system

Lavender aromatherapy may have beneficial acute effects on coronary circulation.[88] A Korean study investigated the effects of aromatherapy on blood pressure and stress responses of clients with essential hypertension. There were 52 participants divided into an essential oil group, placebo group and control group by random assignment. The application of aromatherapy was the inhalation method of blending oils with lavender, ylang ylang and bergamot once daily for 4 weeks. The results suggested that the inhalation method using essential oils can be considered an effective nursing intervention, which reduces psychological stress responses and serum cortisol levels, as well as the blood pressure of clients with essential hypertension.[89]

Insomnia

Lewith et al.[90] evaluated the efficacy of lavender (*Lavandula angustifolia*) on insomnia. Interventions comprised *Lavandula angustifolia* (treatment) and sweet almond oil as placebo/control. Outcomes appeared to favour the lavender.

Essential oils as antiseptics

Many essential oils and their constituents have antimicrobial properties.[91] Indeed, essential oils have been used externally to eradicate fungal or bacterial infections for hundreds of years.[92] At the time of the

Black Death, apothecaries would wrap scarves soaked in essential oils such as camphor around their necks and over their mouths when visiting sick patients.

In the early years of the twentieth century and following an article in *Nature*, Even, a French pharmacist, impregnated gauze with the essential oils bergamot, geranium, lavender and rosemary.[93] These volatile oils were selected because in his opinion they had the greatest antiseptic value while being the least irritating. The fragranced dressing was used to cover suppurating wounds. Gattefossé is reputed to have used essential oils on the skin as disinfectants for healing wounds.[94] Essential oils that are said to have microbial qualities include cinnamon, salvia (sage), sandalwood and thymus (thyme).[94]

Several other essential oils are said to have antimicrobial qualities, including cinnamon, salvia (sage), sandalwood and thymus (thyme). Essential oils of eucalyptus, lavender and thyme in the proportion 2:2:4 provide an effective disinfectant, and tissues impregnated with the mixture are recommended for wiping toilet seats, baths and basins in areas of uncertain pedigree! A disinfectant suitable for tropical countries has oregano added, the essential oil of which contains up to 15% thymol.

Although lavender oil is often assumed to be 'very antiseptic',[95] studies carried out on a range of commercial lavender oils have shown a wide variation in antibacterial effect.[96] Nevertheless, a few drops of lavender, lemongrass and thyme are reported as being effective in disinfecting mattresses. A wide variation in activity in other essential oils has also been reported.[97]

Peppermint is one of the oldest and best-known European medicinal herbs, and is reputed to produce a gentle disinfectant effect (preventing fermentation) when there are abnormal decomposition processes in the stomach. Both the herb and its oil may be used externally in baths to treat cuts and skin rashes. The oil contains about 50% menthol.

One of the most widely used antiseptic oils in recent years has been tea tree oil.[98] The oil is obtained from the leaves of *Melaleuca* spp., historically used by Australian aboriginals and New Zealand Maoris to treat skin abrasions and infections. The name was invented by Captain Cook, whose crew used the leaves to make tea and to flavour beer. Tea tree oil was distributed to Australian soldiers during military operations as a disinfectant, leading to a high demand for its products locally. In recent years the oil has become widely available in Europe. It contains terpinoids and is effective against fungus and bacteria, including pneumococci, staphylococci,[99] streptococci and those resistant to some orthodox antibiotics.[100] A 3-month single-blind study has shown that topical application of 5% tea tree oil gel in patients suffering from acne is at least as beneficial as 3% benzylperoxide, with fewer side effects.[101] A double-blind study found that a 10% tea tree oil cream was as effective as clotrimazole in the treatment of athlete's foot.[102] It has been pointed out that topical application of a gel or lotion in this fashion does not really constitute true aromatherapy.[103]

The aromatogram[104]

The aromatogram is a laboratory test that allows aromatherapists to analyse in vitro the antibacterial activity of essential oils and to select more accurately those considered to be the most effective in destroying a particular microbial infection. The test is conducted much like the conventional culture test for antibiotic activity.

Safety

One of the concerns with aromatherapy is its marketable strengths, which suggests that the consumer does not have to be an expert aromatherapist to use the oils.[105] Indeed, the availability of essential oils on the high street and advice columns in magazines and newspapers could be interpreted as evidence of total safety.

It is important to view the possibility of side effects in context, because they are only likely to occur with prolonged use of high concentrations and in people with acute hepatic or renal problems. However, clearly some of the chemical groups present in essential oils are potentially toxic and clients should be instructed that essential oils should be used judiciously and according to instructions.

Most of the data on toxicity relate to the ingestion of essential oils. Oral administration is extremely rare in the UK, so the reports available refer to poisoning from accidental or intentional ingestion of large amounts of essential oils, including citronella[106,107] and eucalyptus. Death is usual after consuming about 30 ml of the latter, following severe cardiovascular, respiratory and central nervous effects.[108] There are many recorded cases of poisoning by essential oils in young children.

Camphor and sassafras are claimed to be carcinogenic and their use is generally contraindicated in aromatherapy. Camphorated oil is not an essential oil and so cases of poisoning due to ingestion of this are not included here. In general, toxicity is dose dependent: the more of an oil that is used, the higher the potential toxicity.

Potential toxic effects

Potential side effects include dermal toxicity, skin sensitisation (allergy), phototoxicity and dependence.[109]

Dermal toxicity

Skin irritation is a relatively common reaction to the application of several essential oils, although this risk may be reduced by dilution. Some oils may cause a dermatological reaction after prolonged use. Severely irritant essential oils include horseradish and mustard; moderately or strongly irritant oils include cinnamon, clove, oregano, parsley, rue and wintergreen. Tea tree oil has also been cited as causing dermatitis.[110]

Skin sensitisation (allergy)

Allergies to camomile have been reported,[111] with two cases of nipple dermatis after the application of an OTC product containing the essential oil.[112] The most notorious oils for causing allergies are costus (formerly used widely in perfumes) and verbena. Cinnamon, garlic and laurel leaf oil can also cause sensitisation reactions to varying degrees. Skin rashes and itching have been reported after the application of tea tree oil.[113] Table 9.4 shows a number of commonly used essential oils for which sensitising constituents have been identified.[114] Aromatherapists themselves may be subject to sensitisation, particularly if they are handling significant quantities of oils on a daily basis.[115]

Phototoxicity[116]

Certain essential oils (e.g. verbena, bergamot and the citrus oils, including grapefruit, lemon, lime and orange) may cause increased photosensitivity in some individuals if the skin is exposed to direct sunlight shortly after application (see 'Aromatherapy during pregnancy', below). Substances known to be phototoxic include many with antiseptic properties that are added to toiletries and suntan preparations. Phototoxic components (psoralens or furanocoumarins) are present in a limited number of essential oils and in small amounts, normally < 2%, but nevertheless they are still capable of causing a reaction, even if the essential oil is diluted substantially. One report concerns a woman who was treated for minor burns after 20 min spent on a sunbed immediately after taking a sauna in which a few drops of lemon oil had been added to the burner.

It has been found that the bergapten component of bergamot oil produces abnormally dark pigmentation and reddening of the surrounding skin after exposure to an ultraviolet lamp. This condition is known as berloque dermatitis or bergapten dermatitis. The darkened patches of skin can remain for several years. To ensure that the risk of photosensitivity is reduced to a minimum, maximum-use levels have been set for some common essential oils. These are summarised in Table 9.5.

Dependence

It is possible that the repeated application of rubs and ointments containing large amounts of essential oils (e.g. Vick or Tiger Balm) may lead to some dependence, with the product being used long after it needs to be. Pharmacists should be alert to this possibility.

Interactions with orthodox medicines[117]

There may be interactions between orthodox medicines and essential oils. Possible problems include enhanced transdermal penetration, potentiation effect of warfarin, monoamine oxidase inhibition and the induction of cytochrome P450 (an important detoxifying enzyme that is

Table 9.4 Main sensitising constituent of some common essential oils

Essential oil	Main sensitising constituent
Bergamot	Coumarins
Camphor	Terpene
Dill	Carvone
Eucalyptus	Creole and phellandrene
Fennel	Phellandrene
Lemon	Limonene
Lemongrass	Citral
Pine oil	Borneol
Rose oil	Citronelle
Spearmint	Limonene

Table 9.5 Characteristics and uses of common essential oils

Oil	Characteristic	Examples of indications
Bergamot	Uplifting	Anxiety, appetite loss, skin problems
Camomile	Comforting	Muscle/joints, skin, soothing, calming
Clary sage	Relaxing	Sedative, stress/tension
Clove	Stimulating	Antiseptic, toothache
Eucalyptus	Energising	Antiseptic, respiratory, antiviral
Geranium	Uplifting	Anxiety, skin problems
Ginger	Warming	Cold/flu, stomach problems
Lavender	Relaxing	Muscle/joints, skin problems, soothing
Lemon	Refreshing	Antiseptic, cold/flu/throat, tonic, skin, digestion
Patchouli	Soothing, sensual	Anxiety, skin problems
Peppermint	Stimulating	Anxiety, cooling, feet, insect repellent
Rosemary	Reviving	Circulation, mental processes, lethargy
Sandalwood	Balancing	Urinary, throat, skin problems
Tea tree	Revitalising	Antibacterial, fungal (especially thrush)
Ylang ylang	Relaxing, sensual	Heart rate/respiration regulation, shock, trauma, skin

induced by alcohol and certain drugs, including carbamazepine, diphen-hydramine, nicotine, nitrazepam, phenobarbital, phenytoin and pro-gestogens). Any essential oil taken orally that also induces this enzyme may reduce the effect of a drug.

Common drugs that are incompatible with topically applied oils include aspirin (clove and garlic), paracetamol (basil, camphor, cinna-mon, clove), pethidine (parsley) and warfarin (cinnamon, clove, garlic, wintergreen).

Interaction with homeopathic medicines

Traditionally it is said that homeopathic remedies are inactivated by aromatic oils, so the two should not be used together. There is no firm evidence to substantiate this perception, but it is usual to instruct patients to leave 1–2 h between brushing the teeth with a peppermint toothpaste and taking a homeopathic medicine.

Aromatherapy during pregnancy

Authorities are divided as to the advisability of using aromatherapy oils during pregnancy because there are no reliable data on potential teratogenic and abortifacient risks. However, it is probable that the components of essential oils can cross the placental barrier and a number are contraindicated or should be used with caution during pregnancy (see below).[118]

One of the most versatile essential oils, lavender, is classified by some aromatherapists as emmenagogic (i.e. it may cause menstrual discharge and/or potentially a miscarriage) and is restricted to the later stages of pregnancy or not used at all. Some authorities promote its use throughout pregnancy. Other essential oils said to be emmenagogic are calendula, jasmine, juniper, marjoram, melissa, nutmeg, peppermint and thyme. There is no evidence that, even if these oils were potentially emmenagogic in the small amounts used during aromatherapy, they would necessarily be abortifacients.

Aromatherapists sometimes recommend that new mothers add six to eight drops of lavender oil to bathwater following childbirth, but a study found no evidence that such a practice was effective in reducing perineal discomfort.[119]

There are accounts in the literature of women attempting to bring on menstruation[120] or induce abortions with pennyroyal, an essential oil that is in any case contraindicated in aromatherapy because of hepatotoxicity.[121] Extra care should be taken with topical use of essential oils during pregnancy. For aromatherapy massage over large areas of skin a maximum concentration of 2% essential oil is recommended. The phototoxic risk mentioned above is particularly important in pregnant women, who already have raised melanocyte-stimulating hormone levels and are therefore more likely to burn in strong sunlight. These oils should be used only by qualified practitioners for short periods and mothers advised to keep out of the sun for between 2 and 12 h after therapy, depending on the concentration of oil used.

An example of a special topical formulation for nursing mothers is in use at the Maternity Unit at the Southern General Hospital in Glasgow. It comprises a mixture of three oils – cypress, geranium and lavender – in the proprietary gel known as KY and is applied three times a day to the vaginal area to reduce discomfort after delivery.

The following is a summary of oils that may be used in pregnancy and those that should be avoided:

- Oils that are generally considered safe to use during pregnancy: camomile, ginger, lavender, rose, sandalwood.
- Oils that may be used externally during pregnancy: anise, mace, nutmeg, rosemary, spike lavender.
- Oils that should be avoided during pregnancy: oils rich in apiole, e.g. parsley leaf and seed, and oils rich in sabinyl acetate, e.g. sage.

OTC supply

A list of common aromatherapy oils and their main indications is provided in Table 9.6.

Reducing the risks of adverse reactions

Containers and labelling

Inadequate labelling and lack of appropriate guidance on how the product should be used at the point of sale are two major inadequacies that could be rectified relatively easily. Containers that restrict the delivery of contents to drops, facilitating more accurate dilution, are essential.

Counselling

Clients intending to self-treat should be advised to take the following precautions:[122]

- Never eat or drink essential oils except under medical supervision.
- Never use concentrated essential oils directly on the skin; always dilute with a suitable carrier oil (e.g. almond oil) – a typical dilution for massage is 15 drops of essential oil to 50 ml of a carrier oil.
- Be aware that some oils (e.g. bergamot, lemon and orange) can react with sunlight and burn the skin.
- Clients in an 'at-risk category' (infants, elderly people, pregnant women, or those who have kidney or liver problems, etc.) should seek professional advice before attempting to treat ongoing conditions.
- Do not use homeopathic and aromatherapy remedies concurrently.

Table 9.6 Characteristics and uses of a selection of common oils

Oil	Characteristics	Examples of indications
Bergamot	Uplifting	Anxiety, appetite loss, skin problems
Camomile	Comforting	Muscle/joints, skin, soothing, calming
Clary sage	Relaxing	Sedative, stress/tension
Clove	Stimulating	Antiseptic, toothache
Eucalyptus	Energising	Antiseptic, respiratory, antiviral
Geranium	Uplifting	Anxiety, skin problems
Ginger	Warming	Colds/flu, stomach problems
Lavender	Relaxing	Muscle/joints, skin problems, soothing
Lemon	Refreshing	Antiseptic, colds/flu/sore throat, tonic, skin
Patchouli	Soothing/sensual	Anxiety, skin problems
Peppermint	Stimulating	Anxiety, cooling, feet, insect repellant
Rosemary	Reviving	Circulation, mental processes, lethargy
Sandalwood	Balancing	Urinary, throat, skin problems
Tea tree	Revitalising	Antibacterial, fungal (thrush)
Ylang ylang	Relaxing, sensual	Respiration regulation, shock, trauma

More information

Aromatherapy Council: www.aromatherapycouncil.co.uk
Aromatherapy Organisations – links:
    www.aromacaring.co.uk/uk_aromatherapy.htm
Aromatherapy Organisations Council – Education and Training in Clinical
    Aromatherapy: http://tinyurl.com/2w8e9g
Holistic Medicine Resource Center Aromatherapy internet resources: http://
    tinyurl.com/2vat9x
International Federation of Aromatherapists: www.ifaroma.org/
National Association Holistic Aromatherapy: www.naha.org

Further reading

Davis P. *Aromatherapy A- Z*, revised edn. London: Vermilion, 2005.
Lis-Balchin M. *Aromatherapy Science – A guide for healthcare professionals.*
    London: Pharmaceutical Press, 2006.
Price S, Price L. *Aromatherapy for Health Professionals*, 3rd edn. London:
    Churchill-Livingstone Elsevier, 2007.
Schnaubelt S. *Medical Aromatherapy: Healing with essential oils.* Berkeley, CA:
    Frog Ltd, 1999.

References

1. *Webster's Third New International Dictionary*, Unabridged (CD-ROM 3.0 version). Merriam-Webster, 2002.
2. Price S, Price L. *Aromatherapy for Health Professionals*. London: Churchill Livingstone, 1999.
3. Delgado Ayza C. What is aromatherapy? *Rev Enferm* 2005;**28**:55–8, 61–4.
4. Damian P, Damian K. *Aromatherapy. Scent and psyche*. Rochester, VT: Healing Arts Press, 1995: 3.
5. Gattefossé R-M. *Aromathérapie: Les Huiles Essentielles Hormones Végétales*. Paris: Girardot, 1937.
6. Gattefossé R-M. *Gattefossé's Aromatherapy* (edited by Tisserand R). Saffron Walden: CW Daniel, 1993.
7. Shultz V, Hansel R, Tyler VE. *Rational Phytotherapy. A physicians' guide to herbal medicine*. Berlin: Springer, 1997.
8. Hongratanaworakit T, Buchbauer G. Relaxing effect of ylang ylang oil on humans after transdermal absorption. *Phytother Res* 2006;**20**:758–63.
9. Semple S Dermal exposure to chemicals in the workplace: just how important is skin absorption? *Occup Environ Med* 2004;**61**:376–382.
10. Bowman A, Maibach H. Percutaneous absorption of organic solvents. *Int J Occup Environ Hlth* 2000;**6**:93–5. PubMed
11. Brown EW, Scott WO. Absorption of methyl salicylate by human skin. *J Pharmacol Exp Ther* 1934;**50**:32–50.
12. Bronaugh RL. In vivo percutaneous absorption of fragrance ingredients in rhesus monkeys and humans. *Food Chem Toxicol* 1990;**28**:369–73.
13. Kayne S B. The sweet smell of health. *Chemist Druggist* 1998; 21 March: i–v.
14. Davis P. *Aromatherapy – An A–Z*. Saffron Walden: CW Daniel, 1995: 110–15.
15. Buckle J. Aromatherapy. Does it matter which lavender essential oil is used? *Nurs Times* 1993;**89**:32–5.
16. Morales MR, Simon JE, Charles DJ. Comparison of essential oil content and composition between field and greenhouse grown genotypes of methyl cinnamate basil. *J Herbs Spices Medicinal Plants* 1990;**1**:25–35.
17. Price S, Price L. *Aromatherapy for Health Professionals*, 3rd edn. London: Churchill-Livingstone Elsevier, 2007: 14–17.
18. Tisserand R, Balacs T. *Essential Oil Safety*. Edinburgh: Churchill Livingstone, 1996: 8.
19. Serrentino J. *How Natural Remedies Work*. Washington: Hartley & Marks, 1991.
20. Halva S, Craker LE, Simon JE, Charles DJ. Growth and essential oil in dill, *Anethum graveolens* in response to temperature and photoperiod. *J Herbs Spices Medicinal Plants* 1993;**1**:47–56.
21. Letchmo W. Effect of storage temperatures and duration on the essential oil and flavenoids of chamomile. *J Herbs Spices Medicinal Plants* 1993;**1**:13–26.
22. Davis P. *Aromatherapy: An A–Z*. Saffron Walden: CW Daniel, 1995.
23. Barnes J. Aromatherapy. *Pharm J* 1998;**260**:862–7.

24. Betts T, Fox C, Rooth K, MacCallum R. An olfactory countermeasure treatment for epileptic seizures using a conditioned arousal response to specific aromatherapy oils. *Epilepsia* 1995;**36**(suppl 3):S130.
25. Buckle J. Aromatherapy. In: Novey DW (ed.), *Clinician's Complete Reference to Complementary and Alternative Medicine*. St Louis, MO: Mosby, 2000: 653.
26. BBC News. Essential oils 'combat superbug'. BBC News online, 20 March 1997. Available at: http://tinyurl.com/2wtnut (accessed 18 October 2007).
27. Anon. Aromatherapy. Health. *Which?* 1999; June: 30–31.
28. Damian P, Damian K. *Aromatherapy. Scent and psyche*. Rochester, VT: Healing Arts Press, 1995: 23–4.
29. Mason R. Exploring the potentials of human olfaction: an interview with Alan R Hisch MD. *FACP J Alt Compl Ther* 2005;**11**:135–40.
30. Martin GN. Olfactory remediation: current evidence and possible applications. *Soc Sci Med* 1996;**43**:63–9.
31. Tisserand R. *The Art of Aromatherapy*. Saffron Walden: CW Daniel, 1990.
32. Lin ZP, Hsu J-J, Esposito EN. *Aromatherapy Massage*. Available at: http://tinyurl.com/yrjrdq (accessed 18 October 2007).
33. Kim MA, Sakong JK, Kim EJ, Kim EH, Kim EH. Effect of aromatherapy massage for the relief of constipation in the elderly. *Taehan Kanho Hakhoe Chi* 2005;**35**:56–64. PubMed
34. Gedney JJ, Glover, TL, Fillingim RB. Sensory and affective pain discrimination after inhalation of essential oils. *Psychosom Med* 2004;**66**:599–606.
35. Sadler J. *Aromatherapy*. London: Paragon, 1984.
36. *British National Formulary*, vol. 41. London: British Medical Association/ Royal Pharmaceutical Society of Great Britain, 2001.
37. Somerville KW, Ellis WR, Whitten BH et al. Stones in the common bile duct: experience with medical dissolution therapy. *Postgrad Med J* 1985;**61**: 313–16.
38. Engelstein E, Kahan E, Servadio C. Rowarinex for the treatment of ureterolithiasis. *J Urol* 1992;**98**:98–100.
39. Jandourek A, Vaishampayan J K, Vazquez J A. Efficacy of melaleuca oral solution for the treatment of fluconazole refractory oral candidiasis in AIDS patients. *AIDS* 1998;**12**:1032–7.
40. Zarno V. Candidiasis: a holistic view. *Int. J Aromatherapy* 1994;**6**:20–3.
41. Tisserand R, Balacs T. *Essential Oil Safety*. Edinburgh: Churchill Livingstone, 1996: 35–44.
42. Jager W, Buchbauer G, Jirovetz L, Fritzer M. Percutaneous absorption of lavender oil from a massage oil. *J Soc Cosmet Chem* 1992;**43**:49–54.
43. Kovar KA, Gropper B, Friess D, Ammon HPT. Blood levels of 1.8-cineole and locomotor activity of mice after inhalation and oral administration of rosemary oil. *Planta Med* 1987;53:315–18.
44. Elisabetsky E, Marschner J, Souza D. O. Effects of Linalool on glutamatergic system in the rat cerebral cortex. *Neurochem Res* 1995;**20**:461–5. PubMed
45. Yamada K, Mimaki Y, Sashida Y. Anticonvulsive effects of inhaling lavender oil vapour. *Biol Pharmaceut Bull* 1994;**17**:359–60. PubMed

46. Aoshima, H, Hamamoto, K. Potentiation of GABAA receptors expressed in *Xenopus* oocytes by perfume and phytoncid. *Biosci Biotechnol Biochem* 1999;**63**:743–8. PubMed

47. Wake G, Court J, Pickering A et al. CNS acetylcholine receptor activity in European medicinal plants traditionally used to improve failing memory. *J Ethnopharmacol* 2000;**69**:105–14. PubMed

48. Holmes C, Ballard C Aromatherapy in dementia. *Adv Psychiatr Treat* 2004; **10**:296–300.

49. Bulsing PJ, Smeets MA, van den Hout MA. Positive implicit attitudes toward odor words. *Chem Senses* 2007;**32**:525–34.

50. Howard S, Hughes BM. Expectancies, not aroma, explain impact of lavender aromatherapy on psychophysiological indices of relaxation in young healthy women. *Br J Health Psychol* 2007;Sep 7. [Epub ahead of print] Abstract available at: http://tinyurl.com.4kdjj9 (accessed 10 May 2008).

51. Vance D. Considering olfactory stimulation for adults with age-related dementia. *Percep Motor Skills* 1999;**88**:398–400. PubMed

52. Fitzgerald M, Culbert T, Finkelstein M, Green M, Johnson A, Chen S. The effect of gender and ethnicity on children's attitudes and preferences for essential oils: a pilot study. *Explore (NY)* 2007;**3**:378–85.

53. Buckle J. Literature review: should nursing take aromatherapy more seriously? *Br J Nurs* 2007;**16**:116–20.

54. BBC News. Essential oils 'combat superbug'. BBC News online 20 March 1997. Available at: http://tinyurl.com/2wtnut (accessed 18 October 2007).

55. Cooke B, Ernst E. Aromatherapy: A systematic review. *Br J Gen Pract* 2000; **50**:493–6.

56. Lis-Balchin M. Essential oils and aromatherapy; their modern role in healing. *J R Soc Hlth* 1997;**11**:324–9.

57. Wiebe E. A randomized trial of aromatherapy to reduce anxiety before abortion. *Effect Clin Pract* 2000;**3**:166–9.

58. Muzzarelli L, Force M, Sebold M. Aromatherapy and reducing preprocedural anxiety: A controlled prospective study. *Gastroenterol Nurs* 2006;**29**:466–71. PubMed

59. Cooke M, Holzhauser K, Jones M, Davis C, Finucane J. The effect of aromatherapy massage with music on the stress and anxiety levels of emergency nurses: comparison between summer and winter. *J Clin Nurs* 2007;**16**: 1695–703. PubMed

60. Murakami S, Shirota T, Hayashi S, Ishizuka B. Aromatherapy for outpatients with menopausal symptoms in obstetrics and gynecology. *J Altern Compl Med* 2005;**11**:491–4.

61. Kim HJ. Effect of aromatherapy massage on abdominal fat and body image in post-menopausal women. *Taehan Kanho Hakhoe Chi* 2007;**37**:603–12. PubMed

62. Ching M. Contemporary therapy: aromatherapy in the management of acute pain? *Contemp Nurse* 1999;**8**:146–51.

63. Kim JT, Ren CJ, Fielding GA et al. Treatment with lavender aromatherapy in the post-anesthesia care unit reduces opioid requirements of morbidly obese patients undergoing laparoscopic adjustable gastric banding. *Obes Surg* 2007;**17**:920–5. PubMed

64. Kim JT, Wajda M, Cuff G et al. Evaluation of aromatherapy in treating postoperative pain: pilot study. *Pain Pract* 2006;**6**:273–7.
65. Kane FM, Brodie EE, Coull A et al. The analgesic effect of odour and music upon dressing change. *Br J Nurs* 2004;**13**:S4–12.
66. Thorgrimsen L, Spector A, Wiles A, Orrell M. Aromatherapy for dementia. *Cochrane Database Syst Rev* 2003;(3):CD003150.
67. Brooker DJ, Snape M, Johnson E, Ward D, Payne MBr. Single case evaluation of the effects of aromatherapy and massage on disturbed behaviour in severe dementia. *J Clin Psychol* 1997;36(Pt 2):287–96. PubMed
68. Wolfe N, Herzberg J. Can aromatherapy oils promote sleep in severely demented patients? *Int J Geriatr Psychiatry* 1996;**11**:926–7.
69. MacMahon S, Kermode S. A clinical trial of the effects of aromatherapy on motivational behaviour in a dementia care setting using a single subject design. *Aust J Holistic Nurs* 1998;**52**:47–9.
70. Ballard CG, O'Brien JT, Reichelt K, Perry EK. Aromatherapy as a safe and effective treatment for the management of agitation in severe dementia: the results of a double-blind, placebo-controlled trial with Melissa. *J Clin Psychiatry* 2002;**63**:553–8. PubMed
71. Holmes C, Hopkins V, Hensford C, MacLaughlin V, Wilkinson D, Rosenvinge H. Lavender oil as a treatment for agitated behaviour in severe dementia: a placebo controlled study. *Int J Geriatr Psychiatry* 2002;**17**:305–8. PubMed
72. Smallwood J, Brown R, Coulter F, Irvine E, Copland C. Aromatherapy and behaviour disturbances in dementia: a randomized controlled trial. *Int J Geriatr Psychiatry* 2001;**16**:1010–13. (PubMed)
73. Burns A, Byrne J, Ballard C, Holmes C. Sensory stimulation in dementia. (Editorial) *BMJ* 2002;**325**:1312–13.
74. Lin PW, Chan WC, Ng BF, Lam LC. Efficacy of aromatherapy (*Lavandula augustifolia*) as an intervention for agitated behaviours in Chinese older persons with dementia: a cross-over randomized trial. *Int J Geriatr Psychiatry* 2007;**22**:405–10.
75. Bowles EJ, Griffiths DM, Quirk L et al. Effects of essential oils and touch on resistance to nursing care procedures and other dementia related behaviours in a residential care facility. *Int J Aromatherapy* 2002;**12**:22–9. PubMed
76. Nguyen QA, Paton C. The use of aromatherapy to treat behavioural problems in dementia. *Int J Geriatr Psychiatry* 2008;**23**:337–46.
77. Burns E, Zobbi V, Panzeri D, Oskrochi R, Regalia A. Aromatherapy in childbirth: a pilot randomised controlled trial. *Br J Obstet Gynaecol* 2007;**114**:838–44.
78. Burns E, Blamey C, Ersser SJ et al. The use of aromatherapy in intrapartum midwifery practice: an observational study. *Compl Ther Nurs Midwifery* 2000;**6**:33–4.
79. Mousley S. Audit of an aromatherapy service in a maternity unit. *Compl Ther Clin Pract* 2005;**11**:205–10.
80. Stevenson C. The psychological effects of aromatherapy massage following cardiac surgery. *Compl Ther Med* 1994;**2**:27–35.
81. Evans B. An audit into the effects of aromatherapy massage and the cancer patient in palliative and terminal care. *Compl Ther Med* 1995;**3**:229–41.

82.   Wilkinson S. Aromatherapy and massage in palliative care. *Int J Palliat Nurs* 1995;**1**:21–33.
83.   Corner J, Cawley N, Hildebrand S. An evaluation of the use of massage and essential oils on the wellbeing of cancer patients. *Int J Palliat Nurs* 1995;**1**: 67–73.
84.   Stevensen C. Aromatherapy. In: Micozzi MS (ed.), *Fundamentals of Complementary and Alternative Medicine.* Edinburgh: Churchill Livingstone, 1996: 137–48.
85.   Wilkinson SM, Love SB, Westcombe AM et al. Effectiveness of aromatherapy massage in the management of anxiety and depression in patients with cancer: a multicenter randomized controlled trial. *J Clin Oncol* 2007;**25**: 532–9.
86.   Kyle G. Evaluating the effectiveness of aromatherapy in reducing levels of anxiety in palliative care patients: results of a pilot study. *Compl Ther Clin Pract* 2006;**12**:148–55.
87.   Cohen BM, Dressler WE. Acute aromatics inhalation modifies the airways. Effects of the common cold. *Respiration* 1982;**43**:285–93.
88.   Shiina Y, Funabashi N, Lee K et al. Relaxation effects of lavender aromatherapy improve coronary flow velocity reserve in healthy men evaluated by transthoracic Doppler echocardiography. *Int J Cardiol* 2007;Aug 7. [Epub ahead of print] Abstract available at: http://tinyurl.com/4ver8x (accessed 12 June 2008).
89.   Hwang JH. The effects of the inhalation method using essential oils on blood pressure and stress responses of clients with essential hypertension. *Taehan Kanho Hakhoe Chi* 2006;**36**:1123–34.
90.   Lewith GT, Godfrey AD, Prescott P. A single-blinded, randomized pilot study evaluating the aroma of *Lavandula augustifolia* as a treatment for mild insomnia. *J Altern Compl Med* 2005;**11**:631–7.
91.   Knobloek K, Pauli A, Iberl B et al. Antibacterial and antifungal properties of essential oil components. *J Essent Oil Res* 1989;**1**:119–28.
92.   Valnet J. *The Practice of Aromatherapy.* Saffron Walden: CW Daniel, 1982.
93.   Gattefossé R-M. *Gattefossé's Aromatherapy* (edited by Tisserand R). Saffron Walden: CW Daniel, 1993: 107.
94.   Lis-Balchin M. *Aromatherapy Science.* London: Pharmaceutical Press, 2006.
95.   Cornwell S, Dale A. Lavender oil and perineal repair. *Modern Midwife* 1995;**5**:31–5, 97.
96.   Lis-Balchin M. *Aroma Science: The chemistry and bioactivity of essential oils.* Surrey: Asherwood Publishing, 1995.
97.   Lis-Balchin M, Hart S L, Deans SG, Eaglesham E. Comparison of the pharmacological and antimicrobial action of commercial plant essential oils. *J Herbs Spices Medicinal Plants* 1994;**4**:69–86.
98.   Schuyler W, Lininger DC, Gaby A R et al. *The Natural Pharmacy.* Rocklin, CA: Prima Publishing, 1999: 463–4.
99.   Raman A, Weir U, Bloomfield SF. Antimicrobial effects of tea-tree oil and its major components on *Staphylococcus aureus, Staph. epidermidis* and *Propionibacterium acnes. Appl Microbiol* 1995;**21**:242–5.
100.   Carson CE, Cookson BD, Farrelly HD, Riley T. Susceptibility of methicillin-resistant *Staphylococcus aureus* to the essential oil of *Melaleuca alterifolia. J Antimicrob Chemother* 1995;**35**:421–4.

101. Bassett IB, Pannowitz DL, Barnetson RS. A comparative study of tea tree oil versus benzoylperoxide in the treatment of acne. *Med J Aust* 1990;**153**: 455–8.

102. Buck DS, Nidorf DM, Addino JG. Comparison of two topical preparations for the treatment of onychomycosis: *Melaleuca alternifolia* (tea tree oil) and clotrimazole. *J Fam Pract* 1994;**38**:601–5.

103. Barnes J. Aromatherapy. *Pharm J* 1998;**260**:862–7.

104. Damian P, Damian K. *Aromatherapy. Scent and psyche*. Rochester, VT: Healing Arts Press, 1995: 45–8.

105. Mackereth P. Aromatherapy – nice but not 'essential'. *Compl Ther Nurs Midwifery* 1995;**1**:4–7.

106. Temple WA, Smith NNA, Beasley M. Management of oil of citronella poisoning. *J Toxicol Clin Toxicol* 1991;**29**:257–62.

107. Mant AK. A case of poisoning by oil of citronella. In: Tisserand R, Balacs T (eds), *Essential Oil Safety*. Edinburgh: Churchill Livingstone, 1996: 51.

108. Gurr FW, Scroggie JG. Eucalyptus oil poisoning treated by dialysis and mannitol infusion with an appendix on the analysis of biological fluids for alcohol and eucalyptol. *Aust Ann Med* 1965;**14**:238–49.

109. Tiran D. Aromatherapy in midwifery: benefits and risks. *Compl Ther Nurs Midwifery* 1996;**2**:888–92.

110. DeGroot AC, Weyland JW. Systemic contact dermatitis from tea tree oil. *Contact Dermatitis* 1992;**27**:279–80.

111. Van Ketel WG. Allergy to *Matricaria chamomilla*. *Contact Dermatitis* 1982;**24**:139–40.

112. McGeorge BC, Steele MC. Allergic contact dermatitis of the nipple from Roman chamomile. *Contact Dermatitis* 1991;**24**:139–40.

113. Knight TE, Hansen BM. Melaleuca oil (tea tree oil) dermatitis. *Med J Aust* 1994;**30**:423–7.

114. Packham C. Re: Essential oils and aromatherapy: their role in healing – letter to the editor. *J R Soc Hlth* 1997;**117**:400.

115. Selvaag E, Holm J-O, Thune P. Allergic contact dermatitis in an aromatherapist with multiple sensitisations to essential oils. *Contact Dermatitis* 1995; **33**:334–5.

116. Tisserand R, Balacs T. *Essential Oil Safety*. Edinburgh: Churchill Livingstone, 1996: 83–5.

117. Tisserand R, Balacs T. *Essential Oil Safety*. Edinburgh: Churchill Livingstone, 1996: 41–3.

118. Tiran D. Aromatherapy in midwifery: benefits and risks. *Compl Ther Nurs Midwifery* 1996;**2**:86–92.

119. Dale A, Cornwell S. The role of lavender oil in relieving perineal discomfort following childbirth: a blind randomised clinical trial. *J Adv Nurs* 1994; 19:89–96.

120. Tisserand R, Balacs T. *Essential Oil Safety*. Edinburgh: Churchill Livingstone, 1996: 93–4.

121. Balacs T. Safety in pregnancy. *Int J Aromather* 1992;**4**:12–15.

122. Anon. Aromatherapy. *Health Which?* 1999;June:30–31.

10

Flower remedy therapy

Steven B Kayne

Flower remedies do not fit in with the homeopathic or herbal systems of classification, having a unique method of preparation and use. It should not be confused with flower therapy where flowers are used as a source of colour and aroma to foster wellbeing (see Chapter 17).

It has been acknowledged that, although homeopathy and flower remedy therapy are clearly different, some common ground exists and they may have a complementary role, which is perhaps insufficiently recognised.[1] They are currently included in the *British Homeopathic Pharmacopoeia*.[2] However, many homeopaths consider this inappropriate for the following reasons:

- Flower remedies are not prepared by trituration or alcoholic extraction.
- There is doubt as to whether the manufacturing process of flower remedies includes standard potentisation.
- The flower remedies have not undergone provings.
- Prescribing is based on accurate perception of archetypes with a psyche (i.e. mental state) rather than matching symptoms to a drug picture.
- Flower remedies have a wide spectrum of activity and are not known to be negatively affected by aromatic agents, tea, coffee, etc.

Currently the remedies fall outwith either group's licensing system. Although still known as 'remedies' in Europe, they are called 'essences' in the USA and other countries, causing some confusion with certain aromatherapy products that bear a similar description.

Definition

Flower remedy therapy is a form of therapy that treats predominantly mental and emotional manifestations of disease, relying on the administration of remedies derived from the flowering parts of plants.

History

There are many variants of flower remedies, but the original and best known are the Bach flower remedies discovered by the English bacteriologist and physician Edward Bach, who was born in Moseley, Birmingham on 24 September 1886. Dr Bach (whose name is usually pronounced 'Batch' although the gutteral 'ch' as in the Scottish 'loch' is also used) trained in medicine and, during time spent at the London Homoeopathic Hospital as a bacteriologist and pathologist, he became inspired by the teachings of Hahnemann about homeopathy, especially not healing the disease, but the diseased, although he found the complexity of homeopathic prescribing rather difficult. He developed seven Bach nosodes. He was a profoundly religious man and took up medicine from a desire to heal. Bach took his holidays in Wales and Norfolk, enjoying long walks in the countryside either alone, or latterly with his companion and assistant Nora Weeks. It is claimed that he was intuitively drawn towards certain wild flowers which he was able to associate with particular emotions. Thus, if he experienced a sudden adverse emotion and went outside to seek fresh air and exercise he would always be drawn inextricably towards a particular plant or tree. Simply being in its presence would relieve his emotional state. He believed that these were not just chance occurrences, but indications that he had been led divinely towards a new method of healing. But his breakthrough came when he used the flowers in a new kind of preparation that used fresh dew exposed to the sun.

Initially Bach described 12 original 'healers':[3]

- Agrimony (*Agrimonia eupatoria*), for those who hide their trouble behind a brave face
- Centaury (*Centaurium umbellatum*), for those who are averse to saying 'no' and are always anxious to please
- Cerato (*Ceratostigma willmottiana*), for those who doubt their ability to make decisions
- Chicory (*Cichorium intybus*), for those who are overprotective of others
- Clematis (*Clematis vitalba*), for lack of interest in present circumstances
- Gentian (*Gentiana amarella*), for those who are easily discouraged or who may become despondent following a set-back
- Impatiens (*Impatiens glandulifera*), for those who may become irritable and frustrated as a result of impatience

- Mimulus (*Mimulus gluttatus*), for the timid and shy
- Rock rose (*Helianthemum nummularium*), for those suffering from terror
- Scleranthus (*Scleranthus annuus*), for those who are indecisive in the face of two clear options
- Vervain (*Verbena officinalis*), for those with fanatical opinions
- Water violet (*Hottonia palustris*), for those who prefer to be alone.

In 1934 Dr Bach established a healing centre in a small house at Mount Vernon, England, where many of the plants used in his remedies could be grown or were available as wild specimens in the immediate vicinity. He subsequently completed his collection with a further 26 remedies, and considered the final total of 38 to be sufficient to treat the most common negative moods that afflict the human race. He then republished his earlier book, keeping the title similar so as not to confuse and making it clear that all 38 remedies were of equal status.[4]

The remedies are: aspen, beech, cherry plum, chestnut bud, crab apple, elm, gorse, heather, holly, honeysuckle, hornbeam, larch, mustard, oak, olive, pine, red chestnut, rock water, star of Bethlehem, sweet chestnut, vine, walnut, white chestnut, wild oat, wild rose and willow. All Bach's remedies can be found growing naturally in the British Isles, with the exception of olive and vine.

Development of other flower remedies[5,6]

California essences

For many years after Edward Bach died no new flower remedies were created. Then in 1982, over 200 essences were produced from the native plants of California according to the methods of Bach, to the opposition of some practitioners who maintain that Bach finished the system when he died. The main themes of the Californian essences are sexuality, social integration, work, life and growth (http://tinyurl.com/2dhetu).

Alaskan essences

These were first produced commercially in the summer of 1983 from the native plants of that state; they are mainly focused on mental and spiritual ideas, considered to be abstract by many (http://alaskanessences.com).

Australian Bush essences

These were created in the early 1980s and have a strong focus on the issues of healing relationships and sexuality, aiming to bring out and cultivate people's positive qualities. This group contains remedies derived from a wide range of Australian plants and trees, including banksia, bottlebrush, jacaranda, paw paw and waratah (http://tinyurl.com/ys6mxg).

North American essences

These comprise a range of 103 essences. There are also some combination products including a five-flower essence for stress and trauma (http://tinyurl.com/2hsrzd).

Other essences

Bailey flower essences are a group of 45 flower essences that were developed over a period of 20 years in Yorkshire (www.baileyessences. com). Another range of related essences are the Green Man group, covering 74 trees grown in the British Isles and offering separate male and female forms where the trees are sexed. The first essence made was from the flowers of the hazel tree, whose qualities encourage the growth of new skills and information (www.greenmantrees.demon.co.uk).

There is currently great interest in essences from the flowers of tropical, subtropical and equatorial regions, e.g. the Himalayan tree and flower essences (http://tinyurl.com/2db9qc), the Amazon orchid essences and the Hawaiian essences (http://tinyurl.com/ypqjdl), and the New Millennium essences from New Zealand offer a range of flowery essences and essential oils (www.nmessences.com).

Theory

Dr Bach's explanation for the healing power of his medicinal herbs was quite simple: he believed that they were divinely enriched. The remedies are not used directly for physical symptoms, but for the state of mind, the rationale being that the state of mind may hinder recovery and also may be the primary cause of certain diseases. This emphasises the idea that all true healing must come from a spiritual level.

Monvoisin has stated that the basic principles of Bach's theory are settled on ungrounded, deeply intuitive hypotheses, belong to magical thinking, and promote philosophical approaches that weaken patients/ consumers, particularly with regard to sectarian trends.[7]

Preparation of Bach remedies

There are two methods of preparation:

1. The sun method is used to prepare remedies from flowers that bloom during late spring and summer, when the sun is at its strongest. The procedure is carried out where the plants or trees have been gathered, commencing around 9.00 am on a calm settled day. Fifty parts of pure spring water are added to a glass container until the level reaches just below the brim. One part of flower heads is floated on the surface of the water. The container is then left in the sunshine for 3 hours, after which the flowers are removed and the remaining solution strained into a glass bottle. It is mixed with an equal quantity of grape brandy, vigorously shaken and stored in a cool dark place.
2. The boiling method is used to prepare remedies from flowers and twigs of trees, bushes and plants that bloom early in the year, before there is much sunshine. The material is gathered as before, and one part is added to 10 parts of water in a glass vessel. The resulting mixture is boiled for half an hour and allowed to cool before being diluted with grape brandy and vigorously shaken.

According to the *British Homeopathic Pharmacopoeia* (BHomP)[2] in both cases the resulting mother tinctures should be diluted to the equivalent of the fifth decimal homeopathic dilution (5x) using 22% ethanol. In reality 2 drops of the mother tincture are added to 30 ml brandy (brandy at 27%, termed grape alcohol in order to comply with regulations) to make the finished product (Chapman K, personal communication, 2006). The potential confusion here is first the difference between 22% w/w (weight per weight) and 27% v/v (volume per volume), and second confusion with the methodology for conventional homeopathic medicines.

Bach flower therapy in practice

The 38 Bach remedies can be split into seven groups according to their principal use:

1. Despondency or despair (crab apple, elm, larch, oak, pine, star of Bethlehem, sweet chestnut, willow)
2. Fear (aspen, cherry plum, mimulus, red chestnut, rock rose)
3. Loneliness (heather, impatiens, water violet)
4. Oversensitivity to influences and ideas (agrimony, centaury, holly, walnut)
5. Insufficient interest in present circumstances (chestnut bud, clematis, honeysuckle, mustard, olive, white chestnut, wild rose)
6. Overcare for the welfare of others (beech, chicory, vervain, vine, rock water)
7. Uncertainty (cerato, gentian, gorse, hornbeam, scleranthus, wild oat).

For full details on the subtleties of how the remedies are used within each group the reader is referred to more specialised literature from the manufacturers (www.bachflower.com). However, as a guide the most useful remedy from each group is listed in Table 10.1.

One of the difficulties of using Bach remedies is that, during the resolution of disease, mental symptoms are likely to change, requiring the administration of different treatments. In order to deal with this there is an extremely useful combination of five Bach flower remedies, known as five-flower remedy or **Rescue Remedy**. It was so named for its stabilising and calming effect on the emotions during a crisis. The remedy comprises cherry plum (for the fear of not being able to cope mentally), clematis (for unconsciousness or the 'detached' sensations that often accompany trauma), impatiens (for impatience and agitation), rock rose (for terror) and star of Bethlehem (for the after-effects of shock). This remedy is often used in place of arnica, where the mental symptoms resulting from a traumatic episode or overwork are more evident than the physical.

Table 10.1 Examples of useful Bach flower remedies

Emotion	Bach flower remedy indicated
Confidence, lack of	Larch
Energy, lack of	Olive
Envy	Holly
Indecision or uncertainty	Scleranthus
Over-enthusiasm	Vervain
Terror	Rock rose

The practice of blending flower remedies appears to be growing. One range of products includes nine combination remedies with names such as 'male essence', 'bowel essence' and 'night essence'.

Bach rescue cream is a skin salve that is claimed to help a wide range of skin conditions. The cream contains the same five remedies as the Rescue Remedy drops plus crab apple (for a sense of uncleanliness). It is broadly used for conditions similar to those for which arnica might be applicable. However, it is difficult to understand how topical use in this way fits in with the concept of treating mental symptoms.

Administration

Frequency of administration depends to a large extent on each individual patient. If the mood is transient only one dose might be appropriate, whereas if the condition persists repeated dosing could be appropriate.

Patients should add two drops of the single flower remedies or four drops of Rescue Remedy to a beverage of their choice (fruit juice or still mineral water are both acceptable) and the mixture sipped every 3–5 min for acute problems until the feelings have subsided. For ongoing problems a dose may be taken four times daily.

The remedy should be held in the mouth for a moment before swallowing. If no suitable beverage is available, four drops of the remedy may be placed under the tongue.

Bach remedies, particularly Rescue Remedy, are added to animals' drinking water by owners at similar dose levels during stressful times, e.g. firework displays, travelling or showing.

Supply of flower remedies

Flower remedies are usually sold in individual bottles or sets (Figure 10.1). The manufacturers provide charts that can be consulted to help with choosing the correct remedy. Rescue Remedy is the easiest to counter prescribe because it has clear indications. Retailers in the southern part of the UK may receive requests from visitors from continental Europe, particularly Germany, where the remedies are expensive and generally in short supply.

Evidence

Howard explored the potentiality of Bach flower remedies as a means of pain relief through a retrospective case study analysis.[8] Of the 384

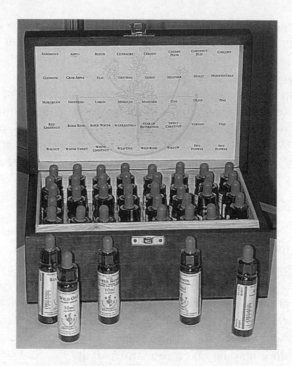

Figure 10.1 Flower remedy set.

individuals, 41 suffered pain. Of these, 46% felt that treatment had relieved their pain; in 49% the physical outcome was unknown. About 88% of all participants reported an improvement in their emotional outlook. The author suggests that the flower therapy shifted the focus from physical pain to emotional outlook. The client–practitioner relationship and belief in the therapy were also important. The conclusion was that Bach flower remedies may be effective in the relief of pain. Much of the other published literature is negative. A randomised double-blind clinical trial of 100 university students who had previously suffered from examination nerves, in which participants took one to four doses daily of Rescue Remedy or identical placebo, revealed no benefit from taking the remedy.[9]

Ernst carried out a systematic review of flower remedy therapy and concluded, from the four studies that merit his inclusion criteria, that any hypothesis that flower remedies are associated with effects beyond a placebo response is not supported by data from rigorous clinical trials.[10]

A double-blind, prospective, controlled study involving 40 children with attention deficit hyperactivity disorder (ADHD), aged 7–11 years, has shown that there is no statistically significant difference between the effects of Bach flower remedies compared with placebo in the treatment of children with ADHD.[11]

Despite these largely negative results, there are numerous anecdotal reports in the literature supporting the view that Rescue Remedy is of benefit in stressful situations for both human and veterinary patients.[12]

More information

Flower Essence Therapy: http://tinyurl.com/339hqj

Further reading

Chancellor P. *Illustrated Handbook of Bach Flower Remedies*. London: Random House Books/Vermillion, 2005.

Boericke W, Dewey WA. *The Twelve Tissue Remedies of Scheussler*. Sittingbourne: Homoeopathic Book Service, 2001.

References

1. van Haselen RA. The relationship between homeopathy and the Dr Bach system of flower remedies: a critical appraisal. *Br Homeopath J* 1999;**88**:121–7.
2. British Association of Homeopathic Manufacturers. *British Homeopathic Pharmacopoeia*, 2nd edn. Ilkeston, Derbyshire: British Association of Homeopathic Manufacturers, 1999.
3. Bach E. *The Essential Writings of Edward Bach. The twelve healers and heal thyself*. London: Random House, 2005.
4. Bach E. *The Twelve Healers and Other Remedies*. Wappingers Falls, NY: Beekman Books, 1996.
5. Harvey CG, Cochrane A. *The Encyclopaedia of Flower Remedies*. London: Thorson's, 1995.
6. Mansfield P. *Flower Remedies*. London: Optima, 1995.
7. Monvoisin R. Bach flower remedies: a critic of the pseudoscientific, pseudomedicinal concepts and philosophical postures inducted by Dr Bach theory. *Ann Pharm Fr* 2005;**63**:416–28. PubMed
8. Howard J. Do Bach flower remedies have a role to play in pain control? A critical analysis investigating therapeutic value beyond the placebo effect, and the potential of Bach flower remedies as a psychological method of pain relief. *Compl Ther Clin Pract* 2007;**13**:174–83.
9. Armstrong NC, Ernst E. A randomised double blind placebo controlled clinical trial of a Bach flower remedy. *Perfusion* 1999;**12**:440–6.

10. Ernst E. Flower remedies: a systematic review of the clinical evidence. *Wien Klin Wochenschr* 2002;**114**:963–6. PubMed
11. Pintov S, Hochman M, Livne A, Heyman E, Lahat E. Bach flower remedies used for attention deficit hyperactivity disorder in children – a prospective double blind controlled study. *Eur J Paediatr Neurol* 2005;**9**:395–8. PubMed
12. Vlamis G. *Rescue Remedy. The healing power of Bach flower Rescue Remedy*. London: Thorson's, 1994.

Part 3

Traditional medicine

11

The traditional healthcare environment

Steven B Kayne

> Foolish the doctor who despises the knowledge acquired by the ancients.
> Hippocrates

More than 25 years ago the World Health Organization (WHO) estimated that in 'many countries, 80% or more of the population living in rural areas are cared for by traditional practitioners and birth attendants'.[1] It has since revised its view, adopting a rather safer position, now stating: 'most of the population of most developing countries regularly use traditional medicine.'[2] Whereas most people use traditional medicine in developing countries, only a minority have regular access to reliable modern medical services.[3]

Countries in Africa, Asia and Latin America use traditional medicine (TM) to help meet some of their primary healthcare needs. In Africa, up to 80% of the population uses TM for primary healthcare. In industrialised countries, adaptations of TM are termed 'complementary' or 'alternative' (complementary and alternative medicine – CAM). Over a third of the population in developing countries lack access to essential medicines. The provision of safe and effective TM therapies could become a critical tool to increase access to healthcare. In 2004 the South African Health Minister Manto Tshabalala-Msimang suggested that the use of African traditional medicines may eventually replace antiretrovirals in the treatment of HIV and AIDS.

Definition

The WHO defines TM as referring to health practices, approaches, knowledge and beliefs incorporating plant-, animal- and mineral-based medicines, spiritual therapies, manual techniques and exercises, applied singularly or in combination to treat, diagnose and prevent illnesses or maintain wellbeing.[2]

This is a similar definition to those quoted for CAM in general and makes no mention of the fact that TM is usually considered to be associated with discrete populations or geographical locations. In fact the WHO does include all CAM disciplines as TM. The definition offered by Wikepedia (http://tinyurl.com/ywyr6b) is:

> The term traditional medicine describes medical knowledge systems, which developed over centuries within various societies before the era of modern medicine.

Traditional medicines that are described in this section of the book are traditional Chinese and Tibetan medicine (see Chapter 12) and Ayurvedic and Unani medicine (see Chapter 13). Other examples not covered in this edition include:

- Australian Bush medicine (http://tinyurl.com/2pwumu)
- Japanese kampo medicine (http://tinyurl.com/2ox973)
- Korean medicine (http://medcity.com/kom/)
- Native American medicine (http://tinyurl.com/2ghytc)
- New Zealand Maori (Rongoa) Medicine (http://tinyurl.com/4wzfho)
- Southern African muti (http://en.wikipedia.org/wiki/Muti)
- South American traditional herbal medicine (http://tinyurl.com/29dtj5)
- West African yoruba (http://tinyurl.com/39slgw) and ifá medicine (http://tinyurl.com/2wud3t).

Traditional medicine in practice

Traditional medicine has maintained its popularity in all regions of the developing world and its use is rapidly spreading in industrialised countries.

- In China, traditional herbal preparations account for 30–50% of the total medicinal consumption.
- In Ghana, Mali, Nigeria and Zambia, the first line of treatment for 60% of children with high fever resulting from malaria is the use of herbal medicines at home.
- The WHO estimates that in several African countries traditional birth attendants assist at most births.
- Some traditional therapies, in particular traditional Chinese medicine and ayurveda, have become popular in industrialised nations, spreading out from immigrants into the host community.

The following two examples serve to illustrate the use of TM. A study was aimed at highlighting the new or lesser known medicinal uses of plant bioresources along with a validation of traditional knowledge that is widely used by the tribal communities to cure four common ailments in the Lahaul-Spiti region of the western Himalayas.[4] The study area inhabited by Lahaulas and Bodhs (also called Bhotias) is situated in the cold arid zone of the state of Himachal Pradesh (HP), India. During the ethnobotanical explorations (2002–6), observations on the most common ailments such as rheumatism, stomach problems, liver and sexual disorders among the natives of Lahaul-Spiti were recorded. As a result of a strong belief in a traditional system of medicine, people still prefer to use herbal medicines prescribed by local healers. A total of 58 plant species belonging to 45 genera and 24 families have been reported from the study area to cure these diseases. Maximum use of plants is reported to cure stomach disorders (29), followed by rheumatism (18), liver problems (15) and sexual ailments (9). Among plant parts used, leaves were found used most widely in herbal preparations (20), followed by flowers (12) and roots (11), respectively. Most of these formulations were prescribed in powder form, although juice and decoction forms were also used. Plants having more than one therapeutic use were represented with 24 species; however, 34 species were reported to be used against a single specific ailment. Validation of observations revealed 38 lesser known or new herbal preparations from 34 plant species, where 15 species were used to cure stomach disorders, 7 for rheumatism, 10 for liver disorders and 6 for sexual problems. Mode of preparation, administration and dosage are discussed together with the family and local names of plants and plant parts used.

The use of traditional herbal medicine by AIDS patients in Kabarole District, western Uganda has been studied.[5] Using systematic sampling, 137 AIDS patients were selected from outpatient departments of 3 hospitals and interviewed via questionnaire. The questions related to such areas as type and frequency of herbal medicine intake, concomitant herb–pharmaceutical drug use (including herb–antiretroviral drug co-therapy), and the perceived effectiveness of herbal medicine. Overall, 63.5% of AIDS patients had used herbal medicine after HIV diagnosis. Same-day herbal medicine and pharmaceutical drugs use was reported by 32.8% of AIDS patients. Patterns of traditional herbal medicine use were quite similar between those on antiretroviral therapy and those who received supportive therapy only. The primary conclusion is that AIDS outpatients commonly use herbal medicine for the treatment of HIV/AIDS.

When many people from developing countries emigrate they continue to seek medical advice from traditional practitioners working in their own communities, even in countries where all citizens have free access to good-quality western medicine.[6] They have difficulties adjusting to a new lifestyle, let alone to a new system of medicine. It is not surprising that they turn to their own healers, who emigrated before them and practise their trade much the same as they did in their home countries. Although the main reasons for this are probably cultural and linguistic, the role of mistrust and fear should also be acknowledged.

The ethnic medical systems embrace philosophies very different from those of the West. They are derived from a sensitive awareness of the laws of nature and the order of the universe. Practised according to traditional methods, their aim is to maintain health as well as restore it. The ideas are complex and require much study to grasp their significance and the nuances of practice.

Traditional medical systems are challenging because their theories and practices strike many conventionally trained physicians and researchers as incomprehensible. Should modern medicine dismiss them as unscientific, view them as sources of alternatives hidden in a matrix of superstition or regard them as complementary sciences of medicine?[7]

It is appropriate to look at the ways in which traditional (ethnic) medicine and western medicine exist side by side in the countries from which immigrant practitioners can be expected, because it gives us an understanding of how they may approach their profession in the UK and other host communities.

Key policy issues in integration have been outlined by Commonwealth health ministers.[8] Ministers established the Commonwealth Working Group on Traditional and Complementary Health Systems to promote and integrate traditional health systems and complementary medicine into national healthcare.

Medical pluralism – the use of multiple forms of healthcare – is widespread in Asia. Consumers practise integrated healthcare irrespective of whether integration is officially present. In Taiwan, 60% of the public use multiple healing systems, including modern western medicine, Chinese medicine and religious healing. A survey in two village health clinics in China's Zheijang province showed that children with upper respiratory tract infections were being prescribed an average of four separate drugs, always in a combination of western and Chinese medicine.[8] The challenge of integrated healthcare is to generate evidence on which illnesses are best treated through which approach. The

Zheijang study found that simultaneous use of both types of treatment was so commonplace that their individual contributions were difficult to assess.

Asia has seen much progress in incorporating its traditional health systems into national policy. Most of this began 30–40 years ago and has accelerated in the past 10 years. In some countries, such as China, the development has been a response to mobilising all healthcare resources to meet national objectives for primary healthcare. In other countries, such as India and South Korea, change has come through politicisation of the traditional health sector and a resultant change in national policy.

Two basic policy models have been followed: an integrated approach, where modern medicine and traditional medicine are integrated through medical education and practice (e.g. China), and a parallel approach, where modern medicine and traditional medicine are separate within the national health system (e.g. India).

Unfortunately, at the present time it is generally recognised that regulation of traditional systems of medicine, the products used in traditional systems and the practitioners of these systems is very weak in most countries.[9] This leads to misuse of the medicines by unqualified practitioners and loss of credibility of the system. In TM, practitioners and manufacturers (particularly the small ones) usually oppose any steps to strengthen regulation by the health administration. Their fears are that regulation such as that applied to allopathic medicine is not suitable for TM. The WHO has initiated an effort in this direction and may be the appropriate body to help countries not only to develop a regulatory system but also to take steps to meet the obligations under the Trade-related Intellectual Property Rights Agreement, when this became applicable in the developing countries in 2005. It means that traditional healers (hakkims) who have come to the UK may practise within a culture that is oblivious to the highly regulated status of western medicine. Healthcare providers should be vigilant to ensure that any risks to patients are minimised.

All the foregoing may seem to indicate that integrating traditional and western medicine is at best difficult and at worst impossible. Most of the remarks in this chapter have been directed to Chinese and Indian medicine, these two systems being the two traditional disciplines that pharmacists are most likely to meet in the UK. It should be noted that traditional medicines in other cultures also flourish and many are integrated into local healthcare. In their own countries Australian

Aboriginals,[10] New Zealand Maoris,[11] North American Indians,[12,13] Africans,[14,15] Pacific Islanders[16] and the peoples of Latin America[17] continue to make important contributions to their national cultures.

Each culture has its own range of remedies, although some elements are common to all. One notable success to cross the cultural divide is tea tree oil, known as melaleuca in Australian bush medicine and manuka in New Zealand. It has become a popular and effective remedy in Europe (see Chapter 14).

Traditional healers may be called shamans. They practise a method of healing that is supplemented by rituals and explanatory systems appropriate to their particular culture and environment. The healing often includes meditation, prayer, chanting and traditional music (e.g. Celtic drumming), together with the administration of herbal, and occasionally orthodox, remedies.

Safety

The following safety matters are a source of concern in ethnic medicine: training, uncontrolled products and concurrent therapy.

Training

Practitioners' training varies widely, raising concerns for the quality of the treatment being offered. Little is being done currently to regulate the delivery of traditional healthcare.

Uncontrolled products

Large amounts of traditional medicines are imported into the UK, legally and illegally, and use of such medicines is frequently not admitted when serious illness forces patients to consult western medical practitioners. These medicines carry with them a risk of adverse reactions; the risk needs to be quantified and as far as possible minimised.

An issue under discussion by European regulatory authorities is whether the proposed Herbal Medicines Directive (see Chapter 5) should extend to traditional medicines containing non-herbal ingredients, such as those used in Chinese and ayurvedic medicine.

The UK Medicines and Healthcare products Regulatory Agency (MHRA) has established an ethnic medicines forum. This is to encourage and assist the UK ethnic medicines sector to achieve improvements in safety and quality standards in unlicensed ethnic medicines, in advance of any improvements to the statutory regimen that might emerge from current policy initiatives. Representatives of ayurvedic and traditional Chinese medicine suppliers, manufacturers and practitioners in the UK form part of this forum, as well as other bodies in the herbal medicines sector with experience of operating self-regulatory arrangements.

One issue identified by the forum is the lack of understanding of existing law by some of those operating in the ethnic medicines sector. The document *Traditional Ethnic Medicines: Public health and compliance with medicines law*, published on the MHRA website, highlights problem areas.[18] It aims to help consumers make an informed choice and seeks to assist businesses and practitioners to understand certain aspects of medicines law.

Concurrent therapy

Patients with chronic or recurrent conditions are particularly vulnerable because they tend to lose confidence in conventional medicine and resort to self-medication without informing their general practitioner.

What needs to be done to ensure the safety of traditional medicine?

There can be no doubt that safety issues are of extreme concern as the use of traditional therapies increases in a largely uncontrolled manner. Travel by tourists and business people to long-haul destinations has brought increasing numbers of people into contact with other cultures.

Immigration brings different cultures to enrich our own. Whether you consider TM to have a part to play in modern medicine is for you alone to decide. The fact is that it has arrived without seeking your permission! Healthcare is an emotive subject. The holistic and spiritual qualities associated with oriental medicine appeal to the public, leading to the HYGSE ('Have you got something else?') syndrome.

The risks of participating in traditional Chinese medicine or ayurveda are certainly outweighed by the many benefits that are reported. Adverse reactions are relatively rare, although when they do happen they can be very severe. Perhaps the best solution is to control the practice, improve training and license the medicines. However, there are problems in establishing these ideals.

Practitioners of TM certainly need to be more aware of the problems of toxicity. In particular, they must learn that infrequent adverse drug reactions will not be recognised without a formal system of reporting. They must participate in such a scheme, and consideration should be given by the Medicine and Healthcare products Regulatory Agency (MHRA – now the MCA) in the UK to making such reporting compulsory, as it is in Germany. This is an important deficiency and, until a formal mandatory system of reporting adverse reactions for TM becomes available, all healthcare professionals should be aware of the potential difficulties, advise the public of the dangers whenever necessary, and record and report any problems promptly in mainstream literature.

All practitioners of orthodox and traditional medicine need to be aware of the occurrence and dangers of dual treatment. Patients need to appreciate that they must disclose exactly what they are taking; such information should be recorded carefully because, as stated above, there is a risk that patients will receive simultaneous western and traditional treatments, particularly when self-treating. This may require a sympathetic non-judgemental approach to questioning. Purchasers of traditional medicines should be advised accordingly.

All practitioners who offer traditional medicines need thorough training and continuing education.[2] Great attention has been paid to the quality of training and further education in orthodox western medicine, and it is time to police more carefully the practice of TM in the UK. For European herbal medicine this should be easy. The training establishments are situated in the UK, which makes guaranteeing standards and limiting the right to practise to those who are thoroughly trained relatively straightforward. It is much more difficult in the case of traditional Chinese and Indian medicine, because full training cannot currently be obtained in the UK. Verifying the quality of the training given in China and India by identifying appropriate qualifications and recognising them seems prudent. Practitioners who are not qualified should be barred from practice in the UK, and policing this would clearly require a powerful registration body. Ultimately, the creation of academic establishments in the UK, where such training could be given under appropriate regulation, should be considered.

Evidence

Scientific evidence is available only for many uses of acupuncture, some herbal medicines and some manual therapies. Further research is urgently needed to ascertain the efficacy and safety of several other practices and medicinal plants.

The limited scientific evidence about the safety of TM and efficacy, as well as other considerations, make it important for governments to:[2]

- formulate national policy and regulation for the proper use of TM/CAM and its integration into national healthcare systems in line with the provisions of the WHO strategies on traditional medicines
- establish regulatory mechanisms to control the safety and quality of products and of TM/CAM practice
- create awareness about safe and effective TM/CAM therapies among the public and consumers
- cultivate and conserve medicinal plants to ensure their sustainable use.

Traditional medicine and the healthcare provider

It is recognised that many healthcare providers will not relish the thought of taking a proactive interest in the highly complicated world of TM unless they share the origins of their clientele. However, given their healthcare role within the multicultural society in which most of us live, the possibilities of coming into contact with traditional Chinese medicine and ayurvedic medicine are possible for a number of reasons:

- Concern over interactions between traditional remedies and orthodox medicine
- Concern over using traditional remedies during pregnancy
- Concern over intrinsic toxicity of traditional remedies and cosmetics, and the safety of some procedures
- The necessity of considering and understanding a patient's total healthcare status when designing pharmaceutical care plans.

This puts pharmacists firmly into the frame as the healthcare professional whom the public sees most. The opportunities to provide assistance and counselling should not be lost. The significant proportion of pharmacists of Asian origin within the profession should be of great benefit in helping to break down barriers of suspicion between new immigrants and established medical practice.

The practice of TM involves concepts with which we in the West are generally unfamiliar. It may be that, with more understanding of the therapies involved, some can be incorporated into our own procedures, e.g. our focus on treating illness could be shifted more towards maintaining health, a process that has already started. We may be able to understand better the needs of our immigrant communities and perhaps use approaches with which they feel more comfortable.

Biodiversity and sustainability[19]

Environmental awareness

Up to 40% of all pharmaceuticals in industrialised countries are derived from natural sources. In the USA about 2% of prescriptions are for drugs that have natural ingredients, are synthetic copies or have artificially modified forms of natural chemicals. The search continues for more therapeutically active plant-sourced materials, not always to the satisfaction of host communities.

Two centuries ago, orthodox medicine was offering digitalis, and laudanum, but now there are thousands of powerful, efficacious drugs that save lives somewhere almost every second of the day.[20] However, modern drugs struggle to make much impact on the rise in cancer, heart disease and other afflictions of the industrialised world.

This lack of efficacy, together with patients' growing unease over side effects of synthetic drugs, has coincided with an international growth in environmental awareness, particularly concern about the depletion of natural resources. In turn, this has led to a greater sensitivity to the delicate symbiotic balance that exists in nature.

Disappearing rainforests

It was said at a British Herbal Medicine Association Symposium that rainforests offer the greatest chance of discovering new potent drugs. Unfortunately the forest is being destroyed at such a rate that thousands of species may become extinct before their medicinal potential can be examined. Five thousand years ago the rainforest covered two billion hectares, or 14% of the earth's land surface. Now only half remains, but it is inhabited by 50% of all the plants and animals found on the globe.[21] Humans are continuing to destroy an area equivalent to 20 football fields every day, a rate that if maintained will cause the rainforest to vanish by 2030. Slash-and-burn agriculture accounts for 50% of the annual loss. This is a primitive system that involves cutting down a patch of forest and setting the timber alight to release phosphorus, nitrogen, potassium and other nutrients. The resulting ash fertilises the sod, which will then support crops for 2 or 3 years. After this time the land becomes barren, necessitating the clearing of another patch of forest. Logging is a second major cause of forest destruction. In 1990, 3.5 billion cubic metres of tropical wood were felled throughout the world, more than half for fuel sources.

Trees are also consumed for their important products, e.g. India earns $US125m annually from its production of perfumes, essential oils, flavourings, resins and pharmaceuticals. The petroleum nut tree yields an oil that can power engines as well as provide a homeopathic remedy. Other examples are the bark of the cinchona tree which gives the antimalarial quinine (also known as *china*), products of immense historical significance to homeopathy. In Madagascar, common *Cantharanthus* (*Vinca*) species are exploited for the anti-cancer drugs vinblastine and vincristine, two naturally occurring alkaloids isolated in the early 1960s by the pharmaceutical company Eli Lilly. Although there is no fear of these particular plants becoming extinct, serious damage has been done to the ecosystem of which they are a part.

Growing demand

Curare, the South American poisonous vine extract, is a muscle relaxant. In fact, the Amazon Indians use at least 1000 plants medicinally. In Malaysia and Indonesia more than twice this number of plant materials are used to make jamu, the traditional medicine. But it is not only in the developing world where there are problems. Germany, the largest European medicinal plant importer, is also a major exporter of finished herbal products, accounting for at least 70% of the European market.

A patent taken out by a US company in 1999 angered Indian scientists and ecology experts greatly. They were furious at what they considered to be the raiding of their country's storehouse of traditional knowledge.[22] The Americans were granted a patent on a composition of bitter gourd, eggplant and jamun, the fruit of the rose-apple tree, which is abundant all over India during the summer months. The use of these substances to treat diabetes dates back many centuries and is mentioned in many ancient texts on healing. Other indigenous Indian herbal products on which patents have been taken out include mustard seeds (used for bronchial and rheumatic complaints), Indian gooseberry (coughs, asthma, jaundice and wounds) and neem (pesticidal, dermatological, antibacterial properties). The last has attracted dozens of patent applications. It is probably the most celebrated medicinal tree in India.

A Worldwide Fund for Nature (WWF) report warns that the enormous market demand could have an irreversible impact on many species unless action is taken to regulate trade.[23] For example the terpenoid taxol can be made semisynthetically from one or more of the constituents of *Taxus baccata*, a yew tree that grows among pine forests at around 3000 m in the Himalayas. Taxol is of use in the treatment of ovarian and breast cancer. Pharmaceutical companies have stripped forest areas of this species and available trees in a bid to meet the demand for this drug. One cause of the problem was an earlier unconsidered arbitrary decimation of the yew tree population. In 1977 the plant was not considered important enough even to be included in a book on trees, but within 15 years it had become an endangered species.

According to a newspaper report more South Africans are using traditional muti made from plants or animals, driving some species to extinction and pushing up prices.[24] The traditional medicine trade in South Africa is a large and growing industry, the authors of the report said. There are 27 million consumers of traditional medicines and the trade contributes an estimated R2.9bn ($US0.43bn) to the national economy. At least 771 plant species are known to be used for traditional medicine including scarce species that fetch up to R4800 a kilogram. It is estimated that 86% of the plant parts harvested will result in the death of the plant with significant implications for the sustainability of supply.

The WWF report reviews the data available on medicinal plant trade and cites the urgent need for further investigation. One problem is that it is often difficult to decide whether the medicinal plant imports are derived from cultivated or wild specimens. Brazil, China and Nepal have conservation programmes, but India and Pakistan still harvest from the wild, and little is known of the ecological impact of such trade.

Climatic changes

As well as the direct threat to plants through the actions of humans on the habitat or by exhausting the plant stock, there are other more natural factors such as climate, although it has to be said that this may well have been changed as a result of human actions too. Scientific tests at Canberra's Australian National University have proved a link between stunted plant growth and higher ultraviolet radiation caused by depletion of the earth's protective ozone layer. This depletion is being caused by synthetic chemicals, especially chlorofluorocarbons (CFCs), found in products such as air-conditioners and foam packaging.[25] Since the late 1970s the use of CFCs has been heavily regulated. In 1990, diplomats met in London and voted to call for a complete elimination of CFCs by the year 2000. By the year 2010 CFCs should also be completely eliminated from developing countries as well.

Changes in climate from global warming as a result of the greenhouse effect are also important. However, we cannot be sure how long-term changes in the composition of the mix of atmospheric gases, soil structure or pest and disease patterns are going to affect the capacity of plants to manufacture the important active principles upon which we currently rely. *Arnica montana* usually grows in alpine regions, but has been known to flourish in milder climates too. Following the increased use of natural gas and low sulphur fuels, the amount of sulphur dioxide in the atmosphere has fallen.

At the same time, ammonia concentrations have risen, having the effect of changing the pH of rootwater and directly affecting the chances of this plant surviving in some habitats.[26]

Tackling the problem

Awareness

In Britain, John Evelyn (1620–1706) was the first to warn about the fact that its native trees were disappearing faster than they could grow. Evelyn's *Sylva*, published in 1664, became the tree growers' handbook for two centuries.[27] Collecting is a threat to some rare plants; others are affected by the trampling feet of hikers or climbers. At risk from this danger are plant species on the sea coast and hilly areas. The greatest number of endangered species (38) are those of lowland pasture, open grassland and other natural open habitats.[28] Examples of UK-endangered or vulnerable species with herbal or homeopathic applications include species of rock cinquefoil *(Potentilla)*, Jersey cudweed *(Gnaphalium)*, gentians *(Gentians spp)*, rough marshmallow *(Althaea)* and purple spurge *(Euphorbia)*.

Working with local populations

So how can the problem be tackled? Perhaps the most important way to conserve resources is to work closely with the people who live in and use the forest, the indigenous population, rubber tappers, ranchers, loggers, etc. to strike a balance between the extremes of conservation and exploitation that will protect species and threatened environments while still fostering economic development and reducing poverty. Finding alternative uses for crops is one solution – the town of Aukre in Brazil is making money harvesting Brazil nut oil for the late Anita Roddick's Body Shop.

Redevelopment

Another solution is finding use for the deforested areas. The return of large-scale cattle ranching is even a possibility, provided that grass can be grown for fodder. Programmes of continuing education encourage better forestry management and appropriate legislation such as the US Endangered Species Act 1973 or the British Wildlife and Countryside Act 1981. A total of 332 plants was either listed or proposed for listing, under the latter, from 1985 to 1991. It has been suggested that companies should fund forest protection schemes by putting cash up in exchange for exploitation rights. $USlm has been invested by an American drug company in a pilot scheme in Costa Rica. However, the costs are enormous, running into billions of dollars just to preserve resources solely for the pharmaceutical industry.

Some of Britain's rarest wild flowers are likely to be encouraged to make a return as a result of an EC Set Aside scheme.[29] The reduction in the cropped area of over 450 thousand hectares between 1992 and 1993 was mainly as a result of the impact of EC Set Aside Schemes, which were established to reduce the amount of agricultural land in arable production. The first of these schemes, the Five-Year Scheme, was introduced in 1988. This scheme was superseded in 1992 by the Arable Area Payments Scheme (AAPS), which included a compulsory set-aside requirement except for the smallest farmers. A reduction in the area of land set aside in the UK in 1996–7 was generally attributed to the reduction in payments made to farmers under the Set Aside Scheme; however, between 1998 and 1999 the amount of set aside increased by over 250 000 hectares as a result of the reintroduction of the grants. Other agri-environment schemes make payments for the adoption of agricultural practices to conserve wildlife habitats, historic, archaeological and landscape features, and to improve opportunities for countryside enjoyment. Support is also provided for a variety of capital works.

With reforms to the EU Common Agricultural Policy which were agreed by the member states in March 1999 the principle of compulsory set aside was retained with a rate set at 10% for the 2000–2006 period. However the rate for any particular year can be altered by the agreement of the Commission and a qualified majority of member states. With food shortages there is pressure to scrap the scheme.

Strategic approach

The WHO launched its first-ever comprehensive TM strategy in 2002.[2] The strategy is designed to assist countries to:

- develop national policies on the evaluation and regulation of TM practices
- create a stronger evidence base on the safety, efficacy and quality of the traditional products and practices
- ensure availability and affordability of TM including essential herbal medicines
- promote therapeutically sound use of TM by providers and consumers
- document traditional medicines and remedies.

Plant alternatives

Chemical synthesis would cut down the amount of plant material consumed in extraction processes. Ideally, pharmaceutical companies require novel, single active molecules that can be made in a laboratory. Although this may be possible for some allopathic drugs, the activity of most crude extracts can seldom be attributed to a single molecule but is usually the result of several compounds acting in synergy, making production of synthetic copies extremely difficult. Medical herbalists are obliged to use the original source material to protect this unique mix of active principles. Furthermore, the holistic principles of herbal medicine suggest that the relative concentrations of useful plant chemicals achieved by mixing different species together in individualised prescriptions are important in treating patients despite the general lack of standardisation. We know little about the interactive abilities of naturally occurring chemicals, much to the consternation of our orthodox colleagues whose demands are for purified, fully characterised medicines given in regulated doses. Homeopaths need to use naturally occurring source materials too, complete with any inherent impurities, so that modern drug pictures can be assumed to match exactly with Hahnemann's own work.

There is also the possibility of creating a problem of another kind by following the synthesis strategy. The isolation of the chemical diosgenin from the Mexican *Dioscorea* species in the 1940s led to a booming steroid industry in that country. As sophisticated isolation, separation and elucidation techniques developed, the requirement for this particular raw material fell away completely and with it went the accompanying industry, causing widespread local social deprivation.

Dioscorea species continue to be used by homeopaths. There is some irony in the fact that the largest pharmaceutical companies in the world are scouring the South American rainforests increasingly, seeking natural sources for drug products.[30] Estimates of the 'hit' rate from random screening programmes vary widely, but are put between 1 in 1000 and 1 in 10 000. The chances of finding active plant extracts is greatly increased by studying the use of plants by various cultures, and the discipline of 'ethnobotany' is growing slowly. Table 11.1 lists a number of common drugs that came to scientific attention as a result of ethnobotanical studies.

Success story

Certainly it is not all doom and gloom! There have been successes. *Ginkgo biloba* (Figure 11.1) is one such example.

It is the only survivor from the Jurassic dinosaur era some 190 million years ago, all of its related species having long since died out. The tree survived in cultivation because of its valuable fruit and wood and possibly because of temple plantings. It was introduced to Europe from its native China in 1730. *Gingko biloba* was heading for extinction until fortuitous intervention saved it. Its extracts are used in Chinese herbalism under the name baguo to treat hypertension.

It is no consolation that complementary practitioners are the cause of the problems, because our uses are but a fraction of the total

Table 11.1 Common orthodox drugs derived from plants

Medicine	Plant
Atropine	*Atropa belladonna*
Cocaine	*Erythoxylum coca*
Colchicine	*Colchicum autumnale*
Digoxin	*Digitalis purpurea*
Ephedrine	*Ephedra sinica*
Hyoscymine	*Hyoscymus niger*
Morphine	*Papaver somniferum*
Pilocarpine	*Pilocarpus jaborandi*
Quinine	*Cinchona legeriana*
Strychnine	*Strychnos nux vomica*
Theobromine	*Theobroma cacao*

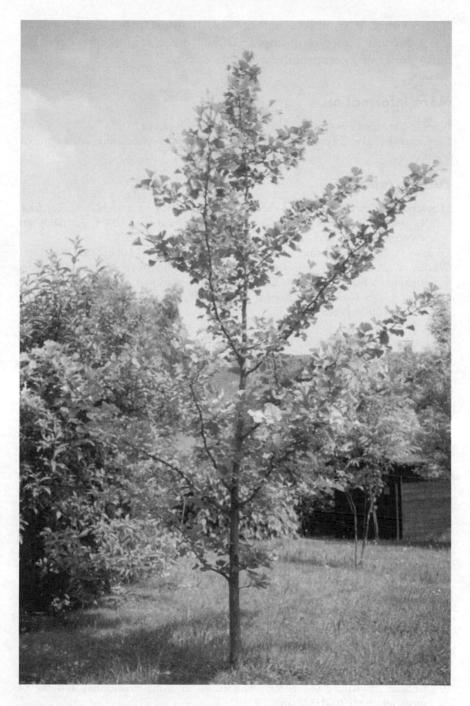

Figure 11.1 *Gingko biloba* tree.

requirements. It would be unforgivable if future generations were to suffer because remedies disappeared due to the actions of others. We must work out a compromise in plenty of time

More information

Botanic Gardens Conservation International: www.bgci.org
European Herbal and Traditional Medicine Practitioners Association: www.ehpa.eu

Further reading

Hawkins B. *Plants for Life: Medicinal plant conservation and botanic gardens.* Richmond: Botanic Gardens Conservation International, 2008. Available at: www.bgci.org/medicinal/medplants (accessed 10 May 2008).
Okpako D. African medicine: tradition and beliefs. *Pharm J* 2006;**276**:239–40.
Waylen K. *Botanic Gardens: Using biodiversity to improve human well-being.* Richmond: Botanic Gardens Conservation International, 2006.
Williamson E. Systems of traditional medicine from South and South East Asia. *Pharm J* 2006;**276**:539–40.

References

1. Bannerman RH. *Traditional Medicine and Healthcare Coverage.* Geneva: World Health Organization, 1983.
2. World Health Organization. *Traditional Medicine.* WHO Fact Sheet N134, Revised. Geneva: WHO, 2003. Available at: http://tinyurl.com/5mrd5 (accessed 11 December 2007).
3. Bodeker G. Lessons on integration from the developing world's experience. *BMJ* 2001;**322**:164–7.
4. Singh KN, Lal B. Ethnomedicines used against four common ailments by the tribal communities of Lahaul-Spiti in western Himalaya. *J Ethnopharmacol* 2008;**115**:147–59.
5. Langlois-Klassen D, Kipp W, Jhangri GS, Rubaale T. Use of traditional herbal medicine by AIDS patients in Kabarole District, western Uganda. *Am J Trop Med Hyg* 2007;**77**:757–63. PubMed
6. Atherton D J. Towards the safer use of traditional remedies. *BMJ* 1994;**308**:673–4.
7. Loizzo JJ, Blackhall LJ, Rabgyay L. Tibetan medicine: A complementary science of optimal health. *Ann NY Acad Sci* 2007; 28Sep. [Epub ahead of print] Abstract available at: http://tinyurl.com/2gjcwh (accessed 10 May 2008).
8. Bodeker G. Traditional (i.e. indigenous) and complementary medicine in the Commonwealth: new partnerships planned with the formal health sector. *J Altern Compl Med* 1999;**5**:97–101.
9. Chaudhury RR. Commentary: challenges in using traditional systems of medicine. *BMJ* 2001;**322**:167.

10. Low T. *Bush Medicine*. North Ryde, NSW: Collins/Angus & Robertson, 1990.
11. Riley M. *Maori Healing and Herbal*. Paparraumu: Viking Sevensen NZ, 1994.
12. Cohen K. Native American medicine. In: Jonas WB, Levin J (eds), *Essentials of Complementary and Alternative Medicine*. Baltimore, MD: Lippincott/ Williams & Wilkins, 1999: 233–51.
13. Nauman E. Native American medicine. In: Novery D (ed.), *Clinician's Complete Reference to Complementary Alternative Medicine*. St Louis, MO: Mosby, 2000: 293–308.
14. Sofowora A. Plants in African traditional medicine – a review. In: Evans WC (ed.), *Trease and Evans' Pharmacognosy*, 14th edn. London: WB Saunders, 1996: 511–20.
15. van Wyk B-E, van Oudtshoorn B, Gericke N. *Medicinal Plants of South Africa*. Pretoria: Briza Publications, 1997.
16. Weiner MA. *Secrets of Fijian Medicine*. Berkeley: Quantum Books, 1983.
17. Feldman J. Traditional medicine in Latin America. In: Novery D (ed.), *Clinician's Complete Reference to Complementary Alternative Medicine*. St Louis, MO: Mosby, 2000: 284–92.
18. Medicine and Healthcare products Regulatory Agency. *Traditional Ethnic Medicine: Public health and compliance with medicines law*. MHRA Available at: http://tinyurl.com/2olbvg (accessed October 31 2007).
19. Kayne S. Plants, medicines and environmental awareness. *Hlth Homoeopath* 1993;**5**:12–14.
20. Huxtable RJ. The pharmacology of extinction. *J Ethnopharmacol* 1992; **27**:1–11.
21. Holloway H. Sustaining the Amazon. *Sci Am* 1993;**269**:77–84.
22. Orr D. India accuses US of stealing ancient cures. *The London Times* Saturday, 31 July 1999.
23. Worldwide Fund for Nature. *International Report – Booming medicinal plant trade lacks controls*. Godalming, Surrey: WWF, 1993
24. Ferreira A. Muti is killing off South Africa's flora and fauna. *South Africa Times* 7 December 2007. Available at: http://tinyurl.com/2sbpkn (accessed 11 December 2007).
25. Anon. Ozone hole cuts plant growth. *Independent* 11 June 1993.
26. Dueck ThA, Elderson J. Influence of ammonia and sulphur dioxide on the growth and competitive ability of *Arnica Montana* and *Viola canina*. *New Phytol* 1992;**122**:507–14.
27. Bellamy D. Something in the air. *BBC Wildlife* 1993;**11**(7):31–4.
28. Sitwell N. *The Shell Guide to Britain's Threatened Wildlife*. London: Collins, 1993.
29. Anon. Threatened wild flowers saved by EC's arable farm policy. *Independent* 19 July 1993.
30. Fellows L. What can higher plants offer the industry? *Pharm J* 1993;**250**:658.

12

Traditional Chinese medicine

Steven B Kayne

The English phrase 'traditional Chinese medicine' (TCM) was created in the 1950s by the People's Republic of China in order to export Chinese medicine. There is no equivalent phrase in Chinese.

Definition

Traditional Chinese medicine is a generic term used to describe a variety of medical practices that originated in China but have now spread throughout the world. It includes not only acupuncture, moxibustion and Chinese herbal medicine (CHM), but also a number of other disciplines including dietary therapy, mind and body exercise (including tai c'hi) and meditation.

History

The earliest Chinese medical treatise known, *The Huang di Neijing* or *The Yellow Emperors Classic of Internal Medicine*, is considered the highest authority on TCM.[1] The *Neijing* is attributed to the highly esteemed Yellow Emperor (Huangdi) who, according to legendary history, ascended to the throne of China around 2698 BC.[2] However, Huangdi is a semi-mythical figure, and the book probably dates from later, around 300 BC and may be a compilation of the writings of several authors. Whatever its origin, the book has proved influential as a reference work for practitioners of TCM well into the modern era. The book takes the form of a discussion between Huangdi and his physician, in which Huangdi enquires about the nature of health. It consists of two separate texts: *The Suwen* or 'simple questions' and *The Lingshu*, a book on acupuncture and moxibustion.

The origins of what might be called modern TCM can be traced back to Zhang Ji, who practised in the Qing Chang mountains close to Chengdu, Szechuan province, in the early years of the third century AD, although it was known to exist in various forms for more than 1000 years before this date.[3]

In 1849 the Gold Rush in California brought a large influx of Chinese people to the western USA. They brought their traditional medicine with them and it proved to be popular among the prospectors and their families, particularly as western medicine was largely unavailable in these remote areas. The steady expansion of interest in TCM in the past 35 years in the USA has been attributed to media interest during President Nixon's visit to the People's Republic of China in the early 1970s (see 'Acupuncture', below).

Theory

As with most forms of traditional medicine, the theoretical and diagnostic basis of TCM cannot be explained in terms of western anatomy and physiology. It is rooted in the philosophy, logic and beliefs of a different civilisation, and leads to a perception of health and disease that is alien to western scientific thinking. But it is an entirely coherent system, with internal logic and consistency of thought and practice.[4] The Chinese approach to understanding the human body is unique. It is based on a highly sophisticated set of practices designed to cure illness and to maintain health and wellbeing.[5] These practices also represent an energetic intervention designed to re-establish harmony and equilibrium for each patient according to the holistic principle. Whenever the practitioner uses acupuncture or herbal medicine, prescribes a set of exercises or proposes a new diet, his or her activities are all considered to be mutually interdependent and necessary to restore (or maintain) health.

There are five basic principles associated with TCM:

1. Yin and yang
2. The five elements
3. The five substances
4. The organs
5. The meridians.

Yin and yang

According to TCM practitioners, the world and all life within it comprises pairs of opposites, each giving meaning to the other. These are known as yin and yang:

- Yin is a negative state associated with cold, dark, stillness and passiveness: its symbol can be represented by the dark side of a mountain.
- Yang is a positive state associated with heat, light and vigour: its symbol can be represented by the sunny side of a mountain.

They are reflected in the well-known entwined symbol (the *tai ji* symbol), depicted in Figure 12.1.

The relationship between the two elements of yin and yang is dynamic; nature constantly moves between the two. An analogy might be provided by considering a cup of coffee that starts as yang; as it cools the yang changes to yin, passing through an equilibrium that is just right for drinking. At any stage the application of heat will cause a flow back into yang. This element of change involving energy flows (see below) is seen as a fundamental quality of life.

As the organs of the body were discovered they were deemed to be yin or yang. Yin organs are vital and solid, including the heart, spleen, lungs, kidneys and liver. Yang organs are hollow and functional, and include the stomach, intestines and bladder. Each organ also has a yin and yang element within it, and it is the overall imbalance that leads to disease.

An example of the yin–yang principle in therapeutics may be provided by considering a patient suffering from a fever, i.e. an excess of yang. Only when the opposites are in equal balance is life in harmony. Too much or too little of either element results in disharmony. Treatment would therefore be seen as the ability to promote the conversion of excess yang into yin, allowing restoration of the equilibrium between the two and a consequent resolution of the fever.

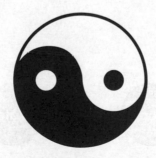

Figure 12.1 The symbol used to depict yin and yang.

The five elements

According to Chinese philosophy, the body organs are related to one of the five phases (or elements): wood, fire, earth, metal and water. These are said to represent the circle of life. The five phases have a flow in which they move called the 'generating cycle' (Figure 12.2):

1. Water generates wood (by nourishing trees)
2. Wood generates fire (rubbed together to generate fire)
3. Fire generates earth (ashes fall to support the soil)
4. Earth generates metal (ore)
5. Metal generates water (when molten resembles water).

The five phases are at the core of a complex system of relationships (Table 12.1), an imbalance in which causes ill health. They are applied to the practice of TCM in a number of ways including the following examples.

The cosmological sequence considers water to be the most important element. Water corresponds to the kidney and reflects the importance that Chinese prescribers place on this organ. It is viewed as the centre of all yin and yang energy in the body and its health is therefore vital.

There may be a supporting or familial relationship between organs, e.g. the kidney may be considered as a fire or 'mother' organ

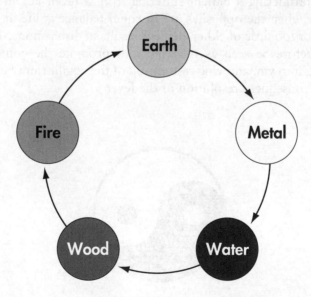

Figure 12.2 The generating cycle.

Table 12.1 Relationships of the five phases

	Wood	Fire	Earth	Metal	Water
Seasons	Spring	Summer	Late summer	Autumn	Winter
Environment	Wind	Heat	Damp	Dry	Cold
Zang organs (yin)	Liver	Heart	Spleen	Lung	Kidney
Fu organs (yang)	Gallbladder	Small intestine	Stomach	Large intestine	Bladder
Directions	East	South	Middle	West	North
Tastes	Sour	Bitter	Sweet	Pungent	Salty
Senses	Eye	Tongue	Mouth	Nose	Ear
Tissues	Tendon	Vessel	Muscle	Skin, hair	Bone
Emotions	Anger	Joy	Worry	Grief	Fear

and the liver an earth or 'son' organ. Treating the 'mother' organ might provide a route to improving the health of a deficient 'son' organ. The spleen may be considered to nourish, similar to the function of earth in nature; thus it is described as being an earth organ and malfunction may be associated with soft tissue problems and worry (Table 12.1)

There may also be a degree of control, as when water 'controls' fire. When an organ is weak it is unable to exert the control necessary to assist other organs. Thus, if the lungs are weak the liver may become too strong, leading to headaches or hypertension.

The five substances

In TCM five substances encompass both tangible and intangible elements within the body. The first three, qi, jing and shen, include qualities such as energy and spirit, and are known as the three treasures. They are believed to be the essential components of an individual's life. The other elements, blood and body fluids, are rather easier for the scientifically trained health professional to understand, although these too have essentially intangible properties.

Qi (chee or chi)

Qi is a type of vital energy responsible for the following day-to-day body functions:

- Movement, both conscious (voluntary) and unconscious (involuntary)
- Transforming food and drink into blood, body fluids and energy
- Containment: holding organs, blood vessels and body tissues in their proper places
- Protection, from external environmental factors including heat, cold and dampness
- Maintenance of body heat.

A number of qi disharmonies may be identified during illness, e.g. a deficiency in qi will lead to debilitation and slowed recovery from ill health. An excess of qi is not considered to be detrimental unless it is blocked or is over-acting on another organ system, e.g. in the case of a migraine headache where the qi of the liver is blocked and in excess, to clear itself it invades the stomach and causes vomiting; with this release of energy the intensity of migraine symptoms is often reduced.

Feng shui is an ancient Chinese practice believed to use the Laws of both Heaven (astronomy) and Earth (geography) to help one improve life by receiving positive qi. Most of today's feng shui schools teach that it is the practice of choosing a place to live or arranging objects and using colour, to achieve harmony with one's environment.

Essence (jing)

The concept of jing is translated as 'essence' and underpins all aspects of organic life. If jing is plentiful life itself is good, and full of harmony and vitality. If jing is lacking then qi will be weak, life will be dull and the person will be susceptible to contracting disease.

Jing is responsible for the following:

- Governing growth, reproduction and development
- Production of bone marrow
- Promotion of kidney qi
- Determination of the basic constitutional strength.

Deficiency of jing is the only disharmony and is said to be more prevalent in men than in women. It can cause:

- developmental disorders, including physical, mental and learning problems, and kidney-related disorders
- poor memory and concentration.

Shen

Shen is both mind and spirit. It is based in the heart and governs spiritual, mental and emotional health. Disharmony can range from mild confusion and insomnia to substantial psychiatric disturbances accompanied by irrational behaviour.

Blood

In TCM blood is much more than simply a physical transport system, as in western medicine. It is closely linked to qi.

Three imbalances may be identified:

1.   Deficiency shows in pale face, dry skin, light-headedness and emaciation.
2.   Stagnation produces stabbing pains and purple lips and tongue.
3.   Excessive heat in the blood can cause bleeding skin conditions and fever.

Body fluids

Body fluids include external light and watery fluids, such as saliva and tears (known as jin), and the dense thicker fluids that circulate inside the body, e.g. gastric juices and joint fluids (known as ye). The function of all the body fluids is to nourish and lubricate the body. They are essential for the maintenance of healthy qi. Deficient body fluids result in dryness of the eyes, lips and hair, a dry cough and excessive thirst. Excess body fluids can lead to problems known as dampness and phlegm in TCM, characterised by productive coughs, weeping skin rashes and vaginal discharge.

The organs

The organs (*Zangfu*) detailed below have a special status in TCM, being the creators and storers of the five substances. They are considered to be closely related to specific emotions and virtues and, if their essential requirements are not fulfilled, ill health will result.

Each organ also has a yin and yang element within it, and it is the overall imbalance that leads to disease. Rather like the constitutional patient in homeopathy, many ailments may be described as being yin or yang. Thus a yin-deficient patient may be hot and feverish, restless and stressed out. A yang-deficient patient will feel cold and be pale and lethargic.

The following vital organs are known as the solid or *Zan* organs and are associated with yin:

- The **heart** governs the circulatory system, but is also the centre of shen. It is positively associated with compassion, love and affection, and negatively with overexcitement. Symptoms of ill health include insomnia and hyperactivity.
- The **lungs** relate to qi and require confidence to function effectively. They are positively associated with conscientiousness and negatively with sadness. Symptoms of ill health include irregular breathing, coughs and susceptibility to colds.
- The **liver** ensures that qi flows smoothly. When the liver is in harmony, a person will feel relaxed and optimistic but when out of balance the person will feel irritable and unable to move forward positively. Symptoms of ill health may be irregular periods, premenstrual syndrome, headaches, irritable bowel syndrome and a bad temper.
- The **spleen** creates qi. Its health depends on a good diet and a non-stressful lifestyle. It is positively associated with empathy and negatively with obsession. Symptoms of ill health include poor appetite and diarrhoea.
- The **kidneys** store jing and are associated with long-term growth. Their positive emotion is courage; their negative emotion is fear. Symptoms of ill health include lethargy, diarrhoea, infertility and oedema.

The following functional organs are known as the hollow or *Fu* organs and are associated with yang:

- The gallbladder
- Large and small intestines
- Bladder
- Stomach
- *San jiao*, also known as the 'triple burner' or 'triple heater', roughly corresponds to the thoracic, abdominal and pelvic regions. It coordinates transformation and transportation of fluids in the body.

The meridians or channels

Qi is said to circulate through the body along specific interconnected channels called meridians. They form an invisible network close to the surface of the body, which links together all the fundamental textures and organs and are named for the organs or functions to which they are attached. Kaptchuk mentions 14 meridians in his book;[6] other writers refer to different numbers ranging from 11 to 20. As the meridians unify all parts of the body and energy can pass along the channels, they are essential for the maintenance of harmonious balance. Set along the meridians are a number of points used by acupuncturists (see below).

There is no physically verifiable anatomical or histological proof of their existence. They are considered to form an invisible network close to the surface of the body, which links together all the fundamental textures and organs. Set along the meridians are a number of points used by acupuncturists (see below).

Practice of TCM

Whenever the practitioner uses acupuncture or herbal medicine, prescribes a set of exercises or proposes a new diet, his or her activities are all considered to be mutually interdependent and necessary to restore (or maintain) health. It is common practice to treat patients using a combination approach. This differs somewhat to how Chinese medicine is practised in China where doctors tend to specialise in acupuncture, herbal medicine or massage.

Diagnosis

A diagnosis is achieved using four traditional methods:[7]

1. Listening carefully to the sound and quality of the patient's voice, (auscultation) and evaluating any breath or body odours (olfaction)
2. Asking questions to ascertain the features of the illness (enquiry)
3. Observing the patient's general demeanour and emotional state, and assessing the quality and texture of the skin and the shape, colour and coating of the tongue (inspection)
4. Palpation of the pulses and body.

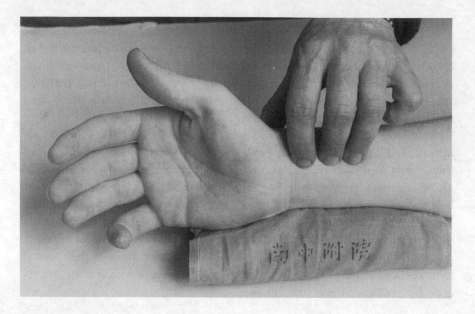

Figure 12.3 Reading the pulse (courtesy T. Booker).

Reading pulses

The experienced practitioner can deduce much information on the patient's past and present health status from reading the pulses and palpating the body. Following the taking of a full history, pulses will be read (Figure 12.3). Chinese medicine recognises up to 28 pulses, which are palpable on the right and left wrists. The right-hand pulses represent conditions of the lung, spleen and kidney yang, whereas the left-hand pulses represent conditions of the heart, liver and kidney yin.

The pulse is assessed in seven criteria: depth, fluency, rhythm, size/shape, speed, strength and tension. The aim is to determine which organ or organs might be out of balance by considering all the many elements outlined above, and to take appropriate action to rectify the problem according to the various principles outlined above. Treatment is by a range of different therapies (see below).

Evidence

There are a number of difficulties in assembling the evidence of effectiveness for TCM. Much research has been carried out in China but is considered inadmissible because of problems associated with:

- poor translation of studies
- the quality and design of the research not being up to western standards
- the use of unvalidated methods and other methodological deficiencies.

In addition:

- It is vital that correct plant species are used when researching traditional herbal medicine and that tests are carried out on material prepared ethnically.[8]
- The charisma and seniority of the practitioner may introduce a significant element of placebo response that cannot be quantified.

Modern Chinese medicine

Since the 1950s, the Chinese government and the government of Taiwan have put great efforts into promoting the modernisation of Chinese medicine. This has been in response to national planning needs to provide comprehensive healthcare services. Previously, TCM had been viewed as part of an imperial legacy, to be replaced by a secular health-care system. Integration was guided by health officials trained in modern medicine; harmonisation with modern medicine was the goal. This was accomplished by a science-based approach to the education of TCM and an emphasis on research. In an article discussing the research priorities in TCM, there are now Chinese professionals trained in both TCM and modern western medicine who conduct research on the development of Chinese medicine. Western science methodologies have been employed to analyse the effectiveness of herbs and treatment on various individuals. Many of the differences between TCM and western scientific practices are now being studied for their synergistic potential.

Acupuncture

The term 'acupuncture' is of western origin, derived from Latin and meaning 'puncturing with needles'. It was first used by the Dutchman Wilhelm Ten Rijn, who wrote on the subject at the end of the seventeenth century.

Practitioners of acupuncture generally follow one of two broad approaches to the discipline, using either TCM with all its many ramifications for maintaining health or the simpler symptom-oriented western acupuncture. This section gives an outline of both.

Definition

Acupuncture is a technique involving the insertion of fine needles into the skin at selected points over the body.

History

The oldest known text to include a reference to acupuncture is attributed to *The Yellow Emperor's Classic of Internal Medicine* (*The Neijing*), which developed over the centuries until a definitive version appeared in the first century BC. The names and reputed functions of all the acupuncture points were established by about AD 259 when *The Classic of Acupuncture* (*Zhen Jiu Jia Jing*) was published. Acupuncture continued to flourish in China, especially throughout the Ming period (1368–1644). Subsequently, it went into gradual decline until 1822, when it was finally banned by Emperor Dao Guang, who disapproved of its practices. In the early part of the twentieth century acupuncture became part of the ongoing debate as to whether Chinese culture should be overtaken by western influences or maintain its own traditions. With the arrival of western medicine, acupuncture was increasingly relegated to rural and remote backwaters.

In the 1950s the discipline was reintroduced by the communist authorities, who saw TCM as a solution to the problem of providing healthcare to an ever-growing population. Acupuncture developed once again as people were quickly trained and pressed into service. Today it is practised alongside western medicine.

News of the success of acupuncture was brought to the west in 1683 by Dr Willen Ten Rhijn, a physician working for the Dutch East Indies Company in Japan. Dr Rhijn's report was not the first, but it was the most reliable. Usage of the English word 'acupuncture' is attributed to him.

Acupuncture was widely practised in France in the late eighteenth century with Dr Berlioz, a Parisian doctor, becoming the first western practitioner of acupuncture in the early nineteenth century. John Churchill, the first British acupuncturist, used the technique in the treatment of rheumatism in 1821. Acupuncture was even mentioned in the first edition of *The Lancet* in 1823 as being chiefly used in 'diseases of the head and lower belly'.[9]

When China opened up to visitors shortly after President Nixon went to the country in 1971, physicians and others from the west made visits to witness how acupuncture was being used.[9]

Theory

In addition to the classic principles of Chinese medicine outlined under the general heading TCM above, there is one key aspect of practice still to consider. This is the theory of acupuncture points that are stimulated usually by the superficial insertion of needles into the skin. Other methods of stimulation include the application of pressure (see below) and the passing of a weak electrical current.

Patterns of disharmony (i.e. bad health and emotional disorders) that are recognised in the body are thought to be caused by disruptions of the body's energy flow along the meridians. To correct those disruptions, specific points on the meridians called acupoints are stimulated via needles, burning incense cones (moxa), applying pressure or other means.

It is suggested that acupuncture may work by stimulating the nervous system, leading to the release of opiate peptides (endorphins), compounds that are closely involved with the mechanisms by which the body controls its perception of pain. Thus, acupuncture can be used in the treatment of intractable pain without the attendant traditional Chinese theory.

Practice of acupuncture

Traditional acupuncture

The meridians   The Standard Acupuncture Nomenclature published by the World Health Organization[10] lists 20 meridians connecting most of the acupuncture points (see below). The 20 meridians comprise 12 standard meridians, with each meridian corresponding to an organ, and 8 extraordinary meridians, 2 of which have their own sets of points, and the remaining ones connect points on other channels.

Meridians are divided into yin and yang groups. Examples include:

- the yin meridians of the arm are lung, heart and pericardium
- the yin meridians of the leg are the spleen, kidney and liver

- the yang meridians of the arm are the large intestine and small intestine.

Acupuncture points   A basic 365 mapped acupuncture points ('acupoints') are situated along the meridians detailed above. A further 1000 extra points and special use points may also be identified on the hand, ear and scalp. It is not known how these points were discovered. Acupoints cannot be identified by their appearance and no consistent features of their anatomy have been found that distinguish them from other tissues. It has been suggested that the points may be sites of tenderness.[11] The study of an acupoint known as spleen 6 found that there was no strong evidence to support the hypothesis that acupuncture points were more tender than control points.[12]

Figure 12.4 shows an acupuncture doll with acupoints on the head and neck marked.

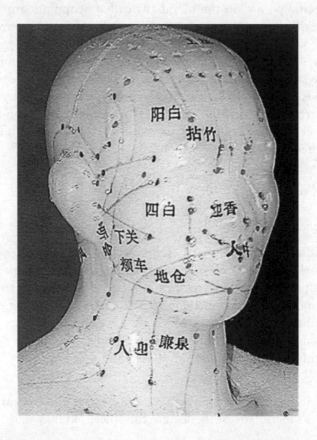

Figure 12.4 Acupuncture doll showing acupoints on the head and neck.

Needling procedure   There is archaeological evidence that shows that the earliest acupuncture needles date back to the Stone Age, when instruments called bian were thought to have been used in China.[13] By the Bronze Age acupuncture was already well developed and needles were made of bronze. Needles were subsequently made of many different metals: gold, silver, copper, etc. Modern acupuncturists use solid sterile disposable needles of narrow bore, about 3 cm long (although longer needles may be used at different sites). The patient is usually treated lying down to minimise any tendency to faint. As many as 15–20 needles may be inserted superficially at the appropriate point or points. The practitioner then gently introduces the needles a little more deeply into the muscle, rotating them between finger and thumb. Qi and blood flow throughout the meridians and this is where manipulation of the needle is critical in properly moving this flow.

The arrival of qi is signified by a dull ache or tingling sensation and slight inflammation. Some practitioners may use electrical stimulation, connecting the needles to a small piece of equipment powered by batteries.

Needles are left in place for up to 20 min: the patient is invited to lie back and relax. Occasionally a needle may be left in place for several days, normally situated in the ear; these so-called indwelling needles should not be used in patients with heart valve disease or those who are immunocompromised.

Number of sessions   Usually 10–12 sessions constitute a single course of treatment. Two or three courses may be required for the treatment of chronic conditions. Acupuncture point selection may vary at each treatment, depending on the patient's response. If significant improvement is achieved, the patient will be discharged at the end of the treatment but will normally be instructed to continue with other elements of TCM, e.g. dietary control and perhaps exercises.

Minimal acupuncture (western or medical acupuncture)[14]

The traditional theory of meridians and acupoints is either ignored altogether or is radically reinterpreted in western acupuncture. Some general practitioners (GPs) and physiotherapists with orthodox backgrounds find it difficult to accept the intangible nature of traditional acupuncture, which relates to the flow of qi. Many dispute the existence of meridians or acupuncture points,[15] preferring to link their practice to trigger points instead.[16,17]

Practice may be linked to trigger points, small hyperirritable areas in skeletal muscle known as nodules that have been strained or injured and not healed. This variant, which involves very brief needling and lasting no more than a few seconds at trigger points with few needles, has been termed 'minimal acupuncture'. Exponents of minimal acupuncture commonly treat musculoskeletal pain, arthritis and symptoms of stress, including tension headaches, gastrointestinal problems and nausea.

Other simplified ways of choosing where to needle exist, and there are also many techniques of electroacupuncture (mostly developed by Japanese and European acupuncture researchers).

Western acupuncture lends itself to use in a busy practice where there is little time to spend on each patient. It also has the advantage that it can be learned much more easily than traditional acupuncture by modern health practitioners, such as doctors, physiotherapists, osteopaths, chiropractors and podiatrists.

Evidence

Evidence of effectiveness is largely restricted to case studies, although randomised controlled trials (RCTs) are available for western acupuncture (see below). The findings of many of these randomised trials have caused much debate. Positive trials have been criticised because of inadequate blinding, and negative trials have been criticised because the intervention was not administered by properly trained practitioners or control interventions may have had analgesic effects.[18]

There are problems with designing trials for acupuncture associated with the control arm of an RCT. The most usual placebo method is sham acupuncture, when needles are inserted outside acupuncture points with a minimum of interaction between practitioner and patient.

Cautious approval of some applications of acupuncture was given by the US National Institutes of Health consensus development meeting in 1997.[19] The 12-member panel was asked to evaluate current evidence for the efficacy of acupuncture and concluded that there is 'clear evidence' of efficacy in the control of nausea and vomiting occurring in some patients postoperatively and in association with chemotherapy, and for the relief of postoperative dental pain. The panel said that acupuncture was 'probably' also effective in the control of nausea in early pregnancy. The British Medical Association reached a similar conclusion in their report on acupuncture.[20] A number of correspondents to the *British Medical Journal* criticised this support, claiming that the evidence was not sufficient to reach a positive conclusion.[21]

Safety

Adverse reactions

Examples of potential dangers during needling and trauma include the following:

- **Pain and dizziness** is commonly reported by patients.[22]
- **Infection** during needling: non-sterile needles or poor hygiene may lead to infection. Reuse of needles with inadequate sterilisation has been the source of hepatitis in a number of patients, although the literature refers mainly, but not exclusively, to the 1980s and before.[23–25]
- **Trauma**: traumatic damage to blood vessels may produce a haematoma or result in serious injuries.[26,27]
- **Allergic reactions** caused by the metal of the needles, particularly chrome and nickel, are possible.[28,29]
- **Other adverse effects**: other possible adverse reactions to acupuncture include cardiac arrhythmias,[30] the triggering of asthma[31] and the exacerbation of symptoms.[32]

Contraindications

Acupuncture is contraindicated or must be used with extreme care in patients who:

- are unwilling to be needled; they should not be pressurised to undergo treatment
- have a tendency to bleed excessively
- have a pacemaker; it might be affected by the electrical stimulation of acupuncture needles.

Precautions

A number of precautions may be suggested when practising acupuncture:

- Patients should lie down during treatment.
- Disposable sterile needles should be used.
- Needles should be counted before and after treatment so that all may be accounted for.
- Patients should be carefully observed for excessive bleeding.

Applications of acupuncture

Therapeutic areas in which acupuncture has been used include the following:

- Pain: back,[33,34] dental,[35] headaches and migraine,[36,37] knee,[38,39] neck[40,41]
- Drug dependence[42,43]
- Gastrointestinal disorders[44]
- Insomnia[45]
- Nausea and vomiting[46]
- Osteoarthritis[47,48]
- Smoking cessation[49]
- Weight loss.[50]

Variants of acupuncture

Acupressure

Acupressure is a form of acupuncture in which fingers, thumbs and elbows are used to stimulate the body's acupuncture points. Acupressure relieves muscular tension, facilitating blood flow and therefore distributing more nutrients and oxygen throughout the body as well as removing waste products.

Acupressure has been used to relieve mental tension, for tired and strained eyes, headaches, menstrual cramps and arthritis as well as to promote general healthcare. Elasticated travel bands used to combat motion sickness have a small raised bead that presses on a wrist acupressure pint.

Moxibustion

Moxibustion is similar to both acupuncture and acupressure in its effects but uses a glowing moxa or wick of dried herbs (e.g. *Artemisia vulgaris*) instead of needles or fingertips as the source of stimulation for the acupoints. The glowing moxa rolls are usually held about 2 cm from the acupoint. Moxibustion tones, stimulates and supplements energy in the meridians. It is claimed to be an effective treatment for arthritis and menstrual problems.

Availability of acupuncture to patients

The United Kingdom

In the UK the practice of acupuncture is not legally restricted to medically qualified doctors as it is in many other European countries (e.g. France, Hungary, Italy, Poland and Portugal), so the market may be partially satisfied by non-medically qualified practitioners (NMQPs). There are more than 5500 acupuncturists in the UK, of whom 3500 are statutorily registered health professionals. A government report (Pittilo report 2008) has called for acupuncturists to be statutorily registered (http://hdl.handle.net/10059/176).

The United States of America

Acupuncture has been increasingly embraced by practitioners and patients in the USA since the appearance of an article describing experience with successful post-appendectomy pain management using acupuncture needles.[51] California became the first state to license acupuncture as an independent healthcare profession in 1976. Since then, 40 states and the District of Columbia have adopted similar laws.

Chinese herbal medicine

Like other TCM disciplines, CHM is based on the concepts of yin and yang and of qi energy. The herbs are ascribed qualities such as 'cooling' (yin) or 'stimulating' (yang), and are often used in combination according to the deficiencies or excesses of these qualities in the patient. They may also be combined with zoological or mineral materials.

Definition

Chinese herbal medicine is a traditional therapy that uses a combination of plant material (crude drugs and pieces of prepared drugs), minerals and animal products in the promotion and maintenance of good health and the treatment of ill health.

History

China's greatest materia medica (*Pen Ts'ao*) was published by Li Shizhen in 1578.[52] The culmination of 26 years' work, it comprised

1892 species of drugs of animal, vegetable and mineral origin, and included 8160 prescriptions.

Secret recipes (also known as 'prepared medicines') were the equivalent of modern patent medicines. A variety of dose forms were available including pills, liquids and honey boluses. By the time of the Ming dynasty (1368–1644) more than 60 000 formulae had been recorded in the 1406 book entitled *Formulas of Universal Benefit* (*Pu Ji Fang*). In recent years many of these formulae have passed into public usage, but there may be as many as 5000 licensed patent medicines still circulating in China.

Classification of Chinese herbal medicines

Chinese herbal medicines may be classified in a number of different ways:[53]

- **The four energies**: this reflects the degree of yin and yang, ranging from cold (extreme yin), cool, neutral to warm and hot (extreme yang). Following a determination of the state of balance of a patient's yin and yang the appropriate herb can be chosen. Examples include sheng di huang (rehmania root – cold), ron gui (cinnamon bark – warm/hot) and fu ling (poria – neutral).
- **The five tastes**: the five tastes are pungent, sweet, sour, bitter and salty, each of which has different functions and characteristics, e.g. pungent herbs are used to generate sweat and vitalise qi whereas sour and astringent herbs absorb body substances and control the functions of the organs. Bitter herbs reduce qi.
- **The meridians**: these refer to organs on which the herb is considered to be active. Individual herbs are thought to enter specific meridians moving towards the associated organs, e.g. da zan (Chinese date) is thought to enter the spleen and stomach meridian to tone the spleen and augment its qi.
- **The movement of herbs**: some herbs are said to move in different directions through the body. Ascending herbs influence the upper parts of the body, e.g. jie geng (platycodi root) acts on the lungs whereas herbs that descend and sink influence the lower part of the body, e.g. da huang (rhubarb) used for the relief of constipation.

CHM in practice

The prescription

Chinese medicinal substances are combined in a herbal formula that is often a complex mixture of energetic qualities, function and foci. The main aims are to:

- increase therapeutic effectiveness by synergy
- reduce toxicity or adverse reactions
- accommodate complex clinical situations
- alter the actions of the substances.

The formula

The prescription may be individualised, compounded according to a standard 'patented' formula (see below) or sold as a pre-packaged over-the-counter (OTC) product. In all cases it is usual for the formula to comprise at least four components:[54]

1. The main ingredient, which treats the main disease
2. The associate ingredient, which assists the main ingredient
3. The adjuvant, which acts as an enhancer of the main ingredient, and moderates or eliminates the toxicity of other ingredients; it may also have an opposite effect to the main ingredient to produce supplementary benefits
4. The guide ingredient (or envoy), which focuses the actions of the formula on certain meridians or areas of the body or harmonises and integrates the actions of the other ingredients.

Preparation of herbs

In preparing traditional Chinese medicines it is important that the appropriate procedures are followed carefully, otherwise the final medicine may not have the desired effect. Processing herbs to alter their properties is an ancient method used in TCM and has the following aims:

- To enhance the curative effect
- To reduce toxicity
- To change the curative properties (e.g. from cooling to warming).

For both internal and external use herb preparation may involve drying, grinding, extraction with water alcohol or oil, baking, boiling, roasting, steaming or stir frying with or without ancillary liquids (e.g. honey, ginger juice or vinegar).

Presentation

Presentations available for internal use include:

- extracts and alcoholic tinctures
- teas (boiled from 10 minutes to an hour)
- pills (made with both traditional and modern processes)
- powders, most often taken as drafts (stirring the powder into water and drinking the mix) or as large pills (6–9 g) made by mixing in honey.

Presentations available for external use (bruising, burns, sprains and wounds, etc.) include:

- liniments
- pastes (made by mixing powders with a binder, e.g. sesame oil)
- creams and ointments
- medicated plasters.

Chinese 'patent' medicine

Chinese patent medicines are standardised herbal formulae. Several herbs and other ingredients are dried and ground, mixed into a powder and then formed into little black pills using honey as a binder. Chinese patent medicines are not easy to individualise on a patient-by-patient basis. They are best used when a patient's condition is not severe and the medicine can be taken as a long-term treatment.

These medicines are not 'patented' in the western sense of the word. No one has exclusive rights to the formula. Instead, 'patent' refers to the standardisation of the formula. All Chinese patent medicines of the same name will have the same proportions of ingredients. An example is the Chinese herbal formula known as 'four gentleman decoction' (si jun zi tang).[55] This is used for fatigue, reduced appetite, loose stools, pale tongue and weak pulse, which occur because of the deficiency of spleen and stomach qi and 'dampness in the digestive system' (see Table 12.1). The formula comprises the following:

- Main herb: *Radix ginseng* (ren shen), to enhance spleen qi
- Associate: *Rhizoma atractylodis macrocephalae* (bai zhu), to strengthen the spleen and dry off the 'dampness'
- Adjuvant: *Sclerotium poriae coco*s (fu ling), to assist the main and associate herbs
- Guide: *Radix glycyrrhizae uralensis* (zhi gan cao), to harmonise the other three herbs and regulate spleen qi.

Examples of Chinese herbs used in the UK

Examples of herbs used in TCM formulae in the UK are listed in Table 12.2.

Regulatory affairs

Chinese herbalism is the most prevalent of the ancient herbal traditions currently being practised in the UK.[56] About 500 different herbal materials worth several million pounds each year are imported.[57] In addition

Table 12.2 Examples of common Chinese herbs

Source and Chinese name	Parts used	Clinical use
Agastache rugosa Hua xiang	Herb	Digestive stimulant, antiemetic
Cinnamonium spp. Rou gui	Bark	Warms, circulatory stimulant
Clematis chinensis Wei ling xian	Root	Antirheumatic, stimulant, expels wind and damp
Glycyrrhiza uralensis Gan cao	Root	Expectorant, tonic, detoxifier
Lonicera japonica Jin yin hua	Flowers	Cooling and disinfecting, antipyretic, detoxifier
Magnolia spp Xin yi hua	Bark	Digestive stimulant, expectorant
Panax ginseng Ren shen	Root	Sedative, tonic
Phellodendron amurensei Po-mu	Bark	Bitter digestive, diuretic, antipyretic
Taraxacum mongolicum Pu gong ying	Whole plant	Anti-infective, antipyretic

an unquantified amount of material enters the country illegally through smuggling in luggage.

As in western herbal medicine (Chapter 8) the regulatory framework for traditional Chinese herbal medicines includes the Medicines Act 1968 and the EU Directive for Traditional Herbal Medicinal Products (2004/24/EC).[58] The latter provides for the setting up of a Traditional Herbal Medicines Registration Scheme (THMRS) and was implemented in the UK in November 2005. Manufacturers are required to demonstrate product quality, safety and evidence of at least 30 years' traditional use for specified conditions, at least 15 years of which must have been in the EU. Products registered under the scheme are subject to pharmacovigilance requirements (Directive 2001/83/EC). Manufacturers with unlicensed products on the market before the new arrangements have until April 2011 to comply. Registration is available for traditional herbal medicines that are taken orally, for external use or inhalation. Herbal medicines intended for injection are ineligible under the scheme. The scheme allows traditional herbal remedies to be combined with vitamins and minerals, where there is evidence of safety and the action of the nutrient is ancillary to the herb, but products containing other non-herbal ingredients, other than excipients, are not covered by the THMRS.

There are a number of herbal ingredients that have accepted usage in a range of different regulatory categories besides medicines, including food, cosmetics and general consumer products. If a product is currently sold legally as a food, cosmetic or general consumer product, companies can continue to sell their products under these regimens.

In the USA, legislation now allows the import of Chinese herbal materials, as the Food and Drug Administration (FDA) has lifted earlier restrictions that limited imports to ethnic groups. This has prompted the wider availability of prepared medicines.

The use of animal parts is a controversial issue in western communities and it is currently illegal in the UK to use anything other than plant material in herbal decoctions. In China and other Asian countries the practice is still widespread, but it has been largely discontinued elsewhere after action by regulatory authorities whose enthusiasm may occasionally be misplaced.

Western CHM

In many western cities the Chinatown districts support herb shops and practices with remedies imported directly from Asia, and practitioners trained by the old system of long apprenticeship. Increasingly, local western practitioners are training in their home countries to satisfy the growing interest in CHM. In particular, acupuncturists seem to be extending their practice. There are a substantial number of traditional Chinese patent medicines, some of which have found their way to ethnic sellers in the west.

Safety

There are a number of important safety issues associated with CHM.

Competence of practitioners

Most patients who seek treatment are unable to distinguish between adequately and inadequately trained practitioners. No data exist on exactly how many practitioners now offer Chinese herbal treatment in the UK, and only some of them will belong to a professional body. The main body is the Register of Chinese Herbal Medicine (RCHM), which maintains minimum standards of training and practice. Another organisation, the Association of Traditional Chinese Medicine (ATCM), also exists to represent mainly ethnic Chinese practitioners of both acupuncture and CHM. There have been calls for statutory regulation of practitioners in the UK (Pittilo report).

Intrinsic toxicity

It is estimated that there are 7000 species of medicinal plants in China and, of the 150 species most frequently used, 10 are toxic.[59] In Hong Kong most cases of serious poisoning are related to the use of the roots of cao wu (*Aconitum kusnezoffii*), fu zi and chuan wu (*Aconitum carmichaeli*). These herbs contain variable amounts of highly toxic alkaloids, including aconitine, which activates sodium channels and causes widespread excitation of cellular membranes. Several other herbal preparations containing aconitine alkaloids, e.g. monkshood (*Aconitum* spp.), are commonly used in Chinese medicine to treat arthritic, rheumatic and musculoskeletal pain.

Quality problems

Some traditional Chinese medicines have already caused serious health problems in the UK and other developed countries and, despite initiatives from both the Medicines and Healthcare products Regulatory Agency (MHRA) and some representatives from the Chinese herbal medicine sector, problems with the quality of traditional Chinese medicines continue to arise.[60] A warning that there can be no guarantee of the safety or quality of traditional Chinese medicines was issued by the MHRA in 2004 (http://tinyurl.com/2olbvg), following a similar warning 3 years earlier. The warning was circulated again in the light of clear evidence that problems with traditional Chinese medicines containing toxic, and often illegal, ingredients persist, with the ingredients not always being declared on labels.

The herbs prescribed by practitioners of TCM in the UK are generally purchased from wholesale companies that specialise in this trade. These companies import herbs from the People's Republic of China either directly or through dealers in Hong Kong. The quality of imported herbs varies considerably, and great skill is needed to ensure that the correct herbs are provided to the practitioner. Some substitution of herbs is acceptable in China but can lead to problems if the wholesaler or practitioner is unaware of the substitution (see below). Confusion may arise over the precise identity of the herb being ordered; no standardised nomenclature exists for herbs. Fortunately, the best wholesalers and properly trained practitioners are able to make fairly reliable checks, at least visually. Unrecognised contamination by other herbs, drugs and various chemicals (including heavy metals or insecticides) is another possible hazard.

The following quality issues continue to give cause for concern:

- Inferior and incorrectly identified raw materials
- Poor storage of raw materials leading to the appearance of mycotoxins
- Intentional adulteration with orthodox drugs and other chemicals. Several examples of such practices have been reported[61] including four cases of severe acute liver injury resulting from ingestion of a slimming product[62]
- Poor processing leading to adulteration with impurities
- Deficient packaging resulting in spoilage.

The MHRA in the UK offers safety advice to potential users of herbal medicines at http://tinyurl.com/6k7q9c.

Administration during pregnancy

A number of herbs, e.g. pennyroyal (*Mentha pulegium*, *Hedeoma pulegoides*) and valerian (*Valerian wallichi*), have abortifacient properties and should be avoided during pregnancy. Their action is thought to be due to the presence of volatile oils, which can induce uterine contractions.

Administration to children

Infants are at greater risk of possible poisoning from Chinese herbal medicines than adults because of their inadequate biotransformation processes. Chinese infants are frequently given huang lian (*Coptis chinensis*) by their mothers to clear up 'products of pregnancy'. The main alkaloid of this herb is berberine and it can displace bilirubin from its serum-binding proteins, causing a rise in free bilirubin concentration and a risk of brain damage. Yin-chen hao (*Artemisia scoparia*) is used for the treatment of neonatal jaundice and has a similar effect.

Concurrent use with orthodox medicines

There are two problems here: an enhanced activity from the herbal medicine or the orthodox medicine, or both, and an intrinsic toxicity, real or threatened, from the allopathic ingredient.

Pharmacovigilance – Yellow Card ADR reporting schemes

RCHM

The Register of Chinese Herbal Medicine's Yellow Card scheme was established in order to gather safety data on Chinese herbal medicines, through identifying suspected adverse drug reactions (ADRs) to herbs. Although Chinese herbs have a long established history of use there is still relatively little present-day information on herbal safety.

MHRA

The Yellow Card scheme operated by the MHRA has been widened to encourage reporting of suspected ADRs in association with herbal medicines, including unlicensed products. Patients are now able to report suspected ADRs direct.

Evidence

A small number of RCTs in TCM have been carried out; most are of poor quality.[63] The situation may result partly from methodological difficulties, such as design and implementation of placebo-blinded trials of individualised treatments. There is also the problem of different perceptions of disease and outcome measures. In the absence of robust outcome studies of effectiveness, protagonists will continue to rely almost exclusively on circumstantial evidence obtained from case studies. Research in China has shown that CHM can be effective in several disorders and supports its provision in state hospitals throughout China, alongside conventional medicine.[64] Conditions that have been treated with TCM include atopic dermatitis[65] and the management of side effects from some chemotherapeutic agents.[66]

Other elements of TCM[67]

Chinese massage

Massage has been an important element of TCM for at least 2000 years. There are two types:

1. Tui na focusing on pushing, stretching and kneading the muscle
2. Zhi ya focusing more on pinching and pressing at acupressure points.

Chinese massage may be used to balance yin and yang and to regulate the function of qi, blood and the organs, as well as to loosen joints and relax muscles and tendons.

Dietary therapy

Chinese dietary therapy is an important part of life in the country as well as being included in many practitioners' prescriptions. Knowledgeable Chinese housewives often prepare special meals for common family ailments. Thus a patient suffering from insomnia due to a disharmony of heart and kidney might be advised to make a soup of *Lotus plumule* (lian zi xin) to nourish the heart and include morus fruit (sang shen zi) to enhance kidney essence. These measures would be in addition to other TCM treatments, e.g. CHM and/or acupuncture.

Nutritional interventions may be of three types:

1. **Supplementation**: as well as various vitamins and minerals, the range may contain animal and plant products (e.g. algae or kelp).
2. **Dietary modification**: this involves changes in dietary habits to exclude elements not considered nutritious or to establish better eating patterns.
3. **Therapeutic systems**: the inclusion (or exclusion) of foods considered to have a contributory role to the patient's health.

Examples of diets with properties beneficial to health include the following:[68]

- **White rice porridge**: this regulates the bowels (constipation and diarrhoea), for nausea and loss of appetite.
- **Sweet and sour sauce**: considered to be an important constituent of diet because of its antiseptic properties.
- **Sweet and sour crispy noodles**: noodles are a good source of nutrients for athletes and growing children. The vinegar in the sauce has antiseptic properties.

Examples of dietary remedies for common illnesses include the following:

- **Acne**: infusion of the flowers of peach (*Prunus persica*) or almond (*P. amygdalus*) in water daily.
- **Arthritis**: cinnamon tea (*Cinnamonum cassia*); for cold arthritis, sage steeped in rice wine sipped daily and for warm arthritis infusion of purslane (*Portalaca oleracea*) in water.
- **Constipation**: fig wine, stewed pears and bananas eaten cold with honey.
- **Flatulence**: seeds of mandarin orange chewed.
- **Haemorrhoids**: simmer a mixture of almonds, peach kernels, pine nuts and sesame seeds in water and drink as a soup.
- **Halitosis**: a few leaves of peppermint or the peel of a mandarin orange chewed.

Martial art therapy

This approach uses movements and exercises adapted from martial arts, such as tai ji quan and kung fu.

Qigong

This is a meditative therapy that is often combined with body movement and breathing exercises to achieve a balance of energy. Qigong is mostly taught for health maintenance purposes, but there are also some who teach it as a therapeutic intervention.

Tai ji quan (tai c'hi)

Tai c'hi consists of a series of slow flowing exercises inspired by the movement of animals, as reflected in the names given to the movements, e.g. 'white stork spreading wings'. The focus and calmness cultivated by the meditative aspect of tai c'hi are seen as necessary in maintaining optimum health (in the sense of relieving stress and maintaining homeostasis) and in application of the form as a soft style martial art.

Traditional Tibetan medicine

Tibetan medicine is reputed to be the most comprehensive form of Eurasian healthcare and the world's first truly integrative medicine. Incorporating rigorous systems of meditative self-healing and ascetic self-care from India, it includes mind–body and preventive medicine together with elements of religion and astrology.

More information

British Acupuncture Council: http://tinyurl.com/2hb9zo
British Medical Acupuncture Society: http://medical-acupuncture.co.uk/
Medical Toxicology Unit (Guy's and St Thomas' NHS Foundation Trust London), Chinese Medicine Advisory Service: http://tinyurl.com/yrmcg3
The Register of Chinese Herbal Medicine: www.rchm.co.uk

Further reading

Bensky D, Clavey S, Stoger E, Gamble A, Bensky L. *Chinese Herbal Medicine: Materia Medica*, 3rd edn. Vista, CA: Eastland Press, 2004.
Fan J-WA. *Manual of Chinese Herbal Medicine: Principles and practice for easy reference.* Boston, MA: Shambhala Publications Inc., 2003
Ho PY, Lisowski A. *Brief History of Chinese Medicine*, 2nd edn. Singapore: World Scientific Publishing Co. Pty, 1998.
Kaptchuk TJ. *Chinese Medicine: The web that has no weaver.* London: Rider (Ebury Press), 2000.
Maciocia G. *The Foundations of Chinese Medicine: A comprehensive text*, 2nd edn. London: Churchill-Livingstone Elsevier, 2005.

Teng L. Shaw D, Barnes J. Traditional Chinese herbal medicine. *Pharm J* 2006; **276**:361–3.
Williams T. *The Complete Illustrated Guide to Chinese Medicine*. Shaftsbury: Element Press, 1999
Williamson E. Systems of traditional medicine from South and South East Asia. *Pharm J* 2006;**276**:539–40.

References

1. Curran J. The Yellow Emperor's Classic of Internal Medicine. *BMJ* 2008; **336**:777.
2. Bliss B. *Chinese Medicinal Herbs*. San Francisco, CA: Georgetown Press, 1980: 3.
3. Hoizey D, Hoizey M. *A History of Chinese Medicine*. Vancouver: University Press, 1993: 42.
4. Hesketh T, Zhu WX. Health in China: Traditional Chinese medicine: one country, two systems. *BMJ* 1997;**315**: 115–17.
5. Williams T. *Chinese Medicine*. Shaftsbury: Element Books, 1996.
6. Kaptchuk TJ. *Chinese Medicine*. London: Rider, 2000: 105–41.
7. Lao L. Traditional Chinese medicine. In: Jonas WB, Levin J (eds), *Essentials of Complementary and Alternative Medicine*. Baltimore, MD: Lippincott/ Williams & Wilkins, 1999: 222–3.
8. Houghton P. The role of plants in traditional medicine and current therapy. *J Altern Compl Med* 1995;**1**:131–43.
9. Kaplan G. A brief history of acupuncture's journey to the West. *J Altern Compl Med* 1997;**3**:5–10.
10. World Health Organization Regional Office for the Pacific. *Standard Acupuncture Nomenclature*, 2nd edn. Manila: WHO Regional Office for the Pacific, 1993. Available at: http://tinyurl.com/yunc49 (accessed March 2008).
11. MacDonald AJR. *Acupuncture: From ancient art to modern medicine*. Boston: George Allen & Unwin, 1982.
12. Janovsky B, White AR, Filshie J et al. Are acupuncture points tender? A blinded study of spleen 6. *J Altern Compl Med* 2000;**6**:149–55.
13. Fulder S. *The Handbook of Alternative and Complementary Medicine*. Oxford: Oxford University Press, 1996: 126.
14. Filshie J, White AR, eds. *Medical Acupuncture, a Western Scientific Approach*. Edinburgh: Churchill Livingstone, 1998.
15. Macdonald AJR. Acupuncture and analgesia and therapy. In: Wall PD, Melzack R (eds), *Textbook of Pain*, 2nd edn. Edinburgh: Churchill Livingstone, 1989.
16. White A. The principles behind acupuncture. *Health Matters Magazine* 1999;May:30–1.
17. Ernst E, White A. Acupuncture: safety first. *BMJ* 1997;**314**:1362.
18. Herbert R, Fransen M. Management of chronic knee pain. (Editorial) *BMJ* 2007;**335**:786.
19. Marwick C. Acceptance of some acupuncture applications. *JAMA* 1997;**278**:1725–7.
20. Silvert M. Acupuncture wins BMA approval. *BMJ* 2000;**321**:11.

21.   Moore RA, McQuay H, Oldman AD, Smith LE. BMA approves acupuncture. *BMJ* 2000;**321**:1220.
22.   Chen F, Hwang S, Lee H et al. Clinical study of syncope during acupuncture treatment. *Acupunct Electrother Res* 1990;**15**:107–19.
23.   Rampes H, James R. Complications of acupuncture. *Acupunct Med* 1995;**11**:26–33.
24.   Boxall EH. Acupuncture hepatitis in the West Midlands. *J Med Virol* 1978; **2**:377–9.
25.   Hussain KK. Serum hepatitis associated with repeated acupuncture. *BMJ* 1974;**278**:41–2.
26.   Ernst E. Adverse effects of acupuncture. In: Jonas WB, Ernst E (eds), *Essentials of Complementary and Alternative Medicine*. Baltimore, MD: Lippincott/Williams & Wilkins, 1999: 172–5.
27.   MacPherson H. Fatal and adverse events from acupuncture: allegation, evidence and the implications. *J Altern Compl Med* 1999;**5**:47–56.
28.   Fisher AA. Allergic dermatitis from acupuncture needles. *Cutis* 1976;**38**:226.
29.   Castelain M, Castelain PY, Ricciardi R. Contact dermatitis to acupuncture needles. *Contact Dermatitis* 1987;**16**:44.
30.   White AR, Abbot NC, Ernst E. Self reports of adverse effects of acupuncture included cardiac arrhythmias. *Acupunct Med* 1996;**14**:121.
31.   Ogata M, Kitamura O, Kubo S, Nakasono Q. An asthmatic death while under Chinese acupuncture and moxibustion treatment. *Am J Forensic Med Pathol* 1992;**13**:338–41.
32.   Abbot NC, White AR, Ernst E. Complementary medicine. *Nature* 1996; **381**:361.
33.   Ernst E, White AR. Acupuncture for back pain: a meta analysis of randomised controlled trials. *Arch Intern Med* 1998;**158**:2235–41.
34.   van Tulder MW, Cherkin DC, Berman B et al. The effectiveness of acupuncture in the management of acute and chronic low back pain. *Spine* 1999; **24**:1113–23.
35.   Ernst E, Pittler MH. The effectiveness of acupuncture in treating acute dental pain: a systematic review. *Br Dental J* 1998;**184**:443–7.
36.   Melchart D, Streng A, Hoppe A et al. Acupuncture in patients with tension-type headache: randomised controlled trial *BMJ* 2005;**331**:376–82.
37.   Vickers A J, Rees RW, Zollman CE et al. Acupuncture for chronic headache in primary care: large, pragmatic, randomised trial *BMJ* 2004;**328**:744.
38.   Milgrom C, Finestone A, Eldad A, Shlamkovitch N. Patellofemoral pain caused by overactivity. A prospective study of risk factors in infantry recruits. *J Bone Joint Surg Am* 1991;**73**:1041–3.
39.   White A, Foster NE, Cummings M, Barlas P. Acupuncture treatment for chronic knee pain: a systematic review. *Rheumatology (Oxford)* 2007; **46**:384–90.
40.   Irnich D, Behrens N, Molzen H et al. Randomised trial of acupuncture compared with conventional massage and 'sham' laser acupuncture for treatment of chronic neck pain. *BMJ* 2001;**322**:1574–9.
41.   White AR, Ernst E. A systematic review of randomised controlled trials of acupuncture for neck pain. *Rheumatology (Oxford)* 1999;**38**:143–7.

42. Avants SK, Margolin A, Holford TR, Kosten TR. A randomised controlled trial of auricular acupuncture for cocaine dependence. *Arch Intern Med* 2000;**160**:2305–12.
43. Margolin A, Avants SK. Should cocaine abusing, buprenorphine maintained patients receive auricular acupuncture? Findings from an acute effects study. *J Altern Compl Med* 1999;**5**:567–4.
44. Diehl D. Acupuncture for gastrointestinal and hepatobiliary disorders. *J Altern Compl Med* 1999;**5**:27–45.
45. Chen HY, Shi Y, Ng CS, Chan SM, Yung KKL. Auricular acupuncture treatment for insomnia: A systematic review. *J Altern Compl Med* 2007;**13**:660–76.
46. Vickers AJ. Can acupuncture have specific effects on health? A systematic review of acupuncture antiemesis trials. *J R Soc Med* 1996;**89**:303–11.
47. Ernst E. Acupuncture as a symptomatic treatment for osteoarthritis – a systematic review. *Scand J Rheumatol* 1997;26:444–7.
48. Foster NE, Thomas E, Barlas P et al. Acupuncture as an adjunct to exercise based physiotherapy for osteoarthritis of the knee: randomised controlled trial. *BMJ* 2007;**335**:436.
49. White AR, Rampes H, Ernst E. Acupuncture for smoking cessation. *Cochrane Library* 1999;**4**:1–10.
50. Ernst E. Acupuncture/acupressure for weight reduction? A systematic review. *Wien Med Wochenschr* 1997;**109**:6–62.
51. Reston J. Now about my operation in Peking. *The New York Times* 1971;July 26:1,6.
52. Unschuld PU. *Medicine in China. A history of pharmaceuticals*. Berkeley, CA: University of California Press, 2000.
53. Williams T. *The Complete Illustrated Guide to Chinese Medicine*. Shaftsbury: Element Press, 1999: 164–5.
54. Lao L. Traditional Chinese medicine. In: Jonas WB, Levin J (eds), *Essentials of Complementary and Alternative Medicine*. Baltimore, MD: Lippincott/ Williams & Wilkins, 1999: 215.
55. Lao L. Traditional Chinese medicine. In: Jonas WB, Levin J (eds), *Essentials of Complementary and Alternative Medicine*. Baltimore, MD: Lippincott/ Williams & Wilkins, 1999: 215.
56. Vickers A, Zellman C. ABC of complementary medicine – herbal medicine. *BMJ* 1999;**319**:1050–3.
57. Houghton P. Traditional Chinese medicine: does it work? Is it safe? *Chemist Druggist* 1999;**20**:vi–vii.
58. Teng L, Shaw D, Barnes J. Traditional Chinese herbal medicine *Pharm J* 2006;**276**:361–3.
59. Chan TVK, Chan JCN, Tomlinson B, Critchley JAH. Chinese herbal medicine revisited: a Hong Kong perspective. *Lancet* 1993;**342**:1532–4.
60. Barnes J, Teng K. TCM: balancing choice and risk? *Pharm J* 2004;**273**:342.
61. Gould M. Patients warned of dangers of Chinese medicines. *BMJ* 2001; **323**:770.
62. Lai V, Thorburn D, Raman VS. Severe hepatic injury and adulterated Chinese medicines *BMJ* 2006;**332**:304.
63. Tang JL, Zhan SY, Ernst E. Review of randomised controlled trials of traditional Chinese medicine. *BMJ* 1999;**319**:160–1.

64. Dharmananda S. *Controlled Clinical Trials of Chinese Herbal Medicine: A review*. Oregon: Institute for Traditional Medicine, 1997.
65. Hon KLF, Leung TF, Ng PC et al. Efficacy and tolerability of a Chinese herbal medicine concoction for treatment of atopic dermatitis: a randomized, double-blind, placebo-controlled study. *Br J Dermatol* 2007;**157**:357–63.
66. Zhang M, Liu X, Li J, He L, Tripathy D. Chinese medicinal herbs to treat the side-effects of chemotherapy in breast cancer patients. *Cochrane Database System Rev* 2007, Issue 2. Art. No.: CD004921.
67. Lao L. Traditional Chinese medicine. In: Jonas WB, Levin J (eds), *Essentials of Complementary and Alternative Medicine*. Baltimore, MD: Lippincott/ Williams & Wilkins, 1999: 226–7.
68. Windridge C. *Tong Sing, The Chinese Book of Wisdom*. London: Kyle Cathie, 1999: 211–19.

13

Indian ayurvedic medicine

Steven B Kayne

Ayurveda and traditional Chinese medicine (TCM) have many com-
monalities. The focus of both the systems is on the patient rather than
on the disease. Both systems fundamentally aim to promote health and
enhance the quality of life, with therapeutic strategies for treatment of
specific diseases or symptoms in a holistic fashion. Almost half of the
botanical sources used as medicines have similarities; moreover, both
systems have similar philosophies geared towards enabling classification
of individuals, materials and diseases. [1]

There are about 25–30 qualified ayurvedic physicians in the UK
who are registered with the Ayurvedic Medical Association UK, which
holds malpractice insurance and maintains a code of ethics. Most of the
physicians are based in London but some of them are in areas that have
a large Asian community such as Leicester, Birmingham and Bradford.
In the USA legal licensure for any healthcare profession, including
ayurveda, is under the jurisdiction of each individual state. Currently,
none of the US states licenses ayurvedic physicians as primary care
physicians. However, many ayurvedic physicians utilise their education
and knowledge in combination with their other healthcare-related
licensed credentials.

Definition

The indigenous system of medicine in India is termed ayurveda (*ayu*
means life or longevity and *veda* means knowledge) whereas that of
Pakistan is called unani-tibb or unani for short. The two systems have
much in common and are not considered separately in this chapter.

Disease is considered to be an imbalance and its treatment involves
diverse procedures to restore optimum function and balance.
Practitioners use nutrition, yoga, exercise, complex herbal medicines
and surgical techniques reactively as therapies and proactively for the
preservation of health.

History

The origins of 'the science of life' have been placed by scholars of ancient Indian ayurvedic literature at somewhere around 6000 BC.[2] The teachings were orally transmitted for thousands of years and then written down in melodic Sanskrit poetic verses known as shlokas. Ayurveda in its first recorded form (literature known as vedas) is specifically called atharveda.

Indian medicine spread across the eastern world to Tibet, central Asia, Indo-China, Indonesia and Japan, filling the same role in Asia as Greek medicine did in the west. The surgical and medical aspects of ayurveda developed separately around the eighth century BC, and were recorded in great detail in texts (samhitas). The surgical principles of ayurveda were explained by Sushruta, considered to be the father of surgery in his particular samhita, a text known as the *Sushruta Samhita*. He described a number of techniques and instruments familiar to modern-day surgery: pre- and postoperative care, asepsis, suturing and sterilisation. He also described 141 types of surgical instruments and a number of surgical procedures, including the treatment of cataracts, haemorrhoids and bone problems, as well as techniques involved in cosmetic surgery such as rhinoplasty.[3]

The early medical aspects of ayurveda were collected and revised by Charak around the first century AD in his samhita and this work has provided the basis for future practice over the centuries. Charak's text described the significance of the vata, pitta and kapha doshas, elements that form the basis of tridosha physiology (see below), the seven tissues (dhatus) and the three excretions (malas), as well as giving information on the treatment of disease and the preparation of drugs. Other important compendia were written during the first and second centuries by Susruta and Vagbhata, who together with Charak are considered to be the great three fathers of ayurveda.

Eight specialities have developed within ayurveda:

1. General surgery (shalya tantra)
2. Ear, nose and throat (shalkya)
3. Medicine (kaya chikitsa)
4. Psychiatry (bhutvidya)
5. Obstetrics, gynaecology and paediatrics (kumar-bhritya)
6. Toxicology (agada tantra)
7. Geriatrics (rasayans)
8. Fertility and sterility (vajikaran).

Theory

Ayurvedic philosophy is based on the samkhya philosophy of creation. The word *samkhya* is derived from the Sanskrit *sat* (truth) and *khya* (to know). The main beliefs are as follows:

- There is a close relationship between humans and the universe.
- Cosmic energy is manifest in all things, both living and non-living.
- There are 24 elements of the universe.
- Cosmic consciousness is the source of all existence present as male (shiva, purusha) and female (shakti, pakritt) energy.

The general ayurvedic approach is threefold:

1. Determine the elemental constitution of the patient.
2. Identify the cause of the illness.
3. Apply therapeutic recommendations to balance any disharmonies.

Determining the constitution and the cause of illness

Ayurveda embraces certain fundamental doctrines, known as the darshnas. The body is thought of as being composed of five basic concepts:

1. The five basic elements of life
2. The three doshas (or humours), made up of the five basic elements of life
3. The seven tissues (dhatus)
4. The three waste products (malas)
5. The gastric fire.

Health is believed to comprise a balanced state of the doshas (made from five basic elements and senses), the dhatus, the malas and a gastric fire (agni), together with the clarity and balance of the mind, senses and spirit.

The basis of Ayurvedic theory is summarised in Figure 13.1.

The five basic elements and senses of life

Ayurveda considers that the universe is made up of combinations of the five elements (pancha mahabhutas). These are akasha (ether), vayu (air), teja (fire), aap (water) and prithvi (earth). The five elements can be seen to exist in the material universe at all levels of life and in both

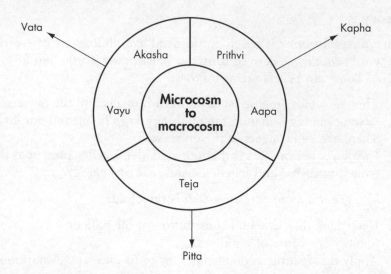

Figure 13.1 Ayurvedic principles.

organic and inorganic things. The five basic elements join together in different combinations to make up the three doshas (or humours):

1. Ether (space), represented in the hollow spaces of the mouth, nose, gastrointestinal tract, thorax, capillaries and tissues – associated with the sense of hearing (ear and speech)
2. Air, represented by movement of the various organs, i.e. expansion, contraction and pulsation – associated with touch (hand)
3. Fire, the source of heat and represented by metabolism, digestion, body heat and intelligence – associated with sight (eyes)
4. Water exists as secretions of the salivary glands and mucous membranes – associated with taste (tongue)
5. Earth, represented by solid structures of the body, i.e. bones, cartilage and muscles – associated with smell (nose).

Ether and air are said to be the vata dosha (where *dosha* means a 'principal' that is protective in health or disease producing in ill health), fire and water combine as the pitta dosha, and earth and water combine as the kaph dosha. Collectively they control all biological and psychological functions of the body, mind and consciousness. They are also responsible for emotions, including anger, compassion, fear, greed and love.

The three doshas (humours)

In biological systems, such as humans, the five basic elements outlined above are coded into three forces, which govern all life processes. These three forces (kapha, pitta and vata) are known as the three doshas or collectively the tridosha:

1. Vata (air principle) is responsible for all body movement; it represents the nervous system and controls the emotions of fear and anxiety. Vata areas include the large intestine, pelvic cavity, skin and ears.
2. Pitta (bodily fire principle) governs digestion, absorption, nutrition, skin colour, intelligence and understanding. It arouses hate and jealousy. Pitta areas include the small intestine, stomach, blood, eyes and skin. It governs all heat, metabolism and transformation in the mind and body.
3. Kapha (biological water principle) is present in the throat, chest, head, sinuses, nose, mouth, etc. It governs body resistance and biological strength, promotes wound healing and supports memory. Psychologically kapha governs greed, envy and love.

A balance of the doshas is necessary for optimal health. In childhood kapha elements associated with growth predominate; in adulthood pitta is more important, whereas as the body deteriorates in old age vata becomes more important. When there is an imbalance or disharmony in health more than one dosha may be present.

Physical constitution An individual may have one of seven different constitutions, known as *prakriti*. It is believed that prakriti (*pra* means before and *akriti* means conception) is determined at conception and depends on the permutation and combination of the doshas. Bodily features may be characterised in terms of the doshas, e.g. a person having a vata prakriti would be light-weight, tall and ill-nourished, a pitta prakriti would be characterised by moderate weight and a well-nourished appearance, and a kapha prakriti would be typically associated with a heavily built person. Examples of prakriti are presented in Table 13.1.[4]

Mental constitution Three guras or temperaments correspond to the humours that determine physical constitution, as described above, and are responsible for a person's behaviour patterns. They are, with brief examples of the main characteristics:

Table 13.1 Examples of prakriti characteristics

Characteristic	Pitta	Vata	Kapha
Body size	Medium	Slim	Large
Body weight	Medium	Low	High
Eyes	Sharp, bright, grey–green	Small, sunken, black or brown	Big, blue
Nose	Long, pointed	Uneven shape	Short, round
Skin	Oily, smooth, warm	Thin, dry, cold	Thick, oily, cool
Teeth	Medium, tender gums	Protruding, thin gums	Healthy Strong gums
Appetite	Strong	Irregular, scanty	Slow, steady
Digestion	Quick with burning	Irregular with wind	Prolonged with mucus
Taste preference	Sweet, bitter	Sweet, sour, salty	Bitter, pungent
Emotions	Anger, jealousy	Anxiety, fear	Greedy
Intellect	Accurate	Quick, careless	Slow, exact
Finance	Spends on luxuries	Poor wastes money	Thrifty, astute

1. Satvas: people with a satva temperament have healthy bodies and pure behaviour. They are often very religious, compassionate and loving.
2. Rajas: people who are interested in business, prosperity, power and prestige. They enjoy wealth and are extroverts.
3. Tamas: people who are ignorant, lazy, selfish and show little respect for others.

The seven tissues (dhatus)

The seven tissues are as follows:

1. Plasma or cytoplasm (ras), which contains nutrients from digested food
2. Blood (rakata), which governs oxygenation
3. Muscles (mamsa), which maintain the physical strength of the body
4. Bone and cartilage (asthi), which give support to the body
5. Bone marrow and nerves (majja), which fill bony spaces and facilitate communication
6. Fat (medas), responsible for body bulk
7. The sex hormones and immune system (shukra).

Each of the dhatus depends on its predecessor for good health. For good health all must function correctly.

The three waste products (malas)

These are sweat (svet), faeces (poorish) and urine (mutra). These must be produced in appropriate amounts and eliminated through their respective channels.

The gastric fire (Agni)

The final element important for healthy life is *agni*, the 'fire' that sustains vitality. Agni covers whole sequences of chemical interactions and changes in the body and mind. It has been compared with the digestive enzymes but is considered to be responsible for more than just the biochemical processes because it also maintains the health of the immune system, and destroys microorganisms and toxins in the gut.

Practice of ayurveda

Choice of treatment

After a diagnosis has been made as to the particular dysfunction or disharmony present, there are several different types of treatment available to the ayurvedic practitioner. These may all be used alone or to complement each other and include:

- dietary advice
- administration of medicines
- aromatherapy
- enemas
- massage
- mind–body interventions
- surgery.

An example of an ayurvedic treatment regimen is known as *pancha karma*.[5] It consists of five very intensive techniques designed to direct body toxins to specific sites for elimination. The five techniques are:

1. Therapeutic vomiting
2. Purgation
3. Enemas
4. Nasal aspiration of herbs
5. Therapeutic release of toxic blood.

Despite its long history, ayurveda has not been averse to change. The Indian subcontinent has been subject to countless invasions during its history, with diseases being imported from other geographical locations and techniques absorbed from other cultures.[6] During the Middle Ages, for example, heavy metals, particularly mercury, entered the ayurvedic armamentarium and were used in the treatment of syphilis, which was brought by the Portuguese. The invention of new remedies is encouraged by modern practitioners.

Dietary advice

Just as with TCM, Indian medicine places an importance on diet. Diet is considered to be particularly important for both its direct effect on the individual's physiological state and its influence on the medicine. Inadequate digestion will result in the formulation of intermediary products. It is suggested that a build-up of these intermediate products, collectively known as ama, might lead to disease. Ayurveda stresses the importance of avoiding this possibility through maintaining a diet appropriate to one's constitution and recommends the application of measures to ensure correct digestion. Food should be clean and fresh, taken in small quantities and chewed well before swallowing.

Ayurveda identifies six tastes and says that each taste is associated with an organ in the body and, when found in excess, will adversely affect the organ. The six tastes are:

1. Sweet: spleen, pancreas
2. Salty: kidney
3. Sour: liver
4. Pungent: lungs
5. Bitter: heart
6. Astringent: colon.

People are encouraged to take food appropriate to their constitution, for example:

- Vata is aggravated by astringent, bitter and pungent tastes, and balanced by salty, sour and sweet tastes. Generally most sweet fruit (including dates, figs and papaya) are found to be beneficial.
- Pitta is aggravated by pungent, salty and sour, and balanced by astringent, bitter and sweet. Sweet fruit (e.g. apples, cherries and ripe mangoes) are beneficial here too.
- Kapha is aggravated by salty, sour and sweet, and balanced by astringent, bitter and pungent. Cranberries and other astringent or sour fruit are beneficial.

Each person eats according to his or her own state of health in order to maintain harmony within the body. Thus an individual showing a pitta prakriti would benefit from 'cool' spices such as cardamom, mint or turmeric. Turmeric is especially beneficial to the liver because this is considered to be a pitta organ. Like their Chinese counterparts, Indian housewives choose – or perhaps 'prescribe' would be a better word – their dinner menus carefully with reference to prevailing environmental conditions and family activities, thus ensuring that their relations are kept in the best of health, both physically and mentally. Knowing this aim, one can appreciate the origin of the delicate balance of herbs and spices so characteristic of Indian cuisine. A number of dietary incompatibilities are recognised: milk is incompatible with bananas, fish with bread, and melons are claimed to be incompatible with most other foods.

For hypertension, the instructions might be to drink one cup of mango juice, followed an hour or so later by half a cup of warm milk, a pinch of cardamom and nutmeg, and a teaspoonful of ghee. Ghee is a butter curd product that increases the *agni* and improves assimilation. Cucumber raita may also help if taken with a meal. Cucumber is a diuretic and raita is a yoghurt-based spicy condiment that often features in Indian recipes. Ayurveda prescribes specific diets for several psychiatric disorders and for different drug therapies. For anxieties almond milk may be prescribed. It is made by soaking 10 raw almonds in water overnight, then peeling and blending them with a cup of warm milk. While in the blender a small pinch of nutmeg and saffron is added.

Administration of medicines

It should be noted that, as with Chinese herbal medicine (CHM) the term 'herbal medicine' includes animal and mineral products as well as products derived from vegetable sources. In common with other complementary and alternative therapies the type and dose of medicine chosen are influenced by the individual's constitution as well as by the nature of the disease. Other factors governing the choice of medicine include the age and strength of the patient, digestive capacity, degree of tolerance and psychological state.

There are detailed descriptions of the methods by which medicines should be prepared. One technique, known as samskara (refinement), eliminates the toxicity of the source materials, rather like the aim of serial dilution in homeopathy. Mixtures of medicines (*sumyoga*) may be administered to achieve a balanced preparation, one principle balancing another through synergism or antagonism, as with CHM. Some ingredients enhance the action, whereas others reduce the toxicity. The ayurvedic formula chyavanprash combines more than 25 finely powdered herbs in a base of honey and ghee. It is taken with food as a tonic.

Plant-based medicines   These are used by ayurvedic practitioners in a number of ways, among which are the following examples:

- In the treatment of a gastric disturbance in a person exhibiting a pitta prakriti the usual remedies black pepper (*Piper rotundum*) and ginger (*Zingiber officinale*) would be administered judiciously or not at all, because they are both considered to increase pitta and may exacerbate the imbalance.
- Tonification, or supplementation therapy, uses herbs and foods that build and nourish tissues. This is prescribed for individuals who are elderly, malnourished, chronically ill or emaciated. The timing of administration is also seen as being important. The particular formula given depends on the constitution of the patient.
- There is a range of herbal preparations available for treating women's problems. The Chinese herb dong quai (*Angelica sinensis*) is used in the treatment of many gynaecological ailments. It is said to regulate menstruation, 'tonify' the blood and relieve constipation. Again, there are various herbal mixtures tailored to the constitutional type. Table 13.2 illustrates remedies suitable for cramps in women.[7] One of the most popular herbal mixtures is known as triphala ('the three fruits'). This product is rejuvenating and strengthening for all three doshas and all seven dhatus. It is

Table 13.2 Example of constitutional treatments for cramping in women

Vat	Pit	Kapha
Blue cohosh	Camomile	Black cohosh
Cramp bark	Cramp bark	Blue cohosh
Ginger	Peppermint	Camomile
Pennyroyal	Skullcap	Cramp bark
Valerian	Squaw vine	Ginger
	Yarrow	

also a mild laxative. Triphala comprises three of the most popular ayurvedic herbs: amalaki, bibbitakiu and haritaki. It is normally taken alone, mixed with honey or as a tea an hour after the evening meal. However, being a mild diuretic, some people prefer to take it in the morning.

The medicines are supplied as mixtures of herbs in dried form, or more usually with a suitable vehicle (*anupana*) to facilitate absorption. The most usual vehicles are water, milk, honey, aloe vera and ghee. People with high cholesterol levels should be wary about taking large amounts of ghee. Herbal oils are made by introducing active principles (cloves, garlic, etc.) into a suitable oily vehicle. Herbal oils, fine powders or ghee may be administered intranasally (nasya).

Until a few years ago most traditional Asian remedies used in the UK were imported from India. Only a few local hakims (traditional healers) produced their own remedies, using imported raw materials. However, there are now several companies producing ayurvedic medicines in the UK. Many of these remedies may be purchased over the counter, by mail order through Asian and English language newspapers and the internet, or brought back from visits to the subcontinent. Licensing of the herbal remedies will be similar to CHM (see Chapter 12). A range of ayurvedic toiletries, including soap and shampoo, has appeared on the UK market.

Animal products   There is some controversy about using animal products. However, finely ground deer horn as a paste may be applied to the thoracic region and is said to be of benefit in angina.

Metals For medicinal use metals are traditionally taken internally after undergoing rigorous purification to neutralise any toxic effects. The metals are boiled in water that is then reduced in volume by evaporation. Typically 5 ml of this water is taken orally two to three times daily. The following are some examples of the medical uses of metals:

- Copper is a good tonic for the liver, spleen and lymphatics.
- Gold strengthens the nervous system.
- Silver has cooling properties and is beneficial in the treatment of excess pitta.
- Iron is beneficial for bone marrow and helps in anaemia.

Treatment with aromatherapy (see Chapter 9)

Sweet warming aromas such as musk and camphor can balance vata, whereas pitta is soothed by calming aromas such as sandalwood, jasmine and rose. Kapha is pacified by warming stimulating oils together with pungent oils such as eucalyptus, sage and thyme.

Treatment with an enema (basti)

Basti introduces medicinal remedies, including sesame oil or herbal decoctions, in a liquid medium into the rectum. Medicated enemas pacify vata and alleviate many vata disorders, such as constipation, backache, arthritis and various nervous disorders.

Treatment with massage

Nauli is a method of massaging the internal organs, particularly the colon, intestines, liver and spleen. It also helps to maintain abdominal 'fire' and keep the colon clean. A warm ayurvedic oil massage is prescribed for anxiety. Vatas should use sesame oil, pittas sunflower or coconut oil and kaphas corn oil.

Indian head massage is another specialised form of massage, sometimes known as champissage from its Indian name *champi*, which is part of the wider ayurvedic medical approach. The head, neck and facial areas are massaged with the purpose of manipulating energy channels. The goal is to clear blocks in these energy channels that cause a build-up of negative energy, which are purported to cause ailments. It claims to help stress, insomnia, ridding the body of toxins and promoting hair growth.

Mind–body interventions (see also Chapter 17)

Colour therapy Ayurvedic treatments make use of colour in their healing procedures. As the colours of the rainbow are perceived as correlating with the body tissues (dhasus) and the doshas, the vibratory energy of the colours may be used to establish psychological harmony and peace of mind. As colour is so important, patients are told to illuminate themselves and their environment in the appropriate coloured lighting. An appreciation of the colours of nature is also considered to be important.

Colours have particular properties:

- Red is stimulating and warming (kapha).
- Orange is also warming; it gives energy and strength and is stimulating (kapha).
- Yellow relieves excess vata and kapha.
- Gold is a warming colour beneficial to vata and kapha.
- Silver is cooling and soothes pitta.

Treatment with precious and semiprecious stones Gems are thought to have healing properties that can be harnessed by wearing them as jewellery or by placing them in a suitable liquid overnight and drinking the solution. It is believed that gems absorb the vitality of their owners, for example:

- Diamond strengthens immunity.
- Pearls have a cooling effect on wakening.
- Ruby strengthens concentration.
- Sapphire (blue) calms vata and kapha and stimulates pitta.

Treatment with meditation Meditation, the art of bringing harmony to body, mind and consciousness, is used to soothe the body and reduce stress. Meditation is not concentration, quite the opposite. There should be no conscious effort – the mind should be allowed to relax completely ('float') as one listens to every sound.

Treatment with yoga This is believed to calm the nervous system and balance the body, mind and spirit, as well as providing exercise. It is thought by its practitioners to prevent specific diseases and maladies by keeping the energy meridians open and maintaining life energy.

Treatment with surgery   The 'Father of Indian Surgery' is said to be Sushruta.[8] Controversy exists about the time when Sushruta lived, with estimates ranging from 1000 BC to the tenth century AD. Sushruta compiled his knowledge as the *Sushruta Samhita* (Sushruta's compendium). The book provides minute details of preoperative and postoperative care as well as other aspects of ayurvedic practice. Sushruta described surgery under eight headings:

1.   Incision (bhedana)
2.   Excision (chedana)
3.   Scarification (lekhana)
4.   Puncturing (vedhya)
5.   Probing (esana)
6.   Extraction (ahrya)
7.   Drainage or evacuation (vsraya)
8.   Suturing (sivya).

Safety

Safety of administered medicines

Intrinsic toxicity[9]

The following examples illustrate the toxicity problems of certain medicines used in traditional Indian medicine.

Khat **(Catha edulis)**   Khat is a herbal product consisting of the leaves and shoots of the shrub *Catha edulis*.[10] It is cultivated primarily in east Africa and the Arabian Peninsula, harvested and then chewed to obtain a stimulant effect. There are many different varieties of *Catha edulis* depending upon the area in which it is cultivated. The herb is chewed, smoked or drunk as an infusion. The active principles are the two alkaloids: norpseudoephedrine (cathinine) and cathinone. Khat produces a feeling of wellbeing and lessens fatigue. Although users say that the herb is not addictive, withdrawal has been known to cause lethargy and nightmares. In 1980 the World Health Organization classified khat as a drug of abuse that can produce mild-to-moderate psychological dependence, and the plant has been targeted by anti-drug organisations. It is a controlled/illegal substance in many countries. Khat is not currently controlled under the UK Misuse of Drugs Act 1971, but cathinone and cathinine are classified as class C drugs under the Act. An offence is committed if cathinone or cathinine is extracted from the plant. Although this offence has been identified there have been no successful prosecutions to date. Khat is currently licensed as a medicinal product under the Medicines Act 1968. To date khat has never been imported as a medicinal product. It can be imported legally to the UK when declared as a vegetable.

Betel **(Piper betle)**   A betel quid comprises tobacco, *Areca catechu*, saffron and lime wrapped in a leaf from the plant *Piper betle*. The quid is placed in the buccal cavity, where it stimulates salivation. It is considered to have beneficial digestive properties. A number of the ingredients are reported to be carcinogenic.

An associated practice involves chewing betel nuts, often together with tobacco, and this too is known to cause buccal carcinoma.

Heavy metals   Practitioners of traditional medicine from the Indian subcontinent have generally received 5 years' training in academic establishments. They understand well their patients' beliefs about disease, and great benefits undoubtedly arise from their practice. However, their medicines – and some cosmetics too[11] – may be hazardous due to the presence of heavy metals or other adulterants, by accident or by design.

Ayurvedic medicine uses arsenic, mercury[12] and lead[13] as active ingredients. Lead is regarded as an aphrodisiac, and has been used to counteract impotence in men with diabetes. The following are other examples:

- The product al kohl is applied as an eye cosmetic; its main ingredient is lead sulphide.
- Suma powders contain over 80% lead and are applied as a cosmetic to the conjunctival surface of infants and children, from where they may be transferred to the mouth by the hands.
- Sikor is rich in lead and arsenic; it is used as a remedy for indigestion.

Kales et al.[14] compared the relative haematopoietic toxicity of ayurvedic lead poisoning with a common form of occupational lead poisoning They found that ayurvedic poisoning produces greater haematopoietic toxicity than paint-removal poisoning. Ayurvedic ingestion should be considered in patients with anaemia. The author recommends that these patients should be screened for lead exposure and strongly encouraged to discontinue metal-containing remedies.

Following a systematic strategy to identify all stores 20 miles or less from Boston City Hall that sold ayurvedic products, Dr Robert Saper and colleagues at Harvard Medical School estimated that one of five ayurvedic products produced in south Asia and available in the area under study contained potentially harmful levels of lead, mercury and/or arsenic.[15] It is suggested that users of ayurvedic medicine may be at risk for heavy metal toxicity, and testing of ayurvedic products for toxic heavy metals should be mandatory.

Drugs   Some years ago a report appeared of a patient presenting at a hospital in Birmingham with powders from the Punjab individually wrapped in newspaper, which he was using to self-treat psoriasis.[16] High-performance liquid chromatography analysis of the powders revealed the presence of prednisolone, a prescription medicine that is potentially dangerous.

Identification of medicines

A number of problems that pharmacists and other health professionals may experience in identifying ingredients and assessing their potential toxicity in Asian remedies have been identified:[17]

- typographical errors on the label
- phonetic transliteration
- changes in nomenclature
- absence of generic names on the label
- undeclared ingredients and adulterants
- assessing the literature and finding information – *Trease and Evans' Pharmacognosy*,[9] to which frequent references are made in this chapter, provides an excellent and readily available source of information for traditional medicine practices.

Potential interactions

There is a substantial risk that patients will receive simultaneous western and traditional treatments. Patients seldom volunteer information concerning any traditional medicines being taken. A case has been reported in which a woman receiving chemotherapy for Hodgkin's disease supplemented her treatment with at least nine different ayurvedic medicines.[18] She suffered a thrombosis thought to result from an interaction between the orthodox and traditional medicines. Pharmacists can provide an extremely valuable function in this respect by intervening with advice whenever they consider it to be appropriate.

An interaction between the fruit karela (*Momordica charantia*), an ingredient of curries, and chlorpropamide has been reported.[19] Although this particular drug has been largely superseded, it serves to flag up a possible difficulty with concurrent treatment. Karela improves glucose tolerance and is therefore hypoglycaemic. There are a number of other close relatives of this plant that are also used by hakims to treat diabetes, including crushed seed kernels of the marrow (*Curcubita pepo*) and the honeydew melon (*Cucumis melo*). There is a danger that some patients may be treating their diabetes with both allopathic and traditional remedies without realising the risk of interaction.

Betel nut (see above) is prescribed by hakims either alone or in mixtures. There may be a risk of interactions between this herbal medicine and orthodox drugs.

Safety of surgical and manipulative procedures

The inclusion of surgical techniques adds another potential danger from non-sterile instruments and consulting environments, and incompetent procedures. There is also a risk from undue pressure or incorrect manipulation by inexperienced practitioners.

Evidence

As stated in Chapter 11, there are difficulties in applying western methods to proving the effectiveness of traditional therapies. The best that can be said is that ayurveda has stood the test of time and appears to have some impressive successes. Its complex nature means that practitioners require extensive training, and a proper integrated ayurvedic treatment is not something that can be bought off the shelf in a health store or, for that matter, a pharmacy.

The Indian Council of Medical Research has set up a unique network throughout India for carrying out controlled clinical trials of herbal medicines.[20] The programme is monitored by a scientific advisory group consisting of people from the ayurveda, unani and modern allopathic systems of medicine. This group contains experts in pharmacognosy, toxicology, pharmacology and clinical pharmacology, as well as clinicians and experts in standardisation and quality control. Trials are planned and protocols prepared by the whole group. All trials are comparative, controlled, randomised and double blind unless there is a reason for carrying out a single-blind study. The trials are planned by the whole group but carried out at the centres of allopathic medicine with established investigators. There are over 20 clinical trial centres throughout the country for carrying out the multicentre studies. Using this network the council has shown the efficacy of several traditional medicines, including *Picrorhiza kurroa* in hepatitis and *Pterocarpus marsupium* in diabetes.[21] As a result of these trials these traditional medicines can be used in allopathic hospitals.

The Central Council of India systems of medicine oversees research institutes, which evaluate treatments. The government is adding 10 traditional medicines into its family welfare programme, funded by the World Bank and the Indian government. These medicines are for anaemia, oedema during pregnancy, postpartum problems such as pain, uterine and abdominal complications, difficulties with lactation, nutritional deficiencies and childhood diarrhoea.[22]

New regulations were introduced in July 2000 to improve Indian herbal medicines by establishing standard manufacturing practices and quality control. The regulations outline requirements for infrastructure, labour, quality control and authenticity of raw materials, and absence of contamination. Of the 9000 licensed manufacturers of traditional medicines, those who qualify can immediately seek certification for good manufacturing practice. The remainder have 2 years to comply with the regulations and to obtain certification.

The government has also established 10 new drug-testing laboratories for Indian systems of medicine and is upgrading existing laboratories to provide high-quality evidence to the licensing authorities of the safety and quality of herbal medicines. This replaces an ad hoc system of testing that was considered unreliable. Randomised controlled clinical trials of selected prescriptions for Indian systems of medicine have been initiated. These will document the safety and efficacy of the prescriptions and provide the basis for their international licensing as medicines rather than simply as food supplements.[23]

A randomised, double-blind, placebo-controlled, parallel group monocentre trial with 182 patients investigated the efficacy and toxicity of an orally administered ayurvedic formulation for rheumatoid arthritis.[24] It was concluded that the preparation was not significantly superior to a strong placebo response except for joint swelling, although improvement in the group taking active medicine was numerically superior at all evaluation time points. Other trials have shown some promise in the treatment of bronchial asthma[25,26] and angina.[27] It is claimed that ayurveda, can be used effectively in combination with modern medicine to provide better treatment of cancer.[28]

Integration with western medicine

The Indian Medicine Central Council was established by a 1970 Act to oversee the development of Indian systems of medicine and to ensure good standards of training and practice. Training for Indian medicine is given in separate colleges, which offer a basic biosciences curriculum followed by training in a traditional system. Recently the Department of Indian Systems of Medicine has expressed concern over the substandard quality of education in many colleges, which in the name of integration have produced hybrid curricula and graduates unacceptable to either modern or traditional standards. The department has made it a priority to upgrade training in Indian systems of medicine.[29]

Purists in ayurveda and unani oppose this trend to modernise their systems, particularly when such integration is carried out by experts in allopathy.[30] They have no objection to the use of modern concepts of the methodology of clinical trials in evaluating the efficacy and side effects of herbal preparations used in the traditional systems. Such clinical evaluation is essential because the remedies used in these systems will not be used in allopathic hospitals in a country such as India unless these have shown efficacy in well-controlled trials. However, carrying out randomised, double-blind multicentre trials with standardised extracts is a slow and laborious process. Furthermore, not all herbal medicines need to undergo this rigorous trial because these preparations are already in use. The situation is still further complicated because the randomised trial may not be totally appropriate for the evaluation of medicines from the traditional systems, where the prakriti (ayurveda system) or mijaj (unani system) of the individual determines the specific therapy to be used.

Examples of common ayurvedic medicines

Some examples of herbal ingredients used in the preparation of common ayurvedic medicines in the UK are provided in Table 13.3.[31]

Table 13.3 Examples of herbs used in the UK for ayuverdic medicines

Source material	Indian name	Parts used	Main constituent	Example of use
Azadirachta indica	Neem	Seeds, oil	Alkaloids Glycosides	Anthelmintic, antiseptic, astringent
Abrus precatorius	Ghungchi rati	Root, seeds	Alkaloids	Abortifacient Eye inflammation, oral contraceptive
Allium cepa	Tukhm piyaz	Seeds	Volatile oils (allyl sulphate)	Diuretic, expectorant Poultice
Artemesia absinthium Artemesia indica	Afsentin roomi Nagdoona	Leaves	Sesquiterpines, lactones, bitters	Anthelmintic, tonic
Bombax celba	Mush simbhal	Gum, root	Glycosides, tannins	Hepatic dysfunction Menorrhagia
Cassia absus	Chaksu	Seeds	Alkaloids	Astringent Eye inflammation Ringworm
Crocus sativus	Zafran (saffron)	Flower styles	Volatile oil	Catarrh Enlarged liver
Cyperus rotundus	Nutgrass	Root, seeds	Sesquiterpenes	Antiemetic Anti-inflammatory Antipyretic
Ferula galbaniflua	Jawashir	Oleo gum resin	Sesquiterpenes	Asthma, bronchitis Dysentery Menstrual irregularities
Ficus benghalensis	Anjir jangli	Root Bark	Glycosides Triterpenes	Bark: tonic, diuretic Root: diarrhoea and hypoglycaemic
Hedera nepalense	Bikh tablab	Fruit	Triterpenoid saponins	Rheumatism
Mallotus philippensis	Kamala	Fruit	Resin	Anthelmintic Oral contraceptive Red dye
Mentha piperita	Paparaminta	Leaves	Volatile oil	Cough and fever Diarrhoea, flatulence Nausea and vomiting
Quercus infectoria	N/A	Galls	Tannins	Haemorrhoids – ointments and suppositories
Rosmarinus officinalis	Rusmari	Leaves	Volatile oil	Pulmonary infections Oil – toothache, rheumatism
Salvia officinalis	Bahaman surkh	Leaves	Volatile oil	Gargle, gingivitis Treatment of thrush

Table 13.3 Continued

Source material	Indian name	Parts used	Main constituent	Example of use
Solanum indicum	Bari-khatai, barhanta	Fruiting plant	Steroidal alkaloids	Chest and urinary infections Skin conditions (paste)
Tephrosia purpurea	Sarphunkha	Whole plant	Flavonoids	Cystitis Dysentery Facial oedema
Vitex agnus castus	Remuka	Fruit	Flavonols	Diuretic Stimulant
Zingiber officinalis	Zanjibil	Rhizome	Oleo resin	Antiemetic, bronchitis, rheumatism

Examples of common ayurvedic treatments[32]

By the very nature of the philosophy surrounding the practice of ayurvedic medicine it should not really be possible to treat conditions purely symptomatically. However, Table 13.4 gives a brief list of treatments to illustrate the general approach to herbal treatment.

Table 13.4 Examples of ayurvedic treatments for some common conditions

Condition	Typical herbal treatment	Other treatments
Acne	Herbs – kutki, guduchi, shatavari Aloe vera juice Tea – cumin, coriander and fennel	Apply melon to the skin Yoga postures Breathing exercises
Anxiety	Calming tea – valerian, musta	Relaxing bath Almond milk Acupressure
Athlete's foot	Tea tree oil Aloe vera gel and turmeric	Wash with neem soap Neem oil applied
Boils	Neem powder paste Triphala wash For diabetics: neem, turmeric, kutki taken orally	Cooling, healing paste of sandalwood and turmeric Poultice of cooked onions to draw Liver cleanser (aloe vera gel)
Diarrhoea	Ghee, nutmeg, ginger, sugar Ginger powder with sugar. Mix and chew	
Eye problems		Cool water wash Gaze into the flame of a traditional ghee lamp

Table 13.4 *Continued*

Condition	Typical herbal treatment	Other treatments
Jet lag	One hour before flight – ginger On flight – drink water After flight – rub warm sesame oil on scalp	
Sore throat	Gargle – turmeric and hot water Ginger–cinnamon–liquorice tea	Avoid dairy produce Yoga postures Breathing exercises

More information

National Ayurvedic Medical Association: www.ayurveda-nama.org
National Institute of Ayurvedic Medicine: http://tinyurl.com/2qd89j
The Ayurvedic Institute: www.ayurveda.com
Unani Herbal Healing: http://www.unani.com/
Ayurvedic Medical Association UK, 59 Dulverton Road, Selsdon, South Croydon, Surrey CR2 8PJ. Tel: 0208 657 6147; fax: 0208 333 7904; email: Dr.N.S.Moorthy@ayurvedic.demon.co.uk

Further reading

Godagama S. *Ayurveda*. London: Kyle Cathie, 2001.
Williamson E. Ayurveda: introduction for pharmacists. *Pharm J* 2006;**276**:108–10.

References

1. Patwardhan B, Warude D, Pushpangadan P, Bhatt N. Ayurveda and traditional Chinese medicine: A comparative overview. *eCAM* 2005;**2**:465–473. Available at: http://tinyurl.com/yo8b32 (accessed 22 October 2007).
2. Sodhi V. Ayurveda: the science of life and mother of the healing arts. In: Pizzorno J Jr, Murray M T (eds), *Textbook of Natural Medicine*, 2nd edn. Edinburgh: Churchill Livingstone, 1999: 257–8.
3. Rana RE. Arora history of plastic surgery in India. *J Postgrad Med* 2002;**48**: 76–8.
4. Lad V. *The Complete Book of Ayurverdic Home Remedies*. London: Patkus, 1999: 18–19.
5. Packard CC. *Pocket Guide to Ayurvedic Healing*. Freedom, CA: Crossing Press, 1996: 111.
6. Glazier A. A landmark in the history of ayurveda. *Lancet* 2000;**356**:1118–22.
7. Jonas W B, Ernst E. *Essentials of CAM. Introduction: Evaluating the safety of complementary and alternative products and practices*. Baltimore, MD: Lippincott/Williams & Wilkins, 1999: 89–107.

8. Tewari M, Shukla HS. Sushruta: 'The Father of Indian Surgery'. *Indian J Surg* 2005;**67**:229–30.

9. Aslam M. Asian medicine and its practice in Britain. In: Evans WC (ed.), *Trease and Evans' Pharmacognosy*, 14th edn. London: WB Saunders, 1996: 489–91.

10. *Report of the Advisory Council On The Misuse of Drugs*. London: The Home Office, 2005. Available online at http://tinyurl.com/6h7zck (accessed 1 May 2008).

11. Aslam M, Davis SS, Healy MA. Heavy metals in some Asian medicines and cosmetics. *Public Hlth* 1979;**93**:274–84.

12. Kew J, Morris C, Athie A et al. Arsenic and mercury intoxication due to Indian ethnic remedies. *BMJ* 1993;**306**:306–7.

13. Keen RW, Deacon AC, Delves HT et al. Indian herbal remedies for diabetes as a cause of lead poisoning. *Postgrad Med* 1994; 70: 113–14.

14. Kales SN, Christophi CA, Saper RB. Hematopoietic toxicity from lead-containing Ayurvedic medications. *Med Sci Monit* 2007;**13**:CR295–8.

15. Saper RB, Kales SN, Paquin J et al. Heavy metal content of ayurvedic herbal medicine products. *JAMA* 2004;**292**:2868–73.

16. Barnes AR, Paul CJ, Secrett PC. Adulteration of Asian alternative medicines. *Pharm J* 1991;**247**:650.

17. Aslam M. Problems of identity with traditional Asian remedies. *Pharm J* 1992; **248**:20–1, 23.

18. Fletcher J, Aslam M. Possible dangers of Ayurvedic herbal remedies. *Pharm J* 1991;**247**:456.

19. Aslam M, Stockley IH. Interaction between curry ingredient (Karela) and a drug (chlorpropamide). *Lancet* 1979;i:607.

20. Indian Council of Medical Research. *Annual Report of Council 1998–99*. New Delhi: Indian Council of Medical Research.

21. Atherton DJ. Towards the safer use of traditional remedies. *BMJ* 1994;**308**: 673–4.

22. Kumar S. India's government promotes traditional healing practices. *Lancet* 2000;**335**:1252.

23. Hoizey D, Hoizey M. *A History of Chinese Medicine*. Vancouver: University BC Press, 1993: 42.

24. Chopra A, Lavin P, Patwardhan B, Chitre D. Ayurvedic medicine reduces joint swelling in patient with rheumatoid arthritis. *J Rheumatol* 2000;**27**:1365–72.

25. Sekhar AV, Gandhi DN, Rao NM, Rawal UD. An experimental and clinical evaluation of anti-asthmatic potentialities of Devadaru compound (DC). *Indian J Physiol Pharmacol* 2003;**47**:101–7. PubMed

26. Gupta I, Gupta V, Parihar A, Gupta S, Ludtke R, Safayhi H. Effects of *Boswellia serrata* gum resin in patients with bronchial asthma: results of a double-blind, placebo-controlled, 6-week clinical study. *Eur J Med Res* 1998; **3**:511–14. PubMed

27. Kumar PU, Adhikari P, Pereira P, Bhat P. Safety and efficacy of Hartone in stable angina pectoris – an open comparative trial. *J Assoc Physicians India* 1999;**47**:685–9. PubMed

28.   Garodia P, Ichikawa H, Malani N, Sethi G, Aggarwal BB. From ancient medicine to modern medicine: ayurvedic concepts of health and their role in inflammation and cancer. *Oncology* 2007;**5**:25–37.

29.   Department of Indian Systems of Medicines and Homoeopathy. *Annual Report 1999–2000*. Department of Indian Systems of Medicines and Homoeopathy, 2000. Available at: http://mohfw.nic.in/ismh/ (accessed 25 October 2000).

30.   Chaudhury RR. Commentary: challenges in using traditional systems of medicine. *BMJ* 2001;**322**:167.

31.   Aslam M. Asian medicine and its practice in Britain. In: Evans WC (ed.), *Trease and Evans' Pharmacognosy*, 14th edn. London: WB Saunders, 1996: 491–504.

32.   Lampert N. Letter. *Lancet* 2001;**357**:802.

Part 4

Other therapies and
diagnostic techniques

14

Naturopathy and its associated therapies

Steven B Kayne

Naturopathy is not widely practised in the UK, but the therapy is very popular in many other English-speaking countries, including Australia, New Zealand, South Africa and North America, where naturopathic physicians have either 'licensure' or state-mandated 'registration' in 13 US states. In Canada, naturopathic medicine is an emerging profession that is gaining formal recognition, including regulation in four provinces so far. Although naturopathic medicine has undergone significant growth and legitimisation, it still faces substantial challenges to acceptance as a fully fledged healthcare profession within the Canadian healthcare system.[1]

Definition

Naturopathy is a multidisciplinary approach to healthcare that recognises the body's innate power to heal itself. It is primarily a preventive discipline with education in the basics of healthcare as one of its most important goals. The philosophy of naturopathic medicine also includes the treatment of disease through the stimulation, enhancement and support of the inherent healing capacity of the person.

History

Naturopathy can trace its origins back to doctors Bernard Lust and Robert Foster, who worked in the USA around the turn of the nineteenth century. American doctors disillusioned with contemporary procedures were joined by a number of European immigrants involved in natural cures. In the following years the popularity of naturopathy became cyclical, with periods of intense interest and scepticism. At one time there were thousands of practitioners, numerous journals and much informed debate. In recent years the discipline has enjoyed a revival, particularly in the countries stated above. In the UK there are currently around 400 practitioners, with qualifications recognised by the General Council and Register of Naturopaths.

Theory

Naturopaths work from the premise that the body needs certain basics to function properly: the correct nutrients, adequate rest and relaxation, appropriate exercise, fresh clean air, clean water and sunlight. They are skilled in adapting natural health programmes to patients' unique requirements.

There are considered to be six important principles for naturopathic practice:[2]

1. The healing power of the body (*vis medicatrix naturae*) has the ability to establish, maintain and restore health.
2. The cause of the illness must be identified and treated (*tolle causam*) – underlying causes of a disease must be discovered and removed; symptoms are not the cause of a disease, and the causes of diseases include physical, mental, emotional and spiritual factors, which all must be dealt with.
3. First do no harm (*primum no nocere*) – therapeutic action should be complementary to and synergistic with the healing process.
4. Treat the whole person.
5. The physician as teacher (*docere*) – he or she should create a healthy interpersonal physician–patient relationship.
6. Prevention is the physician's aim and the best cure; naturopathy is the building of health rather than fighting the disease.

Professor Hans Selye of Montreal was the first to postulate the concept of a general adaptation syndrome, by which an individual reacts positively to an episode of injury or disease. According to Selye the body's response to any physical or emotional stress initiates a three-phase sequence:

1. Alarm: there is pain from an injury
2. Shock: from bad news
3. Inflammation: due to friction.

Naturopaths attach great importance to the body's adaptive capacity and recognise that symptoms such as inflammation, fever and pain are signs of the defences at work and should not be suppressed. Furthermore, the process of recovery from chronic ailments may necessitate a return to the stage of resistance, known in natural therapy as the healing crisis. As the body adjusts to the crisis, there is a stage of resistance in which the body adapts to withstand the stimulus. If the stresses are prolonged and the body is no longer able to adapt, it becomes exhausted and collapse or degeneration occurs.

The contribution of emotions to the cause of physical illness is considered carefully by many naturopaths, with a variety of counselling and psychological approaches being adopted.

Practice of naturopathy

While recognising the limitations of our modern world, the naturopath seeks to assist patients to create a healthier diet and lifestyle that will help their health return. Thus, a cold might be considered as being self-limiting and not treated directly, but the patient will be supported in a return to good health using various naturopathic measures. In degenerative disease the body may be supported in its compensatory reorganisation of function.

Information is gathered during a consultation by the usual complementary techniques of listening, observing, questioning and physical examination, so that an overall impression of the patient and his or her particular requirements may be obtained. Factors such as hereditary tendencies, constitution and previous treatments are considered to be particularly important in choosing an appropriate course of action. Iridology (see Chapter 16) is a valuable diagnostic tool of the naturopath. Some therapists use iridology as a basis for recommending dietary supplements and/or herbs.

Naturopaths use a variety of treatments, including dietary advice, nutritional supplements, detoxification, hands-on work (such as osteopathy and massage), herbs, homeopathic remedies and hydrotherapy, which can be summarised as follows:

- Nutrition: dietetics, nutritional supplements and the maintenance of optimum health through good wholesome food (see below)
- Hydrotherapy: hot and cold water treatments to encourage circulation (see below)
- Detoxification: cleansing programmes that allow healing to take place (see below)

- Physical therapy: to restore structural balance and improve tissue tone; may include gentle manipulation, massage and ultrasound, and exercise (see Chapter 16)
- Administration of homeopathic or herbal medicines (see Chapters 7 and 8)
- Minor surgery: in some countries naturopaths may perform simple surgical procedures, e.g. removal of warts.

The particular portfolio of therapies chosen will depend on factors other than those found during the consultation process, e.g. when treating diabetes naturopathic physicians prescribe comprehensive therapeutic lifestyle change recommendations – dietary counselling, stress reduction techniques and exercise. In addition patients receive prescriptions for botanical and nutritional supplementation, often in combination with conventional medication. Naturopathic medicine as a whole medical system supplies evidence-based lifestyle recommendations as suggested in management guidelines for diabetes, hypertension and hyperlipidaemia, set forth by the respective national organisations. The authors recommend that there should be an increased research effort to determine the safety and efficacy of combinations of supplements or medications and supplements if warranted.[3]

The time spent with a naturopath is variable. Typically a first consultation can take 1–2 h. Subsequent repeat sessions may last only half an hour.

Evidence

As a result of the complex nature of naturopathy, research on its practice as a complete therapy has rarely been studied. A paper by Jagtenberg et al.[4] presents the voices of tradition-sensitive naturopathic practitioners in response to what they perceive as an ideological assault by advocates of evidence-based medicine (EBM) on the validity and integrity of natural medicine practice. Those natural medicine practices, which have tradition-based paradigms articulating vitalistic and holistic principles, may have significant problems in relating to the idea of EBM as developed in biomedical contexts. The paper questions the appropriateness of imposing a methodology that appears to minimise or bypass the philosophical and methodological foundations of natural medicine, and itself seems primarily driven by political considerations.

Qualifications

Membership of the British Naturopathic Association is open to any practitioner who has a Naturopathic Diploma after completing a course in naturopathy accredited by the General Council and Register of Naturopaths and who is registered with that body. Such courses are currently offered by the British College of Naturopathy and Osteopathy and the College of Osteopaths Educational Trust. There is also a modular postgraduate course available from the British Naturopathic and Osteopathic Association.

Naturopathic physicians (NDs) in North America are primary care providers trained in conventional medical sciences, diagnosis and treatment, and experts in natural therapeutics. They diagnose and treat conditions typically seen in a 'first contact' setting. They are not trained in the advanced use of highly technical conventional therapies for life-threatening diseases. Rather, they focus primarily on health issues encountered in outpatient ambulatory care settings. Although some tools of naturopathic practice differ from those of conventional practice, the goals of naturopathic medicine parallel those of family medicine in providing for and maintaining the wellbeing of both the patient and the healthcare system as a whole.[5]

In the absence of universal regulation of naturopathy, another group of practitioners (the so-called 'traditional naturopaths') has emerged. Traditional naturopaths are guided by the same naturopathic philosophies and principles as board-licensed naturopathic physicians and often prescribe similar treatments, but do so as alternative or complementary practitioners rather than as primary care providers. Some may voluntarily join a professional organisation, but these organisations do not accredit educational programmes in any meaningful way or license practitioners as such. The training programmes for traditional naturopaths can vary greatly, are less rigorous and do not provide the same basic and clinical science education as naturopathic medical schools do.[6]

Therapies used in naturopathy

Detoxification therapy

In naturopathy it is believed that a common cause of all diseases is the accumulation of waste and poisonous matter in the body resulting from overeating. Most people eat too much and follow sedentary occupations that do not permit sufficient and proper exercise for the utilisation of this large quantity of food. The surplus food overburdens the digestive and assimilative organs and clogs up the system with impurities or poisons.

On the basis of a comprehensive dietary anamnesis, it is often possible to identify foodstuffs and eating behaviour capable of aggravating the patient's symptoms.[7] The underlying basic principle of treatment is that the gastrointestinal tract first undergoes a temporary period of rest before being gradually re-accustomed to a biologically high-quality diet. Digestion and elimination become slow and the functional activity of the whole system is deranged A central approach includes various forms of fasting therapy, in particular in the case of severe conditions, which can usefully be supported by additional relaxation techniques, psychotherapy, hydrotherapy, massage and special manual techniques.

Practice of detoxification therapy[8]

Detoxification programmes are often used to assist a transition from an unhealthy lifestyle to a healthier one. There are a number of stages involved:

- Initiating the cleansing process through elimination of the offending substances and application of a formal cleansing procedure through dietary modification and fasting
- Facilitating elimination through normal excretion (e.g. colonic cleansing and increased fluid intake to stimulate urine flow)
- Nutritional supplementation
- Return to healthier lifestyle and diet.

Safety

Detoxification over extended periods can lead to a risk of nutritional deficiencies.

Chelation therapy

Chelation therapy is used to rid the body of toxic metals (e.g. arsenic, cadmium, lead, mercury and nickel), which can cause disruption of basic cell function. Signs of metal poisoning include headaches, dizziness, memory impairment, irritability and weight loss. Chelation is the incorporation of a metal ion into a heterocyclic ring structure. More than 10 000 chelating agents exist, but only 7 or 8 are available for administration to humans by intravenous infusion.

Lead, cadmium and nickel may be removed with calcium disodium ethylenediaminetetra-acetic acid (disodium EDTA, a synthetic amino acid with chelating properties), meso-2,3-dimercaptosuccinic acid (DMSA) or D-penicillamine. DMSA is also used for removing arsenic and mercury. Treatment is usually associated with the administration of various supplements (vitamins, minerals, etc.).

Chelation therapy may be useful in various coronary and vascular diseases.[9]

Hydrotherapy[10]

Water has been used as a valuable therapeutic agent since time immemorial. In all major ancient civilisations, bathing was considered an important measure for the maintenance of health and prevention of disease. It was also valued for its remedial properties.

History

The ancient vedic literature in India contains numerous references to the efficacy of water in the treatment of disease. In modern times, the therapeutic value of water was popularised by Vincent Priessnitz, Father Sebastian Kneipp, Louis Kuhne and other European water-cure pioneers. They raised water cure to an institutional level and employed it successfully for the treatment of almost every known disease. There are numerous spas and *Bads* in most European countries where therapeutic baths are used as a major healing agent. Water exerts beneficial effects on the human system. It is claimed to have beneficial effects on circulation, to boost muscular tone and to aid digestion and nutrition. Hydrotherapy may also be of great value in restoring a better range of joint motion through a combination of pain relief, muscle relaxation and stretching exercises.[11]

Practice of hydrotherapy

The main methods of water treatment that can be employed in the healing of various diseases are described below.

Enemas Rectal irrigation or enema involves the injection of 1–2 l of warm water into the rectum and is used for cleaning the bowels. After

5–10 min, the water can be ejected together with the accumulated morbid matter.

A cold-water enema is helpful in inflammatory conditions of the colon, especially in cases of dysentery, diarrhoea, ulcerative colitis, haemorrhoids and fever.

A hot-water enema is beneficial in relieving irritation caused by inflammation of the rectum and painful haemorrhoids. It also benefits women in leukorrhoea.

Compresses

Cold compresses

A cold compress is claimed to be an effective means of controlling inflammatory conditions of the liver, spleen, stomach, kidneys, intestines, lungs, brain and pelvic organs. It is also advantageous in cases of fever and heart disease. It is generally applied to the head, neck, chest, abdomen and back.

Heating compresses

A heating compress consists of three or four folds of linen cloth wrung out in cold water, applied to the affected area, and then completely covered with a dry flannel or blanket to prevent the circulation of air and help accumulation of body heat. A compress is sometimes applied for several hours. A heating compress can be applied to the throat, chest, abdomen and joints. A throat compress relieves sore throat, hoarseness, tonsillitis, pharyngitis and laryngitis. An abdominal compress helps those suffering from gastritis, hyperacidity, indigestion, jaundice, constipation, diarrhoea, dysentery and other ailments relating to the abdominal organs. A chest compress, also known as a chest pack, relieves cold, bronchitis, pleurisy, pneumonia, fever, cough, etc. whereas a joint compress is helpful for inflamed joints, rheumatism, rheumatic fever and sprains.

Baths   The common water therapy temperature chart is cold 10–18°C, neutral 32–36°C and hot 40–45°C. Above 45°C, water loses its therapeutic value and is destructive.

Hip baths

A hip bath involves only the hips and the abdominal region below the navel. A special type of tub is used for this purpose. A cold hip bath (10–18°C) is a routine treatment in many diseases. It relieves constipation, indigestion and obesity, and helps the eliminative organs to function properly.

A hot hip bath (40–45°C) is generally taken for 8–10 min. It helps to relieve painful menstruation, pain in the pelvic organs, painful urination, inflamed rectum or bladder, and painful piles. It also benefits an enlarged prostatic gland, painful contractions or spasm of the bladder, sciatica, and neuralgia of the ovaries and bladder. It is recommended that a cold shower be taken immediately after the hot hip bath.

A neutral hip bath (32–36°C) is generally taken for 20–60 min. It helps to relieve all acute and subacute inflammatory conditions, such as acute catarrh of the bladder and urethra and subacute inflammations in the uterus, ovaries and tubes. It also relieves neuralgia of the fallopian tubes or testicles, and painful spasms of the vagina. It is used as a sedative treatment for sexual hyperactivity in both sexes.

In an alternative hip bath, also known as a revulsive hip bath, the patient sits in a hot tub for 5 min and then in a cold tub for 3 min. The duration of the bath is generally 10–20 min. The head and neck are kept cold with a cold compress. The treatment ends with a dash of cold water to the hips. This bath relieves chronic inflammatory conditions of the pelvic viscera such as salpingitis, inflammation of the ovaries, cellulitis and various neuralgias of the genitourinary organs, sciatica and lumbago.

Spinal bath

A spinal bath is another important form of hydrotherapy treatment. This bath provides a soothing effect on the spinal column and thereby influences the central nervous system. It is given in a specially designed tub with a raised back in order to provide proper support to the head. The bath can be administered at cold, neutral and hot temperatures. The water level in the tub should be 4–5 cm and the patient should lie in it for 3–10 min.

A cold spinal bath relieves irritation, fatigue, hypertension and excitement. It is beneficial in almost all nervous disorders, such as hysteria, fits, mental disorders, loss of memory and tension. The neutral spinal bath is a soothing and sedative treatment, especially for the hyperactive or irritable patient. It is the ideal treatment for insomnia and also relieves tension of the vertebral column. The duration of this bath is 20–30 min.

A hot spinal bath, on the other hand, helps to stimulate nervous individuals, especially when they are in a depressed state. It also relieves vertebral pain in spondylitis and muscular backache. It relieves sciatic pain and gastrointestinal disturbances of gastric origin.

Foot baths

In this method, the patient keeps his or her legs in a tub or bucket filled with hot water at a temperature of 40–45°C. Before taking this bath, a glass of water should be taken and the body should be covered with a blanket so that no heat or vapour escapes from the foot bath. The head should be protected with a cold compress. The duration of the bath is generally 5–20 min. The patient should take a cold shower immediately after the bath.

A hot foot bath stimulates the involuntary muscles of the uterus, intestines, bladder, and other pelvic and abdominal organs. It also relieves sprains and ankle joint pains, headaches caused by cerebral congestion and colds. In women it helps restore menstruation, if suspended, by increasing the supply of blood, especially to the uterus and ovaries.

For a cold foot bath, 7–10 cm of cold water is placed in a small tub or bucket and the patient's feet completely immersed in the water for 1–5 min. Friction is continuously applied to the feet during the bath, either by an attendant or by the patient by rubbing one foot against the other. A cold foot bath, taken for 1–2 min, helps in the treatment of sprains, strains and inflamed bunions when taken for longer periods.

Steam bath

A steam bath is one of the most important time-tested water treatments and induces perspiration in a natural way. The patient first takes one or two glasses of water and then sits on a stool inside a specially designed cabinet. The duration of the steam bath is generally 10–20 min or until perspiration takes place. A cold shower is taken immediately after the bath.

A steam bath helps to eliminate morbid matter from the surface of the skin. It also improves the circulation of the blood and tissue activity. It relieves rheumatism, gout, uric acid problems and obesity. A steam bath is helpful in all forms of chronic toxaemias. It also relieves neuralgias, chronic nephritis, infections, tetanus and migraine.

Immersion bath

An immersion bath, also known as a full bath, is administered in a bath tub that can be neutral, hot, graduated or alternative.

A cold immersion bath may last from 4 s to 20 min at a temperature ranging from 10°C to 23.8°C. This bath helps to bring down fever. It also improves the skin when taken for 5–15 s after a prolonged hot bath, by exhilarating circulation and stimulating the nervous system. This bath should not be given to young children or very elderly people, or taken in cases of acute inflammation of some internal organs such as acute peritonitis, gastritis, enteritis and inflammatory conditions of the uterus and ovaries. The literature reveals three randomised controlled trials (RCTs) of the use of hydrotherapy in the treatment of chronic venous insufficiency.[12] Two applied cold-water stimuli alone, or in combination with warm water, and suggested beneficial effects for the condition.

In a graduated bath the patient enters the bath at a temperature of 31°C. The water temperature is gradually lowered at the rate of 1°C/min until it reaches 25°C. The bath continues until the patient starts shivering. A graduated bath is intended to avoid the nervous shock caused by a sudden plunge into cold water. This bath is often administered every 3 h in cases of fever. It effectively brings down the temperature, except in malarial fever. It also produces a general tonic effect, increases vital resistances and energises the heart.

A neutral bath is given for 15–60 min at a temperature of 26–28°C. It can be given over a long duration, without any ill effects, because the water temperature is akin to body temperature. A neutral bath diminishes the pulse rate without modifying respiration. As a neutral bath excites activity of both the skin and the kidneys, it is recommended in cases relating to these organs. It helps those suffering from chronic diarrhoea and chronic afflictions of the abdomen.

A hot bath can be taken for 2–15 min at a temperature of 36.6–40°C. Before entering the bath, the patient should drink cold water and also wet the head, neck and shoulders with cold water. A cold compress should be applied throughout the treatment. This bath can be advantageously employed to relieve capillary bronchitis and bronchial pneumonia in children. It is also invaluable in the treatment of chronic rheumatism and obesity.

Epsom salt bath

The immersion bath tub should be filled with about 135 l of hot water at 40°C. Epsom salts (1–1.5 kg) should be dissolved in this water. The patient should drink a glass of cold water, cover the head with a cold towel and then lie down in the tub, completely immersing the trunk, thighs and legs for 15–20 min. The best time to take this bath is just before retiring to bed. It is traditionally claimed to be useful in cases of sciatica, lumbago, rheumatism, diabetes, neuritis, cold and catarrh, kidney disorders, and other uric acid and skin affections.

Balneotherapy (spa treatment, mineral baths)

The term 'balneotherapy' has gradually come to be applied to everything relating to spa treatment, including the drinking of waters (see below) and the use of hot baths and natural vapour baths, as well as of the various kinds of mud and sand used for hot applications.[13] In addition it includes the addition of herbs and aromatherapy oils to bath water. The principal constituents found in mineral waters are sodium, magnesium, calcium and iron, in combination with the acids to form chlorides, sulphates, sulphides and carbonates. Other substances occasionally present in sufficient quantity to exert a therapeutic influence are arsenic, lithium, potassium, manganese, bromine and iodine. The term 'spa treatment' is derived from the name of the town of Spa, Belgium, where since mediaeval times illnesses caused by iron deficiency were treated by drinking iron-bearing spring water.[14]

Traditionally mineral waters would be used or consumed at their source, often referred to as 'taking the waters' or 'taking the cure'. Although many spa towns still exist, in modern times it is more usual to take bottled water of which there are more than 3000 brands worldwide. The US Food and Drug Administration (FDA) classifies mineral water as water containing at least 250 parts per million (p.p.m.) total dissolved solids (TDSs), and is also water coming from a source tapped at one or more bore holes or spring, originating from a geologically and physically protected underground water source. No minerals may be added to this water.

Evidence

In several European countries, balneotherapy is a common treatment for low back pain. One of the aims of the treatment is to soothe the pain and as a consequence relieve patients' suffering and make them feel well. Although they are expensive, the costs are sometimes reimbursed by health insurance systems. Pittler at al.[15] carried out a meta-analysis of these treatments. They found only five RCTs that satisfied their inclusion criteria. Judged by self-reported pain on a visual analogue scale, the data for both balneotherapy and spa therapy suggested modest beneficial effects compared with waiting list control groups for patients with chronic low back pain. Verhagen et al.[16] assessed the effectiveness of balneotherapy for patients with osteoarthritis. They found some weak evidence of the beneficial effects on pain, quality of life and analgesic intake of mineral baths compared with no treatment.

Periodic changes in endocrinological stress markers have been studied in saliva samples collected from 31 women who spent 8 days in a spa resort.[17] Levels of salivary cortisol and chromogranin A (CgA) were evaluated by enzyme-linked immunosorbent assay. To evaluate health-related lifestyle factors, patterns of behaviour, perceived stressors, and stress reactions of the individuals, the authors administered written questionnaires. Individuals who scored poorly on an index evaluating lifestyle health factors, or reported stressful life events, showed a significant increase in CgA levels during the stay. This suggests that, for these people, the long stay in the spa ameliorated stress. These findings are somewhat different from those of studies in which researchers have evaluated the effects of shorter-term leisure trips. A study was carried out in 297 of the 340 certified spa centres in Italy to investigate whether appropriately applied spa therapy in several indications could be associated with a subsequent fall in the need for costly health services and missed working days as a result of sick-leave.[18] Outcomes considered were: frequency and duration of hospitalisation periods; missed working days; regular use of disease-specific drugs; and resort to 'non-spa' rehabilitation therapies. All the considered outcomes appeared to be significantly reduced in the index year in seven of the eight disease subgroups in comparison with the previous year.

Convincing evidence for other applications of balneotherapy (e.g. rheumatism) is limited.

Safety

Certain precautions are necessary while taking therapeutic baths:

- A cold foot bath should not be taken in cases of inflammatory conditions of the genitourinary organs, liver and kidneys.

- Very weak patients, pregnant women, cardiac patients and those suffering from high blood pressure should avoid steam baths.
- Full baths should be avoided within 3 h of a meal and 1 h before it; however, local baths, such as hip and foot baths, may be taken 2 h after a meal.

Women should not take any of the baths during menstruation. They can take only hip baths during pregnancy until the completion of the third month.

Nutritional therapy

Your food shall be your medicine.

Hippocrates

Diet plays a vital role in the maintenance of good health and the prevention and cure of disease. As seen in Part 3, it is extremely important in traditional Chinese medicine and ayurvedic medicine.

The human body builds up and maintains healthy cells, tissues, glands and organs only with the help of various nutrients. The body cannot perform any of its functions, be they metabolic, hormonal, mental, physical or chemical, without specific nutrients. The food that provides these nutrients is thus one of the most essential factors in building and maintaining health.

Nutrition can be important in the cure and prevention of disease. Naturopaths believe that the primary cause of disease is a weakened organism or lowered resistance in the body, arising from the adoption of a faulty nutritional pattern. There is an elaborate healing mechanism within the body, but it can perform its function only if it is abundantly supplied with all the essential nutritional factors.

Nutrition can also be the cause of disease. Environmental factors, including diet and lifestyle, are thought to play a role in the development of most kinds of cancer. Some forms of cancer are more common in some countries than others, and people who migrate from one country to another eventually assume the cancer risks linked to their new neighbours. For example:

- Stomach cancer in parts of Japan is associated with diets that contain substantial amounts of salt, particularly salted dried fish.
- Colorectal cancer is more common in Australia and New Zealand; red meat and alcohol are possible causes.

An expert panel convened by the World Cancer Research Fund and the American Institute for Cancer Research estimated that 40% of cancer cases worldwide could be prevented by taking an appropriate diet.[19]

It is possible that at least 45 chemical components and elements are needed by human cells. Each of these 45 substances, called essential nutrients, must be present in adequate diets. They include oxygen and water. The other 43 essential nutrients are classified into 5 main groups: carbohydrates, fats, proteins, minerals and vitamins. All 45 of these nutrients are vitally important and they work together, so the absence of any of them will result in disease and eventually death.

It has been found that a diet that contains liberal quantities of (1) seeds, nuts, and grains, (2) vegetables and (3) fruit will provide adequate amounts of all the essential nutrients. These foods have, therefore, been aptly called basic food groups and a diet containing these food groups is the optimum diet for vigour and vitality.

Seeds, nuts and grains

These are the most important and the most potent of all foods and contain all the important nutrients needed for human growth. They contain the germ, the reproductive power that is of vital importance for the lives of human beings and their health. Millet, wheat, oats, barley, brown rice, beans and peas are all highly valuable in building health. Wheat, mung beans, alfalfa seeds and soya beans make excellent sprouts. Sunflower seeds, pumpkin seeds, almonds, peanuts and soya beans contain complete proteins of high biological value.

Vegetables

Vegetables are an extremely rich source of minerals, enzymes and vitamins. Faulty cooking and prolonged careless storage, however, destroy these valuable nutrients. Most vegetables are, therefore, best consumed in their natural raw state in the form of salads.

Fruit

Like vegetables, fruit is an excellent source of minerals, vitamins and enzymes. It is easily digested and exercises a cleansing effect on the blood and digestive tract. It contains high alkaline properties, a high percentage of water and a low percentage of proteins and fats. The organic acid and high sugar content of fruit has immediate refreshing effects. Apart from seasonable fresh fruit, dried fruit, such as raisins, prunes and figs, is also beneficial.

Fruit is at its best when eaten in the raw and ripe states. In cooking, it loses portions of the nutrient salts and carbohydrates. It is most beneficial when taken as a separate meal by itself, preferably for breakfast in the morning.

Other items

Milk is an excellent food. It is considered to be nature's most nearly perfect food. Practitioners advise that the best way to take milk is in its soured form, i.e. yoghurt and cottage cheese. Soured milk is superior to sweet milk because it is a predigested form and more easily assimilated. Milk helps maintain a healthy intestinal flora and prevents intestinal putrefaction and constipation.

It is recommended that high-quality unrefined oils be added to the diet. They are rich in unsaturated fatty acids, vitamins C and F, and lecithin. The average daily amount should not exceed two tablespoons. Honey is also an ideal food. It helps increase calcium retention in the system, prevents nutritional anaemia, and is beneficial in kidney and liver disorders, colds, poor circulation and complexion problems. It is one of nature's finest energy-giving foods.

A diet of the three basic food groups and the special foods mentioned above will ensure a complete and adequate supply of all the vital nutrients needed to satisfy the requirements of any complementary disciplines for maintaining health and vitality, and preventing disease.

Animal proteins such as egg, fish or meat are not mandatory in the diet because they may have a detrimental effect on the healing process. Many complementary practitioners believe that a high animal protein intake is harmful to health and may be responsible for many of our common ailments.

Evidence

Naturopathic physicians commonly make dietary and/or dietary supplement recommendations for breast cancer prevention. A placebo-controlled, parallel-arm, pilot study tested the effects of two naturopathic interventions over 5 menstrual cycles on sex steroid hormones and metabolic markers in 40 healthy premenopausal women.[20] Overall, in this pilot study, the naturopathic interventions had no substantial effects on oestrogen measures. Early follicular phase androgens decreased with the botanical supplement.

In a review by Dunn and Wilkinson,[21] evidence is examined in relation to those factors that naturopaths believe are significant contributors to rheumatoid arthritis, and hence the main focus of therapeutic management. These factors include food allergy, increased gut permeability, increased circulating immune complexes, excessive inflammatory processes and increased oxidative stress. Naturopathic treatment attempts to alleviate symptoms by altering these factors through dietary modification, manipulation of dietary fats, and use of antioxidants and proteolytic enzymes.

Nutraceuticals[22]

Increasingly, opportunities are arising for healthcare providers to offer assistance in the maintenance of health using a group of food supplement products collectively known as nutraceuticals. The term was invented in 1989 by Stephen De Felice of the American Foundation for Innovation in Medicine, who defined a nutraceutical as being a 'food, or part of a food, that provides medical or health benefits, including the prevention and treatment of disease'.[23]

Nutraceuticals have also been called medical foods, designer foods, phytochemicals, functional foods and nutritional supplements, and include such everyday products as bioyoghurts and fortified breakfast cereals, as well as vitamins, herbal medicines and even genetically modified foods and supplements such as fatty acids.[24] In the UK the idea is still comparatively new, but in many traditional healing therapies, e.g. ayurvedic and traditional Chinese medicine, nutrition has been used medicinally for centuries. Food-labelling regulations do not allow food labels to carry health claims. This makes it hard for companies marketing nutraceuticals to advertise the exact benefits of their products and may result in some confusion among consumers as to how such products should be used. Furthermore, there is a general perception that one should avoid any food that has the word 'fat' associated with it because it will cause weight gain, disrupt cholesterol readings and generally have an injurious effect on health. In fact there are good fats and bad fats, with consumption of the former often helping to reduce desire for the latter.

Two examples of nutraceuticals used by naturopaths, other healthcare providers and persons wishing to self-treat are considered below. These are essential fatty acids and probiotics.

Essential fatty acids – not all fats are bad for you

Fats help balance the body's chemistry and provide 'padding' as protection for vital organs. They also act as a source of energy for body processes and help with the transportation of vitamins such as A, D, E and K, as well as providing a source of vital nutrients known as essential fatty acids (EFAs).[25]

Definition   Essential fatty acids are vital nutritional components that are required for good health. They are found in the seeds of plants and in the oils of cold-water fish. They cannot be synthesised by the body and must be supplied externally.

There are two main types of EFA: the omega-3 oils and the omega-6 oils; omega-3 and omega-6 fatty acids are named according to the position of the double bond at either carbon-3 or carbon-6 atoms from the last (omega) carbon atom. The importance of nutritional omega-3 oils was realised by British researchers in 1970.[26]

Types of fatty acids

Saturated fats   These are found in red meat, bakery and pastry products, butter, cheese, chocolate, ice-cream, milk and certain oils. They contain single bonds between all the carbon atoms in a chain saturated with hydrogen. They are usually solid at room temperature. When a person's diet is high in saturated fats, these tend to clump together and form deposits with protein and cholesterol that tend to lodge in blood vessels and organs. One of the earliest suggestions that saturated fats and cholesterol could be related to heart disease was proposed by Ancel Keys in the late 1950s, although he was to make a number of inconsistent and contradictory statements about fats and their influence on health during his life.[27] Despite decades of effort and many thousands of people randomised, there is still only limited and inconclusive evidence of the effects of modification of total, saturated, monounsaturated or polyunsaturated fats on cardiovascular morbidity and mortality.[28] The 40-year Framingham study failed to find a relationship of those traditional dietary constituents, saturated fat and cholesterol, known to have an adverse effect on blood lipids, and on the subsequent development of coronary disease end-points.[29] However, a WHO report in 2002 (endorsed by the 2004 World Assembly) concluded that a diet low in saturated fats, sugar and salt, and high in fruit and vegetables, together with an hour a day of exercise, can counter cardiovascular diseases, cancer, diabetes and obesity.[30]

Unsaturated fats   These are said to be either monounsaturated (e.g. oleic acid found in olive and sesame oils) or polyunsaturated (found in corn, soyabean and sunflower oils). The molecules have one or more positions with double bonds between the carbon atoms and have less hydrogen. The lower the number of hydrogen atoms, the more fluid the fat. Almost all the polyunsaturated fats in the human diet are EFAs.

The following are usually recognised as EFAs; some are precursors for others:[31]

- **Linoleic acid**: an omega-6 fatty acid found in evening primrose, sunflower and sesame oils; symptoms such as acne, arthritic pain and skin disorders, which are regularly seen in the pharmacy environment, may be a result of a deficiency of linoleic acid.
- **Gamma-linolenic acid**: found in small amounts in evening primrose, blackcurrant and borage oils.
- **Alpha-linoleic acid**: an omega-3 fatty acid found in flax and walnut oils.
- **Arachidonic acid**: a long-chain unsaturated fatty acid found in beef, pork, chicken and turkey; both arachidonic acid and docosahexaenoic acid (see below) are present in brain and eye membranes, and play an important role in vision and brain cell function.
- **Docosahexaenoic acid**: a long-chain omega-3 unsaturated fatty acid comprising 22 carbon atoms with 6 double bonds bent in a U shape. It is found in anchovies, herring, mackerel, salmon, sardines and tuna. It is necessary for normal function of both the eye and the cerebral cortex, which is responsible for higher functions such as reasoning and memory. A lack of this acid may lead to attention deficit hyperactivity disorder (ADHD – see below).

The EFAs are claimed to have many vital functions, including:

- lowering dietary triglyceride levels in the blood, thus improving mental state
- assisting in the eradication of plaque from artery walls
- lowering blood pressure
- construction of cell membranes
- prolonging clotting time
- nourishing skin, hair and nails

- acting as precursors to the production of prostaglandins, hormone-like substances that act as catalysts for many physiological processes, including neurotransmission
- regulating the body's use of cholesterol.

Fatty acids and diet

The dietary balance of fatty acids is important and usually expressed in terms of ratios, comparing one type with another. It has been suggested that the most beneficial ratio for human brain function is a 1:1 mixture of omega-6:omega-3 oils. In 1990 the Canadian Minister of National Health and Welfare recommended a daily 6:1 ratio of omega-6:omega-3 fatty acids for people between the ages of 25 and 49.[32] Today the ratio for most people in industrialised nations is estimated to be from 20:1 to 30:1 in favour of omega-6 oils. In breast milk the ratio may be as high as 45:1. Infant feeds are estimated to have a ratio of about 10:1.

There is another difficulty affecting fatty acid ingestion, even if a correct balance of food is being achieved. The production of the appropriate oils in plant material is affected by climate. Northern plants, in response to cold weather, produce more omega-3 fats whereas in southern, warmer areas more omega-6 oils are produced. Thus, depending on the source of foodstuffs, the ratio of oils in a person's diet may vary.

Many factors, including stress, allergies, disease and a diet high in fried foods, such as that found in the west of Scotland, may increase the body's nutritional need for EFAs. As solid saturated fats are more stable than liquid unsaturated fats when they are exposed to light, heat and air, they are more desirable than oils for commercial frying. The Chinese method of stir frying is preferred.

The changing ratio of fatty acids appears to have significant implications for brain function and forms a basis for supplementation with nutraceuticals. Modern lifestyle demands mean that optimal diets are not always followed. Advice offered in the pharmacy on nutritional issues is consistent with the extended role and development of pharmaceutical care programmes, which are gaining acceptance throughout the profession.

Evidence

The difficulty for healthcare providers is to know when to recommend EFA supplementation. Published studies cover a wide range of conditions but the validity of some of the work is questionable, because either the preparations used were inadequately standardised or the influence of confounding dietary factors was not recognised. Notwithstanding this criticism, there is scientific and circumstantial evidence that EFA supplementation can be of benefit in both the treatment and the prevention of disease. The following examples of research provide evidence of effectiveness in a number of conditions.

A pilot study of 44 patients started in the 1980s demonstrated that conditions such as dry skin dermatosis, fatigue, bursitis and irritability appeared to respond to omega-3 supplementation as flax seed oil.[33]

Evening primrose oil has been shown to relieve the distressing itching of atopic eczema in most subjects taking Efamol over several months.[34] It contains gamma-linolenic acid, which converts to arachidonic acid.

Other controlled trials have demonstrated the benefit of evening primrose oil[35] and fish oil[36] administered to patients with rheumatoid arthritis. Evening primrose oil has been used in the treatment of premenstrual syndrome.[37]

Linoleic acid has been shown to stimulate fat utilisation and decrease body fat content in mice, but has not yet been tested in humans.[38]

A prospective study found that a higher consumption of fish and omega-3 polyunsaturated fatty acids is associated with a reduced risk of stroke, primarily among women who do not take aspirin regularly.[39]

Population studies have shown that frequent consumption of small amounts of omega-3 oils protects against the development of type 2 diabetes.[40] Gamma-linolenic acid supplementation in diabetes has been shown to improve nerve function and prevent diabetic nerve disease.[41]

Dietary treatment of children with behavioural disorders has had wide public appeal and been a source of controversy since the 1920s. There is some evidence to suggest that imbalances or deficiencies of certain highly unsaturated fatty acids (HUFAs) may contribute to a range of behavioural and learning difficulties including ADHD, dyslexia, dyspraxia and autistic spectrum disorders. This could help to explain the strong familial associations between these conditions and their common overlap within the same individuals.

A short attention span, inattentiveness and hyperactivity are diagnostic features of the syndrome now called ADHD, first described 100 years ago and suffered from by up to 16% of young children.[42] A connection between omega-3 deficiency and ADHD has been suggested by studies in which youngsters with the condition, when compared with non-ADHD children, had much lower blood levels of docosahexaenoic acid (DHA).[43] Children with ADHD may have trouble converting the short EFAs into omega-3 and omega-6 fats; thus these patients will benefit from receiving ready-made DHA, a long-chain fat, in the form of fish oil. Evening primrose oil can provide the omega-6 fat gamma-linolenic acid, bypassing a blocked omega-6 conversion stage. As a combination product these EFAs offer a healthier balance of omega-3 and omega-6 to the brain and body tissue.[44]

There is considerable debate as to how ADHD should be recognised and whether it should be treated.[45] It has been suggested that a specific diagnosis should be deferred until paediatricians are certain that a problem exists. Under these circumstances EFA supplementation may provide parents with a temporary solution to the problem of an apparently overactive child. Children under the age of 2 years should be referred to their general practitioner.

A review found that regular omega-3 supplements may provide some benefits for people with cystic fibrosis with relatively few adverse effects,[46] although the evidence is insufficient to draw firm conclusions or to recommend routine use of supplements of omega-3 fatty acids in people with cystic fibrosis.

Safety

Tolerance of EFAs is usually satisfactory. However, some allergic skin reactions have been reported. Patients with epilepsy or who are taking phenothiazine should be advised to consult their physician before self-treating with EFAs.

EFA supplementation

Essential fatty acids offer the opportunity for healthcare providers to become involved in improving and/or maintaining health through offering advice on nutrition, especially in the following situations:

- Patients with acne, alcoholism, cardiovascular disease, premenstrual syndrome and rheumatoid arthritis may use EFAs with safety to complement orthodox drug treatment.
- Patients with substantial risk factors of developing type 2 diabetes are likely to benefit from taking EFAs.
- EFAs may be of benefit to patients suffering from anxiety, general lethargy and premenstrual syndrome.

- ADHD may respond to EFA supplementation, although this should be an interim measure pending referral for further investigation.

Ingestion of EFAs may be required over extended periods – months rather than weeks – and to improve concordance patients should be informed as fully as possible of the aim of the supplementation.

Reports of children's intelligence quotients increasing with increased intake of essential fatty acids[47] has prompted parents to seek advice from health professionals. Existing evidence from interventional studies is sparse and conflicting and should not lead to supplementation with polyunsaturated fatty acids.[48]

Probiotics – not all bacteria are bad for you

The human intestine is home to more than a trillion live bacteria from about 400 species. The average adult body contains about 20 times more bacteria than it does cells.[49] In the natural environment a delicate symbiosis evolves between these endogenous bacteria and their host. The vital contribution of natural flora to normal intestinal development is underscored by studies of animals raised in a germ-free environment.[50] Exogenous probiotics are given therapeutically in situations where this naturally beneficial symbiosis has been disturbed, in an attempt to restore normal flora.

History

The use of what was formerly called biotherapeutic agents – now generally termed probiotics – is claimed to be a development from folk medicine, when fermented milks and certain fruit were administered prophylactically, in the prevention of disease.[51] It was found subsequently that this apparent beneficial effect was due to the organisms growing in the milk or on the surface of the fruit, and not to the foodstuffs themselves. Fermented milk products and yogurts have a long history.[52] The ancient peoples of the Middle East are said to have eaten yogurt regularly. Written records confirm that the conquering armies of Genghis Khan lived on the food. Their rich fermented milk was called 'kumiss' and it is reputed to have kept the conquering Mongol hoards (and their horses) fit and healthy. Today yogurt is enjoyed worldwide, except in China where fermented soy products are preferred.

The first specific biotherapeutic agent is believed to have been used in 1885, when Cantini sprayed *Bacterium termo* into a patient's lungs to treat pulmonary tuberculosis.[53] A major clue that intestinal flora played a significant role in disease protection was provided by in vitro studies carried out by the Russian biologist Dr Elie Metchnikoff as early ago as 1894.[54] Dr Metchnikoff was instrumental in recognising the process of phagocytosis for which he shared a Nobel Prize. It was not until 1908 that this work came to the attention of the general public following the publishing of his book entitled *The Prolongation of Life*. He was among the first to acknowledge the relationship between disease and what he called 'the poisons' produced in the bowel, and suggested that 'friendly' living bacteria can normalise bowel habits and fight disease-carrying bacteria. His book persuaded many readers that living longer is the result of an intestinal tract that maintains a healthy daily supply of the cultured bacteria found in yogurt. It was Dr Metchnikoff who named one of the two primary yogurt-culturing bacteria *Lactobacillus bulgaricus* in honour of the yogurt-loving Bulgarians. The other bacterium involved is *Streptococcus thermophilus*.

In 1971 van der Waaij[55] defined the term 'colonisation resistance' for the protective effect of normal flora against pathogenic organisims. Although the term 'probiotics' appeared in the literature as early as 1951,[56] Parker[57] was the first person to use it in relation to the interaction of microorganisms with a whole animal or human host. He described the use of living organisms given in animal feed to promote healthy livestock and to reduce mortality caused by diarrhoea. An extension into human medicine was documented by Fuller.[58]

The consumption of probiotics is perceived as being part of a healthy lifestyle by many. In 1998 the European probiotic yogurt market was valued at £520m (€650; $950), with the UK market reported as being the fastest growing. Probiotic use in animals may take the form of powders, tablets, sprays and pastes. In humans the most commonly used vector involves fermented milk products and over-the-counter (OTC) freeze-dried preparations of lactic acid bacteria, although stable tablets containing probiotics have become available in recent years.

Definition

Probiotics are viable bacterial cell preparation or foods containing viable bacteria cultures or components of bacterial cells that have beneficial effects on the health of the host.[59] The term thus includes fermented foods and specially isolated and cultured bacteria and mixtures of bacteria with adjuvants. Most of the common probiotics are lactic acid-producing bacteria including species of *Bifidobacterium, Lactobacillus, Enterococcus* and *Streptococcus*. They are useful in the treatment of disturbed microflora and increased gut permeability conditions that are characteristic of many intestinal disorders. Examples include acute diarrhoea, certain food allergies, colonic disorders and patients undergoing pelvic radiotherapy.

Types of probiotics

Various probiotic microorganisms may be isolated from the mouth, gastrointestinal content and faeces of animals and humans by repetitive subculturing of the microorganisms on appropriate media. Common criteria used for isolating and defining probiotic bacteria and specific strains include the following:

- Bile and acid stability: important to ensure that colonisation occurs.
- Adhesion to intestinal mucosa: adhesion to the intestinal cells is important for many applications.
- Production of antimicrobial components: lactic acid bacteria commonly produce a wide variety of antibacterial substances. These substances promote successful colonisation by improving the competitive advantage of the probiotic bacterial strain against the established normal strain of the gastrointestinal tract.

Products for OTC sale in a pharmacy are prepared from freeze-dried ingredients, obviating the necessity of refrigeration for dairy products and certain other foods.

Practice

There are a number of situations in which probiotics can be suggested, e.g. they may be indicated in several common OTC situations, particularly those involving diarrhoea of a specific nature.

In diarrhoea after antibiotic administration any or all of the following bacteria may be of use:

- *Lacidophyllus rhamnosus, L. bulgaricus*
- *Bifidobacterium longum, Enterococcus faecium.*

For travellers' diarrhoea the following probiotics may be indicated:

- *L. rhamnosus, L. bulgaricus*
- *B. longum, Streptococcus thermophilus.*

Other common uses for probiotics include:

- facilitating digestion
- stimulating the immune system
- relieving symptoms of thrush
- boosting resistance to infectious diseases of the intestinal tract.

A recent novel development has been the appearance of a product that combines three probiotics with the daily required amount of vitamins and minerals in one tablet. This is designed to help the body combat stress by correcting an unbalanced diet as well as supporting other body systems.

It has been pointed out that patients wishing to use this treatment will have to bear the cost themselves because currently British practitioners cannot prescribe probiotic therapy on NHS prescriptions.[60] Furthermore, it is likely that US health insurance companies will not pay for this treatment; this may be a significant barrier to both use and compliance in clinical practice.

Evidence

A major problem with most existing brands of probiotics is that they appear to contain anonymous strains of bacteria, with no documented probiotic properties. Furthermore they are not enteric coated. In this regard Multibionta (Seven Seas) is among the most efficient products available, being enteric coated so ensuring that the active ingredients – three specified bacteria – reach the site of action safely. This latter requirement would seem to be crucial for effectiveness. The target for *Lactobacillus* is the small intestine and for *Bifidobacterium* the large intestine.

Probiotic research was neglected until a revival in health consciousness prompted an increase in interest. There appear to be few well-designed human intervention studies with probiotics. Most of the studies are in vitro, rather dated and have not been replicated. However, probiotics are not alone in having to bear these problems because many complementary disciplines suffer from similar deficiencies. There is no doubt that a considerable amount of positive circumstantial evidence exists based on patient-oriented outcome measures.

The following are some examples of in vitro studies:

- It has been shown that *Bifidobacterium bifidium* acts on macrophages and activates them to produce a substance that suppresses *Escherichia coli*.[61]
- Extracts of *B. longum* have led to the enhanced destruction of *Salmonella* spp.[62]
- *B. longum* is said to have positive effects on cell-motivated immunity, which is known to be responsible for defence against bacterial and viral infections.[63]
- A combination of *Lactobacillus acidophilus* and *B. bifidium* was shown to be effective in reducing the amount of ammonia produced by bacteria such as *Citrobacter clostridiiforme*, *E. coli*, *Proteus vulgaris* and *Citrobacter freundii*. In addition, *B. bifidium* has been shown to suppress the growth of these ammonia-producing bacteria directly.[64]

Researchers at the Institute for Physiology and Biochemistry of Nutrition (IPBN) in Kiel, Germany, designed a trial to test the cold-fighting effectiveness of a probiotic bacteria supplement, combined with supplements of vitamins and minerals (PVM) in doses similar to those found in typical multivitamins.[65] More than 475 healthy men and women who had not received flu vaccines were randomly assigned to receive a placebo or the probiotic and vitamin/mineral combination. Participants received their doses every day for five and a half months during the winter and spring, and each participant reported any symptoms of respiratory infection. Researchers also monitored cellular immune response in 60 individuals from each group before and after the intervention period. Among those who developed respiratory infections:

- symptoms were generally reduced by 19% in the PVM group compared with placebo
- influenza symptoms were reduced by 25%
- number of days with a fever was reduced by more than 50%
- immune response tests showed a 'significantly higher' response in the PVM group, especially during the first 14 days of supplementation.

Among the in vivo studies are some that have suggested a cholesterol-lowering effect from lactobacilli.[66] Lactobacilli may also be useful in managing diarrhoea: 820 travellers aged 10–80 years were recruited before visiting two holiday destinations in Turkey.[67] They were randomised into two groups: one group received *Lactobacillus rhamnosus* powder and the other a placebo powder. The authors conclude that the administration of *Lactobacillus* can diminish the risk of travellers' diarrhoea during trips abroad. However, the design of the trial could not be considered robust. Other trials are reported in the *Handbook of Probiotics*.[68]

A 2004 Cochrane review reported probiotic therapy to be effective in reducing diarrhoea, and a recent report summarising 185 studies found that probiotics successfully treated 68 different conditions in widely diverse populations.[69]

Safety

The concept of willingly ingesting live bacteria remains somewhat counterintuitive. Although probiotic therapy is considered harmless, rare reports of systemic infections involving probiotic bacteria have raised clinical concerns. Safety in human and veterinary use – the safety of lactic acid bacteria used in clinical and functional food – is of great importance.

Lactic acid bacteria have a good record of safety and no major problems appear in the literature. However, cases of infection have occurred with other strains.[70] A review by Hammerman and colleagues[71] concluded that the benefits of probiotics seem to outweigh the potential danger of sepsis. They acknowledged that anecdotal reports of sepsis do exist, and that we should proceed with caution in clinically advancing probiotic therapeutics and concentrate on the use of organisms other than *Lactobacillus*. A call has been made for improvements in labelling and quality assurance procedures for products containing probiotic organisms.[72] The presence of the potential pathogen *Enterococcus faecium* (intentionally or as a contaminant) gives cause for some vigilance.

Apitherapy

History

The use of honey and other bee products can be traced back thousands of years and healing properties are included in many religious texts including the Veda, Bible and Q'uran. These are mostly attributed to nutritional benefits of consumption of bee products and not use of bee venom. The modern study of bee venom as a therapy was initiated through the efforts of Austrian physician Phillip Terc in his published results 'Report about a Peculiar Connection Between the Beestings and Rheumatism' in 1888. More recent popularity can be drawn to Charles Mraz, a beekeeper from Vermont, USA, over the past 60 years.[73]

Definition

Apitherapy is the medical use of honey bee products. This can include the use of honey, pollen, propolis, royal jelly and bee venom.

Evidence

Bee venom therapy is claimed to be of use in arthritis, bursitis, tendonitis, dissolving scar tissue and shingles. Most claims of apitherapy have not been proved to the scientific standards of evidence-based medicine and are anecdotal in nature. A wide variety of conditions and diseases have been suggested as candidates for apitherapy, the most well-known being bee venom therapy for autoimmune diseases and multiple sclerosis.

Honey   The use of honey as a wound dressing material, an ancient remedy that has been rediscovered, is becoming of increasing interest as more reports of its effectiveness are published.[74,75] The clinical observations recorded are that infection is rapidly cleared, inflammation, swelling and pain are quickly reduced, odour is reduced, sloughing of necrotic tissue is induced, granulation and epithelialisation are hastened, and healing occurs rapidly with minimal scarring. The antimicrobial properties of honey prevent microbial growth in the moist healing environment created. Full healing has been reported in seven consecutive patients whose wounds were either infected or colonised with meticillin-resistant *Staphylococcus aureus* (MRSA).[76] Antiseptics and antibiotics had previously failed to eradicate the clinical signs of infection.

A mixture of honey, olive oil and beeswax has been found to be effective for the treatment of nappy rash, psoriasis, eczema and skin fungal infection.[77] The mixture appeared to have antibacterial properties. The authors concluded that the mixture was also safe and clinically effective in the treatment of haemorrhoids and anal fissures.

Propolis   Propolis (also known as bee bread or bee glue) is a resinous substance that bees collect from tree buds or other botanical sources. It is used as a sealant for unwanted open spaces in the hive. Propolis is used for small gaps (approximately 6.35 mm [0.3 inch] or less), while larger spaces are usually filled with beeswax. The composition of propolis will vary from hive to hive, district to district and season to season. Normally it is dark brown in colour, but it can be found in green, red, black and white hues, depending on the sources of resin found in the particular hive area.

Propolis may:

- show local antibiotic and antifungal properties;[78] studies indicate that it may be effective in treating skin burns[79]
- have good plaque-cleaning, plaque-inhibiting and anti-inflammatory effects,[80] and a protective effect against caries and gingivitis.[81]

Royal jelly This is an emulsion of proteins, sugars and lipids in a water base, and is synthesised by the bee from pollen; 82–90% of the protein content is made up of a group of 20 proteins[82] found only in royal jelly and worker jelly. Most of the components of royal jelly seem to be designed to provide a balance of nutrients for the larvae. As a result of its high nutrient levels, particularly B-complex vitamins such as pantothenic acid (vitamin B_5) and vitamin B_6 (pyridoxine), it is used as a food supplement. It can also be found in various beauty products. Royal jelly may lower serum total cholesterol and serum low-density lipoprotein.[83] The presence of antibacterial components in royal jelly has been demonstrated.[84,85]

Royal jelly has been reported as the cause of severe anaphylaxis.[86]

More information

The British Naturopathic Association: www.naturopathy.org.uk
American Apitherapy Society: www.apitherapy.org
UK Food Standards Agency – Probiotics Research: http://tinyurl.com/3yovew

Further reading

Apitherapy

Fearnley J. *Bee Propolis*. London: Souvenir Press, 2001.

Essential fatty acids

Lee D. *Essential Fatty Acids*. Pleasant Grove, UT: Woodland Publishing, 1997.
Rudin D, Felix C. *Omega-3 Oils*. Garden City Park, NY: Avery Publishing Group, 1996.

Nutritional supplements

Skidmore-Roth. *Mosby's Handbook of Herbs and Natural Supplements*. St Louis, MO: Mosby Inc., 2001.

Mason P. *Dietary Supplements*, 2nd edn. London: Pharmaceutical Press, 2001.

Probiotics

Lee Y-K, Nomoro K, Salminen S, Gorbach SL. *Handbook of Probiotics*. New York: John Wiley & Sons Inc., 1999.

References

1. Verhoef MJ, Boon HS, Mutasingwa DR. The scope of naturopathic medicine in Canada: an emerging profession. *Soc Sci Med* 2006;**63**:409–17
2. Oumeish O. The philosophical, cultural and historical aspects of complementary alternative unconventional and integrative medicine in the Old World. In: Fontanarosa PB (ed.), *Alternative Medicine*. Washington DC: American Medical Association, 2000: 136–7.
3. Bradley R, Oberg EB. Naturopathic medicine and type 2 diabetes: a retrospective analysis from an academic clinic. *Altern Med Rev* 2006;**11**: 30–9.
4. Jagtenberg T, Evans S, Grant A, Howden I, Lewis M, Singer J. Evidence-based medicine and naturopathy. *J Altern Compl Med* 2006;**12**:323–8.
5. Dunne N, Benda W, Kim L et al. Naturopathic medicine: what can patients expect? *J Fam Pract* 2005;**54**:1067–72.
6. Wikepedia. Naturopathic medicine. Available at: http://tinyurl.com/ypz6j4 (accessed 24 October 2007).
7. Stange R. Naturopathic dietary treatment in functional disorders. *MMW Fortschr Med* 2006;**148**:34–6.
8. Haas E, Novey D. Detoxification therapy. In: Novey D (ed.), *Clinician's Complete Reference to Complementary and Alternative Medicine*. St Louis, MO: Mosby, 2000: 705–7.
9. Casdorph HR. EDTA chelation therapy, efficacy in arteriosclerotic heart disease. *J Hol Med* 1981;**3**:53–7.
10. Shri HK. *Bakhru. A Complete Handbook of Naturocare*. Available at: www.healthli-brary.com/reading/ncure/index.htm (accessed 10 May 2008).
11. Dieppe P. Fortnightly review: management of hip osteoarthritis. *BMJ* 1995;**311**:853–7.
12. Pittler M. Complementary therapies for chronic venous insufficiency. *Focus Altern Compl Med (FACT)* 2001;**6**:3–5.
13. Wikepedia. Balneotherapy. Available at: http://tinyurl.com/28eczj (accessed 24 October 2007).
14. Wikepedia. Mineral water. Available at: http://tinyurl.com/278khq (accessed 24 October 2007).
15. Pittler MH, Karagülle MZ, Karagülle M, Ernst E. Spa therapy and balneotherapy for treating low back pain: meta-analysis of randomized trials. *Rheumatology* 2006;**45**:880–4.

Untitled

Untitled

Untitled

Untitled

Untitled

Untitled

Untitled

Untitled

Untitled

Untitled

Untitled

Untitled

Untitled

Untitled

Untitled

Untitled

Untitled

Untitled

Untitled

Untitled

Untitled

Untitled

Untitled

Untitled

Untitled

Untitled

Untitled

Untitled

Untitled

Untitled

Untitled

Untitled

Untitled

Untitled

Untitled

Untitled

Untitled

Untitled

Untitled

Untitled

Untitled

Untitled

Untitled

Untitled

Untitled

Untitled

Untitled

Untitled

Untitled

Untitled

16. Verhagen A, Bierma-Zeinstra S, Boers M et al. Balneotherapy for osteoarthritis. *Cochrane Database Syst Rev* 2007 Oct 17;4:CD006864.
17. Toda M, Makino H, Kobayashi H, Morimoto K. Health effects of a long-term stay in a spa resort. *Arch Environ Occup Hlth* 2006; **61**:131–7. PubMed
18. Coccheri S, Gasbarrini G, Valenti M, Nappi G, Di Orio F. Has time come for a re-assessment of spa therapy? The NAIADE survey in Italy. *Int J Biometeorol* 2008;**52**:231–7.
19. World Cancer Research Fund/American Institute for Cancer Research. *Food, Nutrition and the Prevention of Cancer.* New York: World Cancer Research Fund/American Institute for Cancer Research, 1997.
20. Greenlee H, Atkinson C, Stanczyk FZ, Lampe JW. A pilot and feasibility study on the effects of naturopathic botanical and dietary interventions on sex steroid hormone metabolism in premenopausal women. *Cancer Epidemiol Biomarkers Prev* 2007;16:1601–9. PubMed
21. Dunn JM, Wilkinson JM. Naturopathic management of rheumatoid arthritis. *Mod Rheumatol* 2005;**15**:87–90.
22. Kayne SB. Getting to know the bad guys. *Chemist Druggist* 2001;**255**:22–3.
23. Mannion M. Nutraceutical revolution continues at Foundation for Innovation in Medicine conference. *Am J Nat Med* 1998;**5**:30–3.
24. Bull E, Rapport L, Lockwood B. What is a nutraceutical? *Pharm J* 2000;**265**: 57–8.
25. Lee D. *Essential Fatty Acids.* Pleasant Cove, UT: Woodland Publishing, 1997: 5–6.
26. Fiennes RN, Sinclair AJ, Crawford MA. Essential fatty studies in primates: linoleic acid requirements of Capuchins. *J Med Primatol* 1973;**2**:155.
27. Ancel Keys – villain or hero? Available at: www.stop-trans-fat.com/ancel-keys.html (accessed 28 October 2007).
28. Hooper L, Summerbell CD, Higgins JPT et al. Dietary fat intake and prevention of cardiovascular disease: systematic review. *BMJ* 2001;**322**: 757–63
29. Castelli W. Concerning the possibility of a nut . . . . *Arch Intern Med* 1992; **152**:1371–2.
30. WHO Global Strategy on Diet, Physical Activity and Health. Available at: http://tinyurl.com/2qwpb9 (accessed 28 October 2007).
31. Cunnane SC. Problems with essential fatty acids: time for a new paradigm? *Lipid Res* 2003;**42**:544–68. PubMed
32. Canadian National Ministry of Health and Welfare. *Report on Nation's Health.* Ottawa, Canada: Canadian National Ministry of Health and Welfare, 1990.
33. Rudin D, Felix C. *Omega-3 Oils. A practical guide.* New York: Avery Publishing Group, 1996: 39–49.
34. Burton JL. Dietary fatty acids in inflammatory skin disease. *Lancet* 1989;**i**:27.
35. Belch JJ. Effects of altering dietary essential fatty acids on requirements for non-steroidal anti-inflammatory drugs in patients with rheumatoid arthritis: a double blind placebo controlled study. *Ann Rheum Dis* 1988;**47**:96.
36. Fortin PR, Lew RA, Liang MH et al. Validation of a meta-analysis: the effect of fish oil in rheumatoid arthritis. *J Clin Epidemiol* 1995;**49**:1379–90.

37. Burdeiri D, Li Wan Po A, Dornan JC. Is evening primrose oil of value in the treatment of premenstrual syndrome? *Control Clin Trials* 1996;**17**:60–8.
38. Dyck D J. Dietary fat intake, supplements and weight loss. *Can J Appl Physiol* 2000;**25**:495–523.
39. Iso H, Rexrode KM, Stampfe MJ et al. Intake of fish and omega-3 fatty acids and risk of stroke in women. *JAMA* 2001 **285**:304–12.
40. Feskens EJ, Bowles CH, Kromhout D. Inverse association between fish intake and risk of glucose intolerance in normoglycemic elderly men and women. *Diabetes Care* 1991;**14**:935–41.
41. GLA Multicenter Trial Group. Treatment of diabetic neuropathy with GLA. *Diabetes Care* 1993;**16**:8–15.
42. Naveem S, Chaghary B, Collop N. Attention deficit hyperactivity disorder in adults and obstructive sleep apnea. *Chest* 2001;**119**:294–6.
43. Colquhoun I, Bunday S. A lack of EFAs as a possible cause of hyperactivity in children. *Med Hypoth* 1981;**7**:673.
44. Rudin D, Felix C. *Omega 3 Oils*. New York: Avery Publishing Group, 1996: 97–8.
45. Blackman J A. Attention-deficit/hyperactivity disorder in preschoolers. Does it exist and should we treat it? *Pediatr Clin North Am* 1999;**46**:1011–25.
46. McKarney C, Everard M, N'diaye T. Omega-3 fatty acids (from fish oils) for cystic fibrosis. *Cochrane Database Syst Rev* 2007;(4):CD002201.
47. Whalley LJ, Fox HC, Wahle KW, Starr JM, Deary IJ. Cognitive aging, childhood intelligence, and the use of food supplements: possible involvement of n-3 fatty acids. *Am J Clin Nutr* 2004;**80**:1650–7.
48. Dubnov-Raz G, Finkelstein Y, Koren G. Omega-3 fatty acid supplementation during pregnancy: for mother, baby, or neither? *Can Fam Physician* 2007;**53**:817–8. PubMed
49. O'Sullivan GC, Kelly P, O'Halloran S et al. Probiotics: an emerging therapy. *Curr Pharm Des* 2005;**11**:3–10
50. O'Sullivan GC. Probiotics. *Br J Surg* 2001;**88**:161–2. PubMed
51. McFarland LV, Elmer GW. Biotherapeutic agents: Past, present and future. *Microecol Ther* 1995;**23**:46–73.
52. Trenev N. *Probiotics – Nature's internal healers*. New York: Avery Publishing Group, 1998: 9–17.
53. Reid G, Bruce AW, McGroarty JA et al. Is there a role for Lactobacilli in prevention of urogenital and intestinal infections? *Clin Microbiol* 1990;**3**: 335–44.
54. Metchinikoff E. Recherches sur le cholera et les vibrions iv. Sur l'immunité receptivé vis-à-vis du cholera intestinal. *Ann Inst Pasteur* 1894;**8**:529–89.
55. van der Waaij D, Berghuis JM, Lekkerkerk JEC. Colonization resistance of the digestive tract in conventional and antibiotic-treated mice. *J Hyg* 1971;**69**:405–11.
56. Hamilton Miller JMT, Gibson GR, Bruck W. Some insights into the derivation and early uses of the word 'probiotic'. (Letter) *Br J Nutrition* 2003;**90**:845.
57. Parker RB. Probiotics. The other half of the antibiotics story. *Anim Nutr Health* 1974;**29**:4–8.
58. Fuller R. Probiotics in human medicine. *Gut* 1991;**32**:439–42.

59. Lee Y-K, Nomoto K, Salminen S, Gorbach SL. *Handbook of Probiotics.* New York: John Wiley & Sons, 1999, 1.
60. McLaughlin SD, Clark SK, Nicholls RJ, Tekkis PP, Ciclitira PJ. Effective probiotic treatment is rarely cheap. (Letter) *BMJ* 2006;**333**:1272.
61. Honma N. Intestinal bacterial flora of infants and defence mechanism. *Pediatr Clin* 1974;**27**:20–9.
62. Hatcher GE, Lambrecht RS. Augmentation of macrophagocytic activity by cell-free extracts of selected lactic acid-producing bacteria. *J Dairy Sci* 1993;**76**:2485–92.
63. Yamazaki S, Machii K, Tsuyuki S et al. Immunological responses to monoassociated *Bifidobactereium longum* and their relation to the prevention of bacterial invasion. *Immunology* 1985;**56**:43–50.
64. Yamamoto T, Kishida Y, Ishida T et al. Effects of lactic acid bacteria on intestinal putrefaction substance, producing bacteria of human source. *Basics Clin* 1986;**20**:123.
65. Winkler P, de Vrese M, Laue Ch, Schrezenmeir J. Effect of a dietary supplement containing probiotic bacteria plus vitamins and minerals on common cold infections and cellular immune parameters. *Int J Clin Pharmacol Therapeut* 2005;**43**:311–18.
66. Lichtenstein AH, Golden BR. Lactic acid bacteria and intestinal drug and cholesterol metabolism. In: Salminen S, Wright AV (eds), *Lactic Acid Bacteria.* New York: Marcel Dekker Inc., 1993: 232–3.
67. Oksanen PJ, Salminen S, Saxelin M et al. Prevention of travellers' diarrhoea by *Lactobacillus. Ann Med* 1990;**22**:53–6.
68. Lee Y-K, Nomoto K, Salminen S, Gorbach SL. *Handbook of Probiotics.* New York: John Wiley & Sons, 1999: 67–133.
69. Floch M, Montrose DC. Use of probiotics in humans: an analysis of the literature. *Gastroenterol Clin North Am* 2005;**34**:547–70. PubMed
70. Donohue DC, Salminen S. Safety of probiotic bacteria. *Asia-Pac J Clin Nutr* 1996;**5**:25–8. PubMed
71. Hammerman C, Bin-Nun A, Kaplan M. Safety of probiotics: comparison of two popular strains. *BMJ* 2006;**333**:1006–8.
72. Hamilton-Miller JM, Shah S, Winkler JT. Public health issues arising from microbiological and labelling quality of foods and supplements containing probiotic microorganisms. *Public Hlth Nutr* 1999;**2**:223–9. PubMed
73. Metz C. *Health and the Honey Bee.* Cincinnati: Queen City Publications 1995.
74. Molan PC. A brief review of the use of honey as a clinical dressing. Primary Intention. *Aust J Wound Manag* 1998;**6**:148–58. Available at: http://tinyurl.com/2rhlsa (accessed 28 October 2007).
75. Molan PC. Manuka honey as a medicine. Article available at: http://tinyurl.com/2hhj99 (accessed 28 October 2007).
76. Blaser G, Santos K, Bode U, Vetter H, Simon A. Effect of medical honey on wounds colonised or infected with MRSA. *J Wound Care* 2007;**16**:325–8. PubMed
77. Al-Waili NS, Saloom KS, Al-Waili TN, Al-Waili AN. The safety and efficacy of a mixture of honey, olive oil, and beeswax for the management of hemorrhoids and anal fissure: a pilot study. *Sci World J* 2006;**6**:1998–2005.

78. Orsi RO, Sforcin JM, Rall VLM, Funari SRC, Barbosa Luciano III, Fernandes A Jr. Susceptibility profile of *Salmonella* against the antibacterial activity of propolis produced in two regions of Brazil. *J Venom Anim Toxins incl Trop Dis* 2005;11. Available at: http://tinyurl.com/2e24wj (accessed 28 October 2007).

79. Gregory SR, Piccolo N, Piccolo MT, Piccolo MS, Heggers JP. Comparison of propolis skin cream to silver sulfadiazine: a naturopathic alternative to antibiotics in treatment of minor burns. *J Altern Compl Med* 2002;**8**:77–83.

80. Botushanov PI, Grigorov GI, Aleksandrov GA. A clinical study of a silicate toothpaste with extract from propolis. *Folia Med (Plovdiv)* 2001;**43**(1–2): 28–30. PubMed

81. Park YK, Koo MH, Abreu JA, Ikegaki M, Cury JA, Rosalen PL. Antimicrobial activity of propolis on oral microorganisms. *Curr Microbiol* 1998;**36**:24–8. PubMed

82. Schönleben S, Sickmann A, Mueller MJ, Reinders J. Proteome analysis of *Apis mellifera* royal jelly. *Anal Bioanal Chem* 2007;**389**:1087–93.

83. Guo H, Saiga A, Sato M et al. Royal jelly supplementation improves lipoprotein metabolism in humans. *J Nutr Sci Vitaminol (Tokyo)* 2007;**53**:345–8. PubMed

84. Jiang Y, Xu JZ, Shen CY et al. Determination of chloramphenicol in royal jelly by liquid chromatography/tandem mass spectrometry. *J Assn Official Analyt Chemists* 2006;**89**:1432–6. PubMed

85. Ishii R, Horie M, Murayama M, Maitani T. Analysis of tetracyclines in honey and royal jelly by LC/MS/MS. *Shokuhin Eiseigaku Zasshi* 2006;**47**:277–83. PubMed

86. Testi S, Cecchi K, Severino M et al. Severe anaphylaxis to royal jelly attributed to cefonicid. (Short communication) *J Invest Allergol Clin Immunol* 2007;**17**:277–85. PubMed

15

Diagnostic therapies

Steven B Kayne

Iridology

'Iri' and 'iris' are derived from the Greek name for the goddess of the rainbow, Iris; 'ology' also comes from the Greek, meaning 'study of'. Literally translated, therefore, iridology means the study of the coloration of the eye. It is a diagnostic tool, relying on a perceived link between ill health and changes in the iris. It offers practitioners a foresight of certain abnormalities in the body long before symptoms manifest themselves. The prevention of disease is thus seen as a crucial aspect of the iridologist's work. The number of specialist iridologists in western Europe is small – probably fewer than 2000 – although iridology is used quite widely by German Heilpraktikers. The discipline is more popular in Russia, where it is restricted to medically qualified doctors, around 5000 of whom may use the technique. Iridology may be used by specialists who subsequently refer on as appropriate or it may be used by naturopaths and other practitioners as a diagnostic tool before treatment.

Definition

Iridology is the diagnosis of medical conditions and pre-disease states through the study of abnormalities of pigmentation on the iris. It may also yield information on general constitutional and genetic features of individuals.

History[1]

The first reference by a physician to iridology was made by Philipus Meyens in his book *Chiromatica Medica*, published in Dresden in 1670. Meyens accurately mapped out the segments of the iris and described how they represent certain organs and tissue systems. The method was further refined by a Hungarian monk Ignaz (Edmund) von Peczely

(1822–1911). He is said to have accidentally broken the leg of his pet owl as a child and noticed a black shadow on the bird's eye that slowly changed in texture as the leg healed.[2] In a book published in 1880 he describes a method linking the site of certain iridic phenomena to the site of organic disease.[3] Other workers in this field were von Peczely's contemporary, the Swedish naturopath Liljequist, and Felke in the early 1900s.

Modern iridology owes its development to several Germans, including Angerer[4] and Deck.[5] In the USA Jensen, a chiropractor from California, is an active proponent of iridology.[6]

Theory

Iridologists believe that the iris reveals the changing conditions of every part and organ of the body which is represented in the iris in a well-defined area. In addition, through various marks, signs and discoloration in the iris, nature reveals inherited weaknesses and strengths.

A typical iridology map divides the eye into sections, using the image of a clock face as a base. So, for example, to know the condition of a patient's thyroid gland, you need to look in the iris of the right eye at about 2:30 and the iris of the left eye at about 9:30. Discolorations, flecks, streaks, etc. in those parts of the eyes indicate problems. An iridology map may comprise 60 different sectors for the right and left irises, each being related to an organ to which it is connected by multiple nerve connections, or a body function.[7] The exact nature of the manner in which the segments are subdivided is still under discussion.

Iridologists also believe that the pigment deposits indicate that the body is in a defensive state; the colour, density and position of pigmentation may offer clues to the identification of pathogenesis and specific organ involvement. Iridology cannot detect a specific disease, but can tell an individual if he or she has over- or underactivity in specific areas of the body, e.g. an underactive pancreas might indicate a diabetic condition. Ophthalmologists, on the other hand, see no significance in the diversity of iridic pigmentation, attributing it to an individual's normal characteristics.

Some iris diagnoses are of little interest today and some modern diseases are missing in the diagnostic system.

Practice

As already observed in Chapter 14 iridology is an important diagnostic tool for naturopaths. Several US iridologist organisations exist: the National Iridology Research Association is an iridologists' service organisation; the International Association of Iridologists is the leading organisation for European-style iridology and runs training programmes. In the USA, insurance programmes do not normally cover iridology, but in some European countries they do. In Germany, for instance, 80% of the Heilpraktikers (see Chapter 7) practise iridology.

Iridologists investigate the iris by hands-on clinical examination with an illuminated magnifier or study high-definition colour photographs taken with special cameras. Thorough analysis of the results and referral to charts or maps lead to a diagnosis and treatment or referral as appropriate.

Evidence

A systematic review identified eight tests of iridology, of which four were neither evaluator blind nor controlled, or neither and were therefore excluded from the evaluation.[8] One of the remaining four studies involved 23 patients and reported significant differences in the photometric values in the iris of patients with mitral stenosis.[9] However, there were concerns about the methodology. The other three studies were close to random. It was concluded that the validity of iridology as a diagnostic tool was not supported by scientific evaluations and that patients and therapists should be discouraged from using the method. Ernst has stated that iridology is not useful and is potentially harmful.[10]

Another negative conclusion emerged from a prospective case–control study aimed to investigate the value of iridology as a diagnostic tool in detecting some common cancers;[11] 110 individuals were enrolled in the study: 68 had histologically proven cancers of the breast, ovary, uterus, prostate or colorectum, and 42 were controls. Iridology identified the correct diagnosis in only three cases; it was concluded that iridology was of no value in diagnosing the cancers investigated in this study.

Kinesiology

The word kinesiology is derived from the Greek 'kinesis' (motion) + the suffix -ology or -logy from the Greek 'logos' or 'logia'(meaning a field of study).

A key diagnostic component of kinesiology is its use of muscle testing as part of an interactive neurological assessment process that helps the practitioner determine areas of structural, chemical and mental dysfunction. There are around 50 methods of muscle-testing kinesiology in the world today. Applied kinesiology is described in this section.

The treatment phase that follows diagnosis incorporates procedures from many other complementary disciplines including acupressure, chiropractic and osteopathic manipulation, and nutritional therapy.

Definition

Applied kinesiology comprises both a diagnostic tool and a holistic therapeutic modality which, in much the same way as Chinese or Indian medicine, focuses on bodily dysfunction rather than directly on the disease itself.

History

All the different kinesiologies use the same basic muscle-testing principle and a treatment model based on traditional acupuncture theory. Each variant reflects the interests and personality of its developer, e.g. applied kinesiology, created in 1964 by George Goodheart Jr, a chiropractor, has an emphasis on correcting structural problems. Using chiropractic knowledge of the trigger or reflex points on the body and of acupuncture meridians and their relationship to organs and muscle groups, Goodheart developed a consistent diagnosis and treatment system.[12]

Theory[13,14]

The theoretical basis of applied kinesiology rests on the assumption that muscle weakness is the result of the functional state of the nervous system, expressed in the muscle–nerve connections. The organs express their function via nerves to specific muscle groups. Applied kinesiologists believe that structural, chemical and mental dysfunction is associated with secondary muscle imbalance, usually inhibition. The application of appropriate therapy results in normalisation of the inhibited muscle. The therapy may include manipulation of the cranium, spine and extravertebral joints.

Practice

Applied kinesiology is used to detect incorrect joint function, spinal lesions, muscle weakness, psychological problems and allergies. Gentle pressure is applied to a muscle and the response monitored. The normal muscle response is to lock. By placing a limb in a particular position it is possible effectively to isolate an individual muscle (often an arm muscle) and test its response to this pressure. If the muscle gives way or is spongy, it indicates an energy disturbance in the meridian system. If, for example, this occurs when a muscle is tested in the presence of a food, it may mean that the person is allergic to that food. If the muscle unlocks after a question is asked, it indicates a negative answer to that question.

Some branches of kinesiology do not accept the use of muscle testing to obtain yes/no answers to verbal questions, but rely on a system of reflex points and finger modes to identify current stressors. A wide range of applications is listed in applied kinesiology textbooks.[15] These include allergies, arthritis, asthma, constipation, diarrhoea, hypertension, insomnia and musculoskeletal problems.

Evidence

A number of papers that discuss the use and efficacy of applied kinesiology may be found in the literature. The most recent deal with the neurological basis of applied kinesiology.[16]

Studies have also found that practitioners of applied kinesiology are unable to obtain consistent results from duplicate blinded samples.[17]

More information

Iridology

National Council and Register of Iridologists, 40 Stokewood Road, Winton, Bournemouth, Dorset BH3 7NE.

British Society of Iridologists, 998 Wimborne Road, Bournemouth, Dorset BH9 2DE. Tel: 01202 518078

Guild of Naturopathic Iridologists, 94 Grosvenor Road, London SW1V 3LS. Tel: 020 7834 3579

International Association of Clinical Iridologists, Orchard Villa, Porters Park Drive, Shenly, Radlett, Herts WD7 9DS. Tel: 01923 856222

516   Complementary and Alternative Medicine

Kinesiology

Association for Systematic Kinesiology, 39 Browns Road, Surbiton, Surrey KT5 8ST. Tel: 020 8399 3215

Health Kinesiology, Sea View House, Long Rock, Penzance TR20 8JF. Tel: 01736 719030

International College of Applied Kinesiology. Tel: 913 384 5336; website: www.icak@usa.net

Kinesiology Federation, 30 Sudley Road, Bognor Regis, Sussex PO21 1ER.

References

1. Wolf H. Iridology. In: Novey D (ed.), *Clinician's Complete Reference to Complementary and Alternative Medicine*. St Louis, MO: Mosby, 2000: 756–7.
2. Fulder S. *The Handbook of Complementary and Alternative Medicine*. Oxford: Oxford University Press, 1996: 245.
3. Peczely I. *Discoveries in the Field of Natural Science and Medicine: Instruction in the diagnosis from the eye*. Budapest: KgL, 1880.
4. Angerer J. *Handbook of Iridiagnosis*. Saulgen: Haug, 1953.
5. Deck J. *Fundamentals of Iris Diagnosis*. Karlsruhe: Institute for Fundamental Research in Iris Diagnostic, 1965.
6. Jensen B. *The Science and Practice of Iridology*, 14th edn. Escondido, CA: Jensen's Nutritional and Health Products, 1985.
7. Sharan F. *Iridology: A complete guide to diagnosing through the iris and to related forms of treatment*. Wellingborough: Thorson's, 1989.
8. Ernst E. Iridology: a systematic review. *Forsch Komplemed* 1999;**6**:7–8.
9. Popescu MP, Waniek DA. Perfectionarea metodei iridodiagnostica: posibilitati de computerizare a iridologei. *Oftalmologia* 1996;**30**:29–33.
10. Ernst E. Iridology: not useful and potentially harmful. *Arch Ophthalmol* 2000;**118**:120–1.
11. Münstedt K, El-Safadi S, Brück F, Zygmunt M, Hackethal A, Tinneberg HR. Can iridology detect susceptibility to cancer? A prospective case-controlled study. *J Altern Compl Med* 2005;**11**:515–19.
12. Birdwhistle RL. *Kinesics and Context: Essays on body motion communication*. Philadelphia: University of Philadelphia Press, 1970.
13. Fulder S. *The Handbook of Complementary and Alternative Medicine*. Oxford: Oxford University Press, 1996: 226–7.
14. Maffetone P. Applied kinesiology. In: Novey D (ed.), *Clinician's Complete Reference to Complementary and Alternative Medicine*. St Louis, MO: Mosby, 2000: 639–40.
15. Valentine T, Valentine C. *Applied Kinesiology*. Rochester, VT: Healing Arts Press, 1987: 28–35.
16. Schmitt W, Yanuk S. Expanding the neurological examination using functional neurologic assessment. Part 2: neurologic basis of applied kinesiology. *Int J Neurosci* 1999;**97**:77–108.
17. Vickers A, Zollman C. ABC of complementary medicine: Unconventional approaches to nutritional medicine. *BMJ* 1999;**319**:1419–22.

16

Manual therapies

Steven B Kayne

Alexander technique[1-3]

> Every man, woman and child holds the possibility of physical perfection;
> it rests with each of us to attain it by personal understanding and effort.
> FM Alexander[1]

Definition

The Alexander technique is an educational and therapeutic method of encouraging an individual to expend a minimum of effort to achieve the maximum efficient use of muscles and movement with the aim of relieving pain and improving posture and overall health.[4] Put more simply, it is a practical method for finding out what habits of body use a person has and how best he or she can promote the most beneficial actions and prevent the most harmful actions.

History

Born in Tasmania in 1869, Frederick Mathias Alexander found the development of his promising career as a young Shakespearean actor hampered by respiratory and vocal troubles.[5,6] None of the local doctors seemed able to offer much help other than to suggest that he rested his voice. FM, as he was known, suffered from poor health for much of his life and had to give up acting in favour of teaching at home.

Alexander eventually concluded that his problems lay within his own body. He discovered that the principles of physical coordination do not work in isolation from the rest of our functioning. Specifically, the quality of muscle tone and the way that we are supported at rest and in movement is only one aspect of a whole that includes our thought processes and emotional states. In trying to unravel and understand the interrelationship between these different aspects of his organism, Alexander realised that they were inextricably linked with habit patterns that were deep-rooted and connected with his 'intention to act' or his 'will to do'. During several years of painstaking self-observation with the aid of a mirror, he noted that while reciting prose he tended to adopt a posture that depressed his larynx and vocal cords, and shortened his spine. He realised that he needed to train himself into adopting a more appropriate posture if he was going to improve his delivery. His own success prompted him to teach other actors how to improve their technique. Alexander's improvements in voice and general health led him to propose a new approach to the use of the body as a whole. Encouraged by doctors he moved to London at the start of the twentieth century and expounded his ideas in England and the USA until his death in 1955.

The thespian origins of Alexander's technique have been reinforced over the years and the method has received the acclaim of many theatrical people, including such diverse personalities as playwright George Bernard Shaw and actor John Cleese. It is used in performance schools of dance, acting, circus, music, voice and some Olympic sports. Suitable for those starting at any fitness level, it is also used as remedial movement education to complete recovery and provide pain management.

Theory

When Alexander first tried to apply his observational findings to his own behaviour during public performances, he found that he slipped back into his old habits very quickly. Seeking an explanation for this action, he found three fundamental reasons:

1. **End gaining and the means whereby**: Alexander used the term 'end gaining' to describe the tendency to follow some course of action almost automatically without first thinking through one's intended actions carefully. He called the opposite process of waiting, thinking and assessing the most appropriate activity the 'means whereby'.

2. **Faculty sensory appreciation**: with this term Alexander acknowledged the presence of habits of proprioception or feeling underlying habitual actions. This can result in a feeling of uneasiness during the correction of a long-standing incorrect posture because it represents a change from what has been regarded as normal behaviour in the past.

3.   **Inhibition**: the third idea is linked to the second. It represents a natural self-control of unwanted and inappropriate reactions without any sense of suppressing spontaneity.

When Alexander discovered a way of integrating these concepts he found the solution to his problems. By recognising the strength of his old habits and the inappropriateness of end gaining, he was forced to consider the 'means whereby' he could secure the necessary improvements in posture. To do this he had to overcome the faulty sensory perception of how his body should be. This he did by inhibiting his end-gaining behaviour.

Practice

The technique involves a process of psychophysical re-education that engages both mind and body. This learning process is best achieved through a series of one-to-one lessons with a qualified teacher who, using very gentle non-manipulative touch, gives the pupil the necessary new experiences. Modern practitioners recommend up to an hour to enable changes to be made. In group classes the emphasis is more on experiment and observation. Pupils are also encouraged to observe the thought processes and tensions associated with their activities in daily life. As the principles are assimilated, the pupil begins to develop the tools necessary to make his or her own discoveries and can continue to learn independently. Alexander technique may not be effective for everyone. Most teachers consider that 20–40 lessons are required.

Evidence

Research into the Alexander technique was pioneered by Frank Pierce-Jones, who used photographic, mechanical and electromyographical methods to demonstrate that when a person is guided by its teachings the muscles work more effectively and there is less tiredness.[7] Respiratory function has been investigated in a control group and an active group that had received 20 lessons in Alexander technique.[8] A significant, though relatively small, increase of 6–9% in peak flow of the active group was recorded. By reorganising body function in a general way, many specific difficulties are claimed to be alleviated or eliminated. These include chronic pain,[9] repetitive strain injury, back pain[10] and many conditions related to stress, including those related to performing.

520 Complementary and Alternative Medicine

The technique has gained some support among nurses and other workplace groups involved in carrying and lifting activities.

A randomised study has demonstrated a reduction in performance-related anxiety and improved performance quality in musicians following Alexander technique lessons.[11]

A case study reported by Cacciatore et al.[12] showed that the Alexander technique could improve posture and reduce low back pain. However, because the evidence is so limited another author recommends that a wide range of manual therapies including Alexander technique and Feldenkreis (see below) should not be considered for low back pain.[13]

In 2002, Stallibrass et al.[14] published the results of a significant controlled study into the effectiveness of the technique in treating Parkinson's disease. Four different measures were used to assess the change in severity of the disease. By all four measures, Alexander technique was better than no treatment, to a statistically significant degree (both p values < 0.04). However, when compared with a control group given massage sessions, Alexander technique was significantly better by only two of the measures. The other two measures gave statistically insignificant improvements (p values of approximately 0.1 and 0.6). This appears to lend some weight to the effectiveness of the technique, but more studies and data are required. Another paper by Stallibrass et al.[15] described the retention of skills learnt by Parkinson's disease patients: 27 people (96%) said that they were continuing to use the Alexander technique in their daily life, most often while walking, sitting or standing; 24 people (86%) were also practising the Alexander technique while lying down in a semi-supine position; and 10 people (36%) were using the Alexander technique when they needed more control, especially in crowds and social situations and 7 (25%) in stressful situations.

Feldenkreis method

A technique similar to the Alexander technique has been developed by Moshe Feldenkrais (1904–1984) in Israel over a 40-year period.[16] He synthesised his ideas from eastern and western body concepts, combining some aspects of the Alexander technique with knowledge of oriental body training in the martial arts. The result is a series of exercises that facilitate awareness of the body in movement.

The Feldenkreis method (FM) is viewed as an educational system for the development of self-awareness, which relies on the body as the learning instrument.[17] It deals with the question of how to enable the individual to reorganise and recall forgotten movement patterns. Unlike other complementary and alternative manual and touch modalities, FM is not aimed at curing or healing a client but rather at bringing about a change in his or her awareness, self-image and attitude towards the self, and taking responsibility for his or her wellbeing.

Bowen technique[18]

The Bowen technique involves a gentle, rolling motion, with very light touches. The practitioner stimulates sets of points, often with pauses between sets.

History

Bowen therapy was pioneered by Tom Bowen of Victoria, Australia (1916–82) in the 1950s. He was an industrial chemist who developed his system of bodywork with animals.

Theory

It has been suggested that the Bowen technique may introduce specific harmonic frequencies to the body systems.

Practice

The Bowen technique is not a form of massage, although it does claim to release areas of built-up stress in the muscles, and clients usually experience profound relaxation after a session. A typical session takes place over 30–45 minutes, with occasional 2- to 5-minute breaks during the session to allow the body to respond to the treatment.[19] The Bowen technique has been used to treat back pain, neck pain, frozen shoulder, tennis elbow, repetitive strain injury and other musculoskeletal disorders. It has also been used in veterinary practice particularly with horses (http://tinyurl.com/3yv88z).

Evidence

Following Bowen treatment, a significant increase in overall range of motion and shoulder function was seen in a group of patients suffering from frozen shoulder compared with the placebo group. The average range of motion improvement was 23° for the treatment patients and only 8° for the placebo group.[20] Lack of ethical, methodological and analytical detail in this study draws caution to the strength of inference from the findings.

A single, blinded, longitudinal, randomised controlled trial (RCT) was carried out on 116 male and female volunteers.[21] Participants were randomly assigned to a control group or a Bowen group. Three hamstring flexibility measurements were taken from each participant over a week. Significant hamstring flexibility was seen in the Bowen group, the effect lasting for a week without further treatment.

Chiropractic

Chiropractic is gaining in popularity and in the USA its practitioners are third in number to physicians and dentists. The discipline is the most popular example of complementary and alternative medicine (CAM) in that country, with as many as one in three patients with lower back pain being treated in this way.[22] A review of the use of CAM in the UK states that four of five studies considered placed the popularity of CAM disciplines in the order acupuncture, chiropractic, herbalism, homeopathy and osteopathy.[23] The remaining study, by MORI, did not ask about herbalism and recorded faith healers as third choice but was otherwise identical.

A survey of the 481 primary care groups in England and Wales[24] showed that, in 58% of the 60% of groups that responded, CAM was available through primary care services. Chiropractic (available in 23% of respondents) was among the most commonly used therapies.

In Australia chiropractic is used in sports medicine but has faced lack of recognition and acceptance by organised and orthodox sports medical groups.[25]

Surveys conclude that chiropractic is the most widely used practitioner-provided service of all CAM in the USA.[26] Surveys on chiropractic utilisation in rural areas have found that 15–17% of the population undergo chiropractic treatment,[27,28] compared with approximately 10% nationally.[24,29] This may be due to lack of access to medical care or the higher prevalence of injuries and poorer health status of individuals living in rural communities.[30] In a nationally representative sample of US Medicare beneficiaries, Wolinsky et al.[31] examined the extent of chiropractic used, factors associated with seeing a chiropractor and predictors of the volume of chiropractic use among those having seen one. The average annual rate of chiropractic use was 4.6%.

During the 4-year period (2 years before and 2 years after each respondent's baseline interview), 10.3% had made one or more visits to a chiropractor.

Definition

The following definition for chiropractic has been provided:[29]

> Chiropractic is a complementary discipline that focuses on the spine as being integrally involved in maintaining health, providing primacy to the nervous system as the primary coordination for function and thus health in the body. Maintenance of optimal neurophysical balance in the body is accomplished by correcting structural or biomechanical abnormalities or disrelationships through the use of manipulation and adjustment.

Chiropractors specialise in the diagnosis, treatment and prevention of biomechanical disorders of the musculoskeletal system, particularly those involving the spine and their effects on the nervous system.

History[32]

Although manipulation dates back to ancient times, its popularity in modern times is attributed to Daniel David Palmer (1845–1913), a self-educated scientist from Iowa. In 1895 Palmer was waiting in his office for a client when his janitor, Harvey Lillard, who had been deaf for 17 years, walked by. Noticing a small bump on the back of Lillard's neck, Palmer pushed it in. Lillard felt a snap in his back and suddenly declared that he could hear again. This led Palmer to deduce that the nervous system was the ultimate control mechanism of the body and that even minor misalignments of the spine, which he termed subluxations, could significantly impact on a person's health.

In the closing years of the nineteenth century, Palmer produced his theory of musculoskeletal effects on the central nervous system and developed the first manipulative techniques to relieve them. He asked his friend, the Rev Samuel H Weed, for advice. Weed turned to classic Greek and chose the words *chieri*, meaning hand, and *praktikos*, meaning performed; thus chiropractic means performed or done by hand.

Palmer is reputed to have opened his own school in the 1890s; some texts quote 1895 and others 3 years later. The profession celebrated its centenary in 1995 so the earlier date would seem to be the more appropriate!

Daniel's son, Bartlett Joshua (1882–1961), promoted chiropractic enthusiastically, helped by a number of his father's contemporaries and his own students.

Theory

There are four aspects of chiropractic philosophy:

1.   **The importance of the nervous system**: the basis of Palmer's technique is that as many as 31 different pairs of spinal nerves travel through openings in the vertebrae to and from the brain. If one of the vertebrae is partly displaced from its correct position, it can cause an impingement and pressure, or irritate the surrounding nerves. As a result, essential nerve messages are distorted, causing damage to the surrounding tissues.
2.   **The body's inherent ability to heal itself**: this is embodied in the phrase *vis medicatrix naturae*.
3.   **The effect of subluxation or joint dysfunction**: such abnormalities are believed to interfere with the ability of the neuromuscular system to act in an optimal fashion, in turn contributing to the presence of disease.
4.   **The identification and treatment of subluxations.**

Practice

Examination

As spinal manipulation is of such importance to the chiropractor, examination of this area of the body is of particular interest, following an initial history-taking. The acronym PARTS has been suggested as an appropriate way to proceed with this inspection:[33]

Pain: pain and tenderness are identified using observation, palpation and percussion.

Asymmetry: this may be identified by palpation, radiograph analysis or observation of gait.

Range of motion: this includes assessment of different types of motion, including stability of joints using palpation and radiographs.

Tissue characteristics: these include tone, texture and temperature abnormalities; a range of diagnostic techniques may be employed.

Special procedures: EMG, ultrasonography and kinesiology may be considered to augment information obtained from previous tests.

Treatment[34]

Procedures used during chiropractic treatment may include gentle massage, ultrasonic treatment and adjustment. The chiropractic adjustment (often also called manipulation) to joints in the spine or extraspinal regions entails placement of the practitioner's hands on appropriate contact points. This is followed by positioning of the joint, during which the patient may feel tension of the muscles and ligaments; a popping sound may occur. A short sharp thrust may then be delivered. Chiropractors use different parts of the hand to direct the thrust, depending on the joint being adjusted, e.g. the middle or base of the index finger may be used to adjust the neck whereas an area of the wrist bone may be used to adjust the lumbar spine. In cases of injury an indirect thrust may be used. The joint to be manipulated may be gently stretched over a pad or wedge-shaped block until realignment is accomplished.

A typical course of treatment for uncomplicated cases may involve six sessions over a 2- to 3-week period. It has been suggested that effective communication between chiropractors and medical providers is critical to the success of integration of chiropractic services in primary healthcare.[35]

Evidence

In the UK 22 million people suffer from some form of back pain and 310 000 people are absent from work with the complaint every day of the year. Most people who consult chiropractors do so for low back pain, and it is to this application that much of the literature applies.

The literature contains a variety of low back pain research studies, including sham-controlled RCTs, comparative RCTs and meta-analytic reviews. A selection of research information is presented here. For a fuller account the reader is referred to a comprehensive text published by the *Journal of the American Medical Association*.[36]

Some authors emphasise the distinction between spinal manipulation therapy (SMT) and chiropractic whereas others use the terms interchangeably.[37] This complicates the situation for the casual observer who wishes to research the literature. In fact chiropractic is much more than SMT alone, because it includes massage techniques such as myofascial muscle stimulation and rehabilitative medicine procedures such as exercise, bracing, taping, splinting and casting. Herbal medicines are also often prescribed. This confusion may explain the wide range of results obtained from trials; they may not be comparing like with like.

In a systematic review of systematic reviews of spinal manipulation published between 2000 and 2005 it was concluded that spinal manipulation was not substantially more effective than sham treatment in reducing pain, nor was it more effective than non-steroidal anti-inflammatory drugs (NSAIDs) in improving disability in patients with chronic low back pain.[38] Furthermore, its effectiveness was not supported by compelling evidence from RCTs.

Many US health agencies have endorsed chiropractic treatments and many insurance companies now pay for it. Workmen's compensation commissions have provided an opportunity to compare the efficiency of chiropractic and medical treatment in occupational terms. In Oregon, albeit 30 years ago, it was found that 82% of claimants with certain injuries treated by chiropractors returned to work within 7 days – twice as many as those with similar injuries who were treated by conventional doctors.[39]

Thirty-five RCTs of back and neck pain that compared spinal manipulation with other treatments have been evaluated.[40] Unfortunately the methodology was generally of a poor standard (e.g. low numbers, high drop-out rates, doubtful outcome measures) but 51% showed favourable results.

In the UK there are national guidelines on the treatment of low back pain that recommend chiropractic manipulation as a symptomatic treatment for acute uncomplicated cases where pain fails to resolve spontaneously within the first months.[41] However, the evidence base for such advice, largely derived from a meta-analysis of nine studies,[42] has been questioned in a *British Medical Journal* editorial.[43] It was pointed out that there were no chiropractic studies included in the clinical trials that generated favourable data for the treatment of back pain. Other trials systematically reviewed in another paper revealed substantial methodological flaws.[44] The authors of this second paper concluded that the trials did not provide convincing evidence for the effectiveness of chiropractic in the treatment of low back pain.

The editorial and papers generated substantial correspondence in the literature. Morley et al.[45] claimed that they 'contained repeated misuse of references, misleading statements, highly selective use of certain published papers, failure to refer to relevant literature, inaccurate reporting of the contents of published work, and errors in citation'. One study that was excluded showed that significantly more of those patients who were treated by chiropractic expressed satisfaction with their outcome after 3 years than those treated in hospital: 84.7% (127/150) versus 65.5% (76/116) for those referred by chiropractors

($p < 0.0001$) and 79.2% (103/130) versus 60.2% (71/118) for those recruited from hospitals ($p = 0.001$).[46] Breen[27] stated that 'There is substantial scientific evidence that the manipulation that chiropractors (and indeed osteopaths and some physiotherapists) do for back pain is both effective and safe'.

Other contributors also claimed that the editorial was 'misleading'[28] and ignored patients' expressions of satisfaction.[30] One correspondent acknowledged that in various studies patient satisfaction with chiropractic was indeed relatively high.[47] On balance some benefit seems to accrue from using chiropractic to treat low back pain.

In other applications evidence is similarly rather less than robust. There appears to be some evidence that chiropractic may be beneficial for neck pain,[48,49] migraine,[50,51] tension headaches (examples of both positive[52] and inconclusive[53] evidence may be found in the literature) and headaches resulting from neck dysfunction.[54] Other applications include menstrual pain,[55] asthma[56] and colic,[57] but evidence of effectiveness is mixed. Sports applications are growing in usage, e.g. the New Zealand Olympic team appointed a chiropractor some years ago and found his involvement to be beneficial.[58]

A qualitative review that evaluated the direct analgesic effect of spinal manipulation on spinal or referred pain has been published.[59] A total of 11 studies were considered and they were largely consistent with the theory that the sensory input from spinal manipulation results in some form of pain inhibition.

Safety

Potential risks do exist from inappropriate or unskilled manipulation (particularly cervical manipulation[60] and to a lesser extent lumbar spine manipulation[61-63]).

Gouveia et al.[64] reported three cases of serious neurological adverse events in patients treated with chiropractic manipulation. In all three cases there were criteria to consider a causality relationship between the neurological adverse events and the chiropractic manipulation. The authors concluded that the described serious adverse events warrant the implementation of a risk alert system.

Adverse events may be common, with about 12% of users in one study experiencing adverse reactions.[65] In another (prospective) study mild adverse reactions were reported after a third of all treatments.[66] Adverse reactions are rarely severe in intensity. Most of the patients report recovery, particularly in the long term.

The benefits of chiropractic care for neck pain seem to outweigh the potential risks.[67] The risk of a serious adverse event, immediately or up to 7 days after treatment, is said to be low to very low.[68]

A review of the literature to compare the risk of severe complication from NSAIDs with cervical manipulation concluded that 'cervical manipulation for neck pain is much safer than the use of NSAIDs, by as much as an estimated factor of several hundred times'.[69] Notwithstanding this conclusion, severe complications, even death, have been reported, although the incidence of adverse reactions is relatively low when trained personnel are involved.[70] A small prospective study concluded that many so-called adverse reactions are really only an initial mild discomfort that may be reasonably expected from spinal manipulation and that this should be set against the long-term benefits of the treatment.[71] The methodology of this study was subsequently heavily criticised.[72]

The overuse of radiographs by chiropractors has been cited as a potential hazard, but this is disputed by many practitioners.[73] Chiropractic is contraindicated in certain vascular complications, arteriosclerosis, traumatic injuries and arthritis.

Statutory regulation

Osteopathy and chiropractic are the only two complementary therapies that are currently regulated by statute in the UK. An act of parliament passed in the mid-1990s established a General Chiropractic Council with the aim of regulating the profession. The organisation operates in a similar way to the General Medical Council and has the authority to remove practitioners from the register in disciplinary hearings.

Training

At the Anglo-European College in Bournemouth, England, a 5-year full-time course leads to a BSc(Hon) degree in human sciences after 4 years, followed by a further year leading to a postgraduate diploma in chiropractic, validated by the University of Portsmouth and recognised by the European Council for Chiropractic Education.

Most of the chiropractors in the UK are trained in the McTimoney school in Abingdon (identifiable by the letters AMCA, MMCA or FMCA) and the Oxford College of Chiropractic (previously the Witney School). The two schools teach a similar whole-body approach, although there are differences in technique. Both schools are committed to providing a training that is equivalent to the European standards on chiropractic education, and to comply with the requirement for UK national registration. The approach to treatment varies in that the Anglo-European graduates tend to treat only subluxations whereas their colleagues from the McTimoney school tend to treat the whole spine at every session.

In the USA there are 16 chiropractic colleges and there are two in Canada.

Massage

Although remedial massage has its own methods and procedures, at its simplest it may be considered as being the age-old response to a painful stimulus, i.e. rubbing the bit that hurts! Massage enjoys wide acceptance from both patients and physicians, having one of the highest physician referral rates of all the CAM therapies.[74] Physicians rate bodywork in general as the CAM modality most likely to be beneficial. It is used in physical therapy, sports medicine, nursing, and as an adjunct to chiropractic, osteopathy and naturopathy.

The aims of massage are to:

- relieve pain and reduce swelling
- relax the muscles
- encourage the healing process after strain and sprain injuries.

Contrary to popular opinion, it cannot prevent loss of muscle strength or reduce fat deposits.

Definition

Massage is the systematic manipulation of body tissues, performed primarily (but not exclusively) with the hands for therapeutic effect on the nervous and muscular systems, and on systemic circulation. The primary characteristics of massage are touch and movement. It may be performed in association with another therapy or alone.

History

Massage is reputed to have been used more than 3000 years ago by the Chinese. Later, the Greek physician Hippocrates used friction in the treatment of sprains and dislocations, and kneading to treat constipation. Early in the nineteenth century, Per Henrik Ling (1776–1839) of

Stockholm devised a system of massage to treat ailments involving joints and muscles. Ling believed that vigorous massage could bring about healing by improving the circulation of the blood and lymph. In the past 20–30 years complementary therapists have adapted Swedish massage so as to place greater emphasis on the psychological and spiritual aspects of the treatment. The benefits of massage are now described more in terms such as 'calmness' or 'wholeness' than of loosening stiff joints or improving blood flow. In contrast to the vigorous and standardised treatment recommended by Ling, current massage techniques are more gentle, calming, flowing and intuitive.

Ling's Swedish system was popular at European spa towns in the nineteenth century, when it was used in conjunction with hydrotherapy. It was taken to the USA in 1854 by Dr George Taylor and his brother Dr Charles Taylor.[75] Others later extended the treatment to relieve deformities of arthritis and to re-educate muscles after paralysis.

In the 1940s and 1950s massage became associated with the sex industry, and its use in serious medicine fell into decline, a trend exacerbated by the social conservatism of the day, which questioned the propriety of allowing practitioners to touch an unclothed body. Furthermore, there was a growing scepticism at its effectiveness. However, in the 1960s massage regained its popularity, particularly with sports trainers and later physiotherapists. A decade later the 'wellness' movement gained support, and health professionals began to reassess the benefits of therapies involving touch. The use of massage in British hospital physiotherapy departments is currently less than in the past, but for the aromatherapist it has always maintained a high profile. For the sports person massage is also important, as part of the preparation for competition.

Theory

Massage involves two main components: touch and pressure. Attaining a balance between the two is an important skill. Touch with appropriate sensitivity allows the practitioner to gather information about the body. While giving a standard massage, practitioners gather palpatory information, which helps to adapt treatment to individual needs, e.g. a practitioner will devote extra time to massaging an area of increased muscle tension. Touch can also communicate a sense of caring and relaxation, essential elements in the therapeutic process. Pressure and manipulation stimulate blood circulation and reduce muscular tension.

Practice

The most commonly used therapeutic massage is known as Swedish massage, although many other variants exist, including deep-tissue massage (used to release chronic patterns of muscular tension), sports massage (similar to both Swedish and deep-tissue massage) and acupressure (see Chapter 12). Craniosacral massage is designed to deal with cranial and spinal imbalance.

Treatment often involves several different procedures and may last between 15 and 90 min.[23] It starts with the case history, although this is usually relatively short compared with other complementary therapies.

The patient is ideally treated unclothed on a specially designed massage couch. This normally incorporates soft but firm padding and a hole for the face. The treatment room is kept warm and quiet. Soft music may sometimes be played.

Practitioners generally treat the whole body, using oil, lotion or talc to help their hands move over the patient's body smoothly. A variety of strokes are used:

- Effleurage is a deep stroking movement in the direction of the venous flow that relaxes muscles, improves circulation to the small surface blood vessels and is thought to increase the flow of blood towards the heart.
- Pétrissage is a compression procedure that includes kneading, squeezing and friction; it is useful in stretching scar tissue, muscles and tendons so that movement is easier.
- Friction or rubbing is carried out with a slow elliptical or circular movement to increase blood flow and muscle movement.
- Tapotement or percussion uses the sides of the hands to strike the surface of the skin in rapid succession to improve circulation.
- Vibration or shaking is used on the extremities and is said to lower muscle tone.

Massage practitioners who treat sports injuries and musculoskeletal disorders may incorporate techniques derived from physiotherapy, osteopathy and chiropractic. These include deep massage, passive and active stretching, and muscle energy techniques (in which the patient moves against resistance from the practitioner).

Therapeutic uses

Massage is used by practitioners as a method of treatment for many common ailments. The various forms of massage and their usefulness in various diseases are described here in brief.

Massage of the joints

Stiff and swollen joints can be cured by massage combined with mechanical movements. Massage is, however, not recommended in serious inflammatory cases of the joints and in tubercular joints. Sprains and bruises can be cured by massage. In these cases, affected parts should first be bathed with hot water for 15–30 min. Next the massage should be done for a few minutes. Gentle stroking and kneading are recommended on and around the injured tissues. Fractures can also be treated through massage.

Massaging the nerves

Massage benefits many nerve problems. In cases of acute inflammation of the nerves, massage should be done carefully. Light and gentle stroking is recommended. Deep pressure should not be used on swollen nerves because it will increase the inflammation. All that is needed is a gentle tapotement or beating of the nerve.

Abdominal massage

This form of massage is beneficial in constipation. It stimulates peristalsis of the small intestines, tones up the muscles of the abdomen walls, and mechanically eliminates the contents of both the large and the small intestines.

Chest massage

Chest massage is helpful in many ways. It strengthens the chest muscles, increases circulation and tones up the nervous system of the chest, heart and lungs. It is especially recommended in weakness of the lungs, palpitation and organic heart disorders. Bust and mammary glands can be developed by proper massage.

Massage of the back

The purpose of massage of the back is to stimulate the nerves and circulation for treating backache and rheumatic afflictions of the back muscles, and for soothing the nervous system. The patient is made to lie down with the arms at the sides.

Massage of the throat

This helps to overcome headache, sore throat and catarrh of the throat.

Evidence

A number of reviews of the effectiveness of various applications of massage have been published including massage intervention for promoting mental and physical health in infants,[76] massage for mechanical neck disorders,[77] massage for low-back pain[78] and deep transverse friction massage for treating tendonitis.[79] Unfortunately many of the trials displayed methodological inadequacies and firm conclusions could not be drawn.[80] These include establishing what is an adequate dose of massage and questions about the practitioner skills and establishing an appropriate control group. The study was carried out to compare the effects of facial massage with that of foot massage on sleep induction and vital signs of healthy adults.[81] Both treatments were equally effective in reducing subjective levels of alertness during the interventions, with face massage marginally better at producing subjective sleepiness.

A review was carried out to investigate infant massage.[82] This is increasingly being used in the community for low-risk babies and their primary care givers. Anecdotal claims suggest benefits for sleep, respiration, elimination, and reduction of colic and wind. Infant massage is also thought to reduce infant stress and promote positive parent–infant interaction.

Twenty-three studies were included in the review. The only evidence of a significant impact of massage on growth was obtained from a group of studies regarded to be at high risk of bias. There was, however, some evidence of benefits on mother–infant interaction, sleeping and crying, and on hormones influencing stress levels. In the absence of evidence of harm, these findings may be sufficient to support the use of infant massage in the community, particularly in contexts where infant stimulation is poor. Further research is needed, however, before it will be possible to recommend universal provision.

Anxiety

There is some good evidence from RCTs that massage can reduce anxiety in the short term in psychiatric patients who are children or adolescents,[83] and in palliative care.[84] In one study of cancer patients suffering from pain, 60% of the respondents reported a reduction in pain after a 30-minute massage.[85] Massage has been beneficial in intensive care after cardiac surgery,[86] although some concerns about its effect on critically ill patients have been expressed.[87] Long-term elderly hospital patients are reported to have responded to massage with a reduction in anxiety, tension and heart rate.[88]

Premenstrual syndrome

Massage therapy may be an effective long-term aid for pain reduction and water retention, and a short-term aid for decreasing anxiety and improving mood for women with premenstrual dysphoric disorder.[89]

Low back pain

An RCT with four parts sought to compare the effectiveness of massage therapy with other interventions for the treatment of low back pain.[90] The massage provided a benefit to patients in excess of the other interventions.

AIDS

There is some evidence that massage may improve the immune function and quality of life of AIDS patients.[91]

Massage for children

A critical review of the use of massage therapy in children concluded that there was insufficient evidence to support its use without qualification.[92] None the less it is used in both neonates and older children with a variety of medical conditions. Benefits include improved mood (less crying and salivation), increased sleep and reduced pain in children with juvenile rheumatoid arthritis.

Massage in schools was first introduced in Britain in 2000, and is now used in about 100 schools.[93] The sessions start with the teacher reading a story and then pupils take turns to draw patterns on each other's heads, shoulders and backs. Supporters believe that massage has a positive effect on behaviour, concentration and children's respect for each other.

Sports massage; muscular fatigue

Statistics from the British team at the Atlanta Olympics in 1996 revealed that massage formed 47% of all treatments to athletes from all sports. The demand for massage in Albertville (1992) for the winter Olympics and Barcelona (1992) was also significant. Massage also played an important part in the Athens Olympics.

Despite its popular appeal, a consensus as to its benefit is difficult to obtain from the literature because of the wide range of techniques employed and the outcome measures chosen.[94] A New Zealand shooting competitor in the Beijing Olympics 2008 blamed her disappointing performance on a massage the night before her event which was said to have relaxed her too much.

Some clinical trials do exist that are appropriate to mention within the sports context, and a selection have been considered in a review.[95]

Pre-exercise massage   Athletes often use massage before exercise but there is little evidence to support the hypothesis that it will enhance athletic performance. A whole range of liniments and rubs for use with accompanying massage is available. Many have the characteristic 'go faster' pungent aroma of wintergreen, turpentine or other popular essential oils instantly recognisable in a typical changing-room environment. Some of these products are rubifacients, containing constituents that act as an irritant to the skin (e.g. salicylates and capsicum) and cause dilatation of superficial blood vessels, creating a pleasant warm sensation. There is a risk of an allergic reaction to these chemicals.

The effects of pre-exercise massage, warm-up and stretching movements on the joint range of movement and quadriceps and hamstring strength have been investigated.[96] The results showed that warm-up and stretching produced significant increases in all ranges of movement. The only other significant finding was that massage and warm-up, both separately and in combination, appeared to increase the range of movement on the calf. It was concluded that general warm-up and stretching were a better way of increasing flexibility, with the added advantage of being performed by the athlete without the need for expensive equipment or operators.

A psychological evaluation of pre-exercise massage was undertaken in 10 healthy men.[97] Each man was assigned to a group receiving massage or a group receiving no massage before 10 minutes of submaximal exercise. Various parameters were measured, including oxygen consumption and cardiac output. No difference in performance was detected between the two groups. The very low numbers of participants is a major criticism. The difficulty of eliminating bias in the placebo group, who obviously knew that they were not receiving treatment, is always a potential problem in this type of study.

Although massage is widely used, there is no firm scientific evidence that it confers either physical or mental benefits.

Post-exercise massage   Post-exercise massage is often applied in the belief that it will help overcome fatigue and aid recovery.

Delayed-onset muscle soreness   Delayed-onset muscle soreness is a frequent problem after strenuous exercise, particularly among those people unaccustomed to such activity. The condition usually subsides after 3–4 days but can hamper athletes in that it curtails training and can cause a lack of performance. A number of treatments have been tried, including ultrasonography, NSAIDs, homeopathic Arnica and steroids. Massage therapy has also been suggested, but once again considerable uncertainty exists as to its effectiveness.[98] One study evaluated the effects of manual and mechanical massage on recovery from overall muscular and physiological fatigue.[99] It was concluded that there were definite recuperative benefits from the two types of massage, but not from rest alone. The study had several limitations, however. The numbers involved were low, the results were not treated statistically and, most importantly, it was not made clear whether or not the types of massage delivered by the masseur and the machine were comparable.

If one of the reasons for fatigue is a restriction of blood flow to active muscles as a result of muscle contractions it is reasonable to suppose that any action that increases blood flow to allow transport of metabolic by-products would be beneficial. Increased blood flow was thought to be a major advantage of vibratory massage, yet, when this type of massage was studied, it was not shown to help recovery.[100]

Another study was conducted involving nine athletes.[101] Having completed a maximal run, all participants were rested or manually massaged for 17 min or invited to warm down by exercising at a moderate level. Delayed-onset muscle soreness was less pronounced in the massaged individuals, who also showed a more rapid decline in muscle lactate levels. This was encouraging, but the small sample size hampered its conclusiveness.

A systematic review of seven studies on delayed-onset muscle soreness and massage found that most of the methodology described was seriously flawed.[102] However, it was concluded that massage therapy may be a promising treatment for the condition. Further study is warranted.

Muscle fatigue The effects of various massage techniques on muscle soreness and fatigue after intense muscular activity have been studied. Twenty female volunteers received electrical vibration massages for 40 min after maximal muscular activity.[103] The control group received no treatment after the same physical effort. A pain-rating scale and dynamometric measurements were used as end-points. Compared with controls there appeared to be less loss of muscular strength in the massaged thighs after 1 and 3 days. However, in the upper limbs no such difference could be demonstrated; the pain was not significantly different in the control or massage groups.

In a similar study 12 male volunteers performed quadriceps contractions up to the point of exhaustion.[100] Percussive vibratory massage bouts lasting 4 min did not alter the degree of fatigue in repeated series with or without massages.

A group of 16 volunteers were randomised into two groups receiving massage or placebo massage (near-zero applied force), or no massage at all.[104] Dynamometric measurements and soreness perception were evaluated before, 24 h and 48 h after work. There were no effects of massage on any of the variables measured. The use of so-called placebo massage has to be questioned. The participant must be aware that true massage is not being applied and therefore could be biased. On the basis of these findings the effectiveness of massage in preventing muscle soreness and fatigue remains unproven.

In another study 46 patients suffering from fibrositis were treated 19 times in 4 weeks by massage lasting 30–40 min.[105] Effectiveness was evaluated by a fibrositis score during the treatment period. This parameter decreased significantly after massage therapy. Unfortunately, this trial did not include a control group, so one is left to speculate whether the improvement was due to the treatment itself or a placebo effect, or would have occurred spontaneously anyway.

Several studies have compared massage as a therapy applied in the control group when evaluating treatments such as exercise or manipulation for back pain. Results are mixed, with both positive and negative outcomes being reported.[106,107] Unfortunately, there appears to be little convincing evidence of the effectiveness of manipulation with which to make a meaningful comparison.[108]

The effect of treatment with ultrasonography, massage and exercises on myofascial trigger points in the neck and shoulder was assessed in an RCT.[109] The patients were randomised to three groups. The first group was treated with ultrasonography, massage and exercise, the second group with sham ultrasonography, massage and exercise, and the third group was a control group. The study lasted 6 weeks. The outcome measures were pain at rest and on daily function using a visual analogue scale, analgesic usage, global preference and index of myofascial trigger points. The long-term effect of the treatment and control groups was assessed after 6 months using a questionnaire. No difference was detected between the groups given ultrasonography but minor improvement was noted in both test groups over the control. The combined massage and exercise regimen conferred a slight benefit. It is not possible to say whether the exercise or massage element was the more effective.

Sports specificity   Different sports or even different disciplines within the same sport require a different massage regimen. Cycling has traditionally regarded the masseur as an important member of the team, yet the rationale for this is doubtful. In one study six elite cyclists performed a 4-day stage race by race simulation.[110] After each stage the cyclists were given either massage for 20 min or 30 min blind placebo microwave. The race simulation was repeated 18 days later but the post-race treatments were altered. Serum muscle and liver enzymes were measured to detect muscle damage and recovery status. There were no significant differences between massage and placebo at any time during the study. It was concluded that post-event massage did not expedite muscle recovery or improve performance. A second study to test the effect of massage on the cyclists' psychological profiles also revealed no benefit.[111]

Rhythmical massage therapy

Rhythmical massage therapy (RMT) is an important part of anthroposophical medicine (see Chapter 7). It was developed from Swedish massage by Dr Wegman, a physician and physiotherapist. Special techniques include effleurage with light undulating pressure, kneading with circular loop-shaped movements and gentle lifting movements. There are also elements of friction, percussion and vibration. Throughout the massage (which takes about 30 min) the patient is kept warm. At the start of treatment an ointment containing copper or iron may be lightly rubbed into the skin near a major organ to stimulate calm. A total of 5–12 sessions are usually given at the rate of one or two a week.

Observational studies in inpatient settings suggest that RMT can have clinically relevant effects;[112–114] however, the quality of provided evidence is weak mainly because RMT was one of several treatment components that were studied. In a prospective 4-year cohort study focusing on RMT, patients treated with RMT had substantial long-term reduction of chronic disease symptoms and improvement of quality of life.[115]

Conclusion

It seems that much work is required to establish whether or not massage is as effective as people believe. Much of the existing evidence is contradictory and invalidated to some extent by poor methodology. There may be psychological benefit from massage with essential oils.

Safety

Most massage techniques have a low risk of adverse effects. Adverse effects reported in the literature are rare and have usually involved extremely vigorous massage techniques that are highly unusual in the UK. Certain aromatherapy oils may pose a risk (see Chapter 7).

Baby massage is becoming popular and it has been suggested that the oils used in this procedure may pose a hazard.[116] Special-care baby units, such as those serving London's Queen Charlotte's and Chelsea Hospitals, recommend arachis oil for massage of premature babies.[117] However, if tiny babies suck their hands after a hand massage with arachis (peanut) oil they may ingest large quantities of nut products, with potentially serious consequences.[118,119] It could be argued that the potential risks should be indicated on the labels of massage oils and in baby massage books and at classes. Alternative products could also be used to minimise the risk of reaction.

Osteopathy (osteopathic manipulative medicine)

The name 'osteopathy' stems from the Latin words *osteon* and *pathos*, which translates to 'suffering of the bone'. This name has caused confusion in the sense that it makes people believe that an osteopath treats only conditions of the bones. However, the name was chosen because its founder, Dr Andrew Still, recognised that a well-balanced, properly functioning body relies on both the muscular and the skeletal systems of an individual being healthy and well.

The World Health Organization recognises the osteopathic concept of somatic dysfunction as being scientifically proven, and the British Medical Association also recognises osteopathy as a discrete medical discipline. In Australia, osteopaths are statutorily registered practitioners who have a 5-year, full-time university training.

Definition

Osteopathy is a medical discipline that is based primarily on the manual diagnosis and treatment of impaired function resulting from loss of movement. Its philosophy has an emphasis on internal relationships of structure and function, with an appreciation of the body's ability to heal itself. It uses a wide range of techniques to treat musculoskeletal problems and other functional disorders of the body.

History

Osteopathy was developed in the USA in the 1870s by an American frontier doctor, Andrew Taylor Still (1828–1917). Still used his extensive knowledge of anatomy and physiology to develop a method to diagnose and treat the body through palpation and manipulation. He founded the American School of Osteopathy at Kirksville, Missouri in 1892.

Theory

The philosophy of osteopathic medicine is based on the idea that the human body constitutes an ecologically and biologically unified whole. Body systems are united through the neuroendocrine and circulatory systems. In the study of health and disease, therefore, no single part of the body can be considered autonomous. Osteopaths believe that the problems of health and the treatment of disease can be rationally considered only through the study of the whole person in relation to both internal and external environments. The following key principles are involved:[120]

- The body comprises interrelated organs and systems, and functions as a whole unit; disease results from an imbalance in overall health.
- The body has an ability to heal itself and may be assisted in this function by the practitioner; disease represents a breakdown in this capability.
- The body is much more than the sum of its individual parts; nothing exists in isolation and the totality must be considered, e.g. dysfunction in the musculoskeletal system frequently contributes to pain, poor circulation and changes in function leading to constipation, headache, fatigue.
- Treatment is based on the three basic principles of body unity, self-regulation and the interrelationship of structure and function, as stated above.

Practice

Osteopathic treatment is purely and solely based on manual techniques, which are used to adjust and correct mechanical problems in the whole body. The osteopath does not prescribe any medicines, nor does he or she use any invasive techniques (injections, surgery, etc.), although in the USA the scope of treatment may be wider than this. Diagnostic techniques are as for chiropractic and may include radiology.

The aim is not to treat the illness itself but to stimulate the patient's natural healing processes. There are four phases to treatment:

1. Detection of changes in muscles and tissues (by palpation)
2. Observation of any body asymmetry (e.g. leg length), posture and respiratory function
3. Testing of mobility and sensitivity
4. Application of treatment.

Usually, a patient will be asked to be passive during this phase. However, at times there are some techniques for which the patient must actively participate in the movements. The following treatments are examples of the direct and indirect techniques employed by osteopaths:

- Counterstrain techniques achieve release of restriction by placing the affected joint or muscle in a position of comfort, while applying a counter-stretch to the antagonists of the tight muscles.
- Functional techniques involve gentle mobilisation of joints so that barriers to normal movement are identified until a way is found through the restriction.

Osteopathic manipulations are carried out using minimum force levels in order to maximise safety and minimise patient discomfort; manipulation is not the mainstay of most osteopathic treatments. A treatment session lasts approximately half an hour.

- Craniosacral techniques are very gentle release techniques particularly suited to young children and physically frail individuals; this therapy was evolved by the Swiss practitioner William Garner Sutherland (1873–1954) and depends on the suggestion that cranial sutures have the ability to move slightly and their manipulation is thought to improve the circulation of cerebrospinal fluid, which in turn may relieve certain local symptoms.[121]
- Visceral techniques are used in the management of conditions affecting internal organs and involve gentle and rhythmical stretching of the visceral areas.

Apart from low back pain,[122,123] other conditions treated by osteopathy are similar to those addressed by chiropractors and include neck and shoulder pain, sports injuries, repetitive strain disorders and headache. In addition, practitioners also treat arthritis; although they cannot affect disease pathology or progression, they claim to be able to treat secondary symptoms such as pain from associated muscle spasm. Cranial osteopathy has a particular reputation for treating children with conditions such as infantile colic, constant crying and behavioural problems.[124] Osteopathy has been introduced by some general medical practitioners in the UK to a limited extent[125,126] with limited cost implications.[127] Referral to registered osteopaths under the NHS is also possible in some areas and a few NHS hospital trusts have taken on osteopaths to work within hospital physiotherapy departments.

Comparison with other manual disciplines

Chiropractic

Chiropractic always looks for the cause of the complaint in the vertebral column and treats it by means of manipulations, while osteopathy considers all the other body systems. Chiropractors are more likely to push on vertebrae with their hands, whereas osteopaths tend to use the limbs to make levered thrusts. Osteopathic and chiropractic techniques appear to be converging, and much of their therapeutic portfolio is shared.

Physiotherapy

Physiotherapy principally deals with rehabilitation and local treatment whereas osteopathy approaches the patient as a whole. Many physiotherapists use osteopathic and chiropractic techniques.

Manual therapy

Manual therapy is a method of detecting and treating loss of movement in the locomotor system. Osteopathy goes much further by also subjecting all the other tissues to a thorough examination.

Evidence

Although many people have osteopathic manual therapy, few trials have evaluated this therapy; most patients improve within a month, even without treatment, so assessment of any therapy for low back pain is difficult. As a result of the convergence of chiropractic and osteopathy, the evidence for the former (see above) is often applied to the practice of the latter.

In a commentary[128] on a trial, it was reported that a total of 1193 patients were screened to find 178 individuals who had had back pain for at least 3 weeks but less than 6 months.[129] Twenty-three patients later dropped out, leaving 72 patients in the allopathic treatment group and 83 patients in the osteopathic treatment group. Standard treatment included analgesics, anti-inflammatory drugs, active physical therapy and ultrasonography, but no manual therapy. Physicians from the Chicago College of Osteopathic Medicine treated the other group with a number of osteopathic techniques. At the end of a 12-week period, all the patients had improved, but there were no significant differences between treatment groups, except in medication use. In the allopathic group, NSAIDs and muscle relaxants were prescribed at 54.3% and 25.1% of patient visits, respectively. In the osteopathy group, these drugs were prescribed at only 24.3% and 6.3% of visits.

The UK General Osteopathy Council website states that, after a year-long clinical trial at Salford University, researchers revealed that an osteopathic approach has demonstrated up to a 40% improvement in the very severe symptoms of chronic fatigue syndrome.[130] Two groups took part. One group of patients received osteopathy for 12 months, whereas a control group was allowed any therapy of choice, with the exception of osteopathy. A 40% improvement in all symptoms – severe depression, chronic fatigue, back pain, headaches and sleeplessness – in the patient group was registered by the end of the year. Nine patients recorded an improvement of over 50% whereas two felt completely symptom free. Only seven members of the patient group improved by less than the 23% improvement scored by the best result of the control group. The control group's mean result was 1% worse after the 12 months, with one sufferer worsening by 36%.

Osteopathic manipulation has been used as a complementary modality for treating musculoskeletal problems during postoperative surgery. In a prospective, single-blinded, two-matched group outcome study involving a total of 76 patients, patients receiving osteopathic treatment in the early postoperative period negotiated stairs earlier and walked further distances than control group patients.[131]

The positive outcomes noted above are countered by other less encouraging evidence. Placebo-controlled trials have shown that osteopathy is no better than sham treatment for lower back pain[132] or for pain after knee/hip surgery.[133] A systematic review and critical appraisal of the scientific evidence on craniosacral therapy concluded that there is insufficient scientific evidence to recommend craniosacral therapy to patients, practitioners or third party-payers for any clinical condition.[134,135]

Safety

Safety considerations are similar to those for chiropractic (see above). It is contraindicated in patients with brittle bones.

Statutory regulation

Osteopathy and chiropractic are the only two complementary therapies regulated by statute in the UK. The Osteopaths Act 1993 established a General Osteopathic Council (one of the 13 healthcare and social care regulators) with the aim of regulating the profession. The act may be accessed on the internet at the following address: http://tinyurl.com/3bty3q.

The General Osteopathic Council is responsible for regulating, developing and promoting osteopathy in the UK. It has taken over the functions of previous voluntary bodies with regulatory functions that have now ceased. The legislation was fully enacted in May 2000, and it is now an offence for anyone practising in the UK to claim expressly or by implication to be any kind of osteopath unless registered with the

General Osteopathic Council. The General Osteopathic Council operates in a similar way to the General Medical Council and has the authority to remove practitioners from the register in disciplinary hearings.

In the USA a distinction is made between an osteopath and an osteopathic physician. Doctors of Osteopathic Medicine (DOs) are fully licensed medical physicians and surgeons, practising in all clinical specialties along with their physician colleagues. DOs practise the full scope of medicine, but with an emphasis on the role of the neuromusculoskeletal system. They are active in primary care, paediatrics, or family or internal medicine, and are trained to have a more empathetic approach to patient care.

Training

In the UK most osteopaths now take a 4-year full-time course leading to a Bachelors degree (BOst or BSc) and must register with the General Osteopathic Council (see above). In the USA the original qualification offered by Still was a Diploma in Osteopathy, although under state law he could have conferred the degree of MD. Today the degree is Doctor of Osteopathic Medicine, which allows the holder to practise all branches of medicine (see above).

Reflexology

The word 'reflexology' comprises 'reflex', in this case meaning one part reflecting another part, and 'ology', meaning study of. Put together, we get the study of how one part reflects another. However, the discipline involves much more than simply a study of parts. Reflexology is the most popular complementary discipline in Denmark.

Definition

Reflexology may be defined as 'the scientific theory that maps out the reflexes on the feet and hands to all the organs and the rest of the body'. It involves the application of pressure to reflex areas of the hands or feet to produce specific effects in other parts of the body. Figure 16.1 shows a reflexology map; each of the shaded areas represents different areas of the body or organs.

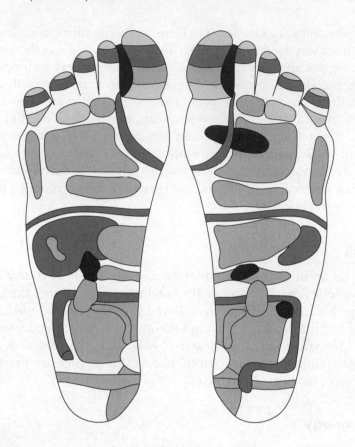

Figure 16.1 Reflexology map. The shaded areas correspond with organs and other areas of the body.

History

A pictograph in the tomb of Ankhmahar, a physician of particularly high esteem, discovered at Saqqara in 1979, revealed that the ancient Egyptians were aware of the benefits of foot and hand reflexology. The pictograph, dating back to around 2500 BC, shows a therapist working on a patient's foot and a second therapist working on another patient's hand. The inscription reads: 'Don't hurt me'. The practitioner's reply is: 'I shall act so you praise me'. Reflexology is also said to have been practised in Chinese and North American Indian cultures.

While working in Vienna in the early 1900s an American ear, nose and throat specialist, Willam Fitzgerald (1872–1942), observed that applying pressure to specific areas of hands and feet caused an anaes-thetising effect on other areas of the body and was useful in the treatment of pain. When he returned to the USA he divided the body into five longitudinal zones on each side of the body. These terminated in the toes and fingers. Fitzgerald suggested that a direct link existed between the areas and organs within each of the zones. This idea was developed by Eunice Ingham (1879–1974), who charted reflex areas in the foot that appeared to correspond to areas of the entire body. Several other charts have been produced since this early work, incorporating various refinements.

Theory

It is suggested that, when the reflexes are stimulated, the body's natural electric energy works along the nervous system and meridian lines to clear any blockages on those lines and in the corresponding zones. A treatment seems to break up deposits (felt as gritty areas under the skin) that may interfere with the natural flow of the body's energy.[136]

Practice

Unlike some other complementary disciplines, reflexologists do not seek to diagnose medical conditions, nor do they prescribe medicines, although the topical use of oils or herbal preparations is often recommended.[137] Dietary advice may also be given.

Most reflexologists work on the feet, although the hands may also be involved. A treatment session lasts around 40 min. Practitioners usually advise their patients that the effects of a treatment may last up to a week. The need for further treatment will vary according to the severity of the condition and the patient.

The following benefits are possible:

- Improved urination
- Improved digestion
- Heightened sense of energy
- Reduction in pain.

Evidence

A review of literature on the effectiveness of reflexology splits the evidence into anecdotal and scientific.[138] Examples of each are presented below. They do not add up to much more than just an impression that reflexology is of benefit.

Anecdotal evidence

There are a number of conditions for which case study reports are available. These include stress-related conditions (anxiety, migraine), back pain, gastrointestinal complaints and arthritis. As well as these specific conditions, patients report an improvement in their ability to relax and this may encourage self-healing.[139] Other benefits include a pleasant warming sensation in an injured area and improved sleep patterns.

While acknowledging that there was no scientific evidence to support the statement, it has none the less been suggested that reflexology may provide some relief from postnatal problems after caesarean section and forceps delivery.[140] Cases have also been presented that demonstrate the apparent benefit of reflexology in midwifery.[141] Reflexology may also be of use during labour.

Scientific data

The first placebo-controlled RCT was reported in an investigation of the use of reflexology in premenstrual syndrome.[142] The trial began with 83 patients but, due to a high drop-out rate, only 35 completed the 6-month protocol. Treatment comprised eight weekly reflexology or placebo treatments. The verum was application of pressure to areas of the hands and feet appropriate to the condition being treated, whereas placebo reflexology was uneven light or heavy pressure to areas considered to be inappropriate to the conditions being treated. The results were in favour of reflexology. However, the type of reflexology used was not stated. This is significant because a number of different schools of thought on reflexology practice have been proposed. These reflect variations in the exact location of some of the reflexes and the methods of treatment. It is thus important that, when outcomes from any particular set of treatments are discussed, the researcher states exactly which approach has been employed. Furthermore, the placebo points chosen in the study were acupressure points and may have been stimulated by the pressure applied to them.[143]

Low back pain was investigated in a double-blind RCT using a total of 91 patients assigned to treatment and placebo groups.[144] The authors report a statistically significant positive outcome with reduction in pain and improvements in muscular contractibility and mobility.

A number of other small-scale studies of reflexology used in the treatment of anxiety states, back pain and chest pain have been reported.[138]

Safety

Concerns may be expressed over the use of reflexology in diabetic patients due to the possibility of damage to the feet that will not be noticed by the patient. Furthermore, it is theoretically possible that stimulation of the reflexes could lead to the increased release of insulin from the pancreas in type 1 diabetes, upsetting patients' calculations as to how much insulin they need to administer. Other common foot diseases may preclude the use of reflexology.

Areas of injury, e.g. fractures and areas corresponding to internal organs that are diseased (e.g. the heart or gastrointestinal system), should be avoided.

Rolfing

> When the body gets working appropriately the force of gravity can flow through then, spontaneously, the body heals itself.
>
> Dr Ida P Rolf

Definition

Rolfing is a comprehensive system of hands-on, connective tissue manipulation and movement education that releases stress patterns in the human organism.

As with other similar techniques (e.g. Feldenkrais), rolfing seeks to organise and integrate the body in relation to gravity by manipulating the soft tissues or by correcting inappropriate patterns of movement. The final goal is that the client can move and function with greater freedom, and effortlessly maintain a more upright posture.

History

Rolfing is the creation of Dr Ida Rolf, a biochemist and physiologist who established the Rolf Institute for Structural Integration in 1970.[145] She believed that, for optimum health, the body must be in alignment with gravity: any deviation from the norm requires extra energy for movement and imposes unnecessary strain on the muscles. She contended that, as the muscles work to compensate for failing efficiency over the passing years, the fascia surrounding them tend to bunch up and harden, creating even more strain. Ultimately, she said, the cumulative stress can interfere with normal breathing and impair circulation, digestion and the nervous system.

Theory

The deep massage techniques employed in rolfing seek to loosen and relax the fascia – the membranes that surround the muscles. (Rolfers believe that the fascia toughen and thicken over time, subtly contorting the body and throwing it out of healthy alignment.)

Practice

To break up knots in the fascia and 'reset' the muscles, rolfers apply slow, sliding pressure with their knuckles, thumbs, fingers, elbows and knees. The treatments are not mild and relaxing – indeed, they can cause a degree of pain. However, practitioners view this temporary discomfort as a sign that the treatment is achieving the changes necessary to bring the body back into proper alignment. During each session, the rolfer will concentrate on a different set of muscles, starting with those nearest the surface and moving on to those deep within the body. To maximise the benefits of treatment, the therapist may also teach self-help exercises known as movement integration. Sessions usually last 60–90 min. The basic sequence of rolfing consists of 10 sessions through which a new structural order and a more efficient movement pattern are developed.

Evidence

Rolf published a total of 13 papers, mainly on the subject of children with poor coordination and disorganised movement patterns.[146] The children established improved muscle tone, improved language skills and social responsiveness after rolfing. A study of neurologically compromised individuals with cerebral palsy found significant improvements in locomotion after rolfing.[147] The facilitation of greater ease of motion has also been shown after rolfing.[148]

More information

Alexander technique

Society of Teachers of the Alexander Technique, 20 London House, 266 Fulham Road, London SW10 9EL. Tel: 020 7352 0828; website: www.stat.org.uk

Chiropractic

British Chiropractic Association, Blagrave House 17 Blagrave Street Reading Berks RG1 1QB. Tel: 0118 950 5950; fax: 0118 958 8946; website: www. chiropractic.org.uk

British Association of Applied Chiropractic, The Old Post Office, Cherry Street, Stratton Audley, Nr Bicester, Oxon OX6 9BA. Tel/fax: 01869 277111

McTimoney Chiropractic Association, 21 High Street, Eynsham, Oxon OX8 1HE. Tel: 01865 880974; fax: 01865 880975

The Oxford College of Chiropractic (formerly the Witney School), c/o The Old Post Office, Cherry Street, Stratton Audley, Nr Bicester, Oxon OX6 9BA; website: www.lifesciences.napier.ac.uk/courses/projects/backpain/chircar.htm

Scottish Chiropractic Association, 16 Jenny Moores Road, St Boswells TD6 0AL. Tel: 01835 823645; fax: 01835 823930; email: Carlahow@scotborders.co.uk

American Chiropractic Association, 1701 Clarendon Blvd, Arlington, VA 22209, USA. Tel: +1 800 986 4636; website: www.amerchiro.org

Massage

British Massage Therapy Council, 17 Rymers Lane, Oxford OX4 3JU. Tel: 01865 774123; website: www.bmtc.co.uk

Osteopathic medicine

The General Osteopathic Council, Osteopathy House, 176 Tower Bridge Road, London SE1 3LU. Tel: 020 7357 6655; website: www.osteopathy.org.uk

British Osteopathic Association, Langham House, East Luton, Bedfordshire LU1 2NA. Tel: 01582 488455; website: www.osteopathy.org

American Osteopathic Association, 142 East Ontario Street, Chicago, IL 60611, USA. Tel: +1 800 621 1773; fax: +1 312 202 8200; website: www.am-osteo-assn.org

Reflexology

Association of Reflexologists, 27 Old Gloucester Street, London WC1N 3XX. Tel: 0870 567 3320; email: aor@reflexology.org

British Association of Reflexology, Monks Orchard, Whitbourne, Worcester WR6 5RB. Tel: 01886 821207; email: bra@britreflex.co.uk

Research sites

www.pacificreflexology.com/res.htm
www.reflexology-research.com
www.internethealthlibrary.com/Therapies/Reflexology-Research% 20.htm#top

Rolfing

The Rolf Institute, 205 Canyon Blvd, Boulder, CO 80302, USA. Tel: +1 303 449 5903;
website: www.rolf.org
UK contact: Simon Wellby, PO Box 14793, London SW1 V2WB. Tel: 020 7834 1493

References

1. Alexander FM. *The Use of the Self*. London: Gollancz, 1985: 42.
2. Stevens C. *Alexander Technique*. London: Vermilion, 1966.
3. McDonald G. *The Complete Illustrated Guide to the Alexander Technique*. Boston: Element Books, 1998.
4. Jonas W, Levin JS, eds. *Essentials of Complementary and Alternative Medicine*. Baltimore, MD: Lippincott/Williams & Wilkins, 1999: 576.
5. Fulder S. *The Handbook of Complementary and Alternative Medicine*. New York: Oxford University Press, 1996: 143.
6. Heaton J, Fisher V. Alexander technique. *Health Which*? 1999;April:26–7.
7. Jones F P. *Freedom to Change: The development and science of the Alexander technique*. London: Mauritz, 1997.
8. Austin JHM, Ausubel BA. Enhanced respiratory muscular function in normal adults after lessons in proprioceptive musculoskeletal education without exercise. *Chest* 1992;**162**:486–90.
9. Fischer K. Early experience of a multi-disciplinary pain management programme. *Holistic Med* 1988;**3**:25–9.
10. Caplan D. *Back Trouble: A new approach to prevention and recovery based on the Alexander technique*. Gainesville, FL: Triad Communications, 1987.
11. Valentine ER, Fitzgerald DFP, Gorton TL, Hudson JA, Symonds ERC. The effect of lessons in the Alexander technique on music performance in high and low stress situations. *Psychol Music* 1995;**23**:129–41.
12. Cacciatore TW, Horak FB, Henry SM. Improvement in automatic postural coordination following Alexander technique lessons in a person with low back pain. *Phys Ther* 2005;**85**:565–78.
13. Maher CG. Effective physical treatment for chronic low back pain. *Orthop Clin North Am* 2004;**35**:57–64. PubMed
14. Stallibrass C, Sissons P, Chalmers C. Randomized controlled trial of the Alexander technique for idiopathic Parkinson's disease. *Clin Rehabil* 2002;**16**:695–708. Available at: http://tinyurl.com/2k49w6 (accessed 29 October 2007).
15. Stallibrass C, Frank C, Wentworth K. Retention of skills learnt in Alexander technique lessons: 28 people with idiopathic Parkinson's disease. *J Bodywork Movement Therap* 2005;**9**:150–7. Available at: http://tinyurl.com/2k49w6 (accessed 29 October 2007).
16. Feldenkrais F. *Awareness Through Movement: Health exercises for personal growth*. New York: Harper & Row, 1972.
17. Ben-Arve E. Katz I, Hermani D. Exploring Feldenkreis practitioners' attitudes toward clinical research. (Letter) *J Altern Compl Med* 2007;**13**:593–4.
18. Wikepdia. Bowen technique. Available at: http://tinyurl.com/2uolj5 (accessed 21 November 2007).

19. European College of Bowen studies website http://tinyurl.com/ypnhnc (accessed 21 November 2007).

20. Kinnear H, Baker J. European College of Bowen Studies Frozen shoulder research programme. Available at: http://tinyurl.com/ytfpfg (accessed 21 November 2007).

21. Marr M, Lambon N, Baker J. Effects of the Bowen technique on flexibility levels: implications for facial plasticity. Presented at the First International Fascia Congress, Boston, October 2007. Available at: http://tinyurl.com/3xwzks (accessed 21 November 2007).

22. Deyo RA, Tsui-Wu Y J. Descriptive epidemiology of low-back pain and its related medicinal care in the United States. *Spine* 1987;**12**:264–8.

23. Zollman C, Vickers A. *ABC of Complementary Medicine. Massage therapies.* London: BMJ Books, 2000: 32–5.

24. Bonnet J. *Complementary Medicine in Primary Care – What are the key issues?* London: NHS Executive, 2000.

25. Pollard H, Hoskins W, McHardy A et al. Australian chiropractic sports medicine: half way there or living on a prayer? *Chiropr Osteopath* 2007;**15**:14. PubMed

26. Eisenberg DM, Kessler RC, Foster C et al. Unconventional medicine in the United States: Prevalence, costs, and patterns of use. *N Engl J Med* 1993; **328**:246–52.

27. Breen A. Chiropractic for low back pain. (Letter) *BMJ* 1999;**318**:261.

28. Leerberg E. Efficacy of spinal manipulation for low back pain has not been reliably shown. (Letter) *BMJ* 1999;**318**:261.

29. Jonas W, Levin JS (eds) *Essentials of Complementary and Alternative Medicine.* Baltimore, MD: Lippincott/Williams & Wilkins, 1999: 577.

30. Meade TW. Patients were more satisfied with chiropractic than other treatments for low back pain. *BMJ* 1999;**319**:57.

31. Wolinsky FD, Liu L, Miller TR et al The use of chiropractors by older adults in the United States. *Chiropr Osteopath* 2007;**15**:12. PubMed

32. Maeri JE. *Alternative Health Medicine Encyclopedia.* Detroit: Visible Ink Press, 1995: 6–7.

33. Bergmann TF, Peterson D, Lawrence DJ. *Chiropractic Technique.* New York: Churchill Livingstone, 1993.

34. Freeman LW, Lawlis GF. *Mosby's Complementary and Alternative Medicine. A Research-based Approach.* St Louis, MO: Mosby, 2001: 297.

35. Davis MA, McDevitt L, Alin K. Establishing a chiropractic service in a rural primary health care facility. *J Altern Compl Med* 2007;**13**:697–702.

36. Kaptchuk T, Eisenberg DM. Chiropractic. In: Fontanarosa P B (ed.) *Alternative Medicine. An Objective Assessment.* Washington DC: *JAMA*, 2000;**284**:514–15.

37. Wright GT. Confusing a profession with a treatment modality again. *BMJ* online 1999;20 July.

38. Ernst E, Canter PH. A systematic review of systematic reviews of spinal manipulation. *J R Soc Med* 2006;**99**:192–6. Review.

39. Martin RA. A study of time loss back claims: workmen's compensation boards (Medical Director's report, State of Oregon). *Arch Calif Chiropractors' Assn* 1975;**4**:83–97.

40. Koes BW, Assendelft WJJ, van der Heijden J et al. Spinal manipulation and mobilisation for back and neck pain: a blinded review. *BMJ* 1991;**303**:1298.

41. Waddell G, Feder G, McIntosh A *et al. Clinical Guidelines for the Management of Acute Low Back Pain: Low back pain evidence review.* London: Royal College of General Practitioners, 1996.

42. Shekelle PG, Adams AH, Chassin MR et al. Spinal manipulation for back pain. *Ann Intern Med* 1997;**117**:590–8.

43. Ernst E, Assendelft W JJ. Chiropractic for low back pain. *BMJ* 1998;**317**:160.

44. Assendelft WJJ, Koes BW, van der Heijden GJ, Bouter LM. The effectiveness of chiropractic for treatment of low back pain: an update and attempt at statistical pooling. *J Manipulative Physiol Ther* 1996;**19**:499–507.

45. Morley J, Rosner AL, Redwood D. A case misrepresentation of the scientific literature: recent reviews of chiropractic. *J Altern Compl Med* 2001;**7**:65–78.

46. Meade T W, Dyer S, Browne W, Frank AO. Randomised comparison of chiropractic and hospital outpatient management for low back pain: results from extended follow up. *BMJ* 1995;**311**:349–51.

47. Ernst E, Assendelft WJJ. Reply to correspondence. *BMJ* 1999;**318**:261.

48. Jordan A, Bendix T. Intensive training, physiotherapy or manipulation for patients with chronic neck pain. A prospective single-blinded randomised clinical trial. *Spine* 1998;**23**:311.

49. Rogers RG. The effects of spinal manipulation on cervical kinaesthesia in patients with chronic neck pain: a pilot study. *J Manipulative Physiol Ther* 1997;**20**:80.

50. Nelson CF, Bronford G. The efficacy of spinal manipulation, amitriptyline and the combination of both therapies for the prophylaxis of migraine headache. *J Manipulative Physiol Ther* 1998;**21**:511.

51. Tuchin PJ, Pollard H, Bonello R. A randomised controlled trial of chiropractic spinal manipulative therapy for migraine. *J Manipulative Physiol Ther* 2000;**23**:91–5.

52. Boline PD, Kassak K. Spinal manipulation vs amitriptyline for the treatment of chronic tension type headaches: a randomised clinical trial. *J Manipulative Physiol Ther* 1995;**18**:148.

53. Bove G, Nilsson N. Spinal manipulation in the treatment of episodic tension-type headaches. *JAMA* 1998;**280**:1576.

54. Nilsson NH, Christiansen HW, Hartvigsen J. The effect of spinal manipulation in the treatment of cervicogenic headache. *J Manipulative Physiol Ther* 1997;**18**:435.

55. Kokjohn K, Schmid DM, Triano JJ, Brennan PC. The effect of spinal manipulation on pain and prostaglandin levels in women with primary dysmenorrhoea. *J Manipulative Physiol Ther* 1992;**15**:279.

56. Balon J, Aker PD, Crowther ER et al. A comparison of active and simulated chiropractic manipulation as adjunctive treatment for childhood asthma. *N Engl J Med* 1998;**339**:1013.

57. Klougart N, Nilsson N, Jacobsen J. Infantile colic treated by chiropractors: a prospective study of 316 cases. *J Manipulative Physiol Ther* 1989;**12**:281.

58. Hill CL. Barcelona Olympics – chiropractic report. *NZ J Sp Med* 1993;**21**:8.

59. Vernon H. Qualitative review of studies of manipulation-induced hypoalgesia. *J Manipulative Physiol Ther* 2000;**23**:134–8.

60. Powell FC, Hanigan WC, Olivero WC. A risk/benefit analysis of spinal manipulation for relief of lumbar or cervical pain. *Neurosurgery* 1993;**33**: 73–8.

61. Halderman S, Rubinstein SM. Cauda equina syndrome following lumbar spine manipulation. *Spine* 1992;**17**:1469–73.

62. Assendelft W, Bouter L, Knipschild PG. Complications of spinal manipulation – a comprehensive review of the literature. *J Fam Pract* 1996;**42**:475–80.

63. Triano J, Schultz A B. Loads transmitted during lumbosacral manipulative therapy. *Spine* 1997;**22**:1955–64.

64. Gouveia LO, Castanho P, Ferreira JJ, Guedes MM, Falcão F, Melo TP. Chiropractic manipulation: Reasons for concern? *Clin Neurol Neurosurg* 2007;**109**:922–5. PubMed

65. Abbot NC, White AR, Ernst E. Complementary medicine. *Nature* 1996;**381**: 361. PubMed

66. Senstad O, Leboeuf-Yde Ch, Borchgevink F. Side-effects of chiropractic spinal manipulation: types, frequency, discomfort and course. *Scand J Prim Health Care* 1996;**14**:50–3. PubMed

67. Rubinstein SM, Leboeuf-Yde C, Knol DL, de Koekkoek TE, Pfeifle CE, van Tulder MW. The benefits outweigh the risks for patients undergoing chiropractic care for neck pain: a prospective, multicenter, cohort study. *J Manipulative Physiol Ther* 2007;**6**:408–18.

68. Thiel HW, Bolton JE, Docherty S, Portlock JC Safety of chiropractic manipulation of the cervical spine: a prospective national survey. *Spine* 2007; **32**:2375–8. PubMed

69. Dabbs V, Lauretti WJ. A risk assessment of cervical manipulation vs NSAID for the treatment of neck pain. *J Manipulative Physiol Ther* 1995;**18**:530–53.

70. Terrett AG. Misuse of the literature by medical authors in discussing spinal manipulative therapy injury. *J Manipulative Physiol Ther* 1995;**18**:203–10.

71. Barrett AJ, Breen AC. Adverse effects of spinal manipulation. *J R Soc Med* 2000;**93**:258–9.

72. Ernst E. Commentary. *Focus Altern Compl Ther* 2000;**6**:206.

73. Wright GT. Confusing a profession with a treatment modality again. *BMJ* online 1999;20 July.

74. Astin JA, Marie A, Pelletier KR et al. A review of the incorporation of complementary and alternative medicine by mainstream physicians. *Arch Intern Med* 1998;**158**:2303–10.

75. Freeman LW, Lawlis GF. *Mosby's Complementary and Alternative Medicine. A research-based approach*. St Louis, MO: Mosby, 2001: 363–6.

76. Underdown A, Barlow J, Chung V, Stewart-Brown S. Massage intervention for promoting mental and physical health in infants aged under six months. *Cochrane Database Syst Rev* 2006;(4):CD005038. Review.

77. Ezzo J, Haraldsson BG, Gross AR et al Massage for mechanical neck disorders: a systematic review. *Spine* 2007l;**32**:353–62. PubMed

78. Furlan AD, Brosseau L, Imamura M, Irvin E. Massage for low back pain. *Cochrane Database Syst Rev* 2002;(2):CD001929.

79. Brosseau L, Casimiro L, Milne S, Robinson V, Shea B, Deep transverse friction massage for treating tendinitis. *Cochrane Database Syst Rev* 2002;(4): CD003528.

80. Ezzo J. Education, initiatives, and information resources. *J Altern Compl Med* 2007;**13**:291–5.

81. Ejindu A. The effects of foot and facial massage on sleep induction, blood pressure, pulse and respiratory rate: Crossover pilot study. *Compl Ther Clin Pract* 2007;**13**:266–75. PubMed

82. Underdown A, Barlow J, Chung V, Stewart-Brown S. Massage intervention for promoting mental and physical health in infants aged under six months. *Cochrane Database Syst Rev* 2006;CD005038.

83. Field T, Morrow C, Valdeon C. Massage reduces anxiety in child and adolescent psychiatric patients. *J Am Acad Child Adolesc Psychiatry* 1992;**31**: 125–31.

84. Wilkinson S. Aromatherapy and massage in palliative care. *Int J Palliat Nurs* 1995;**1**:21–30.

85. Ferrel-Tory T, Glick OJ. The use of therapeutic massage as a nursing intervention to modify anxiety and the perception of pain. *Cancer Nurs* 1993;**16**: 93–101.

86. Stevenson C. The psychophysiological effects of aromatherapy massage following cardiac surgery. *Complement Ther Med* 1994;**2**:27–35.

87. Hill CF. Is massage beneficial to critically ill patients in intensive care units? A critical review. *Intens Crit Care Nurs* 1993;**9**:116–21.

88. Fraser J, Kerr JB. Psychological effects of back massage on elderly institutionalised patients. *J Adv Nurs* 1993;**18**:238–45.

89. Hernandez-Reif M, Martinez A, Field T et al. Premenstrual symptoms are relieved by massage therapy. *J Psychosom Obstet Gynaecol* 2000;**21**: 9–15.

90. Preyde M. Effectiveness of massage therapy for subacute low-back pain: a randomised controlled trial. *Can Med Assn J* 2000;**162**:1815–20.

91. Birk TJ, McGrady A, MacArthur RD, Khuder S. The effects of massage therapy alone and in combination with other complementary therapies on immune system measures and quality of life in human immunodeficiency virus. *J Altern Compl Med* 2000;**6**:405–14.

92. Ireland M, Olson M. Massage therapy and therapeutic touch in children: state of the science. *Altern Ther Hlth Med* 2000;**6**:54–63.

93. Payne S Mother protests at 'massage' in class. *Daily Telegraph* 11 May 2005.

94. Callaghan MJ. The role of massage in the management of the athlete. A review. *Br J Sports Med* 1993;**27**:28–33.

95. Ernst E, Fialka V. The clinical effectiveness of massage. *Forsch Komplementärmed* 1994;**1**:226–32.

96. Wiktorsson-Moller M, Oberg B, Eksrand J, Gillquvist J. Effects of warming up, massage and stretching on range of motion and muscle strength in the lower extremity. *Am J Sports Med* 1983;**11**:249–52.

97. Boone T, Cooper R, Thompson WR. A psychological evaluation of the sports massage. *Athletic Training* 1991;**26**:51–4.

98. Cafarelli E, Flint F. The role of massage in preparation for and recovery from exercise: a review. *Sports Med* 1992;**14**:1–9.

99. Baike B, Anthony J, Wyatt F. The effects of massage treatment on exercise fatigue. *Clin Sports Med* 1989;**1**:189–96.

100. Carafelli E, Sim J, Carolan B, Libesman J. Vibratory massage and short term recovery from muscular fatigue. *Int Sports Med* 1990;**11**:474–8.

101. Bale P, James H. Massage, warmdown and rest as recuperative measures after short term intense exercise. *Physiotherapy Sport* 1991;**13**:4–7.

102. Ernst E. Does post-exercise massage treatment reduce delayed onset muscle soreness? A systematic review. *Br J Sports Med* 1998;**32**:212–14.

103. Eltze Ch, Hildebrandt G, Johansson M. Über die Wirsankeit der Vibrationsmassage beim Muskelkater. *Z Phys Med Bain Klimatol* 1982;**11**:366–76.

104. Ellison M, Goehrs C, Hall L et al. Effects of retrograde massage on muscle soreness and performance. *Phys Ther* 1992;**72**:100.

105. Danneskiold-Samsoe B, Christianen E, Bach-Anderson R. Myofascial pain and the role of myoglobin. *Scand J Rehabil Med* 1983;**15**:174–8.

106. Hochler FK, Tobis JS, Buerger AA. Spinal manipulation for low back pain. *JAMA* 1981;**245**:1835–8.

107. Godfrey CM, Morgan PP, Schatzker J. A randomized trial of manipulation for low back pain in a medical setting. *Spine* 1984;**9**:301–4.

108. Ernst E. Spinal manipulation for low back pain. *Eur J Phys Med Rehabil* 1998;**8**:1–2.

109. Gam AN, Warming S, Larsen LH et al. Treatment of myofascial trigger points with ultrasound with massage and exercise – a random controlled trial. *Pain* 1998;**77**:73–9.

110. Drews T, Knieder B, Drinkard D et al. Effects of post event massage therapy on repeated endurance cycling. *Int J Sports Med* 1990;**11**:407.

111. Drews T, Krieder RB, Drinkard B, Jackson CW. Effects of post event massage therapy on psychological profiles of exertion, feeling and mood during a four day ultraendurance cycling event. *Med Sci Sport Exerc* 1991;**23**:91.

112. Carlsson M, Arman M, Backman M et al. Evaluation of quality of life/life satisfaction in women with breast cancer in complementary and conventional care. *Acta Oncol* 2004;**43**:27–34

113. Hamre HJ, Becker-Witt C, Glockmann A et al. Anthroposophic therapies in chronic disease: The Anthroposophic Medicine Outcomes Study (AMOS). *Eur J Med Res* 2004;**9**:351–60.

114. Hamre HJ, Witt CM, Glockmann A et al. Health costs in anthroposophic therapy users: A two-year prospective cohort study. *BMC Hlth Serv Res* 2006;6. Available at: http://tinyurl.com/yw46r3 (accessed 29 October 2007).

115. Hamre HJ, Claudia Md, Witt M, Glockmann A, Ziegler R. Rhythmical massage therapy in chronic disease: a 4-year prospective cohort study. *J Altern Compl Med* 2007;**13**:635–42.

116. Joyce R, Frosh A. Baby massage oils could be a hazard. *BMJ* 1996;**313**:299.

117. Vickers A, Ohlsson A, Lacy JB, Horsley A. *Massage therapy for premature and/or low birth-weight infants to improve weight gain and/or to decrease hospital length of stay.* Oxford: Cochrane Library, 1998: issue 3.

118. Sampson H A. Managing peanut allergy. *BMJ* 1996;**312**:1050–1.

119. Ewan PW. Clinical study of peanut and nut allergy in 62 consecutive patients: new features and associations. *BMJ* 1996;**312**:1074–8.

120. Kappler R, Ramey KA, Heinking KP. Osteopathic medicine. In: Novey D (ed.), *Clinician's Complete Reference to Complementary and Alternative Medicine.* St Louis, MO: Mosby, 2000: 326.

121. Holmes P. Cranial osteopathy. *Nurs Times* 1991;**87**:36–7.

122. MacDonald RS. An open controlled assessment of osteopathic manipulation in non-specific low back pain. *Spine* 1990;**15**:364–70.

123. MacDonald RS. Osteopathic diagnosis of back pain. *Manual Med* 1988; **3**:110–13.

124. Vickers A, Zollman C. ABC of complementary medicine. The manipulative therapies: osteopathy and chiropractic. *BMJ* 1999;**319**:1176–9.

125. Pringle M, Tyreman S. Study of 500 patients attending an osteopathic practice. *Br J Gen Pract* 1993;**43**:15–18.

126. Williams N. Managing back pain in general practice – is osteopathy the new paradigm? *Br J Gen Pract* 1997;**47**:653–5.

127. Williams NH, Wilkinson C, Russell I et al. Randomized osteopathic manipulation study (ROMANS): pragmatic trial for spinal pain in primary care. *Fam Pract* 2003;**20**:662–9.

128. Senior K. Is osteopathy the best way to treat low back pain? *Lancet* 1999;**354**:1705.

129. Andersson G, Lucente T, Davies AM. A comparison of osteopathic spinal manipulation with standard care for patients with low back pain. *N Engl J Med* 1999;**341**:1426–31.

130. General Osteopathy Council. Osteopathic research press release, 12 May 2006. Available at: www.osteopathy.org.uk/goc/links/research.shtml (accessed 10 May 2008).

131. Jarski R, Loniewski EG, Williams J et al. The effectiveness of osteopathic manipulative treatment as complementary therapy following surgery: a prospective match-controlled outcome study. *Altern Ther Hlth Med* 2000;**6**: 77–91.

132. Licciardone JC, Stoll ST, Fulda KG et al. Osteopathic manipulative treatment for chronic low back pain: a randomized controlled trial. *Spine* 2003;**28**:1355–62.

133. Licciardone JC, Stoll ST, Cardarelli KM, Gamber RG, Swift JN, Winn WB. A randomized controlled trial of osteopathic manipulative treatment following knee or hip arthroplasty. *J Am Osteopath Assoc* 2004;**104**:193–20.

134. Green C, Martin CW, Bassett K, Kazanjian A. A systematic review and critical appraisal of the scientific evidence on craniosacral therapy. Database of Abstracts of Reviews of Effects (DARE), 2000. Available at: http://tinyurl.com/2f7ey2 (accessed 1 November 2007).

135. Williams NH, Edwards RT, Linck P et al. Cost-utility analysis of osteopathy in primary care: results from a pragmatic randomized controlled trial. *Fam Pract* 2004;**21**:643–50.

136. Bisson DA. Reflexology. In: Novey D (ed.), *Clinician's Complete Reference to Complementary and Alternative Medicine*. St Louis, MO: Mosby, 2000: 437.

137. Wolfe FA. *Reflexology*. New York: Alpha Books, 1999: 50.

138. Botting D. Review of literature on the effectiveness of reflexology. *Compl Ther Nurs Midwifery* 1997;**3**:123–30.

139. Shaw J. Reflexology. *Health Visitor* 1987;**60**:367.

140. Evans M. Reflex zone therapy for mothers. *Nurs Times* 1990;**86**:29–32.

141. Tiran D. The use of complementary therapies in midwifery practice: a focus on reflexology. *Compl Ther Nurs Midwifery* 1996;**2**:32–7.

142. Oleson T, Flocco W. Randomised controlled study of premenstrual symptoms treated with ear, hand and foot reflexology. *Obstet Gynecol* 1993;**82**: 906–11.

143. Vickers A. *Massage and Aromatherapy – A guide for health professionals.* London: Chapman & Hall, 1996.

144. Kovaks FM, Abraira V, Lopez-Abente G, Pozo F. Neuro-reflexology intervention in the treatment of non-specified low back pain. In: *Reflexology Research Report*, 2nd edn. London: Association of Reflexologists, 1994.

145. Guild for Structural Integration. *History of Ida P Rolf.* Available at: www.rolfguilod.org.idarolf.html (accessed 12 June 2008).

146. Freeman LW, Lawlis GF. *Mosby's Complementary and Alternative Medicine. A research-based approach.* St Louis, MO: Mosby, 2001: 448.

147. Perry J, Jones MH, Thomas L. Functional evaluation of Rolfing in cerebral palsy. *Dev Child Neurol* 1981;**23**:717–29.

148. Weinberg R, Hunt V. Effects of structural integration on state–trait anxiety. *J Clin Psychol* 1979;**35**:319–22.

17

Mind and body therapies

Steven B Kayne

In this chapter a number of mind and body therapies are discussed in sufficient detail for readers to understand the basic concepts involved.

Dance and movement therapy

Dance and movement therapy depends on the ability to perform various actions, not necessarily on the skill or talent apparent in doing so.

Definition

Dance and movement therapy are basic forms of authentic communication, and as such are an especially effective medium for therapy. Based on the belief that the body, mind and spirit are interconnected, dance/movement therapy is defined by the American Dance Therapy Association as 'the psychotherapeutic use of movement as a process that furthers the emotional, cognitive, social and physical integration of the individual'.[1]

History

Dance and movement were first practised as a separate therapy in the 1940s in the USA.

Theory

Dance and movement therapy, a creative art therapy, is rooted in the expressive nature of dance itself. Dance is the most fundamental of the arts, involving a direct expression and experience of oneself through the body. Changes that occur during therapy relate directly to the brain's interactive function, physical exercise and neural interplay between motion and emotion.[2]

Practice

Dance and movement therapists work with individuals of all ages who have social, emotional, cognitive and/or physical problems. They work in settings that include psychiatric and rehabilitation facilities, schools, nursing homes, drug treatment centres, counselling centres, medical facilities, crisis centres, and wellness and alternative healthcare centres. They focus on helping their clients to improve self-esteem and body image, develop effective communication skills and relationships, expand their movement vocabulary, gain insight into patterns of behaviour, as well as create new options for coping with problems.

Dance and movement therapy are claimed to be a powerful tool for stress management and the prevention of physical and mental health problems.

A novel use of dance was employed by Dr Pamela Garlick, a biochemist and senior lecturer at the Guy's, King's and St Thomas' School of Medicine, London. She won a Millennium Award for an innovative dance project about sickle cell anaemia. The aim of the project was to increase the awareness and understanding of sickle cell anaemia in her local borough of Haringey, London, by making the video entitled *Sickle Cell Anaemia – An Exploration through Dance*, for use in secondary schools. In the video, 27 10-year-old children from local schools use dance to convey the intricate processes by which a gene is converted, via messenger RNA, into a protein such as haemoglobin, and to show the effects that the sickle cell mutation has on the behaviour of the red blood cell. The children wear specially printed colour-coded T-shirts and baseball caps to identify themselves as the individual DNA bases, amino acids, etc. The use of a high-angle camera enables a unique bird's-eye view of the cellular events underlying this painful disorder to be visualised. The video includes interviews with individuals who have sickle cell anaemia and their families to explain the health issues related to this disorder, and is presented by athlete and Olympic gold medallist Linford Christie. Copies were distributed to all health centres and secondary schools in Haringey and to all the children involved in the project.

Evidence

Meta-analysis has shown dance and movement therapy to be effective in the treatment of psychiatric patients and anxiety.[3] Most other evidence is of an experiential nature.

Reiki

> Just for today, I will let go of anger.
> Just for today, I will let go of worry.
> Just for today, I will give thanks for my many blessings.
> Just for today, I will do my work honestly.
> Just for today, I will be kind to my neighbour and to every living thing.
>
> Dr Mikao Usui[4]

Reiki (pronounced ray-key) is another healing discipline with its origins in the east. It involves the laying on of hands.

Definition

Reiki is an energy-based touch therapy that provides a means for life force energy, or qi, to recharge, realign and rebalance the human energy fields, creating optimal conditions needed by the body's natural healing system. The concept of qi is described in Chapter 12. Reiki, similar to other touch therapies, such as therapeutic touch and healing touch (see below), involves the use of energy directed by the practitioner's hands to strengthen the body's ability to heal, inspiring balance, and involves a mind–body connection

The Japanese compound word *reiki* may be translated simply as 'healing'. However, to followers of the practice it stands for far more than this one English word can imply. *Rei* means 'universal' or 'spiritual' and *ki* is 'life force energy'. Thus, more correctly it should be translated as 'universal life force energy'. It is the coming together of the spiritual dimensions and living energies to awaken a dynamic healing process and release the cause of stress in the body, mind, emotions and spirit.[5] Despite having these religious connotations, reiki is not a religion.

History

It is commonly believed that the origins of reiki may be traced back to early Tibetan teachings from around 3000 BC. It has also been suggested that the method was used by Buddha and Jesus Christ. The methodology employed in modern reiki is known as the Usui natural healing system (sometimes written as Usui shiki ryoho) from the name of Dr Mikao Usui of Kyoto, a Christian theologian who developed the system towards the end of the nineteenth century. Dr Usui spent many years on a quest for the secret of the ancient healing traditions. He went to a mountaintop in Japan and underwent 21 days of purification, fasting and meditation, at the end of which he received enlightenment and the power of healing. He came down from the mountain and spent the rest of his life practising and teaching reiki. He took reiki to the USA in 1936.

Theory

All touch therapies share a common similarity, i.e. an underpinning to eastern ideology and philosophy.[6] These values are consistent with the belief that the human body needs a continuous flow of life force energy for sustained health and wellness. The National Center of Complementary and Alternative Medicine (NCCAM) classifies therapeutic touch, healing touch and reiki as biofield therapies, the medical use of subtle energy fields in and around the body for positive health effects:[7]

> The reiki therapist body's channels Qi energy through his or her hands to the recipient, activating the body's natural ability to heal itself. Reiki energy goes to the deeper levels of a person's being, where many illnesses have their origins. It works wherever the recipient needs it most, releasing blocked energies, cleansing the body of toxins, relieving stress, alleviating pain and working to recreate the natural state of balance.

Practice

Reiki practitioners are said to be attuned to the reiki energy, and develop their abilities in conformance with Usui's original system. The procedures are very simple and non-intrusive. A treatment session lasts about an hour. It is usually carried out with the recipient remaining fully clothed, lying on a therapy couch. The practitioner places his or her hands on to the patient's body at a number of strategic points. Each position is held for up to 3 min. There is no pressure exerted. Energy is said to flow into the body and move to the source of the imbalance, not just to the manifesting symptoms.

Evidence

The use of reiki in chronic pain management as an adjunct to opioid therapy has been investigated.[8] Twenty patients collectively experiencing pain at 55 sites were subjected to reiki treatment by a certified therapist. Pain was measured using a visual analogue scale and the Likert scale before and after treatment. A significant reduction in pain was recorded after treatment.

A pilot study was carried out to compare reports of pain and levels of anxiety state in two groups of women after abdominal hysterectomy.[9] An experimental group of patients ($n = 10$) received traditional nursing care plus three 30-minute sessions of reiki, while the control group ($n = 12$) received traditional nursing care. The results indicated that the experimental group reported less pain and requested fewer analgesics than the control group. Also, the experimental group reported less anxiety than the control group on discharge at 72 hours after the operation.

There is some circumstantial evidence from case studies that reiki may be beneficial in stress, tension, sinusitis, menstrual problems, cystitis, migraines, asthma, psoriasis, myalgic encephalomyelitis, constipation, eczema, arthritis, menopausal problems, back pain, anxiety, depression, insomnia and sciatica. Chronic ailments may also respond well.

Research that examined the effects of reiki on cancer-related fatigue, pain, anxiety and overall quality of life found significant decreases in tiredness ($p < 0.001$), pain ($p < 0.005$) and anxiety ($p < 0.01$),[10] These effects were not seen in a control resting condition.

Other evidence is inconclusive and contradictory. Reiki was administered to 50 patients out of 100 patients with normal left ventricular function scheduled for elective coronary artery bypass grafting.[11] Blood components and inflammatory markers were estimated at various time points. Haemodynamic parameters, psychological analysis, intensive care unit stay, incidence of infection, chest tube drainage and mortality were recorded. This study concluded that reiki is a time-consuming process with no significant clinical benefit.

For a comprehensive review of reiki studies categorised by therapeutic area (stress/relaxation, depression, pain, wound healing) and reiki placebo standardisation the reader is referred to a paper by Vitale.[12] A brief description of the studies is provided, followed by a summary of the category as a whole. Vitale says that energy work with reiki allows a compassionate connection through touch and presence between the provider and recipient with the intent to help or heal. The persistence of the metaphor hands-on to mean touch with intent to heal represents the essence of many of today's holistic nursing practices

Therapeutic touch

Therapeutic touch (also known as healing touch) is similar to reiki in that it is an intentionally directed process of energy modulation during which the practitioner uses the hands as a focus to facilitate healing. It differs from reiki in that the practitioner does not need to be 'attuned' to the patient. It is largely passive in its application and requires no conscious participation by the patient. There are specific techniques for specific illnesses/diseases.

Therapeutic touch is claimed to have three main effects:[13]

1. A rapid relaxation response
2. Improved pain relief
3. An acceleration of the body's own healing process.

After a patient-blinded, controlled trial it was concluded that therapeutic touch cannot be routinely recommended for women at the time of stereotactic core biopsy of suspicious breast lesions to achieve a reduction in anxiety and pain.[14]

A review examined the currently available evidence supporting the use of therapeutic touch in treating anxiety disorders.[15] No randomised or quasi-randomised controlled trials of therapeutic touch for anxiety disorders were identified. The authors stated that there is a need for well-conducted randomised controlled trials (RCTs) to examine the effectiveness of therapeutic touch for anxiety disorders.

Relaxation techniques

Relaxation techniques are used by people who wish to relax, for a wide variety of reasons.

History

Though promoted in self-help books in the 1970s it was a decade later before research demonstrated a link between stress and health and suggested that relaxation could be of benefit. The work was widely reported in the American Press.[16]

Practice

Relaxation techniques involve more than simply sitting quietly in a chair or lying on a bed. They may involve a number of different activities including yoga, prayer and exercise. One example of a 'therapeutic' relaxation technique is sequential muscle relaxation, progressive relaxation or Jacobson relaxation. The individual sits comfortably in a dark, quiet room. He or she then tenses a group of muscles, such as those in the right arm, holds the contraction for 15 s, and then releases it while breathing out. After a short rest, this sequence is repeated with another set of muscles. Gradually, different sets of muscles are combined.

Another technique, the Mitchell method, involves adopting body positions that are opposite to those associated with anxiety (fingers spread rather than hands clenched, for example). In autogenic training individuals concentrate on experiencing physical sensations, such as warmth and heaviness, in different parts of their bodies in a learnt sequence. Other methods encourage deepening and slowing the breath, and a conscious attempt to let go of tension during exhalation.

Relaxation technique has been used for:

- anger management
- anxiety attacks
- cardiac health
- depression
- headache
- hypertension
- insomnia
- pain management
- stress management.

Evidence

Relaxation has been found to be beneficial in the treatment of chronic pain.[17] However, in another trial dynamic muscle training and relaxation training did not lead to better improvements in neck pain compared with ordinary activity.[18] Some GP practices in the UK offer relaxation classes to improve wellbeing in patients with mild anxiety or depression or who suffer from chronic physical complaints for which further treatment options are limited.[19]

A sequence of breathing and relaxation exercises in patients with mild asthma reduced asthma symptoms by a third, according to results from an RCT:[20] 85 people with mild or moderate asthma were recruited from the asthma register of a semirural general practice in the UK. They were randomly assigned to a breathing and relaxation technique known as the Papworth method. in addition to their usual drug, or simply to remain on their usual drug therapy. The Papworth method combines diaphragmatic breathing, breathing through the nose and relaxation exercises to reduce anxiety and symptoms arising from hypocapnia. Patients assigned to the breathing method attended five 1-hour training sessions with a respiratory physiotherapist. Patients using the Papworth method showed a significantly lower score for asthma symptoms after the programme. The improvement in symptoms was maintained at 1 year.

Yoga

Definition

The Sanskrit word yoga is translated as 'union' of mind, body and spirit. Yoga is intimately connected to the religious beliefs and practices of the Indian religions and is also visible in Buddhism.

History

The history of yoga is hotly debated and uncertain. Several seals discovered at Indus Valley Civilization (about 3300–1700 BC) sites are said to depict figures in a yoga- or meditation-like posture. Several different varieties of yoga have emerged.

Practice

Yoga involves postures, breathing exercises and meditation aimed at improving mental and physical functioning. Some practitioners understand yoga in terms of traditional Indian medicine, with the postures improving the flow of prana energy around the body. Others see yoga in more conventional terms of muscle stretching and mental relaxation, with an ability to improve vitality.[21]

Commonly practised yoga methods are pranayama (controlled deep breathing), asanas (physical postures) and dhyana (meditation), which are mixed in varying proportions with differing philosophical ideas. In the west, the most widely taught form of yoga is hatha yoga with classes offering students exercises to stretch and flex the body, develop breath awareness, relaxation and sometimes meditation. Hatha yoga is a particular system of yoga described by yogi Swatmarama, a yogic sage of the fifteenth century in India

Evidence

A number of applications for yoga have been examined including the following.

Geriatric depression

The effects of yoga and ayurveda on geriatric depression were evaluated in 69 people aged over 60 who were living in a residential home.[22] The depression symptom scores of the yoga group at both 3 and 6 months decreased significantly, whereas the other groups showed no change. Hence, an integrated approach of yoga, including the mental and philosophical aspects in addition to the physical practices, was useful for institutionalised older people.

Palliative care

A study by McDonald et al.[23] suggests that yoga can be of benefit to patients (and carers) in palliative care settings.

The impact of yoga, including physical poses, breathing and meditation exercises, has been studied on quality of life (QoL), fatigue, distressed mood and spiritual wellbeing among a multiethnic sample of breast cancer patients.[24] Despite limited adherence, this intent-to-treat analysis suggests that yoga is associated with beneficial effects on social functioning among a medically diverse sample of breast cancer survivors. Among patients not receiving chemotherapy, yoga appears to enhance emotional wellbeing and mood, and may serve to buffer deterioration in both overall and specific domains of QoL.

Psychotic treatment

The efficacy of yoga therapy (YT) has been examined as an add-on treatment to the ongoing antipsychotic treatment.[25] Sixty-one moderately ill schizophrenia patients were randomly assigned to YT ($n = 31$) and physical exercise therapy (PT; $n = 30$) for 4 months. Both non-pharmacological interventions contributed to a reduction in symptoms, with YT having better efficacy.

Renal disease

A simplified yoga-based rehabilitation programme has been shown to be a safe and effective clinical treatment modality in patients with end-stage renal disease, improving pain, fatigue and sleep disturbance associated with haemodialysis.[26]

Sexual disorders

Yoga is claimed to be useful in sexual disorders. It appears to be a feasible, safe, effective and acceptable non-pharmacological option for premature ejaculation.[27]

Stress

Yoga has been used to alleviate stress alone and in combination with other therapies. A self-care programme consisting of yoga, tai c'hi, meditation classes and reiki healing sessions was designed for a university-based hospital.[28] The effectiveness of these interventions was evaluated using self-care journals and analysed using a heideggerian phenomenological approach. Outcomes of the self-care classes described by nurses included: (1) noticing sensations of warmth, tingling and pulsation, which were relaxing; (2) becoming aware of an enhanced problem-solving ability; and (3) noticing an increased ability to focus on patient needs.

Other mind–body interventions

Art therapy

Definition

Art therapy is a form of expressive therapy that uses art materials, such as paints, chalk and markers. It combines traditional psychotherapeutic theories and techniques with an understanding of the psychological aspects of the creative process, especially the affective properties of the different art materials.[29]

History

Visual expression has been used for healing throughout history, but art therapy did not emerge as a distinct profession until the 1940s. In the early twentieth century, psychiatrists became interested in the artwork created by their patients with mental illness. At around the same time, educators were discovering that children's art expressions reflected developmental, emotional and cognitive growth. By mid-century, hospitals, clinics and rehabilitation centres increasingly began to include art therapy programmes along with traditional 'talk therapies', underscoring the recognition that the creative process of art making enhanced recovery, health and wellness. As a result, the profession of art therapy grew into an effective and important method of communication, assessment and treatment with children and adults in a variety of settings.

Theory

According to the American Art Therapy Association (http://www. arttherapy.org/aafaq.html), art therapy is based on the belief that the creative process involved in making art is on a basic level healing and life enhancing. Art therapists use the creative process and the issues that come up during art therapy to help their clients increase insight and judgement, cope better with stress, work through traumatic experiences, increase cognitive abilities, have better relationships with family and friends, and just be able to enjoy the life-affirming pleasures of the creative experience.

Practice

Clients who are referred to an art therapist need not have previous experience or skill in art; the art therapist is not primarily concerned with making an aesthetic or diagnostic assessment of the client's image. The overall aim of its practitioners is to enable a client to effect change and growth on a personal level through the use of art materials in a safe and facilitating environment.

The relationship between the therapist and the client is of central importance, but art therapy differs from other psychological therapies in that it is a three-way process of the client, the therapist and the image or artefact. Thus, it offers the opportunity for expression and communication and can be particularly helpful to people who find it hard to express their thoughts and feelings verbally.

The **art of healing programme**, an initiative that aims to use the arts as a form of therapy to soothe patients' minds and bodies and help them on their path to recovery, was launched in Tan Tock Seng Hospital (TTSH), Singapore on 6 February 2006.[30] Through the arts, the hospital is transformed to a warm, welcoming and enriching environment for patients, families, staff and visitors. The Hospital uses the arts to help distract patients from their ailments, express their feelings and reduce anxiety. Through this, the Hospital aims for there to be an improvement in patients' blood pressure and intake of pain medication, which in turn should translate to faster recovery and a shorter length of hospital stay.

The Hospital believes that replacing fear with hope is the essence of modern medicine and art acts as a complementary medicine. Although conventional medicine focuses on treating the body's diseases, it does not treat the patient's emotions and mind. This is where art exhibitions (paintings, pottery, wire sculptures, etc.) and performances (orchestras, big bands, string quartets, plays, dances, etc.) can help. The Hospital ensures that the art of healing programme is an on-going project where activities are unveiled regularly.

Additional objectives are to promote TTSH as a centre of holistic healing of mind and body, and to transform the hospital environment from a traditionally sterile, cold and fearful one to a warm, non-threatening and welcoming place of healing. Using the arts as a platform for its intrinsic value (art as a healing property and as objects of beauty) and its extrinsic values (symbolic of the TTSH's history of healing honed over the past 160 years), the programme looks towards the holistic healing of patients on all levels. The programme provides an enriching multicultural experience for patients and staff and welcomes artists of all art forms to be a part of these performances. Through the use of art to promote healing of patients, the programme's vision of adding years of healthy life to the community is further strengthened

Evidence

Researchers, in particular Roger Ulrich, a behavioural scientist and professor at the Center of Health Systems and Design in the College of Architecture at Texas A&M University, have uncovered interesting correlations between art and healing.[31] They have conducted experiments in which the effects of art on medical outcomes have been measured. Ulrich makes the important distinction that not all art can benefit patients. Only 'psychologically appropriate art' can benefit patients by improving blood pressure, anxiety, intake of pain medication and length of hospital stay. His study also shows that some art styles are not right in healthcare settings because they can have negative effects on patients. Ulrich reports research on patient anxiety in a dental fears clinic, which showed that patients felt less stressed when a large mural depicting a natural scene was hung on a wall of the waiting room, in contrast to when the wall was blank

Art based on the needs of special patient populations (e.g. cardiac patients, patients in intensive care and children) is claimed to:[32]

- mitigate the stress of the environment
- create a sense of security in the patient
- promote a bond between patient and care giver
- perpetuate an image of excellence for the facility.

Patients recovering from open-heart surgery who were exposed to pictures of nature with water experienced less postoperative anxiety than patients exposed to other types of pictures.[33] Patients exposed to abstract pictures had higher anxiety than patients without any picture at all. Also, 4 days after surgery, patients who had been exposed to any type of visual stimulation were able to complete a visuoperceptual functioning test faster than patients exposed to no art.

It has been suggested that nature imagery reduces anxiety and relaxes patients. This makes them more receptive and responsive to treatment. Viewing nature imagery also reduces systolic blood pressure and pulse, helps to redirect negative thought and sustains interest, while decreasing boredom, and reducing intake of pain medication and length of hospital stays.[34]

Colour therapy

Definition

Colour therapy (also called aura soma) is a natural and non-invasive form of healing using pure light/colour energy for the wellbeing of mind, body and spirit. According to colour therapy, the seven rainbow colours relate to the seven main energy centres (chakras) of the body. Colour has an effect on perception and this therapy seems to have a place in complementary practice, although the attachment of the sobriquet 'therapy' might be questioned by many.

History

Colour was of great importance to the Egyptians. They built temples for colour healing where people would gather to be revitalised and renewed.

It is interesting to look at the different phases in history and how those phases have been reflected in the colours generally worn at those times. During times of severity and propriety the code of dress was dominated by black and grey. The Victorians mainly wore black – influenced by Queen Victoria's long period of mourning, no doubt – and were, in many ways, quite austere and not very colourful. The Puritans too, of course, dressed in black.

Wearing black with another colour can enhance that other colour's energy. Black can also give the space sometimes needed for reflection on an inner searching. It can indicate inner strength and the possibility for change.

Theory

Relationships between various colours and areas of the body, glands or organs (known as chakras) are identified by practitioners. Some of the most common colours and their associated chakras are given below:

- Violet/purple relates to the crown chakra, which is at the top of the head. The related organ to this chakra is the brain and the endocrine gland is the pineal gland. Violet relates to our spiritual awareness.
- Indigo relates to the brow chakra or third eye, which is in the centre of the forehead. The related organs to this chakra are the eyes, lower head and sinuses, and the endocrine gland is the pituitary gland. Indigo relates to self-responsibility, that is to say trusting our own intuition.
- Blue relates to the throat chakra. Organs associated with this chakra are the throat and lungs and the endocrine gland is the thyroid gland. The upper digestive tract can be affected by imbalance in this area. This chakra relates to self-expression.
- Green relates to the heart chakra. Associated organs to this chakra are the heart and breasts. The gland is the thymus gland. Allergies and problems related to the immune system can also be connected with this chakra. This chakra relates to love/self-love.
- Yellow relates to the solar plexus chakra, situated below the ribs. Associated organs are the liver, spleen, stomach and small intestine. The endocrine gland is the pancreas. This chakra relates to self-worth.
- Orange relates to the sacral chakra, which is situated in the abdomen. The organs to which this chakra relates are the uterus, large bowel and prostate. The endocrine glands are the ovaries and testes. This chakra relates to self-respect.
- Red relates to the base chakra, which is situated at the base of the spine. The organs to which this chakra relates are the kidneys and bladder. The vertebral column, hips and legs are also related to

this chakra. The endocrine gland is the adrenal gland. This chakra relates to self-awareness.

Practice

An aura soma treatment begins with an examination of the responses triggered by a selection of colours made by the patient. These responses highlight areas of the physical body that are holding a negative pattern. Flower therapy uses flowers to provide a pleasing design of colour and aroma.

Evidence

In the 1930s it was noted that a lot of red was being worn. Red in its most positive aspect is the colour for courage, strength and pioneering spirit, all of which were much needed by the men and women fighting that war. However, in the most negative aspect, it is the colour of anger, violence and brutality. In the mid-1940s pale blue became a popular colour – an omen of the peace to come, perhaps, and also giving everyone the healing that they must have needed so badly. More recently, in a systematic review of 12 published studies, it was shown that colours affect the perceived action and effectiveness of drugs.[35] Moreover, a relationship exists between the colouring of drugs that affect the central nervous system and the indications for which they are used. Red, yellow and orange appeared to be associated with a stimulant effect, whereas blue and green were related to a tranquillising effect. Furthermore, hypnotic, sedative and anxiolytic drugs were more likely than antidepressants to be green, blue or purple.

Businesses are accepting that their employees may work better given a certain environment, and hospitals and prisons are also becoming aware of the effect that the colour around them can have on patients and prisoners respectively. Paint companies have introduced new colour cards with the therapeutic aspects of colour in mind.

Colour therapy healing can be used in many ways, e.g. wearing silk colour scarves or using a light box with the appropriate colour/colours. Light box therapy is also very helpful for those suffering from seasonal affective disorder.[36] The technique involves sitting in front of a light box with the entire visual angle subtended by the light source – the amount of light is important (up to 10 000 lux compared with average office light, which is up to 300 lux). Three controlled trials were published in the early part of the current century that investigate the effect of bright light on sleep disturbance and behavioural disorders in dementia.[37–39] Some benefits were reported for restlessness, but a particular beneficial effect has been found for sleep disturbances. These results are promising.

Crystal therapy[40]

This is a healing method similar to colour therapy in that it uses crystals and gems for physical, emotional and spiritual balance and healing. The crystals are worn or placed near the body. The body needs seven colour rays – red, orange, yellow, green, blue, indigo and violet – for balanced health (as in colour therapy). Each colour ray is associated with one or more of the chakras. By using crystals associated with the colour ray that supports a particular chakra, one can speed healing of the associated areas and organs, e.g. emerald is the carrier of the green ray. The following are examples of the uses of some crystals:

- Amber is great at lifting the heaviness of burdens, allowing happiness to come through.
- Aquamarine can help one understand difficult situations and may be helpful for people who are experiencing a lot of grief.
- Coral protects and strengthens one's emotional foundation.
- Emerald may help in physical and emotional healing.
- Jade helps cure a sore shoulder or back and is useful in relaxation.
- Opal helps one see possibilities and discover a broader view.
- Ruby opens the heart and allows one to overcome fear.

Humour therapy

The therapeutic effects of humour give patients the opportunity to forget about their anxiety and pain, if only for a short period of time and may improve the patient's frame of mind and quality of life.

Integrating humour and laughter into the healthcare surroundings helps healthcare providers handle the stress of looking after patients who are in pain. Furthermore, it promotes good quality working relationships with colleagues and improves morale. Having a positive outlook at work can also extend to colleagues and support staff.[41]

History

The first documented case of humour affecting disease was when Norman Cousins published *Anatomy of an Illness*.[42] The best-selling book, which ran to several editions, gave an account of how in 1964 humour had assisted in the reversal of ankylosing spondylitis, a painful disease causing the disintegration of the spinal connective tissue.

Definition

The term humour can refer to a stimulus that is intended to produce a humorous response (such as a humorous video), a mental process (perception of amusing incongruities) or a response (laughter, exhilaration). Laughter is the most common expression of humorous experience. Humour and laughter are also typically associated with a pleasant emotional state.[43]

Theory

Laughter is believed to act as a coping mechanism to reduce stress, improve self-esteem and reduce psychological symptoms related to negative life events.[44] Although there is considerable information on the neuronal representation of speech, little is known about brain mechanisms of laughter. We do have some evidence that the supplementary motor area of the brain is involved in this response.[45]

Practice

According to Bennett[46] there are situations in which humour should be avoided. In terms of patient care, ethnic and sexist humour should be avoided, as well as sarcastic humour. Cynical humour has been shown to be less effective than humour that puts things in perspective or reduces seriousness. Also, 'gallows humour', the type of morbid humour used to discuss tragedy and death, should be avoided so that patients do not feel that medical professionals are cruel or uncaring. However fighting death with a smile requires courage.[47]

In addition to the provision of verbal humour by hospital staff (and volunteers) professional artists may be engaged principally for visual humour with children (http://tinyurl.com/yp88d2). Clowns did not have any special training for hospital work until the 1980s. Gradually, certain requirements regarding hygiene and familiarity with the medical environment were instituted. There are two main models of clowns involved: clown-doctors and therapeutic clowns:

- **Clown-doctors** wear little make-up apart from a red nose, communicate verbally and always work in pairs. They are dressed like doctors and misappropriate medical equipment, spraying water from rubber syringes and transforming stethoscopes into smile detectors or musical instruments.
- **Therapeutic clowns** are typically more made up and look more like traditional clowns. They work alone and are often silent, communicating with signs, toys and various gestures.

Evidence

Laughter has been shown to improve antibody activity, supply physical exercise to the muscles, lungs and other organs of the body, oxygenate blood, speed up respiration and blood circulation, steady blood pressure, improve digestion and offer emotional cleansing. It can also reduce pain by stimulating the creation of endogenous opioids such as β-endorphin and enhance the function of the immune system.[48]

An American non-profit organisation interested in the use of humour for healing collaborated with a university to collect preliminary data on a sample of 18 children aged 7–16 years.[49] Participants watched humorous video-tapes before, during and after a standardised pain task that involved placing a hand in cold water. Pain appraisal (ratings of pain severity) and pain tolerance (submersion time) were recorded and examined in relation to humour indicators (number of laughs/smiles during each video and child ratings of how funny the video was). Whereas humour indicators were not significantly associated with pain appraisal or tolerance, the group demonstrated significantly greater pain tolerance while viewing funny videos than when viewing the videos immediately before or after the cold-water task. The results suggest that humorous distraction is useful to help children and adolescents tolerate painful procedures.

Despite these potential benefits of humour, in most instances current research is insufficient to validate such claims. The experiments that claim that laughter has both psychological and physiological benefits have not been carefully performed.[43] Many of these experiments need better control groups and manipulation checks. Experiments that have patients completing self-reports on measurements of humour are poor in reliability and validity. Also, as many of the experiments have methodological problems, firm conclusions cannot be drawn. The empirical evidence is weak because of the inconsistency among experiments.

There is support in the literature for the role of humour and laughter in other areas, including patient–physician communication, psychological aspects of patient care, medical education and as a means of reducing stress in medical professionals.[46]

Hypnotherapy

Definition

Hypnotherapy is an intervention based on the use of hypnosis (literally, 'nervous sleep'), a form of cognitive information processing in which a suspension of peripheral awareness and critical analysis cognition can lead to apparently involuntary changes in perception, memory, mood and physiology.[50] In simpler terms hypnosis may be considered as the induction of a deeply relaxed state, with increased suggestibility and suspension of critical faculties.[51]

History

The French physician Mesmer (1734–1815) was the first person to propose a mechanism for hypnosis that did not have a demonic basis to its theory. He suggested that hypnosis was due to magnetism radiating from himself. There have been many other hypotheses as to how hypnosis may work but none has been accepted as the definitive answer.

Practice

Hypnotherapy is often associated with the induction of a trance-like state during which behavioural modification may be suggested (e.g. stop smoking during pregnancy[52] or reduce eating). In fact it is now more widely used as an adjunct to psychological treatments.[53,54]

Evidence

Hypnosis may be indicated if the patient has a high ability to become hypnotised and a positive attitude towards hypnosis for the treatment of a condition in which alteration of perception, memory and mood can reduce the intensity of a symptom. Thus, it may be used in suitable patients for the reduction of chronic pain, reduction in the memory of past pain and mood enhancement.

Apart from pain and headaches, hypnosis has been used for several other conditions,[55] including asthma and removal of warts, and irritable bowel syndrome. Hypnosis improves a range of objective symptoms of irritable bowel syndrome and produces subjective reductions in distress.[56-58]

A study in Saudi Arabia involving 26 patients showed that, after 12 sessions of hypnotherapy administered over 12 weeks, patients' quality of life had improved significantly, but more in the men than in the women.[59] In particular, dissatisfaction with bowel habits was reduced after treatment, but more in the women than in the men

Safety

It has been pointed out that hypnosis or deep relaxation has the capacity to exacerbate psychological problems by retraumatising those with post-traumatic disorders or by inducing false memories in psychologically vulnerable individuals.[51] Concerns have also been raised that it can bring on a latent psychosis, although the evidence is inconclusive. Hypnosis should be undertaken only by appropriately trained, experienced and regulated practitioners. It should be avoided in established or borderline psychosis and personality disorders, and hypnotherapists should be competent at recognising and referring patients in these states.

Training

The British Society of Medical and Dental Hypnosis runs basic, intermediate and advanced courses for doctors and dentists, and holds regular scientific meetings. There is no standard training in hypnosis for practitioners without a conventional healthcare background.

Magnetic therapy

Magnet therapy, magnetic therapy or magnotherapy is a form of alternative medicine involving magnetic fields.[60] Proponents claim that subjecting certain parts of the body to doses of magnetic fields has a beneficial effect. This belief has led to the popularisation of an industry involving the sale of magnetic-based products for 'healing' purposes:[61] magnetic bracelets and jewellery; magnetic straps for wrists, ankles and the back; and shoe insoles, mattresses and magnetic blankets (blankets with magnets woven into the material). Magnet therapy makes use of the static magnetic fields produced by permanent magnets; the related alternative medicine field of electromagnetic therapy involves the application of electromagnetic waves to the patient.

Magnetic therapy for leg ulcers can be prescribed on the UK NHS[62] in the form of 4Ulcercare (www.ulcercare.co.uk). This is a magnet-containing device designed to be wrapped around the leg. It is worn next to the skin, between the knee and the calf muscle. According to the manufacturer, the device should be worn 24 hours a day and, once the ulcer has healed, the device should be worn at night to prevent the ulcer recurring.

In a double-blind study,[63] 26 patients with chronic leg ulcers used either 4Ulcercare or placebo for 12 weeks and their wounds were assessed every 4 weeks. The patients using the magnetic device had reduced ulcer measurements compared with the control group.

An innovative cancer treatment using microscopic magnets to enable 'armed' cells to target tumours has been developed by researchers funded by the Biotechnology and Biological Sciences Research Council (BBSRC).[64] Research showed that inserting these nanomagnets into cells carrying genes to fight tumours resulted in many more cells successfully reaching and invading malignant tumours. The technique involved inserting nanomagnets into monocytes – white blood cells used to carry gene therapy – and injecting the cells into the bloodstream. Systemic administration of such 'magnetic' monocytes to mice bearing solid tumours led to a marked increase in their extravasation into the tumour in the presence of an external magnet.

Meditation

Meditation is the intentional self-regulation of attention, a systematic focus on particular aspects of inner or outer experience, and has developed in association with religious and spiritual contexts (e.g. Buddhist and Hindu rituals), the aim being to seek a full state of mind embodied in the concept of 'enlightenment'. Meditation can be broadly divided into two groups of practices:

1. Concentration or restrictive practices that emphasise the stabilising of attention when directed to a specific object or focus; typically, meditators concentrate on their breath or a sound (mantra) that they repeat to themselves.
2. Mindfulness practices (e.g. Zen) that involve attention to all emotions, perceptions and sensations rather than focusing on

one particular aspect of life; this is said to cultivate a sense of open-mindedness in life.

In fact, it may be difficult to separate these two groups, because the first may be required before the second can be achieved, e.g. in mindfulness practices individuals are taught to concentrate initially on a simple event, such as breathing, and then allow the mind to wander.

Meditation has been shown to enhance competitive performance in shooting[65,66] and may also modify the suppressive influence of strenuous physical stress on the immune system.[67] Meditation training may also reduce the lactate response to a period of standardised exercise.[68]

Meditation – transcendental

Transcendental meditation (TM) was introduced to the west from the vedic traditions of India by maharishi Mahest Yogi and was popularised by the Beatles in the 1960s. In TM the individual sits with the eyes closed for 20 min each day, focusing on a word or syllable. Whenever distraction occurs the attention is directed back to the word. A refreshing state of restful alertness can be achieved with practice. Transcendental meditation has been used in the reduction of stress and various anxiety states. It has also been used, together with orthodox treatments, in the treatment of carotid artery disease.[69]

A group mindfulness meditation training programme is claimed to reduce symptoms of anxiety and panic, and help maintain these reductions in patients with generalised anxiety disorder, panic disorder or panic disorder with agoraphobia.[69] Meditation has also been used to enhance mood[70] and treat hypertension,[71] and for pain control.[72]

Twelve people who practised transcendental meditation for 30 years were shown to demonstrate up to 50% less brain response to pain, compared with 12 non-meditators.[73] Functional magnetic resonance imaging of the response to thermally induced pain applied outside the meditation period found that long-term practitioners of the TM technique showed a lower pain response in the thalamus and total brain than healthy matched controls. After the controls learned the technique and practised it for 5 months, their response decreased by 40–50% in the thalamus, prefrontal cortex and total brain, and marginally in the anterior cingulate cortex. Until now, research into the effects of TM has indicated only that meditators respond to stress more calmly than non-meditators. These latest findings suggest that this is not simply the result of a shift in approach to stress from meditators, but also a fundamental change in the way the brain actually functions.

Canter and Ernst[74] carried out an independent, systematic review of RCTs of TM for cumulative effects on blood pressure. They concluded that all the RCTs of TM for the control of blood pressure published to date have important methodological weaknesses and are potentially biased by the affiliation of authors to the TM organisation. There is at present insufficient good-quality evidence to conclude whether or not TM has a cumulative positive effect on blood pressure.

Music therapy

Definition

Music therapy is the prescribed use of music by a qualified person to effect positive changes in the psychological, physical, cognitive or social functioning of individuals with health or educational problems.

History

The idea of music as a healing influence that could affect health and behaviour is at least as old as the writings of Aristotle and Plato. Five hundred years before Christ, the followers of Pythagoras developed a science of musical psychotherapy. A daily programme of songs and pieces for the lyre made them feel bright and energetic on rising, and another set of pieces relieved them of the cares of the day and prepared them for agreeable dreams when they retired to sleep. Plato believed that musical training was a more potent instrument than any other because 'rhythm and harmony find their way into the inward places of the soul, imparting grace, and making the soul of him who is rightly educated graceful'. The Bible recounts that young David was summoned to play the harp for a tormented King Saul: 'Whenever the spirit from God came upon Saul, David would take his harp and play. Then relief would come to Saul; he would feel better, and the evil spirit would leave him' (I Samuel 16:23).

Anyone who has played in an orchestra or sung in a choir will know that participating in music with others enhances group solidarity as well as promoting individual wellbeing. The twentieth-century discipline began after World Wars I and II when community musicians of all types, both amateur and professional, went to military hospitals around the country to play for the thousands of combatants suffering both physical and emotional trauma from the wars. The patients' notable physical and emotional responses to music led doctors and nurses to request the hiring of musicians by the hospitals. It was soon evident that hospital musicians needed some prior training before entering the hospital and so the demand grew for a college curriculum. The first music therapy degree programme in the world was founded at Michigan State University, USA, in 1944.

Theory

Studies with electroencephalography suggest that music creates a level of coherence between the electrical activity of different areas of the brain.

Practice

According to the American Music Therapy Association website (www.namt.com) music therapists:

- assess emotional wellbeing, physical health, social functioning, communication abilities and cognitive skills through musical responses
- design music sessions for individuals and groups based on client needs, using music improvisation, receptive music listening, song writing, lyric discussion, music and imagery, music performance and learning through music
- participate in interdisciplinary treatment planning, ongoing evaluation and follow-up.

The following groups are said to benefit from music therapy:

- Children with developmental and learning disabilities
- Elderly people with mental health needs, Alzheimer's disease and other age-related conditions
- People with substance abuse problems
- People with physical disabilities and/or acute and chronic pain
- Women in labour.

Evidence

In a controlled study of 40 infants matched for gestational age, sex and birth weight, half had lullabies sung to them and were massaged once or twice a week until they were discharged.[75] The other 20 served as controls. The hospital stay was shortened by an average of 11 days for female infants and 1.5 days for male infants in the music and massage group compared with the control group. Infants of both sexes gained weight, although the amount was not statistically significant.

Music therapy also has a special place in the treatment of children who cannot easily communicate verbally; this includes autistic children and those with learning disabilities or brain damage. It is likely that music can provide an alternative channel of communication that prevents some children from retreating into, or remaining in, a state of total isolation.[76]

A few years ago, a researcher reported a study that showed that listening to Mozart's *Sonata for Two Pianos* (K448) significantly enhanced the ability of a subject to perform tests of spatial perception.[77] The report was widely publicised, and a number of investigators have since attempted to reproduce the findings with mixed results. According to an article in the *Journal of the American Medical Association*,[78] a much larger study found that it was not Mozart but movement that enhances performance ability. Whether the stimulus is auditory or visual, the key is movement, because movement gets attention and, with attention, performance improves. The *Journal of the American Medical Association* reported that 175 individuals were randomly selected and placed into one of seven groups each containing 25 people. Those in six of the groups performed a spatial ability test before and after 8.5 min of exposure to one of the following: the Mozart sonata; audible rhythmic patterns with a steady pitch; random pitches with steady time intervals; environmental sounds, such as falling rain and singing birds; continually changing geometric patterns, such as those that appear on a computer screen-saver; and colour slides of abstract paintings. The control group sat for 8.5 min without exposure to any auditory or visual stimuli. The first five groups tested performed the spatial ability task equally well and significantly better than the controls and those viewing the abstract paintings. The Mozart listeners fared no better than the others.

A Swedish study investigated the possible influence of attendance at cultural events, reading books or periodicals, making music or singing in a choir as determinants for survival.[79] This was a simple random sample of 15 198 individuals aged 16–74 years. Of these, 85% (12 982) were interviewed by trained non-medical interviewers about cultural activities. They were followed up with respect to survival for approximately 8 years. It was concluded that attendance at cultural events may have a positive influence on survival.

Autobiographical recall in patients with dementia improves significantly when music is played. Foster and Valentine[80] examined the recall of personal facts in 23 older adults with mild-to-moderate dementia. Participants were tested in each of four auditory background conditions presented randomly, 1 week apart: quiet, cafeteria noise, familiar music (first movement of Vivaldi's *The Four Seasons*) and novel music (Fitkin's *Hook*). Questions were drawn from three life eras: remote (up to age 20, e.g. where were you born?), medium remote (approximately ages 20–50, e.g. have you ever been married?) and recent past and present (e.g. where do you live now?). Performance was significantly better with sound (mean percentage recall 67%) compared with quiet (61%), and with music (68%) compared with cafeteria noise (66%). There was no difference between familiar and novel music; recall for both was about 68%. Recall was also positively related to age of memory; it was better for remote past (80%) compared with medium remote (68%) and recent past and present (48%). A typical question that participants were able to answer with the aid of background music but not without it was: 'Can you remember the name of the school your children attended?' – something from the middle period of their lives that they probably had not had occasion to think about much since then. It was concluded that music should be played when physicians are interviewing or attempting to get information from patients with dementia and should also be tried in combination with other treatments for dementia management.

Music therapy is a popular complementary treatment in hospitals in the USA, where randomised trials have supported its use for reducing pain and anxiety in the acute setting.[81,82]

There is some evidence that listening to certain types of music may have the potential to change human stability and promote change in the field of fall prevention and rehabilitation, with a potential to decrease disability.[83]

Data collected in a small ($n = 8$) 52-week pilot study seem to suggest that active music therapy sessions could be of aid in improving autistic symptoms as well as personal musical skills in young adults with severe autism.[84]

Radionics

A type of instrument-assisted healing that attempts to detect disease before it has physically manifested itself. Radionics is based on the belief that everyone is surrounded by an invisible energy field that the prescriber 'tunes' into and then attempts to correct problems that have been identified. Practitioners believe that it can be done remotely over long distances.[85]

Spiritual healing and prayer

There is growing empirical evidence of a positive relationship between religious engagement and better clinical health outcomes.[86]

Healers and their clients assume a cause-and-effect relationship between the application of a healer's intention to heal and any subsequent improvement in symptoms.[87] Healers believe that the power of healing is a therapy in its own right; non-believers are sceptical and reject this suggestion.

Practice

The calming effect or coping strategy of prayer can be beneficial and, especially among those with religious faith, provide the necessary support at times of extreme stress and tension. There are four types of prayer, all of which may contribute to an overall effect:

1. Meditative prayer, which involves focusing on a single word, phrase or sound
2. Ritualistic prayer, which involves repeating passages of prose that form part of a religious service
3. Petitionary prayer, which involves making a request, e.g. for better health
4. Conversational prayer, which involves chatting or informing one's deity.

Evidence

The difficulties of conducting research into the effectiveness of spiritual healing are significant. How, for example, does one know when a patient is better?[88] Some healers would say that some of the most significant changes following healing may not be measurable. The healing approach is to act with love and compassion and support patients during their suffering. Measuring such input is a problem, especially when it is complementary to other more orthodox treatments.

A systematic review identified a total of 59 RCTs comparing spiritual healing with a control intervention on human participants. In 37 of these trials healing was used for existing diseases; the remaining 22 trials were excluded from the review, mainly because no identifiable symptoms were present.[89] The author stated that no firm conclusions could be drawn about the efficacy or otherwise of healing from the diverse group of RCTs reported in the literature. He suggested two possibilities for future healing research: pragmatic trials of healing for undifferentiated conditions on patients based in general practice and larger RCTs of distant healing on large numbers of patients with well-defined measurable illness. A double-blind randomised trial of distant healing for skin warts[90] found no evidence that healing practices had any beneficial effects. Blood pressure measurement offers a method of identifying an effective outcome due to prayer particularly in older people.[91]

Higher levels of spirituality and private religious practices are believed to be associated with slower progression of Alzheimer's disease.[92]

An RCT concluded that chronically ill patients who want to be treated by distant healing and know that they are treated improve in quality of life.[93]

Effects of prayer   A study by Yilmaz et al.[94] sought to determine whether repetitive actions carried out in Islam had a role on knee, hip osteoarthritis and osteoporosis: 46 patients who had been performing the prayer for at least 10 years, and 40 patients who had not performed the prayer, were included in this prospective study. It was concluded that prayer had no effect on knee and hip osteoarthritis, but may be related to hand osteoarthritis. It seems to have a negative effect on lumbar bone marrow density.

Intercessory or third-party prayer   This has been practised since Professor John Tyndall caused much debate in 1872 when he proposed comparing mortality rates in London hospitals between patients who were prayed for and those who were not.[95] Every so often a trial adds to the controversy, e.g. a double-blind RCT with a population of 393 cardiac patients split into an active (prayed-for) group and a control group showed that intercessory prayer appeared to be effective in reducing respiratory and cardiac symptoms.[96] More recently, results from an RCT have suggested that intercessory prayer might be an effective adjunct to standard medical procedures in coronary care.[97]

Chumash healing   Chumash healers treat their patients with prayer, laughter, dreaming, phytotherapy, aromatherapy, healing ceremonies and other techniques. Healing involves first healing the spirit, and then healing the body.[98]

More information

Art therapy

American Art Therapy Association: www.arttherapy.org
British Association of Art Therapists: www.baat.org/art_therapy.html

Colour therapy

International Association of Colour Therapy (IAC), 46 Cottenham Road, Histon, Cambridge CB4 9ES. Tel: 01223 563403; email: mailto.iac@cix.co.uk
Colour Therapy Association (CTA), PO Box 121, Chessington KT9 2WQ. Tel/Fax: 020 8391 2380

Crystal therapy

Further information may be found at the following website: www.gems4friends.com/~lorraine/therapy.html

Music therapy

MusicSpace Trust is a charity devoted to the provision of music therapy and the training of music therapy students
The MusicSpace Trust, The Southville Centre, Beauley Road, Bristol BS3 1QG. Tel: 0117 963 8000; fax: 0117 966 9889; website: www.hants.gov.uk/hampshire-musicspace/Trust.html
The American Music Therapy Association, 8455 Colesville Rd, Silver Spring, MD 20910, USA. Tel: +1 301 589 3300; website: www.musictherapy.org

Reiki

Reiki 4 All UK. Tel: 01283 716465; email: info@reiki4all.co.uk www.psinet.co.uk/reikiuk
Center for Reiki Training: www.reiki.com

Yoga

The British Wheel of Yoga: www.bwy.org.uk

References

1.   American Dance Therapy Association. www.adta.org
2.   Berrol C. The neurophysical basis of the mind–body connection in dance/movement therapy. *Am J Dance Ther* 1992;**14**:19–29.
3.   Cruz R, Sabers D. Dance therapy is more effective than previously reported. *Ann Psychother* 1998;**25**:101–4.
4.   Reiki4All UK. *Principles of reiki.* Available at: http://reiki4all.net/principles.html (accessed 12 June 2008).
5.   Fairblass J. Reiki. In: Novey D (ed.), *Clinician's Complete Reference to Complementary and Alternative Medicine.* St Louis, MO: Mosby, 2000: 435.
6.   Engebretson J, Wardell D. Experience of a Reiki session. *Altern Ther Hlth Med* 2002;**8**:48–53.
7.   National Center of Complementary and Alternative Medicine. www.nccam.nih.gov/health (accessed 1 November 2007).
8.   Olson K, Hanson J. Using reiki to manage pain: a preliminary report. *Cancer Prevent Control* 1997;**1**:108–11.
9.   Vitale AT, O'Connor PC. The effect of Reiki on pain and anxiety in women with abdominal hysterectomies: a quasi-experimental pilot study. *Holist Nurs Pract* 2006;**20**:263–72. PubMed
10.   Tsang KL, Carlson LE, Olson K. Pilot crossover trial of Reiki versus rest for treating cancer-related fatigue. *Integr Cancer Ther* 2007;**6**:25–35
11.   Trehan N, Sharma VG, Sanghvi C, Efficacy of reiki on patients undergoing coronary artery bypass graft surgery. *Ann Card Anaesth* 2000;**3**:12–18.
12.   Vitale A. An integrative review of reiki touch therapy research. *Holist Nurs Pract* 2007;**21L**:167–79.
13.   Krieger D. *Accepting your Own Power to Heal. The personal practice of therapeutic touch.* Sante Fe, NM: Bear, 1993.
14.   Frank LS, Frank JL, March D, Makari-Judson G, Barham RB, Mertens WC. Does therapeutic touch ease the discomfort or distress of patients undergoing stereotactic core breast biopsy? A randomized clinical trial. *Pain Med* 2007; **8**:419–24.
15.   Robinson J, Biley FC, Dolk H. Therapeutic touch for anxiety disorders. *Cochrane Database Syst Rev* 2007;**18**:CD006240.
16.   Coleman D. Relaxation: Surprising benefits detected. *The New York Times* 13 May 1986. Available at: http://tinyurl.com/33287z (accessed 1 November 2007).
17.   Carroll D, Seers K. Relaxation for the relief of chronic pain: a systematic review. *J Adv Nurs* 1998;**27**:476–87.
18.   Viljanen M, Malmivaara A, Uitti J, Rinne M, Palmroos P, Laippala P. Effectiveness of dynamic muscle training, relaxation training, or ordinary activity for chronic neck pain: randomised controlled trial. *BMJ* 2003;**327**: 475.

19. Smith WP, Compton WC, West WB. Meditation as an adjunct to a happiness enhancement program. *J Clin Psychol* 1995;**51**:269–73.
20. Holloway EA, West R. Integrated breathing and relaxation training (the Papworth Method) for adults with asthma in primary care: a randomised controlled trial. *Thorax* 2007;**62**:1039–42.
21. Wood C. Mood change and perceptions of vitality: a comparison of the effects of relaxation, visualization and yoga. *J R Soc Med* 1993;**86**:254–8.
22. Krishnamurthy MN, Telles S. Assessing depression following two ancient Indian interventions: effects of yoga and ayurveda on older adults in a residential home. *J Gerontol Nurs* 2007;**33**:17–23. PubMed
23. McDonald A, Burjan E, Martin S. Yoga for patients and carers in a palliative day care setting. *Int J Palliat Nurs* 2006;**12**:519–23. PubMed
24. Moadel AB, Shah C, Wylie-Rosett J et al. Randomized controlled trial of yoga among a multiethnic sample of breast cancer patients: effects on quality of life. *J Clin Oncol* 2007;**25**:4387–95. PubMed
25. Duraiswamy G, Thirthalli J, Nagendra HR, Gangadhar BN. Yoga therapy as an add-on treatment in the management of patients with schizophrenia – a randomized controlled trial. *Acta Psychiatr Scand* 2007;**116**:226–32. PubMed
26. Yurtkuran M, Alp A, Yurtkuran M, Dilek K. A modified yoga-based exercise program in hemodialysis patients: a randomized controlled study. *Compl Ther Med* 2007;**15**:164–71. PubMed
27. Dhikav V, Karmarkar G, Gupta M, Anand KSJ. Yoga in premature ejaculation: a comparative trial with fluoxetine. *Sex Med* 2007;Sep 21. PubMed
28. Raingruber B, Robinson C. The effectiveness of tai chi, yoga, meditation, and reiki healing sessions in promoting health and enhancing problem solving abilities of registered nurses. *Issues Ment Health Nurs* 2007;**28**:1141–55.
29. Wikepedia. Art therapy. Available at: http://en.wikipedia.org/wiki/Art_therapy (accessed 22 October 2007).
30. Wikepedia. The art of healing. Available at: http://en.wikipedia.org/wiki/The_Art_of_Healing (accessed 23 October 2007).
31. Ulrich RS. How design impacts wellness. *Healthcare Forum J* 1992; September–October. Available at: http://tinyurl.com/3bj3jq (accessed 22 October 2007).
32. Hawthorn K. Therapeutic art programs for special patient populations. A paper presented at the American Society of Healthcare Engineers International Conference on Planning, Design and Construction, Nashville, Tennessee, 8–10 March 2000. Available at: http://tinyurl.com/2zao8 (accessed 15 October 2007).
33. Ulrich RS, Lundén O, Eltinge JL. Effects of exposure to nature and abstract pictures on patients recovering from heart surgery. Paper presented at the Thirty-Third Meetings of the Society for Psychophysiological Research, Rottach-Egern, Germany. Abstract published in *Psychophysiology* 1993;**30**(suppl 1):7. Available at: http://aliveltd.org/rspace/nature.html#_edn5 (accessed 15 October 2007).
34. Malone A. The art of healing. *Medical Construction and Design* 2006;**2**: 47–52.

35. de Craen AJM, Roos PJ, Leonard de Vries A, Kleijnen J. Effect of colour of drugs. Systematic review of perceived effect of drugs and of their effectiveness. *BMJ* 1996;**313**:1624–6.
36. Potkin SG, Zetin M, Stamenkovic V, Kripke D, Bunney Jr WE. Seasonal affective disorder: prevalence varies with latitude and climate. *Clin Neuropharmacol* 1986;**9**(suppl 1):181–3.
37. Haffmanns PM, Sival RC, Lucius SA, Cats Q, van Gelder L. Bright light therapy and melatonin in motor restless behaviour in dementia: a placebo-controlled study. *Int J Geriatr Psych* 2001;**16**:106–10.
38. Lyketsos C, Veiel LL, Baker A, Steele C. A randomised controlled trial of bright light therapy for agitated behaviours in dementia patients residing in long-term care. *Int J Geriatr Psych* 1999;**14**:520–5.
39. Graf A, Wallner C, Schubert V. The effects of light therapy on mini-mental state examination scores in demented patients. *Biol Psychiatry* 2001;**50**:725–7. PubMed
40. Crystal Healing. *The Healing Properties of Gemstones and Crystals.* Available at: http://tinyurl.com/3b77ja (accessed 19 November 2007).
41. Lamprecht M. *Therapeutic Humor Value of Humor to Health Care Professionals and Patients.* Suite 101.com 2007 (August 13). Available at: http://tinyurl.com/2dwn4f (accessed 10 November 2007).
42. Cousins N. *Anatomy of an Illness as Perceived by the Patient.* New York: W Norton & Co., 2001.
43. Martin R. Humor, laughter, and physical health: methodological issues and research findings. *Psychol Bull* 2001;**127**:504–19.
44. Dixon, N. Humor: a cognitive alternative to stress? In: Sarason I, Spielberger C (eds), *Stress and Anxiety*, Vol. 7. Washington DC: Hemisphere, 1980: 281–9.
45. Bennett MP, Lengacher CA. Humor and laughter may influence health. I. History and background. *eCAM* 2006;**3**:61–3. Available at: http://tinyurl.com/299x8t (accessed 10 November 2007).
46. Bennett HJ. Humor in medicine. *South Med J* 2003;**96**:1257–61.
47. Farrah Fawcett. *Fawcett Finds Humour in Cancer Battle.* Available at: http://tinyurl.com/3xvy3j (accessed 10 November 2007).
48. Kadkhodayan, A. Humor and health: Is it effective? *J Pre-health Affiliated Students* 2005;**4**:1. Available at: http://tinyurl.com/2gjosw (accessed 10 November 2007).
49. Stuber M, Hilber SD, Mintzer LL, Castaneda M, Glover D, Zeltzer L. Laughter, humor and pain perception in children: a pilot study. *eCAM* 2007;**10**:93. Available at: http://tinyurl.com/2gqurk (accessed 10 November 2007).
50. Wickramasekera I. Hypnotherapy. In: Jonas W, Levin JS (eds), *Essentials of Complementary and Alternative Medicine.* Baltimore, MD: Lippincott/ Williams & Wilkins, 1999: 426.
51. Vickers A, Zollman C. ABC of complementary medicine. Hypnosis and relaxation therapies. *BMJ* 1999;**319**:1346–9.
52. Vaibo A, Eide T. Smoking cessation in pregnancy: the effect of hypnosis in a randomised study. *Addict Behav* 1996;**21**:29–35.

53. Rhue J, Lynn S, Kirsch I, eds. *Handbook of Clinical Hypnosis.* Washington DC: American Psychological Association, 1993.

54. Kirsch I, Montgomery G, Sapirstein G. Hypnosis as an adjunct to cognitive–behavioral psychotherapy: a meta-analysis. *J Consult Clin Psychol* 1995;**63**:214–20.

55. Wadden TA, Anderton CH. The clinical use of hypnosis. *Psychol Bull* 1982;**91**:215–43.

56. Harvey RF, Hinton RA, Gunary RM, Barry RE. Individual and group hypnotherapy in treatment of refractory irritable bowel syndrome. *Lancet* 1989; i:424–5.

57. Gonsalkorale WM, Miller V, Afzal A, Whorwell PJ. Long term benefits of hypnotherapy for irritable bowel syndrome. *Gut* 2003;**52**:1623–9.

58. Whorwell PJ. Hypnotherapy in irritable bowel syndrome. *Lancet* 1989;i:622.

59. Al Sughayir MA. Hypnotherapy for irritable bowel syndrome in Saudi Arabian patients. *WHO Eastern Mediterranean Hlth J* 2006;**13**(2). Available at: http://tinyurl.com/28nqyl (accessed 16 October 2007).

60. Wikepedia. Magnet therapy. Available at: http://en.wikipedia.org/wiki/Magnet_therapy (accessed 10 May 2008).

61. Jackson B. The resurgence of magnetic therapy. *Pharm J* 2006;**276**:480–1.

62. Wang L-N. Leg ulcers and the first magnetic device available on the NHS. *Pharm J* 2006;**276**:481.

63. Eccles NK, Hollinworth H. A pilot study to determine whether a static magnetic device can promote chronic leg ulcer healing. *J Wound Care* 2005; **14**:64–7.

64. Muthana M, Scott SD, Farrow N et al. A novel magnetic approach to enhance the efficacy of cell-based gene therapies. *Gene Therapy* 2008; advance online publication 17 April 2008. http://tinyurl.com/4opc3s (accessed 18 April 2008).

65. Solberg EE, Berglund KA, Engen O, Ekeberg O, Loeb M. The effect of meditation on shooting performance. *Br J Sports Med* 1996;**30**:342–6.

66. Solberg EE, Halvorsen R, Sundgot-Borgen J, Ingjer F, Holen A. Meditation: a modulator of the immune response to physical stress? A brief report. *Br J Sports Med* 1995;**29**:255–7.

67. Solberg EE, Ingjer F, Holen A, Sundgot-Borgen J, Nilsson S, Holme I. Stress reactivity to and recovery from a standardised exercise bout: a study of 31 runners practising relaxation techniques *Br J Sports Med* 2000;**34**:268–72.

68. Zamarra JW, Schneider RH, Besseghini I et al. Usefulness of the transcendental meditation program in the treatment of patients with coronary artery disease. *Am J Cardiol* 1966;**77**:867–70.

69. Kabat-Zinn J, Massion A O, Kristeller J et al. Effectiveness of a meditation-based stress reduction program in the treatment of anxiety disorders. *Am J Psychiatry* 1992;**149**:936–43.

70. Smith WB, Compton WC, West WB. Meditation as an adjunct to a happiness enhancement program. *J Clin Psychol* 1995;**51**:269–73.

71. Eisenberg DM, Delbanco TL, Berkey CS et al. Cognitive behavioral techniques for hypertension: are they effective? *Ann Intern Med* 1993;**118**:964–72.

72. Kabat-Zinn J, Lipworth L, Burney R. The clinical use of mindfulness meditation for self-regulation of chronic pain. *J Behav Med* 1985;**8**:163–90.
73. Orme-Johnson DW, Schneider RH. Son YD, Nidich S, Cho, Z-H. Neuroimaging of meditation's effect on brain reactivity to pain. *NeuroReport* 2006;**17**:1359–63. Abstract available online http://tinyurl.com/399dgv (accessed 16 October 2007).
74. Canter PH, Ernst E. Insufficient evidence to conclude whether or not transcendental meditation decreases blood pressure: results of a systematic review of randomized clinical trials. *J Hypertens* 2004;**22**:2049–54.
75. Standley JM. The effect of music and multimodal stimulation on responses of premature infants in neonatal intensive care. *Pediatr Nurs* 1998;**24**:532–8.
76. Bunt L. *Music Therapy: An art beyond words.* London: Routledge, 1999.
77. Rauscher FH, Shaw GL, Ky KN. Listening to Mozart enhances spatial–temporal reasoning: towards a neurophysiological basis. *Neurosci Lett* 1995; **185**:44–7.
78. Marwick C. Music therapists chime in with data on medical results. *JAMA* 2000;**283**:731–3.
79. Bygren LO, Konlaan BB, Johansson S-E. Attendance at cultural events, reading books or periodicals, and making music or singing in a choir as determinants for survival: Swedish interview survey of living conditions. *Neurology* 2000;**55**:1935–6.
80. Foster NA, Valentine ER. The effect of auditory stimulation on autobiographical recall in dementia. *Exp Aging Res* 2001;**27**:215–23.
81. Winter MJ, Paskin S, Baker T. Music reduces stress and anxiety of patients in the surgical holding area. *J Post Anesth Nurs* 1994;**9**:340–3.
82. Koch ME, Kain ZN, Ayoub C, Rosenbaum SH. The sedative and analgesic sparing effect of music. *Anesthesiology* 1998;**89**:300–6.
83. Carrick F, Pagnacco G. Posturographic changes associated with music listening. *J Altern Compl Med* 2007;**13**:519–26.
84. Boso M, Emanuele E, Minazzi V, Abbamonte M, Politi P. Effect of long term interactive music therapy on behavior profile and musical skills in young adults with severe autism. *J Altern Compl Med* 2007;**13**:709–12.
85. House of Lords Select Committee on Science and Technology. *Sixth Report (CAM).* November 2000. Available at: http://tinyurl.com/3drr38 (accessed 22 October 2007).
86. Maselko J, Kubzansky L, Kawachi I, Seeman Y, Berkman L. Religious service attendance and allostatic load among high-functioning elderly. *Psychosom Med* 2007;**69**:464–72.
87. Charman RA. Placing healers, healees and healing into a wider research context. *J Altern Compl Med* 2000;**6**:177–80.
88. Brown CK. Methodological problems of clinical research into spiritual healing: the healer's perspective. *J Altern Compl Med* 2000;**6**:171–6.
89. Abbot NC. Healing as a therapy for human disease: a systematic review. *J Altern Compl Med* 2000;**6**:159–69.
90. Harkness EF, Abbot NC, Ernst E. A randomised trial of distant healing for skin warts. *Am J Med* 2000;**108**:448–52.

91. Koenig HG, George K, Hays JC et al. The relationship between religious activities and blood pressure in older adults. *Int J Psychiatry Med* 1998;**28**: 189–213.

92. Kaufman Y, Anaki D, Binns M, Freedman M. Cognitive decline in Alzheimer disease: Impact of spirituality, religiosity, and QOL *Neurology* 2007;**68**: 1509–14.

93. Wiesendanger H, Werthmuller L, Reuter K, Walsch H. Chronically ill patients treated by spiritual healing improve in quality of life: results of a randomized waiting-list controlled study *J Altern Compl Med* 2001;**7**:45–51.

94. Yilmaz S, Kart-Köseoglu H, Guler O, Yucel E. Effect of prayer on osteoarthritis and osteoporosis. *Rheumatol Int* 2008;**28**(5):429–36.

95. O'Mathuna DP. Prayer research: what are we measuring? *J Christian Nurs* 1999;**16**:17–21.

96. Byrd RC. Positive therapeutic effect of intercessory prayer in coronary care unit population. *South Med J* 1988; **81**:826–9.

97. Harris WS, Gowda M, Kolb JW et al. A randomised controlled trial of the effects of remote, intercessory prayer on outcomes in patients admitted to the coronary care unit. *Arch Intern Med* 1999;**159**:2273–8.

98. Adams JD, Garcia C The advantages of traditional chumash healing. *Evidence Based Compl Altern Med* 2005;**2**:19–23.

Index

Note: page numbers in *italics* refer to Figures and Tables.

ABC (Aconite, Belladonna and Chamomilla) mixture 193
abdominal compresses 482
abdominal massage 532
absolutes, aromatherapy 349
accessory olfactory system 345
accreditation of practitioners 32, 35–36
  in naturopathy 479
  see also regulation of CAM; training of practitioners
Aconite *209, 242, 245, 247, 249, 251*
  in Chinese herbal medicine 439
ACT acronym 224–226
acupoints *427, 428*
acupressure 432
acupuncture 5, 425–426
  applications 432
  availability 433
  cost minimisation 56
  evidence 430
  problems with RCTs 134
  history 426–427
  perceived effectiveness 53
  practice
  minimal acupuncture 429–430
  traditional acupuncture 427–429
  safety 431
  theory 427
adaptation syndrome, naturopathy 476–477
adjuvans, herbal teas 281
ADROIT (Adverse Drug Reaction On-Line Information Tracking) 164
adulteration of products
  essential oils 352

herbal products 307–309
  Chinese 440
  supplements 34
advances in CAM 139–140
adverse effects 33, 34, 35, 138, 148
  of acupuncture 431
  of chiropractic manipulation 527–528
  of herbal medicines 302–312
  of homeopathic medicines 220–222
  international monitoring 159–160
  of orthodox medicine, role in choosing CAM 46–48
  reporting 146, 155, 311–312
  advantages and limitations of spontaneous schemes 166–167
  by complementary medicine practitioners 169–171
  improvements in pharmacovigilance 175–177
  by pharmacists 167–169
  UK scheme 160–162
  reporting forms 162–164
  signal detection and assessment 164–165
  of traditional medicines 401–402
  see also interactions
advertising regulations, allopathic drugs 109
Advisory Board on the Registration of Homeopathic Products 209
African prune tree (*Pygeum africanum*) 328
AGE (Arsen iod, Gelsemium and Eupatorium) mixture 193, *245*
aggravations, homeopathic 221–222
agni (gastric fire), ayurveda 451, *455*
agrimony (*Agrimonia eupatoria*) 384

AIDS patients
    use of traditional herbal medicine
        397
    value of massage 534
air, ayurveda 452
Alaskan essences, flower remedy
    therapy 386
alcoholic tinctures, herbalism 283
Alexander technique 517–20
alfalfa (*Medicago sativa*) 306, 308,
    316
alkaloids 279
allergies
    to essential oils 370, *371*
    homeopathic remedies *248, 249, 251*
    RCTs 236, 237, 238
    relationship to hygiene 11–12
    to royal jelly 504
allergodes 199, 211
allersodes 213
Allium cepa 209, *245, 249*
allopathic drugs 107
    regulation in USA *108*–109
allopathy 193
aloe vera 316
    adverse effects 304
alternative approach to healthcare 8, 9
alternative medical systems 96
alternative medicine, definitions 3–4,
    24, 27
analgesia, placebo effect 7–8
anaphylaxis, royal jelly as cause 504
anecdotal evidence 135–136
angelica, toxic constituents 151
animal behaviourism 84
animal material
    use in ayurveda 459
    use in Chinese herbal medicine 438
    use in homeopathy 198
anthroposophical medicine 257–259
    market size 226–228
    rhythmical massage therapy
        538–539
anthroposophy 256–257
anti-inflammatories, herbalism 291
antioxidants, value during oncology
    treatments 33
antiseptics
    essential oils 367–369
    herbal 292–295

anxiety
    aromatherapy 362, 366
    ayurvedic treatments *469*
    herbal medicines 327
    homeopathic medicines *247, 249,*
        250, 251
    massage therapy 534
Apis 192, 198, *249, 252*
apitherapy 502–504
apothecaries 271
applied kinesiology 514–515
appraisal of literature 137–138
arachidonic acid 493
arachis oil, use for baby massage 539
Argent met *251*
Argent nit 243, *245, 247, 249, 250, 251*
Aristolochia species
    safety concerns 175
    toxic constituents 150
Arndt's law, homeopathy 194
Arnica 198, 200, *211*, 229, 243, *249,*
        251, 252, 308
    RCTs 236
aromatherapy 353
    in ayurveda 460
    choice of oil 358–360
    conditions treated 360–*361*
    definition 335
    evidence 361–363
    fragrancing 353–354
    history 342–345
    market value *60*
    massage 354–355, 356
    olfactory remediation 354
    during pregnancy 373–374
    safety 369–371
    theory
        dermal action 345–347
        olfactory stimulation 343–345
    see also essential oils
aromatogram 369
Arsenicum album *211*, 223, 243, *246,*
        251, 252
    RCTs 236
art of healing 6–8
art of healing programme, Tan Tock
        Seng Hospital 571–572
art therapy 570–573
arthritis, aromatherapy *361*
asthma

CAM therapies 65
Papworth relaxation technique 567–568
relationship to hygiene 11–12
astringents, herbal 295
atopy, prevalence in anthroposophical families 257
attention deficit hyperactivity disorder (ADHD), dietary treatment 495–496
attitude and awareness studies, homeopathy 242
attitudes to CAM
GPs 70–74
nurses 76–77
pharmacists 74–76
audit 134–135
in homeopathy 240–241
aura soma see colour therapy
Australia
prevalence of CAM utilization 64
regulation of herbal medicines 153–155
Australia and New Zealand Therapeutic Products Authority (ANZTPA) 155
Australian bush essences, flower remedy therapy 386
autism, music therapy 585, 586
autogenic training 567
autoisopathics 212
ayurvedic medicine 449
evidence 465–466
history 450
integration with western medicine 467
practice 455–456
aromatherapy 460
dietary advice 456–457
enemas 460
herbs used 468–469
medicines 458–460
mind–body interventions 461
surgery 462
treatments for common conditions 469–470
regulation 466
safety 462–465
toxic constituents 151
theory 451–455

babies, osteopathy 542
baby massage 533, 539
Bach flower remedies 384–385
see also flower remedies
Bach rescue cream 388
back pain
anthroposophical treatment 258
Alexander technique 520
balneotherapy 486–487
massage 533, 534
osteopathy 543, 544
reflexology 548
see also chiropractic
Bacterium termo 500
balneotherapy 486–488
balsams 277
Bambusa 258
baths, hydrotherapy 482–486
bee venom therapy 503
see also apitherapy
behavioural and psychological symptoms in dementia (BPSD), aromatherapy 364–365
Belladonna 196, 211, 243, 247, 248, 252
benign prostatic hyperplasia, herbal medicines 328
Benveniste, Jacques, 'memory of water' concept 239
bergamot oil 367, 371, 372, 375
betel (Piper betle) 463, 465
bias 134
in clinical trials 238
practitioner bias 133
publishing bias 132–133
Bifidobacterium species 501
bilberry (Vaccinium myrtilus) 293
biochemic tissue salts 254–255
biofield therapies 564
biologically-based medicine 96
biotherapeutic agents see probiotics
bitters 277
blackcurrant (Ribes nigrum) 293
blood, in traditional Chinese medicine 421
blood pressure
effect of aromatherapy 367
effect of transcendental meditation 582
body fluids, in traditional Chinese medicine 421

Boericke, *Materia Medica and Repertory* 224
boils, homeopathic remedies *248*
Boot, Jesse 272–273
borage *306*
Borax *249*
botanical names, use in homeopathy 196
Bowen technique 521–522
brain, possible effects of essential oils 358
breast-feeding, use of herbal products 297
British Herbal Medicine Association, ADR reporting 171
British Homeopathic Pharmacopoeia 197
Bryonia *211*, 225, 243, *245, 246, 247, 251*
burnet saxifrage (*Pimpinelia saxifraga*) 293
burns, homeopathic remedies *248*

Cactus grandiflorus 196
Calc carb 199, *211*
Calc fluor *255*
Calc phos *255*, 211
Calc sulph *255*
Calendula 198, *199*, 200, *248, 249, 251, 252*
California essences, flower remedy therapy 385
camomile *276*, 279, 291, 299, *317*, 328
    see also Chamomilla
camomile oil 350, *361, 365, 366, 375*
    allergies 370
camphor *308*, 367, 369–370
Canada, prevalence of CAM utilization 64, 99
cancer
    complementary care 27, 33, 65–66
    aromatherapy 366
    magnetic therapy *581*
    role of diet 488–489
Cantharis *209*, 243, *248, 250, 252*
cao wu (*Aconitum kusnezoffii*) 439
Carbo veg *209, 246, 250*
cardiac glycosides 280
carrier oils, aromatherapy 356–357

cascara 328
case studies in homeopathy 241–242
case–control studies 172–173
Caulophyllum 236–237, *250*, 297
Causticum *250*
celery *308*
centaury (*Centaurium umbellatum*) 384
centisimal dilution scale 202, *203*
Centre for Evidence Based Medicine (CEBM) 138
Centre for Pharmacy Postgraduate Education (CPPE) 76
cerato (*Ceratostigma willmottiana*) 384
Chamomilla 196, *211*, 243, *245*
    see also camomile
champissage (Indian head massage) 460
Charak 450
chelation therapy 480–481
chemical material, use in homeopathy 196, 199
chemical–skin interactions 346
chemotypes, essential oils 350–351
chest compresses (chest packs) 482
chest massage 534
chicory (*Cichorium intybus*) 385
childbirth *see* midwifery
children
    aromatherapy 359
    massage therapy 534–535
    osteopathy 542
    use of herbal medicines 298–299
    Chinese 441
China, traditional medicine *see* traditional Chinese medicine
Chinese dietary therapy 442–443
Chinese herbal medicine (CHM) 396, 433
    administration to children 441
    classification 18
    classification of medicines 434
    evidence 441–442
    herbal formula 435
    history 433–434
    patent medicines 436–437
    pharmacovigilance 441
    preparation of herbs 435–436
    presentations 436

regulation 437–438
safety 439–441
treatment of irritable bowel
syndrome 28
use during pregnancy 440–441
in western societies 438–439
Chinese herbs 437
Chinese massage 442
chiropractic 522–523
comparison with osteopathy 542
cost-effectiveness 56
evidence 525–527
history 523–524
insurance reimbursement, effects on
use 104
practice 524–525
regulation 528
safety 527–528
theory 524
training 528–529
chronic fatigue syndrome, value of
osteopathy 543–544
chuan wu (Aconitum carmichaeli) 439
chumash healing 589
Cicero 12
Cinchona 188
cinnamon oil 368
claims development, over-the-counter
homeopathic drugs 112
Clark's rule (paediatric doses) 298
clary sage oil 365, 375
classic homeopathy 216
classification of CAM 17–19
cleansing stage, herbalism 273
clematis (Clematis vitalba) 384
climate change 407
clinical audit 134–135
in homeopathy 240–241
clinical questions 136
clinical trials see evidence; randomised
clinical trials
clove oil 375
clown-doctors 578
Cocculus 223, 246, 250, 252
Cochrane Collaboration 5, 27, 137
Coffea 190, 250, 252
cohort studies 172–173
cohosh, black (Cimicifuga racemosa)
317–318
hepatotoxic reactions 151

cohosh, blue (Caulophyllum
thalictroides) 306, 318
cold, effect on survival after trauma 11
cold baths 482, 483, 484, 485
cold compresses 482
colds
aromatherapy 361, 367
effect of probiotics 501
herbal medicines 329
homeopathic remedies 245
colic
herbal medicines 328
homeopathic remedies 245
Colocynth 243, 245
colonisation resistance 498
colorants, herbal teas 281
colour therapy 573–576
ayurveda 461
coltsfoot 306, 328
comfort, provision of 10
comfrey (Symphytum officinale)
interactions 306
toxicity 303, 308
communication 43
communication problems, integrative
medicine 26
complementary and alternative
medicine (CAM)
classification 17–19
conditions treated 64–67
definitions 3–6, 24, 27
distinction from integrative medicine
23
holistic approach 13–17
integration into UK healthcare
system 80–84
patterns of use 61
perceived effectiveness 53
perceptions of 9–10
prevalence of utilization 30–31,
59–60
European countries 62
in USA 62–63
provision 67–68
by complementary practitioners
77–79
by lay practitioners 79
by medically qualified practitioners
68–74
by nurses 76–77

complementary and alternative
        medicine (CAM) (*continued*)
    by pharmacists 74–76
    reasons for avoidance 58
    reasons for patient choice 44–46
    belief in value of CAM 51–54
    culture 58
    disenchantment with OM 48–50
    dissatisfaction with OM consultation
        50–51
    financial reasons 54–57
    'green' association 57
    media coverage 57
    role models 58
    safety concerns 46–48
    relative popularity of disciplines
        60–61
    self-treatment 80
complementary approach to healthcare
        8–9
complementary medicines
    need for pharmacovigilance 147
    utilisation 147–149
complementary practitioners 77–79
    ADR reporting 169–171
complementary referral guidelines,
        Lewisham Hospital NHS Trust
        54
complex prescribing, homeopathy 217
complexity, herbal medicines 149
compresses 482
confirmation bias 125
Conium *250*
conservation 407–409
CONSORT (Consolidated Standards of
        Reporting Trials) guidelines 177
constipation
    herbal medicines 328
    homeopathic remedies *245*
constitutional homeopathic medicines
        213–214
consultations 14, 15–16, 43–44
    in anthroposophy 258
    costs 55–56
    importance of 10
    in naturopathy 477, 478
    as reason for choice of CAM 50–51
consumerism in healthcare 48–49
containers, homeopathic medicines
        207

contaminants *see* adulteration
corrigens, herbal teas 281
cost-benefit 55, 56
cost-effectiveness analyses (CEAs) 54,
        56
cost minimisation 55–56
cost utility 56
coughs
    aromatherapy *361*
    herbal medicines 328
    homeopathic remedies *246*
coumadin, interactions 35
coumarins 279
counter prescribing of homeopathic
        medicines 222–226
    repertory 244–252
counterstrain techniques, osteopathy
        541
craniosacral massage 531
craniosacral techniques, osteopathy 542
Crataegus (hawthorn) 198, 200, *306*,
        323
Critical Appraisal Skills Program
        (CASP) 138
crude drugs, use in herbalism 280
crystal form, homeopathic medicines
        205, 206
crystal therapy 576
Cullen, William 188
Culpepper, Nicholas 271
culture
    relationship to CAM use 103
    role in choice of CAM 58
curcuminoids, extraction from turmeric
        30
current good manufacturing practices
        (cGMPs) 108
cycling, post-exercise massage 538
cystic fibrosis, omega-3 fatty acid
        supplements 496
cystitis, homeopathic remedies *250*

damiana *306*
dance and movement therapy 561–562
dandelion (*Taraxacum officinalis*) *306*,
        328
Dawson, William 74
decimal dilution scale 202–203
decision-making, patient involvement
        44, 50

decoctions 281
deep-tissue massage 531
definitions of CAM 3–6
delayed-onset muscle soreness, value of
    massage 536–537
dementia
    aromatherapy 364–365
    beneficial effects of music 586
demulcents 291
dentistry, homeopathic remedies 249
dependence on essential oils 371
depression
    herbal medicines 327
    value of yoga 569
dermal action, aromatherapy 345–347
detergents, effect on essential oil
    absorption 347
determinism 8
detoxification, in naturopathy 477,
    479–480
detoxodes 213
devil's claw 306
dexamethasone, presence in herbal
    products 308
dhatus (tissues), ayurveda 451,
    454–455
diabetes, ayurvedic medicines 465
diagnosis, in traditional Chinese
    medicine 423–424
diagnostic therapies
    iridology 511–513
    kinesiology 513–515
diarrhoea
    ayurvedic treatments 469
    herbal medicines 328
    homeopathic remedies 245–246,
    251, 252
    use of probiotics 499–500,
    501–502
Dietary Supplement Regulations, New
    Zealand 155
dietary supplements 107
    regulation in USA 108, 109–110,
    155–156
dietary therapy
    ayurveda 456–457
    naturopathy 477, 488–491
    traditional Chinese medicine
    442–443
    see also nutraceuticals

digestion stimulation, herbalism 273
diluents, homeopathic medicines 239
dilution, homeopathic medicines 191,
    238–239
    see also potentisation
disclosure of CAM utilisation 148, 402
disease, definition 6
disinfectants, herbal 292–295
docosahexaenoic acid 493, 496
doctors, use of CAM 68–74
Doctrine of Similars 271
domains of CAM, NCCAM 18–19,
    96–97
dong quai (Angelica sinensis) 458
dosage, herbal medicines 311
dose forms, homeopathy 112,
    205–207
dose regimens, homeopathic medicines
    225–226
doshas (humours), ayurveda 451, 452,
    453
Drosera 246
drug claims, FDA regulations 108–109
drug pictures, homeopathy 195
duration of treatment, homeopathic
    medicines 230
dynamis, homeopathy 191
dyspepsia, herbal medicines 328

ear problems, herbal medicines 328
earth, ayurveda 452
echinacea 283, 288, 291, 292, 310,
    319, 328
    adverse reactions 161
    evidence 300
Economic Botany Collections, Royal
    Botanic Gardens Kew 314
eczema, homeopathic remedies 248
education, relationship to CAM use
    103
effectiveness 123
efficacy 123
    of herbal medicines 158
effleurage 531
elder 306
elderly people
    depression, value of yoga 569
    use of herbal products 299
emmenagogic essential oils 373
end gaining, Alexander technique 518

endangered plant species 407, 408
endorphins, action of acupuncture
       427
enemas 481–482
   use in ayurveda 460
energy medicine 96
entanglement theory 240
enteric coating, probiotics 500
environmental awareness 404
environmental conditions, effect on
       essential oils 351–352
ephedra 329
epilepsy, aromatherapy 367
Epsom salt baths 486
essence (jing) 420–421
essences 341, 348
   flower remedies 383–384
essential fatty acids (EFAs) 492,
       493–494
   evidence 494–496
   supplements 496–497
essential nutrients 489
essential oils 278–279, 341, 347
   absorption, influencing factors
       346–347
   absorption pathways 359
   antiseptic properties 367–369
   chemotypes 350–351
   choice of oil 358–360
   composition 349–352
   dependence 371
   extraction 348–349
   factsheet for pharmacists 74
   ingestion of 313
   interactions 371–372
   maximum dose levels 372
   metabolism 358
   over the counter supply 374–375
   quality 352
   routes of administration 355–357
   sensitising components 371
   storage 352, 353
   toxicity 369–371
   see also aromatherapy
ether, ayurveda 452
ethnic medicines forum, MHRA
       400–401
eucalyptus oil 350, 361, 367, 375
Euphrasia 211, 243, 249, 251, 295
Europe

CAM utilization 61
   registration of homeopathic
       medicines 208
European Union
   regulation of herbal medicines
       152–153, 283–284
   regulatory framework for
       pharmacovigilance 146
evening primrose 306
evening primrose oil, evidence 495
evidence 7, 28–29, 32–33
   acupuncture 430
   Alexander technique 519–520
   anthroposophy 258–259
   aromatherapy 361–369
   art therapy 572–573
   ayurvedic medicine 465–467
   balneotherapy 486–487
   Bowen technique 521–522
   chiropractic 525–527
   colour therapy 575–576
   essential fatty acids 494–496
   flower remedies 390–391
   herbal medicines 299–302
   homeopathy 111, 230–232
   attitude and awareness studies 242
   audit 240–241
   case studies 241–242
   perception of benefit studies 241
   placebo studies 234–235
   randomised clinical trials 235–238
   studies on mechanism of action
       238–240
   humour therapy 577–579
   hypnotherapy 579–580
   iridology 513
   kinesiology 515
   massage 533–538
   music therapy 584–586
   naturopathy 477
   nutritional therapy 490–491
   osteopathy 543–544
   probiotics 500–502
   problems with clinical trials
       129–130
   quality of 124
   influencing factors 124–126
   reflexology 547–548
   reiki 564–565
   relaxation techniques 567–568

spiritual healing 588
traditional medicine 403
Chinese 424–425, 441–442
yoga 568–570
evidence base for CAM 121
types of outcome measures 123
evidence-based medicine (EBM) 7, 28,
126–128
and CAM 128
evidence sources 133
clinical audit 134–135
literature searches 136–138
observational studies 135–136
randomised clinical trials 133–134
examination nerves, homeopathic
medicines 223, 247
exercise, value of massage 535–538
extraction processes
essential oils 348–349
herbalism 282–283
homeopathic medicines 200
eye problems, ayurvedic treatments 469
eyebright (Euphrasia) 295, 328
eyedrops, homeopathic 207

fabricated oils 352
factsheets, availability from RPSGB 74
faculty sensory appreciation, Alexander
technique 518
faith healing, in veterinary medicine 85
farming practices, anthroposophy 257
fatty acids
essential 492, 493–497
saturated and unsaturated 492–493
fear, homeopathic remedies 247, 249
feedback loop, in development of
homeopathic drugs 113
'feel good factor', herbalism 269
Feldenkreis method 520–521
feng shui 420
Ferrum phos 243, 255
feverfew (Tancetum parthenium)
319–320
toxic constituents 150, 308
fibrositis, massage therapy 537
financial issues in choice of CAM 54–57
fire, ayurveda 452
'fire-fighting' approach, herbalism 273
first aid, homeopathic remedies 248,
252

five elements, ayurveda 451–452
five elements (phases), traditional
Chinese medicine 418–419
five substances, traditional Chinese
medicine 419–421
five tastes, Chinese herbal medicine
434
five-flower remedy (Rescue Remedy)
388, 391
flatulence, herbal medicines 328
flavonoids 279
flower remedies 383–384
evidence 390–391
history 384–386
practice 387–389
preparation 387
theory 386–387
flower therapy 575
follow-up, homeopathic treatment
226, 227
foot baths 484
Formica 258
formula development, homeopathic
drugs 111
formula selection, homeopathic drugs
112
Foundation for Integrated Medicine
83–84
four energies, Chinese herbal medicine
434
'four gentlemen decoction', Chinese
herbal medicine 436–437
fragrancing 353–354
Framingham study 492
French Homeopathic Pharmacopoeia
197
friction, massage 531
frozen shoulder, use of Bowen
technique 521–522
fruit, nutritional value 489–490
fu zi 439
fucus 306, 308
functional techniques, osteopathy 541
funding problems, CAM research
128–129

gamma-linolenic acid 493, 495
gap analysis, homeopathic drugs
110–111
gardening, therapeutic effect 167

garlic (*Allium sativum*) *306*, 320
gastric fire (agni), ayurveda 441,
     455
gastrointestinal problems, homeopathic
     remedies 245–246
Gattefossé, René-Maurice 342–343,
     368
Gelsemium *211*, 223, 243, *245*, 247,
     249
gemstones, use in ayurveda 461
gender differences
  in attitudes to CAM 71
  in utilization of CAM 60, 99–100,
     229
General Osteopathic Council
     544–545
generating cycle *418*
gentian (*Gentiana amarella*) 384
geranium oil *375*
German Pharmacopoeia 197
Germany, homeopathic practitioners
     215–216
ginger (*Zingiberis officinalis*) *306*,
     320–321
ginger oil *375*
Ginkgo biloba 289, 302, 310,
     321–322, 327, 410, *411*
  adverse reactions 161
  interactions 35, 305
ginkgolic acids, variability 150
ginseng 294, 304, *308*, *308*, 322, 327
Glasgow Homeopathic Hospital
     Outcome Scale 123
glycosides 279–280
good practice guidelines, CAM
     disciplines 77
GPs, attitudes to CAM 70–4
GRADE Working group, definition of
     quality of evidence 124
graduated baths 485
grains, nutritional value 489
granule form, homeopathic medicines
     205, 206
grapefruit juice, interactions 35
Graphites *248*
green issues, role in choice of CAM 57
grief, homeopathic remedies 247
growing conditions, effect on essential
     oils 351
guras, ayurveda 453–454

haemorrhoids, herbal medicines 328
Hahnemann, Samuel 188–*190*,
     192–193
Hahnemannian method of
     potentisation 202–203
Hamamelis (*Hamamelis virginiana*)
     243
hatha yoga 568
Hawaii, prevalence of CAM use 63–64
hawthorn (*Crataegus* species) 198,
     200, *306*, 323
hay fever, placebo study in homeopathy
     234
head massage, Indian 460
headaches, homeopathic remedies 247
healing 10
  holistic approach 12–16
  self-healing 10–12, 235, 524
healing crisis, naturopathy 477
healing (therapeutic) touch 565–566
health 6
  social determinants 13–14
  WHO definition 13, 33
health behaviour factors, role in CAM
     use 100–103
Health Belief Model (HBM) 102
healthcare, new approach 48–50
healthcare providers, understanding of
     traditional medicine 403–404
healthcare systems
  integrative medicine 32–33, 80–84
  patients' requirements 43–44
heartburn
  herbal medicines 328
  homeopathic remedies *250*
heat effects, homeopathic treatment
     252
heating compresses 482
heavy metals, use in ayurveda 463–464
Heilpraktikers 78
Helicobacter pylori 36
Hepar sulph *248*
herb bennet (*Geum urbanum*) 293
herbal alchemy (spagyric medicine)
     315
herbal medicines
  active constituents 276–280
  adverse event reporting 164
  improvements in pharmacovigilance
     176–177

prescription event monitoring
      171–172
antipodean 295
ayurvedic 458–459
composition 149–150
contaminants 34, 307–309
counselling patients 296–299
evidence 299–302
market value 60
over-the-counter products 289–95
preparation and presentation
      280–283
regulation
   in Australia 153–154
   in Canada 156–157
   in European Union 152–153
   in New Zealand 154–155
   in United Kingdom 151–152
repertory
   conditions 327–330
   materia medica 316–327
safety 157–158, 302–312
standardization 36, 310
supply 283–284
therapeutic groups 276
toxic constituents 150–151
traditional use 397
utilisation 147, 148–149
herbal poisoning, treatment 312–313
herbal sources of drugs 274–275
herbal teas 281
herbalism 269–270
   applications 285–286
   association with pharmacy 73,
      287–288
   differences from orthodox medicine
      275
   future direction 314–315
   history 270–271
   perceived effectiveness 53
   practitioners 284
   reference sources 274
   regulations 283–284
   theory 273–274
   see also Chinese herbal medicine;
      herbal medicines
herbaria, Royal Pharmaceutical Society
      313–314
Hering's law, homeopathy 194
hierarchy of resort 80

highly unsaturated fatty acids (HUFAs)
      495
hip baths 483
Hippocrates 10–11, 51
HIV
   susceptibility 11
   see also AIDS patients
holistic approach 50
   in CAM practice 13–17, 103
   definition 12–13
   homeopathy 193–194
HomBRex database 240
homeopathic medicine types 210–214
homeopathic medicines 35, 107,
      114
   containers 207
   counter prescribing 222–226
   dispensing 219–220
   dose regimens 225–226
   interaction with essential oils 372
   market size 226–228
   methods of administration 216–217
   nomenclature 195–197
   over-the-counter preparations,
      development and marketing
      110–113
   precautions in taking the medicine
      220
   preparation 201
   dose forms 205–207
   extraction procedure 200
   potentisation 200–205
   regulation 208–210
   in New Zealand 156–157
   in USA 108, 110
   repertory 244–252
   requests for supply 218
   source materials 198–200
   supply 217
homeopathic pharmacopoeias 197
   British Homeopathic Pharmacopoeia
      197
   French Homeopathic Pharmacopoeia
      197
   German Homeopathic
      Pharmacopoeia 197
   Homeopathic Pharmacopeia of the
      United States (HPUS) 106,
      197
homeopathic practitioners 214–216

homeopathy
    attitude of pharmacists 73
    availability in UK healthcare system
        80–81
    cost minimisation 56–57
    definition 187
    evidence 230–232
    attitude and awareness studies 242
    audit 240–241
    case studies 241–242
    perception of benefit studies 241
    placebo studies 234–235
    randomised clinical trials 235–238
    studies on mechanism of action
        238–240
    follow-up 226, 227
    funding withdrawal 81
    history 187–190
    limitations 78
    market value 60
    materia medica 242–244
    perceived effectiveness 53
    postgraduate training 76
    reasons for patient choice 45, 52
    regulation in USA 106–107
    safety 220–222
    theory 191–95
    use by role models 58
    user characteristics 228–230
    veterinary use 253–254
homocysteine, as risk factor for
        cardiovascular disease 36
homotoxicology 255
honey
    nutritional value 490
    as wound dressing 503
    see also apitherapy
hops (Humulus lupulus) 293, 306, 329
horehound (Marubium vulgare) 328,
        330
horse chestnut 308, 328
horseradish 306
horsetail (Equisetum arvense) 293
hospital pharmacies, provision of CAM
        products 75
'hot' medicines 277
hot water therapy 482, 483, 484, 485
House of Lords, classification of CAM
        17–18
House of Lords Report 121–122

huang lian (Coptis chinensis) 441
humour therapy 576–579
hydrotherapy 477, 481
    baths 482–486
    compresses 482
    enemas 481–482
hygiene, relationship to allergic diseases
        11–12
Hypercal 248, 249
Hypericum 211, 248, 252
hyperlipidaemia, herbal medicines 329
hypertension, aromatherapy 367
hypnosis, perceived effectiveness 53
hypnotherapy 579–580
hypothesis tests 129

identification, herbal plants 309
Ignatia 211, 243, 247
immersion baths 485
impatiens (Impatiens glandulifera)
        385
imponderables, homeopathy 199–200
indigestion
    herbal medicines 328
    homeopathic remedies 246, 252
individualized care 28–30
infant massage 533, 539
infants, osteopathy 542
influenza
    aromatherapy 361
    CAM therapies 66
    effect of probiotics 501
    herbal medicines 329
    homeopathic remedies 245
information
    gathering from patients 14–15
    provision to patients 44
information sources 137
infusions 280–281
inhalation of essential oils 355–356,
        358
inhibition, Alexander technique 519
insect bites
    aromatherapy 361
    homeopathic remedies 248, 252
insect material, use in homeopathy 198
insect stings, homeopathic remedies
        249
insomnia
    aromatherapy 367

herbal medicines 329
homeopathic remedies *250, 252*
insurance reimbursement 113, 115
  for allopathic drugs 109
  for chiropractic 526
  impact on CAM use 104
  for iridology 513
  for probiotics 500
integrated healthcare 398–399
*Integrated healthcare – a way forward
  for the next five years?* 82–83
integrative medicine (IM) 23, 35–37,
  80–84
  complementary versus alternative
    therapies 27–28
  definitions 23–25
  history-taking 26
  individualized care 28–30
  integration into healthcare systems
    32–33
  natural products, context of use
    30–31
  practice models 25–26
  practitioners 31
  risks to the patient 33–35
intent-to-treat principle 126
interactions 26, 34, 138, 148
  with ayurvedic medicines 464–465
  with essential oils 371–372
  with herbal medicines 299, 304,
    304–305, *306*
  St. John's wort *326*
  with homeopathic medicines 222
intercessory prayer 588–589
internal locus of control, association
  with CAM use 100–101
Ipecacuanha *211, 243, 246*
iridology 477, 511–513
irritable bowel syndrome
  aromatherapy *361*
  Chinese herbal treatment 28
  placebo effect 15–16
Iscador 257
isodes 213
isopathic medicines 210–212
  use as vaccines 212–213

Japan, definition of CAM 5
jet lag
  ayurvedic treatments *469*

homeopathic treatment *252*
jing (essence) 420–421
joints, massage 532
juniper (*Juniper communis*) 294
juniper oil *361*

Kali mur *255*
Kali phos *255*
Kali sulph *255*
Kampo 5
Kan Jang, use in influenza 66
kapha dosha 452, 453, 454, 457
karela (*Momordica charantia*) 465
kava-kava (*Piper methysticum*)
    323–324, 327
  contaminants 34
  hepatotoxic reactions 151, 152, 175
  UK regulatory response 165–166
  interaction with benzodiazepines
    305
keynotes, polychrests 225
Keys, Ancel 492
khat (*Catha edulis*) 462–463
kinesiology 513–515
knitbone (*Symphytum officinale*) 291
Korsakovian method of potentisation
    203–204

labelling
  ayurvedic medicines 464
  herbal medicines 311
  homeopathic medicines 209, 219
Lac can 212
Lachesis 212
Lactobacillus species 501
laughter 577, 578–579
lavender (*Lavendula angustifolia*), use
    during pregnancy 297
lavender oil 350, *361, 363, 364, 367,
    368, 375*
  use during pregnancy 373
law of minimum action, homeopathy
    195
laws of cure, homeopathy 194–195
lay practitioners 79
lead, use in ayurveda 463
Ledum *248, 252*
leg ulcers, magnetic therapy 581
lemon balm (*Melissa officinalis*) 327
  use in aromatherapy 364

lemon oil *372, 375*
Lewisham Hospital NHS Trust,
    complementary referral
    guidelines *54*
licensing of practitioners 32
    see also regulation of CAM; training
    of practitioners
licensing of products 146
    in United Kingdom 151–152
liferoot (*Senecio aureus*) 150
light box therapy *575*
like cures like principle, . homeopathy
    188–189, 192
limitations of CAM 78
Ling, Per Henrik 530
linoleic acid *493, 495*
liquid extracts, herbalism 282
liquorice (*Glycyrrhiza* species) 328
    adverse effects 305, *306, 308*
literature review, in homeopathic drug
    development 111
literature searches 136–138
LM method of potentisation 204
LOAD acronym 223–224
locus of control theory 100–101

macerates 282
Mag phos *255*
magnetic therapy 580–581
malas (waste products), ayurveda 451,
    455
manipulation
    chiropractic *525*
    osteopathy 542
manual therapies 97
    Alexander technique 517–520
    Bowen technique 521–522
    Feldenkreis method 520–521
    rolfing 549–550
    in veterinary medicine 84
    see also chiropractic; massage;
        osteopathy; reflexology
manual therapy, comparison with
    osteopathy 543
marigold (*Calendula officinalis*) 291
marjoram (*Origanum vulgare*) 293
marjoram oil *361*
market values for CAM *60*
marketing authorisation (MA) 146
martial art therapy 443

massage 529–531
    in aromatherapy 354–355, 356,
        361, 363, 364, 366
    in ayurveda 460
    Chinese 436
    evidence 533–538
    sports massage and muscle fatigue
        535–538
    rhythmical massage therapy (RMT)
        538–539
    safety 539
    therapeutic uses 532–533
materia medica
    herbalism 274
    homeopathy 242–244
Materia Medica, William Cullen 188,
    189
Maury, Margaret 343
means whereby, Alexander technique
    518
mechanism of action, homeopathic
    medicines 238–240
media coverage of CAM *57*
medical education, inclusion of CAM
    therapy 69–70, 73
medical homeopathy 215
medicinal plant trade 405–406,
    409–410
meditation 581–583
    in ayurveda 461
Medsafe, New Zealand 155
'memory of water' concept 239
menopausal symptoms
    aromatherapy 363
    herbal medicines 330
menstrual problems, herbal medicines
    330
menthol 367
Merc sol *249*
meridians, traditional Chinese medicine
    423
    acupuncture 427–428
    herbal medicine 434
Mesmer 579
metal poisoning, chelation therapy
    480–481
metals, use in ayurveda 460, 463–464
Metchnikoff, Elie 498
midwifery
    provision of CAM 83–84

use of aromatherapy 365–366
use of reflexology 548
migraine, aromatherapy 361
migraine prophylaxis, homeopathic
    RCT 236
milk, nutritional value 490
milk thistle (*Silybum marianus*) 289,
    324
mimulus (*Mimulus gluttatus*) 385
mind–body medicine 96
mineral baths (balneotherapy)
    486–488
mineral supplements, value of complex
    mixtures 30
minimal acupuncture 429–430
minimal dose principle, homeopathy
    193
mint oil 361
mistletoe 308
Mitchell relaxation technique 567
mobilisation of circulation, herbalism
    273
monounsaturated fats 493
morning sickness
    herbal medicines 330
    homeopathic remedies 223, 246,
        250
Moschus 212
mother tinctures, homeopathy 200, 207
motion sickness
    elasticated travel bands 432
    herbal medicines 328
    homeopathic remedies 252
mouth ulcers, homeopathic remedies
    249
movement of herbs, Chinese herbal
    medicine 434
moxa 427
moxibustion 432
Mozart listening, beneficial effects 585
MRSA (meticillin-resistant
    Staphylococcus aureus)
    infection, value of honey 483
mullein (*Verbascum*) 328
Multibionta 500
muscle fatigue
    homeopathic treatment 251
    massage therapy 537–538
muscle testing, kinesiology 514–515
musculoskeletal conditions, use of

CAM 66–7
aromatherapy 361
homeopathic remedies 251
music therapy 583–586
Musk, use in homeopathy 198
mycotoxin contamination, herbal
    products 309
myrrh 295, 306

National Center for Complementary
    and Alternative Medicine
    (NCCAM) 93, 94, 129
classification of CAM 18
domains of CAM 96–97
National Health Service (NHS),
    availability of CAM 80–84
homeopathic hospitals 215
national healthcare systems, integration
    of traditional medicine 398–399
National Institute of Health (NIH),
    funding of CAM research
    93–96
National Institute of Medical
    Herbalists 284–285
ADR reporting 170
Natrum mur 211, 247, 255
natural health products (NHPs),
    Canadian regulations 156–157
context of use 30–31, 36
nature imagery, beneficial effects
    572–573
naturopathy 475
accreditation 32
chelation therapy 480–481
detoxification therapy 479–480
evidence 478
history 475–476
iridology 511–513
nutritional therapy 488–491
practice 477–478
qualifications 32, 479
theory 476–477
see also balneotherapy;
    hydrotherapy; nutraceuticals
nauli 460
nausea
aromatherapy 361
herbal medicines 328
homeopathic remedies 246
see also morning sickness

needling procedure, acupuncture
    429
negative outcomes, herbal medicines
    301–302
nerves, massage 532
nettle (*Urtica* species) 192, *248*, *249*,
    252, 293–294, 328
neutral water therapy 482, 483, 485
New Zealand, regulation of herbal
    medicines 154–155
non-medically qualified practitioners
    (NMQPs) 77–79
North American essences, flower
    remedy therapy 386
nosodes 199, 211–212, 217
    legal classification 208
    names 196
    use as vaccines 213
    veterinary use 253
Nottingham Health Profile (NHP) 56
nourishment and repair stage,
    herbalism 273
nurses, attitudes to CAM 76–77
nutraceuticals 491
    apitherapy 502–504
    essential fatty acids 492–497
    probiotics 497–501
nutritional supplements
    contaminants 34
    value of complex mixtures 30
nutritional therapy 488–491
    in ayurvedic medicine 456–457
    in traditional Chinese medicine
        442–443
nuts, nutritional value 489
Nux vomica 198, *211*, 243, *245*, *246*,
    252

objectivism 8
observational studies 28, 29, 125,
    135–136
'off-label' use, veterinary homeopathy
    254
Office of Alternative Medicine , USA
    129
oils, nutritional value 490
olfactory remediation 354
olfactory stimulation, aromatherapy
    343–344
omega-3 oils 492

benefits in cystic fibrosis 496
    see also essential fatty acids (EFAs)
omega-6:omega-3 fatty acid ratio 494
opium poppy (*Papaver somniferum*)
    271
oral administration, essential oils 357,
    358, 369
orange oil *361*
*Organon of the Rational Art of
    Healing*, Samuel Hahnemann
    189
organs, traditional Chinese medicine
    421–422
orthodox drugs, decreased efficacy with
    time 53
orthodox medicine (OM),
        disenchantment with 47, 48–51
Oscillococcinum, use in influenza 66
Osteopaths Act (1993) 544
osteopathy 539–540
    comparison with other manual
        therapies 542–545
    evidence 543–544
    history 540
    perceived effectiveness 53
    practice 541–542
    regulation 544–545
    safety 544
    theory 540–541
    training 545
outcome measures 123, 131
over-the-counter (OTC) products 16,
    147, 148
    homeopathic drugs 229–30
    development and marketing
        110–113
Overall Progress Interactive Chart 123
ozone depletion 406–407

pain control
    aromatherapy 363–364, 365
    Bach flower remedies 390
    humour 578
    reiki 564–565
    transcendental meditation 582
palliative care, value of yoga 569
Palmer, Daniel David 523
pancha karma 456
Panex quinquefolium extract, use in
    influenza 66

Papworth relaxation technique
     567–568
Paracelsus 271, 315
Parkinson's disease, effect of Alexander
     technique 520
PARTS acronym, chiropractic 524
Passiflora 252
patchouli oil 375
patent acquisition, homeopathic drugs
     111
patent medicines, Chinese 436–437
patenting of herbal products 405
patient counselling
     about essential oils 374
     about herbal products 296–299
     about homeopathic medicines
          219–220
patient-led consultations 51
patient–practitioner relationships
     43–44
patients
     characteristics of CAM users, USA
          62–63
     definition 6
     as integrators of therapies 31–32
     reasons for choosing CAM 44–46
     belief in value of CAM 51–54
     culture 58
     disenchantment with OM 48–50
     dissatisfaction with OM consultation
          50–51
     financial reasons 54–57
     'green' association 57
     media coverage 57
     role models 58
     safety concerns 46–48
     reasons for not selecting CAM 58
Patients' Charter 48
PC-SPES, contaminants 34
pennyroyal 373, 440
pentacyclic triterpenoid saponins
     278
peppermint (Mentha piperita) 279,
     295
     adverse reactions 161
peppermint oil 368, 375
perception of benefit studies,
     homeopathy 241
perceptions of CAM 9–10
personality traits 15, 61

association with CAM use 103
pétrissage 531
Petroleum 252
pharmacists
     ADR reporting 167–169
     attitudes to CAM 74–76
pharmacopoeias, herbalism 274,
     301
pharmacovigilance 145–146
     case-control and cohort studies
          172–173
     Chinese herbal medicine 441
     communication of safety information
          172–175
     future initiatives 175–177
     prescription event monitoring
          171–172
     randomised clinical trials 173
     regulations
          in Australia 153–154
          in Canada 156–157
          in European Union 152–153
          in New Zealand 154–155
          in united Kingdom 151–152
          in USA 155–156
     spontaneous reporting schemes
          159–166
          by complementary medicine
               practitioners 169–171
          by pharmacists 167–169
          strengths and weaknesses 166–167
pharmacy record-linkage 176–177
pheromones 345
philosophy, use of the term 7
Phosphorus 246
phototoxicity, essential oils 370–371,
     373
physical therapy
     in naturopathy 478
     see also massage
physiotherapy, comparison with
          osteopathy 543
Phytonet 170–171
phytotherapy 270
PICO questions 136
pitta dosha 452, 453, 454, 457
Pittilo Report 284, 439
placebo effect 7–8, 15–16, 232,
     233–234
     practitioner bias 133

placebo studies
  homeopathy 234–235
  massage 537
  problems in CAM 129–130
placebos, definition 233
plant material, use in homeopathic
      medicines 198
plant maturity, effect on essential oils
      351
pluralist prescribing, homeopathy 217
Podophyllum 246
polychrests 210, 211, 229–30
  keynotes 225
polysaccharides 280
polyunsaturated fats 493
positivism 8
post-exercise massage 536, 538
postoperative pain control,
      aromatherapy 363
postoperative rehabilitation, value of
      osteopathy 544
potency, homeopathic medicines 218
potentisation, homeopathy 193,
      200–202
  effects 204–205
  Hahnemannian method 202–203
  Korsakovian method 203–204
  LM method 204
powdered drugs, use in herbalism 290
powerful others health locus of control
      (PHLC) 101
practitioner bias 133
practitioner–patient interaction, effect
      on placebo response 234
pragmatic clinical studies 28, 29
prakriti, ayurveda 453, 454
prayer 587–590
pre-exercise massage 535–536
pregnancy
  aromatherapy 373–374
  homeopathic remedies 250
  use of complementary medicines
      147–148
  use of herbal products 296–297
  Chinese 440–441
  see also midwifery; morning sickness
premature amnion rupture, RCT of
      Caulophyllum D4 236–237
premature ejaculation, value of yoga
      570

premenstrual syndrome
  herbal medicines 330
  homeopathic remedies 250
  massage therapy 534
  reflexology 548
prescription event monitoring (PEM)
      171–173, 177
prescriptions, for homeopathic
      medicines 218
prevalence of utilization
  in Australia 64
  in Canada 63
prevention of disease 45
primary care groups (PCGs),
      availability of CAM 83
Prince of Wales' Initiative on Integrated
      Medicine 83
principle of similars, homeopathy 106
probiotics 497
  definition 498–499
  evidence 500–502
  history 497–498
  practice 499–500
  safety 502
  types 499
propolis 277, 503–504
prostate cancer, use of CAM therapies
      48
'proving', homeopathy 111, 189, 195
psychosocial drivers to CAM use
      100–104
publishing bias 132–133
Pulsatilla 211, 229, 243, 250
pulse reading, traditional Chinese
      medicine 424
pyridoxine (vitamin B6), high-dose 34

qi (chee, chi) 419–420, 422, 429
qianbai biyan pian 150
qigong 443–444
quality of evidence
  definition 124
  influencing factors 124–126
quality problems, Chinese herbal
      medicines 439–440
quenching, aromatherapy 350

racial differences in CAM utilization
      63
radionics 587

rainforest destruction 404–405
rajas, ayurveda 454
randomised clinical trials 7, 28, 128,
    133–134, 173
  in acupuncture 430
  in aromatherapy 362, 364, 365, 366
  in ayurvedic medicine 465–466
  in chiropractic 525–526
  homeopathic 235, 235–238
  in influenza prevention and
      treatment 66
  in massage therapy 537–538
  quality of evidence 125–126
  in reflexology 548
  relevance to everyday practice 29,
      32–33
  in spiritual healing 588
raspberry leaf products, use during
    pregnancy 297
Reckeweg, Hans-Heinrich 255
rectal administration, essential oils 357
rectal irrigation 481–482
reductionism 8
reflexology 545
  evidence 547–548
  history 546–547
  safety 549
  theory and practice 547
reflexology map 546
Register of Chinese Herbal Medicine
    (RCHM), ADR reporting 170
regulation of CAM 36, 67–68, 78
  in Australia 153–154
  ayurvedic medicine 466
  in Canada 156–157
  Chinese herbal medicine 437–438,
      439
  chiropractic 528
  in European Union 152–153
  herbalism 284–284
  homeopathic medicines 208–210
  House of Lords Report 122
  naturopathy 479
  in New Zealand 154–155
  osteopathy 544–545
  pharmacovigilance 146
  traditional medicine 399, 400–401
  in United Kingdom 151–152
  in USA 105
  homeopathy 106–113

products 105–106, 155–156
veterinary homeopathy 253–254
reiki 563–565
relaxation techniques 566–568
remedium cardinale, herbal teas 281
renal disease, value of yoga 569
repertories
  herbalism 274
  conditions 327–330
  materia medica 316–327
  homeopathic medicines 224–225,
      244–252
rescue remedy (five-flower remedy)
    388, 391
research into CAM
  criticisms 130–133
  problems 128–130
  see also evidence; randomised clinical
      trials
resins 274
responsibility for health 48, 49
revulsive hip baths 483
rheumatological patients, use of CAM
    53–54
  herbal medicines 329
  homeopathic medicines 225
rhubarb (Rheum palmatum) 312, 328
Rhus tox 211, 225, 229, 243, 251
  RCTs 235
rhythmical massage therapy (RMT)
    538–539
risk–benefit ratio, role in choice of
    CAM 46–48
risks of CAM use 138–139
  see also adverse effects; safety
rock rose (Helianthemum
    nummularium) 385
role models, use of CAM 58
rolfing 549–550
rosemary oil 361, 367, 375
royal jelly 504
Royal Pharmaceutical Society of Great
    Britain (RPSGB)
  attitude to CAM 74–76
  herbaria 313–314
rubifacients 535
Ruta 211, 243, 251

safety of CAM 35, 138–139
  of acupuncture 431

of aromatherapy 369–370
potential toxic effects 370–371
of ayurvedic medicine 462–465
of Chinese herbal medicine (CHM)
    439–441
of chiropractic manipulation
    527–528
of detoxification therapy 480
of herbal medicines, lack of
    information 157–158
of homeopathy
aggravations 221–222
inappropriate treatment 220
interactions 222
toxicity 220–221
of hypnotherapy 580
of massage 539
of osteopathy 544
of probiotics 502
of reflexology 549
of traditional medicine 402–403
safety concerns, role in choice of CAM
    46–48
sage (Salvia officinalis) 294, 306
St John's wort (Hypericum perforatum)
    283, 300, 305, 306, 324–325,
    327
adverse reactions 161, 162, 175
communication of information
    174–175
interactions 34, 151–152, 305, 306,
    326
variability of preparations 150
salvia oil 368
Sambucus nigra, use in influenza 66
samkhya philosophy 451
san jiao 422
sandalwood oil 361, 366, 368, 375
saponins 277–278
sarcodes 199, 212, 213
sassafras 369
saturated fatty acids 492–493
satvas, ayurveda 454
savory (Satureja species) 294
saw palmetto (Sabal serrulata) 308,
    326, 328
schizophrenia, yoga therapy 569
Schüssler, Wilhelm Heinrich 254
science of healing 6–8
scleranthus (Scleranthus annuus) 385

screening programmes 45
sedative oils 360
sedatives, herbal medicines 327
seeds, nutritional value 489
self-healing response 10–12, 235, 524
self study materials 57
self-treatment 16, 57, 80
homeopathic medicines 229–30
Senecio species, senecionine 150
senna 328
adverse reaction 161, 306
sensitising components, essential oils
    371
Sepia 211, 250
sequential muscle relaxation
    566–567
Set Aside scheme 408
shamans 400
shen 421
sickle cell anaemia, dance project 562
Silica 248, 255
Silicea comp. 258
silver birch (Betula pendula) 294
single medicine principle, homeopathy
    193
sinusitis, anthroposophical treatment
    258
skin, structure 346
skin conditions
aromatherapy 361, 369
ayurvedic treatments 469
herbal medicines 329
homeopathic remedies 248–249,
    252
use of honey 503
skin occlusion, effect on essential oil
    absorption 347
skullcap (Scutellaria baicalensis) 327
sleep induction, value of massage 533
Smilax myosotiflora products,
    adulteration 309
Smuts, Jan Christian 12
social considerations 16
social determinants of health 13–14
sociodemographic drivers to CAM use
    99–100
sore throat
aromatherapy 361
ayurvedic treatments 469
herbal medicines 329

homeopathic remedies *252*
spa treatment (balneotherapy)
    486–488
Spagynk therapy 74
spagyric medicine 315
speedwell (*Veronical officinalis*) 294
spinal baths 483–484
spinal manipulation therapy (SMT)
    differentiation from chiropractic
        525
    evidence 526, 527
spiritual healing 587–589
Spongia *246*
sports massage 531, 535–538
sportspeople
    homeopathic remedies *251*
    use of herbal products 299
squill *308*
standardisation
    of herbal medicines 150, 310
    problems in clinical trials 130
steam baths 484–485
Steiner, Rudolph 256
steroidal saponins 278
steroids, possible interaction with
        homeopathic medicines 222
Still, Andrew Taylor 539, 540
stimulant oils 360
storage, essential oils *352, 353*
Streptococcus thermophilus 498
stress
    herbal medicines 327
    spa treatment 487
    value of yoga 570
stroke, prevention and treatment 67
study design, effect on quality of
        evidence 124
subjective outcome measures 131
succussion, homeopathy 202,
        204–205
Sulphur *247*
surgery
    in ayurvedic practice 462, 465
    in naturopathy 478
    placebo effects 233
Sushruta 450, 462
Swedish massage 530, 531
synergistic effects
    in aromatherapy 349–350
    in herbalism 275

systematic reviews of research
        124
systems approach to treatment
        51

Tabacum *246, 252*
tablets, homeopathic medicines
        205–206
tai ji quan (tai c'hi) 444
tai ji symbol *417*
tamas, ayurveda 454
Tamus *248*
Tan Tock Seng Hospital, art of healing
        programme 571–572
tangerine oil *361*
tannins 278
tapotement 531
tastes, ayurveda 456–457
tautodes 199, 212
taxol production, effect on yew tree
        populations 406
tea tree oil (*Melaleuca*) 295, 357, *361*,
        368–369, 370, *375*, 400
temperature, effect on essential oil
        absorption 346–347
tennis elbow, homeopathic treatment
        251
thalidomide 47, 145
therapeutic clowns 578
Therapeutic Goods Regulations,
        Australia 153–154
therapeutic groups, herbal medicines
        276
therapeutic touch 565–566
Thomson, Samuel 272
throat massage 533
Thuja *249*
thyme (*Thymus* species) 295, 328
    essential oils 350, 368
Tibet, traditional medicine 444
tinctures, herbalism 282, 283
tissue salts 254–255
tonification, ayurveda 458
topical preparations
    essential oils 356–357, 358
    skin irritation 370
    herbal medicines 291–295
    adulteration 308–309
    homeopathy 207
tormentil root (*Potentilla*) 295

touch therapies
  reiki 563–565
  therapeutic touch 565–566
toxicity of herbal medicines 303–309
  ayurvedic 462–464
  Chinese 150–151, 439
  treatment of herbal poisoning
      312–313
traditional Chinese medicine (TCM)
      27, 415
  Chinese massage 442
  dietary therapy 442–443
  evidence 424–425
  history 415–416
  martial art therapy 443
  modernisation 425
  practice 423–424
  qigong 443–444
  tai ji quan (tai c'hi) 444
  theory 416
    five elements (phases) 418–419
    five substances 419–421
    meridians 423
    organs 421–422
    yin and yang 416–417
    toxic constituents 150, 151
  see also acupuncture; Chinese herbal
      medicine
Traditional Herbal Medicines
      Registration Scheme (THMRS)
      438
traditional medicine 395
  definition 395–396
  evidence 403
  and healthcare providers 403–404
  integration into national healthcare
      systems 398–399
  practice 396–400
  safety 400–402
  WHO strategy 409
  see also traditional Chinese medicine
traditional naturopaths 479
traditional Tibetan medicine 444
traditions, art and science of healing
      6–8
training of practitioners 32, 35–36
  in Chinese herbal medicine 439
  in chiropractic 528–529
  in herbalism 284–285
  in homeopathy 215

  in hypnosis 580
  in osteopathy 545
  traditional practitioners 400, 402
transcendental meditation (TM)
      582–583
trauma, homeopathic RCTs 236, 237
Treuhertz, Francis 72
trigger points, acupuncture 429–430
triphala 458–459
trituration, homeopathy 200
tryptophan supplements, contaminants
      34
turmeric, extraction of curcumoids
      30
Turner, William 271

unicist prescribing, homeopathy 216
United Kingdom
  regulation of herbal medicines
      151–152
  Yellow Card scheme 160–162
unsaturated fatty acids 493
upper respiratory tract infections,
      homeopathic RCTs 237, 238
Uppsala Monitoring Centre (UMC)
      159–160
urinary tract infections, herbal
      medicines 329
Urtica (Urtica urens) 192, 248, 249,
      252, 293–294, 328
USA
  CAM utilization 62–63, 64–65, 93,
      97–99
  chiropractic 522–523
  delivery of CAM 104–105
  drivers to CAM use
  insurance reimbursement 104
  psychosocial 100–104
  sociodemographic 99–100
  future of CAM 115
  homeopathic medicines, terminology
      213
  NCCAM domains of CAM 96–97
  NIH funding of CAM research
      93–96
  registration of homeopathic
      medicines 208–209
  regulation of CAM 105, 155–156
  homeopathy 106–113
  products 105–106

user characteristics, homeopathy
228–230
Usui, Mikao 563–564

vaccines, homeopathic 212–213, 253
vaginal administration, essential oils
357
valerian (*Valeriana officinalis*) 283,
306, 327, 329, 440
adverse reactions 161
Valnet, Jean 343
variability, herbal medicines 149, 310
vata dosha 452, 453, *454*, 457
vegetables, nutritional value 489
vervain (*Verbena officinalis*) 385
veterinary practice 84–85
homeopathy 215, 244, 253–254
vibratory massage 531, 536, 537
visceral techniques, osteopathy 542
vital force (dynamis), homeopathy
191–192
vitamin supplements
complex mixtures, value 30
vitamin B6 (pyridoxine), high-dose
34
vitamin E, high-dose, interactions 35
volatile oils *see* essential oils
vomeronasal system 345
action of homeopathic medicines
240
vomiting
herbal medicines 328
homeopathic treatment *252*
see also morning sickness

warfarin, interactions 35
warts, homeopathic remedies *249*
water
ayurveda 452
effect on essential oil absorption 347
importance in traditional Chinese
medicine 418
see also balneotherapy; hydrotherapy
water violet (*Hottonia palustris*) 385

wild carrot (*Daucus carota*) 308
wild cherry bark (*Prunus serotina*)
328
wintergreen 295
wintergreen oil 352
witch-hazel 278, 295
women's conditions
aromatherapy 363
ayurvedic medicines 458, *459*
herbal medicines 330
homeopathic remedies *250*
massage therapy 534
reflexology 548
see also midwifery; morning sickness;
pregnancy
World Health Organization (WHO)
Commission on Social Determinants
of Health 13–14
definition of health 13, 33
definition of herbal medicines 270
definition of pharmacovigilance 145,
146
definition of traditional medicine
395–396
traditional medicine strategy 409
wormwood (*Artemesia absinthium*)
295

yang organs 422
Yellow Card schemes 159–162, 163,
441
pharmacist reporting 167–169
yin organs 422
yin and yang 416–417
yin-chen hao (*Artemesia scoparia*) 441
ylang ylang oil 345–346, 367, *375*
yoga 461, 568
evidence 568–570
yoghurt 497, 498
yohimbine, adverse effects 303–304
Young's rule (paediatric doses) 298

zoological names, use in homeopathy
196